A SYLLABUS
for the
SURGEON'S SECRETARY

Jeannette A. Szulec, B.S., RRA

Medical Records Administrator
Medical Records Consultant
Hospital Administrator

Z. Szulec, M.D.

Physician and Surgeon

SECOND REVISED EDITION

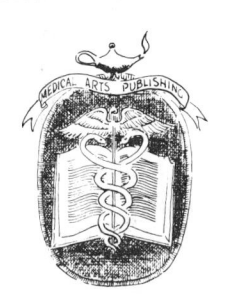

1970

MEDICAL ARTS PUBLISHING COMPANY

P.O. Box 8627 Kensington Station / Detroit, Michigan 48224

Published 1965
Reprinted 1965
Reprinted 1966
Reprinted 1967
Reprinted 1968
Revised 1970
Reprinted 1970
Reprinted 1972
Reprinted 1974
Reprinted 1978

This book may be ordered directly from the publisher:

MEDICAL ARTS PUBLISHING COMPANY
P.O. Box 8627—Kensington Station
Detroit, Michigan 48224

Copyright 1965 and 1970 by Jeannette A. Szulec

in the United States, Canada and countries
outside the United States, under the provisions
of the Universal Copyright Convention.

© Jeannette A. Szulec 1970

Derechos reservados conforme a la ley
para la Republica Mexicana

All rights reserved including the right to
reproduce this book or parts thereof in any form.

Library of Congress Catalogue Number 68-28086

Printed in the United States of America

Dedicated with love
to the memory of my father
DAMIAN SZULEC
and to my mother

For their loving hearts, their gentle nobility, and their delicate aesthetic sensibilities which so enriched my life.

Acknowledgments

An author does not work alone to produce a book of this character and scope. The text develops with the technical assistance and professional guidance of many persons contributing generously of their time and special knowledge. To all who have assisted me in making this technical reference possible, I am deeply indebted.

My gratitude is particularly intended for the following outstanding specialists who worked closely with me in developing those sections which applied to their specialty: Dr. Michael Zylik, radiologist; Dr. John Lucas, biochemist; Dr. Frank E. Check, obstetrician and gynecologist; Dr. Edward R. Heil, otolaryngologist; Dr. J. Chauncey Hipps, plastic surgeon; Dr. J. Anatole Hoski, orthopedic surgeon; Dr. Prescott Jordan, Jr., vascular surgeon; Dr. Philip J. Morgan, anesthesiologist; Dr. Donald R. Simmons, neurologist and neurosurgeon; and, the late Dr. Leo B. Saraf, general surgeon.

I am further grateful to the many specialty surgeons who so graciously consented to contribute descriptions of their operative techniques for use in this book.

My appreciation is also extended to those medical authors through whose courtesy numerous illustrations were obtained for this edition.

Memory of the kindness accorded me by all who have assisted me in this endeavor will remain with me forever.

Jeannette A. Szulec

Preface

Reading maketh a full man; conference, a ready man; and writing, an exact man.

These words should be dedicated to the secretary whose essential role in business and in the professions is indisputable. In the growing field of medicine she is becoming a particularly important member of the physician's staff and hospital team. As medicine becomes more highly specialized, greater demands are made upon her work. She must be prepared through proper training to meet the challenge of tomorrow as well as that of today.

Fluency with the terminology peculiar to one's professional endeavor is an important element in success. The surgeon's secretary has a responsibility to familiarize herself with the terms describing his highly technical equipment. It is for her and for medical records personnel that this book is intended.

I have long felt the genuine need for a comprehensive reference to assist medical secretaries with technical information not usually found in the medical dictionary. For years they have referred to surgical catalogues for assistance with instrument names. These books are seldom accurate enough for use in a secretary's reference library.

Although A SYLLABUS FOR THE SURGEON'S SECRETARY has been designed primarily as a reference source, the author has used it successfully as a training guide.

It is proposed that the student be assigned sections of this book for study. This should include copying of the operative reports from the book repeatedly until the terminology becomes completely familiar.

Too much emphasis cannot be placed on the importance of having the student see the words spelled correctly. She will learn them by actually typing them. Educators agree that it is far more difficult to change erroneous practices than it is to learn correctly from the outset.

It is further recommended that the student's progress be surveyed through periodic progress tests. Terms and operative reports should be dictated by the teacher from the book. These may be recorded on discs or belts for transcription by the student. If page references are given from the book, the student can check her own work. In so doing, she is actually afforded an additional review. Reports should be dated and saved to compare the progress being made.

Only when a satisfactory degree of proficiency has been achieved should a student be given actual work assignments. She thus learns by POSITIVE TUTELAGE as contrasted with the outmoded method of trial and error.

It is sincerely hoped that medical secretaries, medical record librarians and medical records personnel everywhere will find this a valuable reference which fills a long existing need.

If in some small way this book fulfills the purpose for which it is intended, the many years and countless hours invested in the study and research which have made this work possible will not have been in vain.

JEANNETTE A. SZULEC

Detroit, Michigan
January, 1965

Preface to Revised Second Edition

In the three years which have elapsed since publication of the first edition of A SYLLABUS FOR THE SURGEON'S SECRETARY, popularity of the book has continued to grow here at home and abroad. An ever increasing number of schools are using the Syllabus as a textbook. We are particularly pleased that the U.S. Library of Congress has translated the book into Braille and audio tapes for use in rehabilitation programs for the blind. Many blind persons are being successfully employed as medical transcriptionists.

Success of our book coupled with the warm personal response from so many persons in the field of medicine assures us that the book has fulfilled its intended purpose, that of providing transcriptionists and surgical writers with a comprehensive technical reference.

In this revised second edition we have retained almost all of the material which appeared in the original edition; however, each chapter has been expanded in depth and scope to insure a more comprehensive volume.

More than 2,000 listings have been added to the section on surgical instruments and equipment to include all of the latest additions to the surgeon's armamentarium.

A section has been included containing medicolegal consent and release forms designed to cover the various situations which arise in conjunction with surgery.

The sections devoted to laboratory and X-ray examinations have been enlarged to include all examinations in common present day medical practice. A complete discussion of blood typing and immune response in tissue transplantation has been added in addition to a listing of viral, bacterial, fungal, rickettsial and parasitic disease organisms.

A new chapter on the subject of obstetrics has been added with valuable illustrations to supplement the text.

New surgical techniques are discussed which include utilization of the remarkable energy of the laser, use of extreme cold (cryosurgery) for delicate operations, use of the heart lungs by-pass in vascular surgery, control measures in suppressing rejection of transplanted tissues, new uses for radioactive isotopes in diagnosis and treatment, as well as important facts and statistics concerning cancer.

Anatomic plates and illustrations have been added to each specialty chapter to assist the student in an accurate interpretation of the subject matter. In addition, a complete index of diagnoses and operations has been included in each specialty chapter.

Every effort has been made to produce a reference which may justly take its place among the classics in reference literature. To this end will our efforts be consistently dedicated.

Jeannette A. Szulec

Detroit, Michigan
January, 1970

TABLE OF CONTENTS

CHAPTER		PAGE
1	The Surgical Secretary	1
	medicolegal forms related to surgery	
2	Laboratory Examinations	17
3	X-Ray Examinations	73
4	Pre- and Postoperative Considerations	91
	anesthetics, surgical and examining positions, incisions, suture materials, suture techniques, bandages and dressings	
5	Surgical Instruments and Equipment	121
6	Anatomy of Structure, Circulation and Innervation	213
7	General Surgery	261
8	Gynecology	349
9	Neurosurgery	385
10	Obstetrics	411
11	Ophthalmology (Eye)	433
12	Orthopedic Surgery	455
13	Otolaryngology (E.N.T.)	501
14	Plastic Surgery	531
15	Thoracic Surgery	557
16	Urology	577
17	Vascular Surgery	607
18	The Language of Medicine	641
19	A Style Guide	655
	GLOSSARY OF OPERATIVE TITLES	659

INDEX TO PLATES

PLATE	SUBJECT	PAGE
1	OPERATIVE REPORT FORM	4
2	CONSENT TO OPERATE FORM	6
3	CONSENT TO DELIVERY BY ALTERNATE PHYSICIAN	7
4	CONSENT TO OPERATION FOR COSMETIC PURPOSES	8
5	CONSENT TO REMOVAL OF TISSUE FOR GRAFTING	9
6	CONSENT TO OPERATION AND GRAFTING OF TISSUE	9
7	REFUSAL TO SUBMIT TO TREATMENT FORM	10
8	REFUSAL TO PERMIT BLOOD TRANSFUSION FORM	10
9	AUTHORIZATION TO USE EYES (Donor) FORM	10
10	AUTHORIZATION TO USE EYES (by next of kin) FORM	10
11	AUTHORIZATION TO ADMIT OBSERVERS TO OPERATING ROOM FORM	11
12	CONSENT TO TELEVISING OF OPERATION FORM	11
13	CONSENT TO TAKING AND PUBLICATION OF PHOTOGRAPHS FORM	11
14	CONSENT TO TAKING OF MOTION PICTURES OF OPERATION FORM	12
15	RELEASE FORM FOR RITUAL CIRCUMCISION	12
16	REQUEST FOR STERILIZATION FORM	14

INDEX TO PLATES (continued)

PLATE	SUBJECT	PAGE
17	STATEMENT OF NEED FOR THERAPEUTIC ABORTION FORM	14
18	REQUEST FOR MEDICAL INFORMATION FORM LETTER	15
19	PELVICEPHALOMETRY RADIOGRAPHIC EXAMINATION	82
20	X-RAY DETERMINATION OF PELVIC MEASUREMENTS	83
21	DIAGRAM OF FLUOROSCOPE	85
22	SURGICAL AND EXAMINING POSITIONS	94
23	SUTURE TECHNIQUES	106
24	ADDITIONAL SUTURE TECHNIQUES	107
25	ADDITIONAL SUTURE TECHNIQUES	108
26	PRINCIPAL ARTERIES OF THE BODY AND PULMONARY VEINS	220
27	ARTERIES OF HEAD, NECK AND BASE OF BRAIN	221
28	ARTERIES OF THE THORAX AND AXILLA	222
29	ARTERIES OF THE ABDOMEN AND PELVIS	223
30	ARTERIES OF THE UPPER EXTREMITIES	224
31	ARTERIES OF THE LOWER EXTREMITIES	225
32	PRINCIPAL VEINS OF THE BODY	226
33	VEINS OF THE HEAD AND NECK	227
34	SUPERFICIAL VEINS OF THE EXTREMITIES	228
35	ANTERIOR VIEW OF THE HUMAN SKELETON	229

INDEX TO PLATES (continued)

PLATE	SUBJECT	PAGE
36	SKELETON OF ADULT MAN	234
37	MUSCULAR SYSTEM OF MAN	246
38	ANATOMIC LOCATION OF VARIOUS HERNIAS	260
39	THE AXILLARY REGION	277
40	REGION OF THE MOUTH AND SALIVARY GLANDS	282
41	ANATOMY OF THE NECK	285
42	THE ENDOCRINE GLANDS	293
43	INTERNAL ORGANS OF THE BODY	303
44	INTERIOR VIEW OF THE STOMACH	307
45	ANATOMY OF THE COLON	325
46	THE CECUM, VERMIFORM APPENDIX AND ILEUM	327
47	INTERIOR VIEW OF THE CECUM, VERMIFORM APPENDIX AND ILEUM	327
48	RECTUM AND ANUS	332
49	ANUS WITH HEMORRHOIDS	332
50	THE BILIARY SYSTEM AND RELATED STRUCTURES	338
51	THE EXTERNAL FEMALE GENITALIA	351
52	THE INTERNAL FEMALE GENITALIA	353
53	ANATOMY OF THE BRAIN	389
54	THE VENTRICLES OF THE BRAIN	390
55	TRAUMATA OF THE BRAIN	395

INDEX TO PLATES (continued)

PLATE	SUBJECT	PAGE
56	CERVICAL AND THORACIC REGIONS OF THE SPINAL CORD	399
57	LATERAL VIEW OF THE VERTEBRAL COLUMN	401
58	VIEW OF THE THORACIC VERTEBRA FROM ABOVE	401
59	INTERVERTEBRAL DISCS	403
60	THE FOUR BASIC TYPES OF FEMALE PELVES	417
61	EFFACEMENT OF THE CERVIX	418
62	DETERMINATION OF STATION	419
63	LONGITUDINAL LIE (fetal position)	421
64	TRANSVERSE LIE WITH ARM PROLAPSED (fetal position)	421
65	VERTEX PRESENTATION	422
66	BROW PRESENTATION	422
67	FACE PRESENTATION	422
68	PARIETAL PRESENTATION	422
69	FULL BREECH PRESENTATION	423
70	FRANK BREECH PRESENTATION	423
71	SINGLE FOOTLING BREECH PRESENTATION	423
72	KNEE BREECH PRESENTATION	423
73	THE EYE AND RELATED STRUCTURES	435
74	THOMAS CRYOPTOR USED IN CRYOSURGERY	439
75	ANATOMY OF THE HAND	457
76	ANATOMY OF THE FOOT	458

INDEX TO PLATES (continued)

PLATE	SUBJECT	PAGE
77	ANATOMY OF THE SHOULDER	463
78	ANATOMY OF THE ELBOW	464
79	ANATOMY OF THE WRIST	465
80	ANATOMY OF THE HIP	466
81	ANATOMY OF THE KNEE	473
82	ANATOMY OF THE ANKLE	474
83	DISLOCATIONS	479
84	FRACTURES	482
85	TENDON LENGTHENING AND SHORTENING	489
86	THE EAR AND RELATED STRUCTURES	502
87	LARYNGOPHARYNGEAL REGION	520
88	THE PARANASAL SINUSES	526
89	LARYNX, TRACHEA AND BRONCHI	560
90	TRACHEOTOMY	565
91	UROGENITAL SYSTEM, MALE AND FEMALE	576
92	ANATOMY OF THE MALE GENITALIA	594
93	THE MALE PELVIC ORGANS	595
94	PHOTOGRAPH OF TRANSSEPTAL LEFT HEART CATHETERIZATION	609
95	DETAILS OF STRUCTURE OF THE HEART	623
96	PHOTOGRAPH OF HEART-LUNGS MACHINE	625
97	PACEMAKER	638
98	PHOTOGRAPH OF BLOOD VESSEL MICROSURGERY	640

1 | The Surgical Secretary

The surgical secretary is a specialist in the secretarial field and, as such, she is required to be everything that one might expect of an executive secretary and more. In addition to being well versed in the fundamentals of secretarial science, she must have an intelligent concept of her subject matter, whether it be medical terminology in general or, more specifically, the glossology and nomenclature of surgery.

This chapter has been designed to provide a review of the basic considerations in the work of the secretary. It should be of particular value to the student embarking on a medical secretarial career.

Transcription of Dictation

Increasing complexity in the technology of our dictating systems seems to be attended by mounting problems for the secretary. Those of us who have taken dictation directly from the doctor will not argue with the opinion that this is the most satisfactory arrangement. Although shorthand is still used at some facilities, it is fast being replaced by mechanical dictating systems. Without the physician present to whom she might direct her problems with terminology, the secretary must rely on her knowledge of the matter being dictated. It is essential that she be provided with the necessary references to assist her with the more technical phases of her work.

The following books are recommended as basic to the secretary's library.

Webster's Seventh New Collegiate Dictionary.
Medical Dictionary   The large Dorland's or Stedman's are preferred. Taber's Cyclopedic is a good second dictionary. Kimber, Gray, Stackpole & Leavell is popular.
"Human Anatomy and Physiology" by King and Showers
PDR (Physician's Desk Reference)   A directory of drugs and biologicals published annually by Medical Economics of Oradell, N.J.

A secretary who is provided with adequate references can be more productive and efficient than the secretary who must seek out the physician for assistance. Each secretary should have her own references, otherwise desk hopping is inevitable.

Regardless of the proficiency of the secretary, problems with recorded dictations will develop due to poor dictating techniques or failure of the equipment.

Partly inaudible dictations should be salvaged to the extent possible and immediately be brought to the attention of the physican concerned. Any portion of the report may assist him in recalling the case, particularly if he is a very busy surgeon.

Blank spaces which represent difficulties encountered in transcribing do not belong in a medical report. When all measures to obtain the information fail, the physician who dictated the report should be contacted for assistance. Physicians seldom insert the required information when a report is furnished to them for signature.

Corrections cannot be detected prior to transcription with some dictating systems. If there are only a few words involved, erasure might be possible. This should be done with an abrasive eraser, lightly. The error may then be covered over with a soft blackboard chalk. Where colored paper is used for the report form, chalk of a similar color may be used. Where a lengthy error is involved, the report should be retyped. If a doctor habitually makes corrections in his dictations, it might be advisable to listen ahead before transcribing his reports.

It is extremely poor secretarial practice to strike out an error or strike over a character without erasing first. Medical records are permanent documents and therefore require the utmost care in preparation. With the patient's authorization, medical reports are furnished to hospitals, physicians, attorneys and various social agencies. They should always be a credit to the facility from which they are issued.

Judging Your Work Volume

A secretary whose test typing speed is 60 words per minute will usually work at the rate of 50 words per minute. To produce one page of single spaced elite type, which consists of an average of 600 words, in addition to a file copy and three additional carbons, she uses her time as follows:

typing time	12 minutes
proofreading	4 minutes
file & 3 carbons	1 minute each

Typing speed is expressed as words per minute. A word is regarded as five strokes. When a secretary types 60 words per minute, she strikes 300 characters and spaces per minute.

A speed of 30 to 60 words per minute is the usual range of commercial touch typists. Fifty to sixty is considered excellent with ranges to 100. Speed specialists type from 140 to 150 words per minute.

When we speak of typing speed in transcription, we are referring to *lines per hour* rather than words per minute. An experienced secretary should be able to transcribe at the rate of 150 to 180 lines per hour.

Setting Up Your Format

Work will flow much more smoothly if your staff will adopt a particular format for their dictations. In order to implement such a system, a note might be placed at important dictating stations including those in the surgical suite.

The information required to completely identify the patient should be itemized to include the patient's name, case number or out-patient status, room number, name of referring physician and attending physician or surgeon.

On operative reports, the surgeon should also include the name of any assistants. The context of the surgical dictation should contain the pre- and post-operative diagnosis, titles of operations performed, anesthetic and position of the patient, findings at surgery and a description of the actual surgical technique. A paragraph containing a complete report of all positive and negative findings dictated before the actual description of the operation will prove most helpful for future reference.

If the secretary is employed in a hospital, forms will be furnished for the various type reports; however, the secretary in the doctor's office may be required to set up her own formats.

A sample operative report is shown in Fig. 1. Such a report form is usually adequate for most operative dictations.

The secretary in the physician's office will usually be asked to send a medical report to the physician by whom the patient was referred. A carbon copy of the report is retained for the office file.

In the hospital, a carbon copy is prepared for the surgeon, referring physician and the assistants and the original report is filed with the patient's hospital record. When house physicians such as internes and residents serve as assistants, carbon copies are placed in their folders. Responsibility for maintaining folders for house staff copies is usually assigned to the medical records office.

The report of surgery is a vital part of the patient's hospital record. It should be dictated within 24 hours after surgery, while the surgeon can still recall the circumstances clearly. Each report must be an individualized account of what was found and what was done. Under no circumstances should a secretary agree to use routine dictations on certain frequently performed cases in lieu of a specifically dictated report. The requirement for an operative report on the patient's chart was designed to protect the interest of the patient. This interest cannot be well served by simply satisfying the chart requirement. This is a point on which there should be no compromise.

```
                    ST. JOSEPH MERCY HOSPITAL
                         DETROIT, MICHIGAN
                        *Operative Report*
                                              Date_____

Patient's Name_____ Room_____ Case No._____
Surgeon _____ CO-SURGEON _____ Assistant(s)_____
Anesthetist _____ Anesthesia _____
PRE-OPERATIVE DIAGNOSIS:

POST-OPERATIVE DIAGNOSIS:

OPERATION (S):


Procedure:
      FINDINGS:



      TECHNIQUE
```

Figure 1   Operative Report Form

Authorization for Operation and Treatment

For many years hospitals used brief "blanket" consent forms which were so ambiguous as to be worthless in the event of legal proceedings. Physicians likewise performed examinations and treatments with only implied or oral consent. The alarming increase in medical liability claims indicates a need for written agreements which will protect the physician.

Written consent to an operation is not a legal requirement. It is an advisable practice designed to protect the physician in his relationship with the patient. Implied consent is always attended by the possibility that a misunderstanding may develop over the operation agreed upon, or the extent to which the patient authorized the physician to expand the original operative plan.

A form such as that shown in Fig. 2 illustrates a consent to operate form which is comprehensive enough in specific and general authority to permit the physician to pursue good medical practice in any eventuality.

Physicians who practice in hospitals where an informed consent to operate form has not yet been adopted, may protect themselves by requiring the patient to sign such a form in their office.

A provision may be made at the bottom of the form for special instructions to further prevent any future misunderstandings. Patients sometimes desire to have a removed limb turned over to a mortician for burial or place certain limitations on the surgeon. A surgeon may feel justified in proceeding with the operation when these limitations are not inconsistent with good medical practice.

The Valid Consent

A person who has attained legal age and is of sound mind is qualified to give or withhold consent for treatment. Such consent, however, is not valid if the patient is intoxicated, delirious or otherwise unable to exercise rational judgement.

In the case of minors, it is always advisable to obtain the consent of a parent or legal guardian.

In life threatening situations, where the patient is unconscious or unable to consent to treatment, the law will infer consent to cover such treatment as is immediately necessary to preserve life or limb.

To be legally valid, the patient's consent must be an advised and intelligent consent. The release form should be couched in language the patient can readily understand. Simple descriptive statements should be used in lieu of technical terms to identify the treatment or procedure proposed. It is also important that the form indicate that the risks involved had been discussed with the patient.

Just as the patient may consent to treatment, so may he also withhold consent, even in life threatening situations.

CONSENT TO OPERATION, ANESTHETICS, AND MEDICAL SERVICES

1. I hereby authorized Dr. _____
   to perform upon myself (name) _____
   the following operation _____

2. I consent to the performance of other operations and/or procedures, in addition to or different from those now considered which my doctor deems advisable in the course of the operation.

3. I consent to the administration of such anesthetics as are considered advisable by my physician or the anesthesiologist responsible for this service, with the exception of
   _____ (specify or state "None")

4. I consent to the disposal by hospital authorities of any tissues or parts which may be removed.

5. I consent to the photographing or televising of the operation which may include appropriate parts of my body for medical, educational and scientific purposes with the provision that my identity not be disclosed.

6. For purposes of advancing medical education, I consent to the admittance of observers to the operating room.

7. I have been advised that sterility may result from this operation and I understand that this would render me incapable of becoming a parent.

8. My doctor has discussed with me the purpose and nature of the operation, possible alternatives to this treatment, the risks involved, and possible complications. No guarantee or assurance has been given me by any person regarding the results that may be obtained.

SPECIAL INSTRUCTIONS FROM PATIENT: (specify or write "None")

NOTE:
Cross out paragraphs
which do not apply.

Signature of patient or person
authorized to consent for a
minor

Witness _____   Date _____ Time _____
Position _____

Figure 2   Consent to Operate Form

Consent for Delivery by Another Physician

There is a growing trend for obstetricians to practice in groups. Obstetricians who practice without a partner usually designate another obstetrician to substitute for them when they are unable to attend a delivery. The substitute must always be a competent and qualified practitioner. Such substitutions or the possibility that they might be necessary should be explained to the patient in advance. It is advisable to obtain the patient's consent to such an arrangement in writing, and if possible, to also obtain the patient's husband's consent. A form such as the one shown in Fig. 3 may be used for this purpose.

```
                CONSENT TO DELIVERY BY ALTERNATE PHYSICIAN

    Doctor(s) _____

         I hereby agree that you will attend me during my confine-
    ment and delivery. If for any reason you are unable to be
    present, I agree to delivery by a physician whom you  may
    designate for this purpose.

         I free you from any and all liability in conjunction with
    services rendered by the physician who may substitute for you
    at my delivery.


    _____        _____
    Witness                       Signature of patient


    _____        _____
    Date                          Signature of patient's husband
```

Figure 3 Consent to Delivery by Alternate Physician

Special Consent Forms

A variety of situations may develop in the course of patient care which may prove actionable at a later date. The physician's best defense is proof or evidence that he was acting in good faith with the informed consent of the patient. This is best obtained as the patient's signature on an appropriate consent form.

The following forms have been reproduced with the permission of the American Medical Association from their pamphlet Medicolegal Forms with Legal Analysis. Those forms which are used with greater frequency should be prepared in advance by the secretary. These samples are intended as reference formats for use as occasion requires.

CONSENT TO OPERATION FOR COSMETIC PURPOSES

Date_____ Time_____ A.M. P.M.

1. I authorize Dr. _____ to perform an operation upon me for the purpose of attempting to improve my appearance with respect to the following condition: _____

2. The nature and effect of the operation to be performed, risks involved, as well as possible alternative methods of treatment, have been fully explained to me.

3. I also authorize the operating surgeon to perform any other procedures which he may deem desirable in attempting to improve the condition stated in paragraph 1 or any unhealthy or unforeseen condition that he may encounter during the operation.

4. I consent to the administration of anesthetics to be applied by or under the direction of Dr. _____, and to the use of such anesthetics as he may deem advisable.

5. I know that the practice of medicine and surgery is not an exact science and that therefore reputable practitioners cannot guarantee results. No guarantee or assurance has been given by anyone as to the results that may be obtained.

Signed_____
(Patient or person authorized to consent for patient)

Witness_____

Figure 4   Consent to Operation for Cosmetic Purposes

CONSENT TO REMOVAL OF TISSUE FOR GRAFTING

Date_____ Time_____ A.M.
P.M.

1. I authorize Dr. _____, and such assistants as he may designate, to perform an operation upon myself for the purpose of removing the following tissues _____ from my person for
(skin, bone, cartilage, etc.)
donation to _____.
(name of recipient)

The operation is to include such procedures as may be necessary in the judgment of the operating surgeon for the purpose of attempting to graft tissues, and the use of such anesthetics as he may deem advisable.

2. I make this request with full knowledge that this attempt to graft tissue may not be successful. The risks and uncertainties involved as well as the possibility that I may be permanently injured, scarred, or disfigured as a consequence of this operation, have been fully explained to me. Nevertheless, I make this request and grant the authority set forth above, voluntarily and upon my own initiative, and with no assurances from anyone as to the results that may be obtained, either in respect to myself or the recipient.

Signed_____
(Donor)

Witness_____

Figure 5 Consent to Removal of Tissue for Grafting

CONSENT TO OPERATION AND GRAFTING OF TISSUE

Date_____ Time_____ A.M.
P.M.

1. I authorize Dr. _____, and such assistants as he may designate, to perform upon _____
(myself or name of patient)
the following operation _____,
(State nature and extent of operation)
and to do any additional or different procedure that his judgment may dictate during the above operation.

2. I am informed that the above operation will require the grafting of the following tissue _____, and that the tissue to
(skin, bone, cartilage, etc.)
be used will be supplied by _____.
(name of donor or tissue bank)

3. The risks involved in the use of such tissue for grafting, the nature and effect of the operation, and possible alternative methods of procedure or treatment have been fully explained to me. No guarantee or assurance has been given anyone as to the results that may be obtained.

4. I understand that the operating surgeon will be occupied solely with the surgery, and that the administration of the anesthesia is an independent professional function and will be in charge of an anesthetist, whom I authorize to administer such anesthetics as he may deem advisable.

Signed_____
(Patient or person authorized to consent for patient)

Witness_____

Figure 6 Consent to Operation and Grafting of Tissue

REFUSAL TO SUBMIT TO TREATMENT[27]

Date _____ Time _____ A.M. / P.M.

I have been advised by Dr. _____ that it is necessary for me to undergo the following treatment: _____
(Describe operation or treatment)

The effect and nature of this treatment have been explained to me.

Although my failure to follow the advice I have received may seriously imperil my life or health, I nevertheless refuse to submit to the recommended treatment. I assume the risks and consequences involved and release the above-named physician, the hospital and its staff from any liability.

Signed _____

Witness _____

Figure 7   Refusal to Submit to Treatment Form

REFUSAL TO PERMIT BLOOD TRANSFUSION[34]

Date _____ Time _____ A.M. / P.M.

I (We) request that no blood or blood derivatives be administered to _____ during this hospitalization, notwithstanding that such treatment may be deemed necessary in the opinion of the attending physician or his assistants to preserve life or promote recovery. I (We) release the attending physician, his assistants, the hospital and its personnel from any responsibility whatever for any untoward results due to my (our) refusal to permit the use of blood or its derivatives.

Signed _____
Signed _____

Witness _____
Witness _____

Figure 8   Refusal to Permit Blood Transfusion Form

AUTHORIZATION TO USE EYES (DONOR)

Date _____ Time _____ A.M. / P.M.

I authorize, at the time of my death, the removal of both or either of my eyes for donation to any eye bank serving the area in which my death occurs and for such purpose as the eye bank may see fit.

Signed _____
(Donor)

Witness _____

Figure 9   Authorization to Use Eyes (*Donor*) Form

AUTHORIZATION TO USE EYES (NEXT OF KIN)

Date _____ Time _____ A.M. / P.M.

I authorize any member of the medical staff of the _____ Hospital to remove both or either of the eyes of _____ the deceased, for donation to any eye bank serving the area and for such purpose as the eye bank may see fit.

Signed _____
(next of kin)

_____
(relationship to deceased)

Witness _____

Figure 10   Authorization to Use Eyes (*by next of kin*) Form

AUTHORITY TO ADMIT OBSERVERS

Patient_____ Place_____ Date_____

I authorize Dr._____ and the _____Hospital to permit the presence of such observers as they may deem fit to admit in addition to physicians and hospital personnel, while I am undergoing (operative surgery) (childbirth), examination, and treatment.

Signed_____

Witness_____

Figure 11   Authorization to Admit Observers to Operating Room Form

---

CONSENT TO TELEVISING OF OPERATION

Patient_____ Place_____ Date_____

In the interest of medical education and knowledge, I consent to the televising of the operation which is scheduled to be performed upon me on or about _____ 19____. I authorize Dr._____ and the _____ _____ Hospital to admit to the operating room, the cameramen and technicians who are to participate in the televising of this operation, in addition to the usual hospital staff.

Signed_____

Witness_____

Figure 12   Consent to Televising of Operation Form

CONSENT TO TAKING AND PUBLICATION OF PHOTOGRAPHS

Patient_____ Place_____ Date_____

In connection with the medical services which I am receiving from my physician, Dr._____, I consent that photographs may be taken of me or parts of my body, under the following conditions:

1. The photographs may be taken only with the consent of my physician and under such conditions and at such times as may be approved by him.
2. The photographs shall be taken by my physician or by a photographer approved by my physician.
3. The photographs shall be used for medical records and if in the judgment of my physician, medical research, education or science will be benefited by their use, such photographs and information relating to my case may be published and republished, either separately or in connection with each other, in professional journals or medical books, or used for any other purpose which he may deem proper in the interest of medical education, knowledge, or research; provided, however, that it is specifically understood that in any such publication or use I shall not be identified by name.
4. The aforementioned photographs may be modified or retouched in any way that my physician, in his discretion, may consider desirable.

Signed_____
(Patient)

Witness_____

Figure 13   Consent to Taking and Publication of Photographs Form

---

CONSENT TO TAKING OF MOTION PICTURES OF OPERATION

Patient_____ Place_____ Date_____

    1. I consent to the taking of motion pictures of the operation which is scheduled to be performed upon me on or about_____ 19_____. I authorize Dr. _____ and the _____ Hospital to admit to the operating room the cameramen and technicians who will participate in the filming of this operation.

    2. I **waive all rights** that I may have to any claims for payment or royalties in connection with any exhibition, televising, or other showing of this motion picture film, regardless of whether such exhibition, televising, or other showing is under philanthropic, commercial, institutional, or private sponsorship, and irrespective of whether a fee of admission or film rental is charged.

    3. I grant this consent as a voluntary contribution in the interest of medical education and knowledge and subject only to the condition that I will not be identified by name in this motion picture film.

Signed_____

Witness_____

Figure 14   Consent to Taking of Motion Pictures of Operation Form

---

RELEASE FOR RITUAL CIRCUMCISION[24]

Date_____ Time_____ A.M. / P.M.

    We request Dr. _____, the attending physician, and _____ Hospital to permit our son to be circumcised by _____ whom we have selected as a
(person to perform circumcision)
person qualified in the ritual of our faith and by experience to perform this procedure. We assume full responsibility and release the attending physician, the hospital and its staff from liability for any adverse results that may occur.

Signed_____
(Father)

Signed_____
(Mother)

Witness_____

Figure 15   Release Form for Ritual Circumcision

Sterilization Operations

Sterilization is a consideration which the physician weighs in terms of religious, moral and legal factors. Legislation governing such operations varies from state to state. Eugenic sterilization may be performed on sexual deviates, the mentally ill, feebleminded persons and habitual criminals in Alabama, Arizona, California, Connecticut, Delaware, Georgia, Idaho, Indiana, Iowa, Kansas, Maine, Michigan, Minnesota, Mississippi, Montana, Nebraska, New Hampshire, North Carolina, North Dakota, Oklahoma, Oregon, South Carolina, South Dakota, Utah, Vermont, Virginia, West Virginia and Wisconsin. Such persons may be sterilized even over their objection.

In Connecticut, Utah, and Kansas, it is a crime to sterilize a person without medical justification. Sterilization for the sake of convenience is also regarded as a crime in these states.

Sterilization of the male is accomplished by vasectomy requiring a small incision in the scrotum. It is a relatively minor operation in contrast to the operation in the female which requires incision into the abdomen. The female is sterilized by ligation or transection of the fallopian tubes. This is sometimes accomplished incidental to the removal of diseased reproductive organs.

Patients undergoing sterilization operations are usually advised that in all probability they will be unable to become parents. No guarantees are offered when the operation simply consists of tieing off the vas in the male or the fallopian tubes in the female.

Most hospitals have sterilization committees where petitions for therapeutic abortions and sterilizations are reviewed after having been properly submitted in writing with supporting consultations by at least three qualified physicians who are members of the hospital staff.

In those states where sterilization of convenience (non-therapeutic abortion) is a crime (Connecticut, Kansas and Utah), a patient who consents to such a procedure might be denied damages for a bad result on the basis that the patient is in pari delecto in an illegal transaction. This same holding has prevailed in suits involving criminal abortions.

Sterilization does not present any greater exposure to liability in the form of civil damages than other procedures or operations alleged to have been performed negligently. It is advisable, however, to obtain the written consent of the spouse.

The forms shown in Fig. 16 and 17 illustrate the content of recommended forms used in cases of therapeutic abortion and/or sterilization.

STATEMENT OF NEED FOR THERAPEUTIC ABORTION

Date_____ Time_____ A.M. / P.M.

We find from observation and examination of _____ that she is pregnant and that she is suffering from the following ailment or condition:

_____

Further progress of her pregnancy would gravely endanger or imperil her life. Therefore, we are of the opinion that it is medically necessary to perform a therapeutic abortion upon her.

(1) _____
(2) _____
(3) _____

Duly licensed physicians.

Figure 16 Request for Sterilization

REQUEST FOR STERILIZATION

Date_____ Time_____ A.M. / P.M.

We, the undersigned husband and wife, each being more than twenty-one years of age and of sound mind, request Dr. _____, and assistants of his choice, to perform upon _____,
(name of patient)
the following operation: _____
(State nature and extent of operation.)

It has been explained to us that this operation is intended to result in sterility although this result has not been guaranteed. We understand that a sterile person is NOT capable of becoming a parent.

We voluntarily request the operation and understand that if it proves successful the results will be permanent and it will thereafter be physically impossible for the patient to inseminate, or to conceive or bear children.

Signed_____
(Husband)
Signed_____
(Wife)

Witness_____

Figure 17 Statement of Need for Therapeutic Abortion

Request for Medical Information

In the interest of a thorough history it is often necessary to obtain a copy of the patient's medical record from another physician or from a hospital. Such an appeal for information will sometimes include a request for the X-ray films, EKG leads, and/or pathology department tissue slides. A form letter can be very useful in expediting such requests.

Medical information is exchanged between physicians and hospitals without charge. Proper authorization from the patient must accompany all such requests. Provision for the authorizing signature may be contained on the bottom portion of the request letter as exemplified in Fig. 18.

It should be noted that only the patient has the authority to consent to the release of medical information, if that patient is of legal age. A husband may not authorize release of information from his wife's medical record. Where the patient is a minor, either parent must authorize the release. If both parents are deceased, the legal guardian has this authority.

THE SURGICAL SECRETARY

St. Joseph Mercy Hospital
2200 EAST GRAND BOULEVARD
Detroit 11, Michigan

January 24, 1962

PATIENT:
ADDRESS:
BIRTHDATE:

Dear Madame:

Your assistance is requested in furnishing us with the following information regarding the above named patient who is currently under treatment at these facilities.

_____ Medical abstract or photocopy of the medical record particularly _____

_____

_____ Loan of x-ray films

_____ Loan of pathology slides

Your earliest reply in this matter will be appreciated.

Very truly yours,

Jeannette A. Szulec
Jeannette A. Szulec, RRL
MEDICAL RECORD LIBRARIAN

AUTHORIZATION FOR RELEASE OF INFORMATION (patient to complete)

Permission for release of information from my hospital records in accordance with the above request is hereby granted.

I was treated at the _____ Hospital
in (city and state) _____
on (approximate date) _____ by Doctor _____
SIGNATURE OF PATIENT _____
 (name under which hospitalized)

Figure 18   Request for Information Form

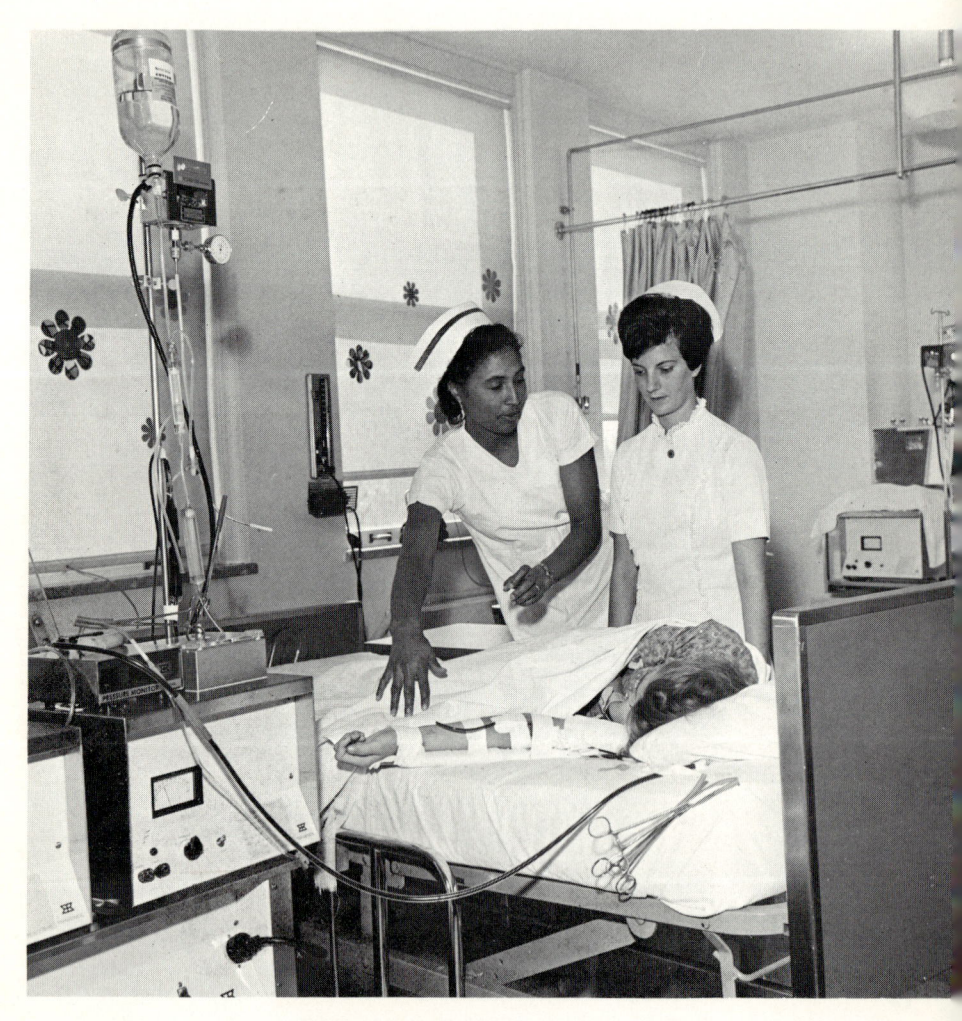

Patient connected to an artificial kidney machine in the modern hemodialysis departme[nt] of the Receiving Branch—Detroit General Hospital (City of Detroit), the university hospital for t[he] Wayne State University College of Medicine.

2 | *Laboratory Examinations*

With advances in our knowledge of physiology and improved technology, laboratory and x-ray examinations have become a valuable diagnostic aid to the physician, helping him to confirm or disprove suspected pathologic conditions. They form an important segment of the diagnostic picture when studied in relation to the clinical findings.

Some of the more commonly used laboratory and x-ray examinations will be discussed in this chapter to provide an understanding for persons engaged in medical secretarial and medical records fields.

Blood

The blood volume of the average person is 5 to 6 quarts (equal to about 5000-6000 ml's or cc.'s). It is broken down and replaced in a healthy individual at a rate of about 50 cc.'s per day. Three types of cells predominate in the composition of the blood; the red corpuscles (RBC's also known as red blood cells or erythrocytes), white corpuscles (also known as WBC's or leukocytes), and platelets. These cells are bathed in a fluid called plasma which serves as a liquid vehicle for their circulation throughout the body.

EXAMINATIONS OF THE BLOOD

Red Blood Count

Normal Values   Male 4,500,000   to 6,000,000 per cu. mm
                             Female 4,300,000   to 5,500,000 per cu. mm

The red blood cells, otherwise known as RBC's or erythrocytes are formed by a cell division in the bone marrow. They are released after approximately seven days into the circulation. The average life of a red blood cell is about 120 days after which it is subjected to a breakdown in the liver and the spleen.

A red pigment known as HEMOGLOBIN is found in the red cells. It possesses the property of carrying oxygen from the lungs to tissues throughout the body.

Red Blood Count (continued)

There is little or no variation in the red blood cell count and hemoglobin during complete rest; however, during hours of activity physiological changes are known to take place. Exercise is known to increase the red blood cell count and hemoglobin level. Fear and excitement may also increase the red blood cell count. High altitudes with their lowered barometric pressure produce anoxemia with a resulting increase in hemoglobin and red blood cells. Dehydration causes a greater concentration of red blood cells while intake of excessive amounts of water may temporarily lower their concentration. A lowered red blood count may be seen in the anemias and after hemorrhage. Adult females have a lower red blood cell count than do adult males.

A complete differential count reports any abnormal features of the cells observed which may include the following:

anisocytosis— variation in size of cells seen in primary and secondary anemias

poikilocytosis— variation in shape of cells seen in advanced anemias

hypochromasia— hemoglobin deficiency seen in hypochromic, sickle cell, and erythroblastic anemia

hyperchromasia— evidence of excessive hemoglobin seen in pernicious anemia

basophilic stippling—forms seen in marked primary and secondary anemias, malaria and lead poisoning

target cell— a form found in Cooley's anemia, sickle cell anemia, hypochromic anemia, and in jaundice

sickle cell— red blood cells assume a sickle shape when deprived of oxygen in persons with sickle cell anemia, a condition seen in about 8% of persons of the Negro race

nuclear remnants— include Cabot's ring bodies, Howell's bodies, chromatin particles, dark staining granules

degenerating red blood cells— include Maragliano body, Ehrlich's hemoglobinemic degeneration

Heinz bodies— may be demonstrated with phase microscopy or dark field examination in patients with hemolytic anemia resulting from certain chemicals or drugs. Also seen in post splenectomy patients, premature infants, and persons addicted to phenacetin or acetanilid

siderocytes— seen in hemolytic anemia and following splenectomy.

A lowered red blood count may be seen in the anemias and after a hemorrhage. An increase may result from dehydration or polycythemia.

Hematocrit

Normal values   Male   38–54%
Female 36–47%

This is a test on the blood which measures the cells compared to the volume of plasma. It is elevated in polycythemia and dehydration and lowered in the anemias and following hemorrhage. The results are inconclusive after an episode of bleeding or soon after a blood transfusion.

Hemoglobin

Normal Values   Male   14-18 Gm.%
Female   12-16 Gm.%
Children 12-14 Gm.%

The red cell component of the blood measures about 2000 ml. and consists of about 600 gm. of hemoglobin which can carry 800 ml. of oxygen from the lungs to the tissues of the body.

The hemoglobin is reduced in anemias and hemorrhage and increased in dehydration and polycythemia. It is studied in relation to the red cell count, which does not always vary with the hemoglobin, when the anemias are differentiated.

Examinations used to determine the hemoglobin content of the erythrocyte include the *Color Index* (normal range 0.9 to 1.1) which is increased over a value of 1 in macrocytic anemia, and the *Mean Corpuscular Hemoglobin* (normal range for adults 27-30; children 26-28). The concentration of hemoglobin in the erythrocyte is determined from examinations which include the *Saturation Index* (normal range 0.9 to 1.1) increased in macrocytic anemias and decreased in microcytic and hypochromic anemias, and the *Mean Corpuscular Hemoglobin Concentration* (normal range adults 32 to 36, and for children 32 to 34.)

White Blood Count (WBC) Normal 5,000-10,000/cu. mm.

The total white blood count (leukocyte count) may vary from one day to the next and be related to a variety of factors such as exercise, state of hydration, high altitudes, meals, hot baths, etc. Healthy persons may demonstrate counts outside the range of normal; however, it is generally accepted that an increase in the leukocytes beyond 10,000 is abnormal.

Abnormal elevation in the white blood count is termed *leukocytosis,* or more specifically designated by the one particular type white blood cell causing the elevated white blood count as *lymphocytic leukocytosis* (lymphocytosis), eosinophilic leukocytosis (eosinophilia), neutrophilic lymphocytosis (neutrophilia), etc.

In order to determine the cause for the elevated white blood count it is important to perform a differential count which distinguishes the various white cells. Generally, one particular cell causes the elevated white count. Some conditions cause an elevation in all of the forms. Much remains to be learned about these cells, but at this stage in our knowledge we have a valuable diagnostic method in the white blood count.

Reduction of the white blood count below the range of normal is called *leukopenia* and usually occurs in the basophiles, eosinophiles or neutrophiles, most commonly in the neutrophiles. A reduction in all white cell forms with anemia and thrombocytopenia is called *pancytopenia*.

White Cell Differential

Several types of white blood cells can be differentiated in the white blood count which furnish a valuable index for detecting certain diseases. The differential is usually based on the percentage of particular white cells found in a sample of 100 white blood cells.

Differentiated Cells	*per cu. mm.*	*%*	*Significance*
Band neutrophiles	150-400	2-5%	Adults
(STABS)	150-300	3-8%	Children (3-10 years)
			Increased in acute infections, with or without an increase in the leukocytes (wbc's).
Basophiles	15-50	0-0.75	Adults
(BASOS)	0-50	0-0.75	Children
			Increased in basophilic and myelogenous leukemia, polycythemia vera and chronic hemolytic anemia. Sometimes also elevated in Hodgkin's disease, chronic infections of bony sinuses, chickenpox, smallpox, and after splenectomy.
Eosinophiles	50-250	1-3%	Adults
(EOSINS)	50-700	1-3%	Children
			Increased in parasitic infections such as trichinosis, schistosomiasis, strongyloidiasis, ancylostomiasis, amebiasis, ruptured hydatid cyst, Taenia solium, Fasciola hepatica, Clonorchis sinensis. Elevated in allergic diseases, some skin diseases, following X-ray irradiation, as a familial anomaly, and in some neoplasms such as carcinoma of the stomach, lung and Hodgkin's disease.
Juvenile neutrophiles	0-100	0-1%	Elevated in severe infections and in myelogenous leukemia.
(POLYS)			
also: metamyelocytes			

LABORATORY EXAMINATIONS

Differentiated Cells	*per cu. mm.*	%	*Significance*
Lymphocytes (LYMPHS) Atypical lymphocytes are found in blood smears of infectious mononucleosis	1500-3000 3250-5000	25-33% 42-48%	Adults Children Increased with elevated WBC in lymphocytic leukemia, infect. mononucleosis, acute infect. lymphocytosis, pertussis, Tbc in persons with good resistance, congenital syphilis, secondary syphilis, thyrotoxicosis, malnutrition and rickets. Increased without elevation of WBC in splenic anemia, pernicious anemia, acute infections such as mumps, German measles, influenza, infect. hepatitis, Typhoid fever, brucellosis, and many viral infections.
Monocytes (MONOS)	285-500 250-700	3-7% 3-5%	Adults Children Elevated in monocytic leukemia, acute infections, SBE (subacute bacterial endocarditis), typhus fever, brucellosis, Rocky Mt. spotted fever, parasitic inf. such as malaria, trypanosomiasis, Kalaazar, leishmaniasis of the skin, and sometimes in Hodgkin's disease, lipoid storage diseases and poisoning by tetrachlorethane.
Myelocytes	0	0%	Presence suggests granulocytic leukemia or pernicious anemia. Metastases to bone in cases of malignancy is suggested.
Segmented neutrophiles (SEGS) Also: mature neutrophiles	3000-5800 3000-8000	54-62% 16-60%	Adults Children Elevated in acute infections by pyogenic cocci. Some bacillary infections cause elevation on lesser scale. Moderate elevation seen in viral diseases as rabies, poliomyelitis, typhus, herpes zoster. Fungal infections of Actinomyces and spirochete infections of Leptospira icterohaemorrhagiae also cause moderate elevation.

Platelets (Thrombocytes)

Normal Range   200,000 to 500,000

Platelet formation is believed to occur from megakaryocytes in the bone marrow during the adult years. Their life span extends from eight to nine days with replacement occurring at the rate of 100,000 per day.

Platelets are important in blood clotting and in clot retraction. An increase in their number above the normal range is called *thrombocytosis* and may result from strenuous exercise, malnutrition, high altitudes, acute infections, hemolytic anemia, myelogenous leukemia, acute hemorrhage, polycythemia vera, after surgery, fractures and during asphyxia.

A decrease in the total platelet count is called *thrombocytopenia* and may be seen in association with reduced prothrombin consumption, increased capillary fragility, prolonged bleeding time, and normal coagulation time. Values are decreased in pernicious anemia, acute leukemia, chronic lymphocytic leukemia, aplastic anemia, thrombocytopenic purpura and septicemia.

BLOOD GROUPS

It is estimated that more than four and a half million transfusions are administered in the United States each year. It is believed that transfusion reactions occur in from three to five per cent of these transfusions, with one death in every 1000-3000 cases. The hazards which attend this form of therapy must be weighed against the particular benefit to be gained.

Many medical authorities question the practice of using a single unit (500 cc.) of blood. Audit committees in hospitals are usually on the alert for abuses in this area.

Extreme care is required in typing and cross matching the blood of donor and recipient when a blood transfusion is indicated. Transfusion with an incompatible blood type causes clumping of the donor red blood cells followed by destruction of these cells. Such transfusion reactions may be severe enough to eventuate in death of the patient.

Human blood types are divided into four groups which make up the ABO system, a universally accepted classification, proposed by Landsteiner in 1900.

Blood Groups	*Percentage Distribution in U.S.A. Population*
A	41%
B	10%
AB (universal recipient)	4%
O (universal donor)	45%

Blood groups are classified on the basis of two factors contained within the red blood cells and two factors present in the plasma or serum. The groups are designated by their red cell factors A & B. Red blood cells may contain one or the other, both or none (type O) of these factors.

The red cell factors A & B act as antigens, provoking the formation of, and being agglutinated by, specific antibodies (agglutinins).

Blood Groups (continued)

The two serum factors are anti-A (alpha agglutinin) and anti-B (beta agglutinin). In addition to these factors, subtypes are also recognized in the blood groupings.

GROUP A—Serum of this type agglutinates (causes clumping) the red cells of types B and AB only. Red cells of this blood type are agglutinated by serum of either types O or B. Subtypes in this group are A_1 and A_2.

GROUP B—Serum of this type agglutinates the red cells of types A and AB only, while its red cells are agglutinated by serum of either types O or A. There are no subgroups.

GROUP AB—This blood type is called the universal recipient because the red cells of the other three groups are not agglutinated (clumped together) by this serum. Persons of this blood type can usually receive any type blood. There is a risk involved, however, if the donor's blood contains a high agglutinin titer. There are no agglutinins (factors causing clumping) in serum of this type. Subtypes are A_1B and A_2B.

GROUP O—This blood type is called the universal donor because red cells of this type are not agglutinated (clumped) by the serum of the other three types. The serums of the other three types are clumped by the serum of this blood type.

In an emergency, group O blood may be given to patients with blood types A, B, or AB provided the anti-A and anti-B titer of the donor is low. There is always a risk factor in such transfusions.

The Rh Factor

Another important and routine factor in blood typing is the Rh factor, an agglutinogen designated as the rhesus factor after the rhesus monkey on which the experiments were carried out.

It is estimated that approximately 85% of the Caucasian race, 94% of the Negroid race and 99% of the Mongoloid race possess this agglutinogen. These persons are classified as Rh positive. Persons who lack this factor in their blood are classified as Rh negative.

Persons with Rh negative blood who are transfused with Rh positive blood by error may produce anti-Rh antibodies. Not all persons are sensitized in this way; however, those who do become sensitized may experience severe hemolytic reactions when given Rh positive blood at some future date. These transfusion reactions may be severe enough to cause death.

The administration of Rh positive blood to an Rh negative female may stimulate antibody formation making it impossible for her to bear normal children to an Rh positive husband. Rh positive blood given to an Rh negative woman before she has become pregnant may result in erythroblastosis fetalis of her offspring.

Recognition of the Rh factor has helped to explain some transfusion reactions and the development of certain hemolytic diseases, particularly erythroblastosis fetalis (hemolytic disease of the fetus and newborn).

An Rh negative woman married to an Rh positive man may conceive an Rh positive child. The blood of the Rh positive fetus escapes into the maternal circulation. Antibodies may be produced in the mother and then enter the fetal circulation through the placenta. These antibodies work to destroy the red blood cells of the fetus. This condition is known as *erythroblastosis fetalis*.

The Rh negative mother sensitized by an Rh positive child doesn't begin to form her dangerous immunity until several weeks after the birth of the child. Once the mother has developed such immunity it is active and permanent. The first child is rarely affected; however, in following pregnancies the mother's antibodies attack the Rh positive blood of the baby endangering its life. Exchange blood transfusions are sometimes necessary to save the infant.

Some physicians routinely test the blood of pregnant Rh negative mothers for determination of possible elevation in titer of anti-Rh antibodies. This information assists the physician, in some instances, of predicting erythroblastosis fetalis in the infant, although it is not necessarily helpful in predicting the severity of the disease. A mother with a high titer may give birth to an infant with the disease manifested only in the mildest form.

In the interest of detecting erythroblastosis fetalis, it is a common practice to perform a direct Coomb's test on the cord blood of all infants and without exception on those born to Rh negative mothers. Although 93% of erythroblastotic infants are born to Rh negative mothers, there is a 7% incidence in Rh positive mothers who have been immunized by a blood factor from the fetus. Diagnostic results may be obtained with the direct Coomb's test in newborns who are seemingly normal at birth. The incidence of this disease is generally believed to be one in every 200 full term deliveries, or one in every 26 pregnancies which terminate short of a living infant.

A new vaccine called RhoGAM designed to prevent erythroblastosis fetalis by inducing passive immunity in the mother was released in June 1968, by Ortho Diagnostics, a subsidiary of Johnson & Johnson. Only one injection of the vaccine is needed after each pregnancy. The hospital or laboratory's cost is $46.60 per dose and therefore the charge to the patient will be somewhat higher.

The vaccine said to be 100 per cent effective in clinical trials was developed by Dr. Vincent J. Freda, assistant clinical professor of obstetrics and gynecology at Columbia University College of Physicians and

The Rh Factor (continued)

Surgeons, working with Dr. William Pollack, research fellow of the Ortho Research Foundation and Dr. John G. Gorman, associate in pathology at Columbia University College of Physicians and Surgeons.

Rh negative mothers who have already been sensitized from a previous delivery, miscarriage or incorrect transfusion of Rh positive blood will not be helped by the vaccine.

Source of the vaccine is the blood of women who have already been sensitized. The blood of the donor is fractionated to yield Immunoglobulin G, the vaccine. The vaccine, actually antibodies, given shortly after delivery to an Rh negative mother neutralize the baby's cells in the maternal circulation before active and permanent immunity is established.

BONE MARROW STUDIES

The bone marrow is a substance found in all bones and made up of adult and young blood cells and their precursors, fat cells, blood vessels, and reticulum. Up to the age of five, all of the marrow is active and functional; however, with maturity, fat cells appear in the marrow of the long bones, rendering the marrow nonfunctional. In the normal adult marrow may be found in the sternum, vertebrae, ribs, skull, and the hip bone (os coxae).

Function of the bone marrow is formation of red blood cells, platelets and granulocytes which pass into the blood stream after maturing.

Examination of the bone marrow is performed by needle aspiration from sites in the sternum, ribs, spinous processes of the vertebrae or iliac crests of the hip bone. The most common biopsy site is the sternum. Aspiration and examination of the material obtained is performed by a hematologist or a clinical pathologist, when there is a strong suspicion that any one of the following conditions may exist: lupus erythematosis, multiple myeloma, aplastic anemia, aleukemic leukemia, leukemia, pernicious anemia, familial splenic anemia (Gaucher's disease), malignant neutropenia, metastatic carcinoma of the bone marrow, thrombocytopenic purpura or leishmaniasis (a protozoan parasitic infection).

Microscopic examination of marrow smears may disclose information regarding certain blood diseases which might not be apparent in studies of peripheral blood samples. The most important information gleaned from this examination is the differential count of marrow cells based on identification and a count of at least 500 to 1000 cells. An important observation is the myeloid:erythroid ratio (M:E ratio, or ratio of nucleated red cell forms to leukocytes). These ranges are normally 4:1 and 2:1.

Ranges of the normal bone marrow cells vary with the investigator. Most hematologists and clinical pathologists adopt a certain standard and furnish their reports on printed forms which list the normal range in one column. The count takes note of the following forms:

Cell Form	Normal Range of Adults by %
Myeloblasts	0.5 - 5
Promyelocytes	1 - 8
Myelocytes	
Neutrophiles	5 - 20
Eosinophiles	0.5 - 3
Basophiles	0 - 0.5
Metamyelocytes (juveniles)	10 - 25
Polymorphonuclear neutrophiles	7.0 - 30.0
Polymorphonuclear eosinophiles	00.5 - 4.0
Band cells	15 - 30
Segmented	
Neutrophiles	10 - 35
Eosinophiles	0 - 5
Basophiles	0 - 1
Lymphocytes	5 - 20
Monocytes	0 - 5
Plasma cells	0 - 1
Nucleated red cells (per 100 leukocytes)	
Megaloblasts	0 - 2
Erythroblasts	1 - 5
Normoblasts	5 - 20
Megakaryocytes	0 - 3
Pronormoblasts (macroblasts)	1.0 - 8.0
Reticulum cells	0 - 2
Myeloid-erythroblast ratio	3.6 to 1.0
Normoblasts (basophilic, polychromatophilic, andacidophilic)	7.0 - 32.0

DIFFERENTIAL COUNT—Normal Bone Marrow

EXAMINATIONS PERFORMED ON THE URINE

Like the blood, the urine yields valuable information to assist the clinician in further assessing the physiologic status of the patient.

The average sized adult urinary bladder usually can hold about 350 cc. of urine before the urge to urinate becomes manifest. In a 24 hour period an adult may void between 1/2 and 2 quarts. Throughout the night urine is secreted into the bladder at the rate of about 40 cc. per hour. The intake of fluids throughout the day influences the amount of urine excreted and the frequency of urination. On an average, about a third of the fluid intake is passed within the first hour.

Urine output is reduced when there is loss of fluid through diarrhea or vomiting. It is also reduced when there is heavy sweating as a result of exercise or an elevated temperature.

Children usually pass three to four times as much urine per kilogram of body weight as do adults.

Urination in excess of approximately 2 quarts per day is regarded as pathologic and is called **polyuria.** This condition may be transient and associated with frequency in nervousness and excitement. There may be excessive urination with a high protein diet or after the intake of alcohol, tea or coffee. The principal organic causes for polyuria are hypertension with renal involvement and chronic nephritis. In diabetes mellitus the patient excretes large quantities of urine of a pale yellow or greenish color.

Oliguria is the name for a condition where there is a decreased urinary output. This may be a normal physiologic response when there is reduced intake of fluids, increased salt consumption, and excessive sweating. Pathological causes may be obstructed ureters, acute nephritis, nephrosis, portal cirrhosis, acute yellow atrophy of the liver, peritonitis, acute intestinal obstruction, cardiac deficiency or poisons which damage the kidneys.

Nocturia is the name for a condition characterized by excessive passage of urine at night. In a healthy individual, under normal conditions, the urine passed during the waking hours is three to four times the amount excreted during the night. Nocturia is seen in nephritis.

Anuria is the term for complete inability to urinate. It may be caused by mechanical obstruction of the ureters, or to a disease process which damages both kidneys.

Color of Urine

Urine is normally yellow to amber in color. Variations in the color may result from drugs, bile, blood, dyes or foods eaten. Pyridium imparts an orange red color to urine. An orange-yellow to greenish-brown may result from bilirubin in obstructive jaundice. Brown or blackish urine may be caused by alkaptonuria or malignant melanoma. A dark brown color may be noted in liver infections, malaria, pernicious anemia or acute infections. Color abnormalities of pathologic significance are comparatively rare.

Cloudiness is usually due to phosphates, urates, carbonates, pus cells or bacteria. Generally turbidity is nonpathologic.

Odor of Urine

An aromatic odor characterizes normal urine. It develops an ammoniacal odor on standing due to decomposition products. A fecal odor suggests a fistulous communication between the intestinal and urinary tracts. An overripe apple odor suggests acetone bodies in the urine, while a fruity or new mown hay odor suggests diabetes. A fishy odor associated with cloudy urine suggests cystitis or pyelitis.

Specific Gravity

Specific gravity of urine is the ratio of the weight of a certain volume of urine to the weight of the same volume of water at a temperature of 4 degrees C. Water has a specific gravity of 1.000 whereas the normal range for urine is from 1.010 to 1.030, reflecting the ability of the kidneys to concentrate urine. Urinary specific gravity is elevated in acute glomerulonephritis, diabetes mellitus, fever, sweating, vomiting and diarrhea. It is low in chronic nephritis and diabetes insipidus.

Microscopic Examination of Urine

No urinalysis is complete without a microscopic examination of the organized sediment for casts, pus cells, red blood cells and epithelial cells. Spermatozoa may be found in the urine of male or female following sexual intercourse. They are sometimes noted in male urine after nocturnal emissions, convulsions and prostatic massage.

A few epithelial cells may be from the bladder or vagina with no pathologic significance. Intelligent recognition of cells may yield valuable information relative to their source of origin. These findings may be useful in diagnosing tumors of the kidney or ulcerative lesions anywhere in the urinary tract.

Red blood cells in the urine, other than those introduced by contamination with menstrual blood or catheter trauma, are considered pathologic, particularly when present in considerable numbers. This condition is called **hematuria** and is found in acute glomerulonephritis, pyelonephritis, tuberculosis of the kidneys, polycystic kidneys, nephrolithiasis, carcinoma of the kidney, tumors of the urinary bladder, leukemia and blood diseases, infarction, prostatitis, urethritis, and collagen diseases such as disseminated lupus erythematosus. It may also develop in patient's undergoing Dicumarol (anticoagulant) therapy.

White blood cells (leukocytes) may be present as contaminants from leukorrhea in the female, or may be due to infection somewhere in the urinary tract in either male or female. Gitter cells may indicate pyelonephritis.

Casts in the urine are tube-like structures that form in the kidney tubules. They may be noncellular such as the hyaline (made up exclusively of protein), waxy, fatty and granular, or cellular casts which include leukocyte (white blood cell) casts, red cell casts, renal failure casts, bacterial casts or epithelial casts.

Hyaline casts may be found in glomerulonephritis, nephritis and nephrosis.

Granular casts may indicate glomerulonephritis or nephrosis, as do waxy casts.

Fatty casts may be found in chronic glomerulonephritis and lipoid nephrosis.

White cell casts suggest pyelonephritis while red cell casts are found in chronic glomerulonephritis and in transfusion reactions with hemolysis.

Bacteriologic Examination of the Urine

The bacteriologic examination may yield valuable information regarding infections of the urinary tract. In pyelonephritis and cystitis the organisms most commonly found include Escherichia coli, Proteus vulgaris, streptococci and staphylococci. Mycobacterium tuberculosis is found in the urine where there is tuberculosis of the kidneys, bladder or prostate, usually secondary to tuberculosis of the lungs. Other pathologic organisms which may be recovered from the urine include Salmonella typhosa, Shigella dysenteriae (dysentery), Brucella abortus and Brucella melitensis (undulant fever), and Leptospira icterohaemorrhagiae (spirochetal jaundice).

Nonpathogenic organisms which may be cultured from the urine include Aerobacter aerogenes, Neisseria catarrhalis, and Pseudomonas aeruginosa.

EXAMINATIONS OF THE CEREBROSPINAL FLUID

In an adult individual, the total cerebrospinal fluid (spinal fluid) amounts to approximately 100-140 cc.'s. It is a clear, colorless fluid which bathes the brain and spinal cord. It is secreted by the choroid plexuses, glandular structures in the lateral ventricles of the brain. The amount secreted in a 24 hour period varies with individuals; however, it is estimated that it may vary from 300 to 1000 cc.'s. The fluid passes through the arachnoidal tissue into the venous circulation.

Samples of cerebrospinal fluid are withdrawn for diagnostic studies by means of a procedure known as a spinal puncture. A long needle is inserted into the vertebral canal through the middle of the space between the third and fourth lumbar vertebrae. Fluid may also be withdrawn by a cisternal puncture by introducing the needle between the first cervical vertebra and the occipital bone.

Pressure readings are usually taken with the patient on his side. In adults the pressure may range from 70 to 200 mm. of water or up to 8 mm. of mercury. In children the normal range may vary from 50 to 100 mm. of water while the range for newborn infants is from 30 to 80 mm. of water. When the puncture is performed in the sitting position, the pressure is increased to almost twice that obtained in the recumbent position. The pressure is increased with coughing or crying. It is also increased in diseases which include cerebral thrombosis, intracranial hemorrhage, edema of the brain, hydrocephalus, some brain tumors, brain abscess, meningitis, and in other inflammatory lesions such as encephalitis and poliomyelitis.

Decreased pressure readings may be obtained in obstructions of the subarachnoid space of the spinal cord, obstructive hydrocephalus, shock and dehydration. Some normal individuals have low spinal fluid pressures which are of no pathologic significance.

In the course of manometer readings, pressure is applied over one jugular vein and then the other. Normally this produces a rise in cerebrospinal fluid pressure and is referred to as a positive Queckenstedt sign. When such jugular compression fails to produce an increased fluid pressure at the lumbar level, the Queckenstedt sign is said to be negative and is usually indicative of obstructed fluid circulation above the level of the puncture. Partial obstruction is characterized by a slow increase in fluid pressure on compression of the jugular veins, with slow return to the resting level.

Cerebrospinal Fluid Examination

EXAMINATION	NORMAL VALUES	SIGNIFICANCE
Sp. Gravity	1.003 - 1.009	
pH	7.35 - 7.40	
Total cells		Increased levels seen in encephalitis, neurosyphilis, meningitis.
Adults:	0 - 10 per cu. mm.	
Infants:	0 - 20 per cu. mm.	
Chlorides	690 - 750 mg.%	Slightly decreased in purulent bacterial meningitis and even lower in tuberculous meningitis.
Cholesterol	0.05 - 0.20 mg.%	
CO_2 combining power	40 - 60 vol.%	
Colloidal Gold	Negative	When a precipitate of colloidal gold is obtained it may suggest multiple sclerosis, neurosyphilis or other diseases of the CNS. It must be evaluated relative to the entire clinical picture.
Proteins, total	20 - 45 mg.%	Increased in hemorrhage. Levels may be elevated as high as 2000 mg.% in meningitis.
Proteins, globulin	4 - 10 mg.%	
Proteins, albumin	16 - 35 mg.%	
Serology	Negative	Positive in neurosyphilis.
Sugar (Glucose)	45 - 75 mg./100 ml.	Absent or low in acute purulent meningitis. Present in ranges from 10 to 20 mg. per 100 ml. in tuberculous meningitis.

EXAMINATION OF THE SPUTUM

Sputum is an exudate which is produced in excessive quantities in bronchial, pulmonary and tracheal infections. Ciliary movements cause these secretions to be brought up from the bronchus into the trachea. The cough mechanism discharges them from the upper trachea into the mouth from which they may be expelled.

Examinations of the sputum take note of the following:

- Amount collected in 24 hours
- Odor
- Color
- Consistency
- Dittrich's plugs
- Curschmann's spirals
- Bronchial casts
- Pneumoliths (concretions or lung stones)

Microscopic Findings

- Elastic fibers
- Crystals
    - Charcot-Leyden
    - Cholesterol
    - Fatty-acid crystals
    - Hematoidin
- Myelin globules
- Heart failure cells (hemosiderin)
- Yeasts

Pathogenic fungi

- Candida albicans (candidiasis)
- Coccidioides immitis (valley fever)
- Cryptococcus neoformans (torulosis)
- Geotrichum (geotrichosis)
- Actinomyces (ray fungus) (sulphur granules)

Bacteria

Search is primarily made for acid-fast bacilli of tuberculosis, Mycobacterium tuberculosis.

Parasites

- Entamoeba histolytica
- Hookworm and Strongyloides (larvae)
- Hooklets and scolices
- Paragonimus westermani eggs (oriental hemoptysis)
- also: Distoma westermani, Distoma ringeri and Distoma pulmonale
- Viruses
- Neoplastic cells (specimen for tumor cells usually obtained directly from bronchi by bronchoscopy)

BACTERIOLOGICAL EXAMINATIONS

Bacterial examination of body secretions, exudates and fluids is carried out through the use of stained smears and cultures. It is sometimes also desirable to determine the virulence of the organism and its sensitivity to various antibiotics. When the disease causing organism cannot be isolated, bacterial agglutination tests with elevated titers assist the physician in establishing the diagnosis.

Blood cultures are often used to identify the causative organism in an infection. Bacteria in the blood may represent a bacteremia or septicemia.

Bacteremia represents a short-lived occurrence of bacteria in the blood with no clinical evidence of infection. This condition may result from abscessed teeth or tonsils.

Septicemia occurs when there is invasion of the blood stream by microorganisms which multiply in this medium and produce toxins causing clinical evidence of infection. Septicemia may develop secondary to an infection in body tissues, or it may cause secondary infections in body tissues.

Organisms are referred to as **gram-positive** or **gram-negative.** This dichotomy is based on whether they retain the stain in Gram's method of staining.

Streptococci

Streptococci, one of the most important groups of pathogenic organisms, are qualified as hemolytic and nonhemolytic depending upon whether or not they produce hemolysis (separation of hemoglobin from the red blood cells) on the blood agar medium on which they are being grown. A more acceptable classification of the streptococci is, Alpha Hemolytic Streptococci, Beta Hemolytic Streptococci, and Gamma Nonhemolytic Streptococci. In the alpha form there is incomplete hemolysis, in the beta there is complete hemolysis, while in the gamma form there is no hemolysis of the blood agar medium.

Staphylococci

Staphylococcic infections are characterized by abscesses, pustules, furuncles (boils), and carbuncles. Although it most commonly produces these lesions of the skin and subcutaneous tissues, it also produces throat infections, bacterial pneumonia with lung abscess and empyema, middle ear infections, paranasal sinus infections, urinary tract infections, and acute bacterial endocarditis.

Staphylococci are classified into three categories on the basis of the colored pigment they produce. Staph. aureus produces a deep golden pigment. Most pathogenic staphylococci are of the aureus group. The other two types are Staph. albus, producing a pure white matter, and Staph. citreus which produces a light yellow pigment.

LABORATORY EXAMINATIONS

Another classification of the staphylococci is whether they are **coagulase positive** or **coagulase negative**. Practically all epidemic or hospital acquired staphylococcic infections are coagulase positive, that is, they cause coagulation of human citrated plasma or rabbit plasma.

Tests for TBC

Examination of the sputum for tuberculosis is performed from smears. These slides are read as negative for acid-fast bacilli, or positive for acid-fast bacilli, specifying them as rare, few or numerous. Another tuberculosis test is the Mantoux skin test. An area of edema and redness greater than 5 mm. in diameter is regarded as positive. In view of the fact that at least 50% of the population at one time or another becomes infected with tuberculosis, the positive skin test has limited diagnostic value.

The following alphabetical listing of bacterial organisms by generic as well as popular name is provided as a spelling reference and makes no effort to classify these organisms.

BACTERIAL MICROORGANISMS

Acid-fast bacilli (usually Mycobacterium tuberculosis)
Actinobacillus lignieresi
Actinobacillus mallei
Aerobacter aerogenes
Alcaligenes faecalis
Alpha streptococcus
Anhemolytic streptococcus
Anthrax bacillus

Bacillus acidilactici
Bacillus aerogenes capsulatus
Bacillus aertryke
Bacillus alvei
Bacillus anthracis
Bacillus botulinus
Bacillus brevis
Bacillus bronchisepticus
Bacillus coli
Bacillus diphtheriae
Bacillus dysenteriae
Bacillus enteritidis
Bacillus faecalis alcaligenes
Bacillus influenza
Bacillus larvae
Bacillus leprae

Bacillus mallei (Glanders bacillus)
Bacillus oedematis maligni No. II
Bacillus oedematiens
Bacillus pertussis
Bacillus pestis
Bacillus pneumoniae
Bacillus polymyxa
Bacillus proteus
Bacillus pseudomallei
Bacillus pyocyaneus
Bacillus subtilis
Bacillus suipestifer
Bacillus tetani
Bacillus tuberculosis
Bacillus tularense
Bacillus typhi
Bacillus typhosus
Bacillus welchii
Bacillus whitmori
Bacterium coli
Bang's bacillus
Bargen's streptococcus
Battey bacilli
Beta streptococcus
Boas-Oppler bacillus
Bordet-Gengou

BACTERIAL MICROORGANISMS (continued)

Bordetella bronchiseptica
Bordetella pertussis
Borrelia duttonii
Borrelia recurrentis
Borrelia refringens
Borrelia vincentii
Brucella abortus
Brucella melitensis
Brucella suis

Calmette-Guerin bacillus
Clostridium bifermentans
Clostridium botulinum
Clostridium butyricum
Clostridium histolyticum
Clostridium perfringens
Clostridium novyi
Clostridium septicum
Clostridium tertium
Clostridium tetani
Clostridium welchii
Coliform organisms
Corynebacterium diphtheriae
Corynebacterium pseudodiphtheriticum
Corynebacterium pseudotuberculosis
Corynebacterium xerosis

Diplococcus pneumoniae
Döderlein's bacillus
Ducrey's bacillus

Eberthella typhi
Enterococcus
Erysipelothrix rhusiopathiae
Escherichia coli (E. coli)

Fehleisen's streptococcus
Fick's bacillus
Flexner's bacillus
Flexner-Strong bacilli
Friedlanders bacillus
Fusobacterium fusiforme

Gaffkya tetragena
Gamma streptococcus

Gärtner's bacillus
Ghon-Sachs bacillus
Glanders bacillus
Gonococcus

Hansen's bacillus
Haverhillia multiformis
Hemolytic streptococcus
Hemophilus aegypti
Hemophilus ducreyi
Hemophilus duplex
Hemophilus influenzae
Hemophilus pertussis
Hofmann's bacillus

Johne's bacillus

Klebs-Löffler bacillus
Klebsiella pneumoniae
Koch-Weeks bacillus

Lactobacillus acidophilus
Lactobacillus bulgaricus
Leptospira canicola
Leptospira hebdomadis
Leptospira icterohemorrhagiae

Malleomyces mallei
Malleomyces pseudomallei
Micrococcus pyogenes var. aureus
Morax-Axenfeld bacillus
Moraxella lacunata
Morgan's bacillus
Mycobacterium bovis
Mycobacterium intracellularis
Mycobacterium kansasii
Mycobacterium leprae
Mycobacterium microti
Mycobacterium paratuberculosis
Mycobacterium phlei
Mycobacterium smegmatis
Mycobacterium tuberculosis

Neisseria catarrhalis
Neisseria gonorrheae
Neisseria intracellularis
    (meningococcus)

BACTERIAL MICROORGANISMS (continued)

Neisseria meningitides
Newcastle-Manchester bacillus
Nocard's bacillus
Nonhemolytic streptococcus

Paracolon bacilli
Paratyphi S.C. (Salmonella hirschfeldii)
Paratyphoid A
Paratyphoid B (Salmonella schottmülleri)
Pasteurella multocida
Pasteurella pestis
Pasteurella pseudotuberculosis
Pasteurella tularensis
Pfeiffer's bacillus
Pneumococcus
Preisz-Nocard bacillus
Proteus morgani
Proteus vulgaris
Pseudomonas aeruginosa
Pseudomonas pseudomallei

Rhinoscleroma bacillus

Salmonella choleraesuis
Salmonella enteritidis
Salmonella paratyphi—A
Salmonella paratyphi—B (schottmülleri)
Salmonella paratyphi—C (hirschfeldii)
Salmonella sendai
Salmonella typhi
Salmonella typhimurium
Salmonella typhosa
Schmitz's bacillus
Schmorl's bacillus
Shiga's bacillus
Shigella alkalescens
Shigella ambigua
Shigella boydii
Shigella ceylonensis
Shigella dysenteriae
Shigella etousae
Shigella flexneri

Shigella madampensis
Shigella paradysenteriae
Shigella schmitzii
Shigella sonnei
Shigella wakefield
Smegma bacillus
Sonne-Duval bacillus
Spirochaeta pallida
Spirochaeta plicatilis
Spirochaeta vincenti
Staphylococcus albus
Staphylococcus aureus
Staphylococcus citreus
Staphylococcus epidermidis
Streptobacillus moniliformis (Actinomyces muris-ratti)
Streptococcus agalactiae
Streptococcus bovis
Streptococcus equi
Streptococcus equisimilis
Streptococcus faecalis
Streptococcus hemolyticus
Streptococcus mitis
Streptococcus of Ostertag
Streptococcus pyogenes
Streptococcus salivarius
Streptococcus viridans
Streptococcus zooepidemicus
Surne rotlauf bacillus

Timothy bacillus
Treponema calligyrum
Treponema carateum
Treponema genitalis
Treponema microdentium
Treponema mucosum
Treponema pallidum
Treponema pertenue
Treponema pintae
Tubercle bacillus
Typhoid bacillus

Vibrio comma (causes cholera)
Vibrion septique
Vincent's organisms

Whitmore's bacillus

RICKETTSIAS

Rickettsias, a form of organism thought to represent an intermediate form between bacteria and viruses, were recognized and described by Howard Taylor Ricketts in 1908. They resemble certain bacteria in form, but are nonmotile. In other characteristics they are more like viruses. They do not appear to have a capsule and grow on living animal matter. Although they live predominantly within the cytoplasm of the cell, they may also be found free in the intestinal lumen or anal canal of lice, fleas, ticks, and mites. It is through these carriers that they are transmitted to man.

Diseases produced by this type organism include Rocky Mountain spotted fever, typhus fever, tsutsugamushi disease, rickettsialpox and trench fever. Rickettsial diseases are manifested by skin rash, severe headache, a steadfast temperature elevation, and possible symptoms of central nervous system involvement.

Like bacteria, they may be demonstrated in infected tissues through proper staining techniques. They have also shown sensitivity to antibiotic therapy.

RICKETTSIAL ORGANISMS

Rickettsia akamushi	Rickettsia orientalis
Rickettsia akari	Rickettsia pediculi
Rickettsia australis	Rickettsia prowazekii
Rickettsia conorii	Rickettsia quintana
Rickettsia diaporica	Rickettsia rickettsii
Rickettsia mooseri	Rickettsia tsutsugamushi
Rickettsia muricola	Rickettsia typhi
Rickettsia nipponica	Rickettsia wolhynica

VIRUSES

Viruses are extremely minute infectious agents which resemble tiny crystals more than they do living organisms. Except for the larger forms such as the poxviruses and psittacosis group, they cannot be observed with an ordinary microscope. An electron microscope is used for this purpose.

Characteristic of this form of organisms is the lack of an independent metabolism. They require a living host in which to live and reproduce themselves. Like most of the rickettsias, they live within the cell or in close relation to it.

One of the principal broad classifications of these agents is based on their host selection, for example, animal viruses, bacterial viruses, and plant viruses. Other classifications are superficial ones based on disease manifestations they produce, mode of transmission, or geographic area from which they were originally isolated.

VIRUSES

Animal viruses
V. animatum
Arbor virus
Attenuated virus
Australian X disease virus

Bacterial viruses
Brunhilde virus
Bunyamwera virus
Bwamba fever virus

C virus (Coxsackie virus)
CA virus (croup virus)
Cache Valley virus
California virus
Chikungunya virus
Coe virus
Colorado tick fever virus
Coryza virus
Coxsackie virus
Croup-associated virus
Cytomegalovirus

Dengue virus

ECBO virus
ECDO virus
ECHO virus
ECHO 28 virus
ECMO virus
ECSO virus
EEE virus
EMC virus
Encephalomyocarditis virus
Enteric virus
Enteric orphan virus
Epidemic keratoconjunctivitis virus
Equine encephalomyelitis virus

Filterable virus
Fixed virus

Guaroa virus

Hemadsorption virus—type 1
Hepatitis virus

Herpangina virus
Herpes virus

Ilheus virus
Inclusion conjunctivitis virus
Insect viruses

Japanese B encephalitis virus
JH virus
Junin virus

Kumba virus
Kyasanur Forest disease virus

Lansing virus
Latent virus
Leon virus
Louping ill virus
Lunyo virus
Lymphogranuloma venerum virus

Masked virus
Mayaro virus
Mengo virus
Murray Valley encephalitis virus

Newcastle disease virus

O'nyong-nyong virus
Ornithosis virus
Oropouche virus
Orphan viruses

Pappataci viruses
Parainfluenza virus
Parrot virus
Pharyngoconjunctival fever virus
Plant viruses
Pneumonitis virus
Poliovirus
Polyoma virus
Powassan virus
Poxvirus
Psittacosis virus

Rabies virus
Respiratory syncytial virus
Rift Valley fever virus

VIRUSES (continued)

RS virus
Russian spring-summer encephalitis virus

St. Louis encephalitis virus
Salivary gland virus
Semliki Forest virus
Sendai virus
Simbu virus
Simian viruses
Sindbis virus
Street virus

Teschen virus
Theiler's virus

Tick-borne virus
Trachoma virus
2060 virus (**ECHO 28 virus**)

Uganda S virus
Unorganized virus
Uruma virus

Vaccine virus
Vaccinicum virus
VEE virus

WEE virus
Wesselsbron virus
West Nile virus

FUNGUS INFECTIONS

Fungi represent a low order of vegetable organisms which are many and varied in type and often bear little resemblance to each other. The over-all percentage of these organisms known to produce disease in man is relatively small.

Diseases caused by fungi are called mycoses (sing: mycosis). Laboratory investigators who make a special study of these diseases are known as mycologists.

The fungus plant develops from a reproductive element called a spore. The germinating spore enlarges sending out branches called germ tubes. These tubes branch out forming filaments which are called hypha. These hyphae are divided into segments by septa. The filaments are collectively called the mycelium. A portion of this mycelium serves the purpose of providing food for the plant by penetrating the surface of its host. It is called the vegetative mycelium as contrasted to the filaments above the surface, called the aerial mycelium, which through spore formation generate new growth.

Fungi may be studied directly under the microscope in most instances from scrapings taken of infected tissues.

The most common fungal infections in man consist of infections involving the nails, hair and hair follicles. These diseases are collectively called the dermatomycoses. Their causative agents are called dermatophytes.

Secondary to a primary fungal lesion, a patient sometimes develops an "id" reaction in the form of cutaneous eruptions. This is believed to be caused by an allergic reaction to mycotic antigens. These secondary lesions are not infected by the fungi. It is interesting to note that when the

LABORATORY EXAMINATIONS

primary infected lesion is successfully treated, the secondary lesions likewise disappear.

Except for the ringworm infections, dermatophytosis (athlete's foot), and certain other dermatomycoses, fungus disease is generally not contagious from man to man. Fungal infections may be picked from the soil, vegetation, or animal dejecta. Infectious fungi are particularly prevalent in certain geographic areas. An example is the Coccidioidomycosis which was once believed to be limited to plants of the San Joaquin Valley, California, but which has spread over much of the southwestern United States. This fungus primarily attacks the lungs (San Joaquin Valley fever) ranging in severity from a mildly benign infection to a rapidly fatal one. Men are more commonly infected than are women. Histoplasmosis is another fungal infection with a particular geographic concentration. It is now believed that as high as 75% of the populace in the central Mississippi Valley and the Ohio Valley develop a benign form of this disease. Blastomycosis is a fungal infection found particularly around Chicago in the United States. The source of this infection or the mode of transmission have not been determined. It is believed that breaks in the skin probably permit invasion by the fungi. This fungus may infect the lungs and almost every site and organ of the body.

Fungi are sometimes divided into groups called false fungi (Actinomyces bovis and Nocardia asteroides), and true fungi. This distinction is based on the observation that the false fungi do not have spores and their filaments are relatively thin and nonseptate. The true fungi usually have spores and thick segmented filaments.

The following list of fungi is an alphabetical one only. Not all of the fungi listed are pathogenic in man.

FUNGI

Achorion
Actinobacillus actinoides
Actinobaccillus actinomycetemcomitans
Actinobacillus equuli
Actinobacillus lignieresii
Actinobacillus mallei
Actinobacillus pseudomallei
Actinomyces baudetii
Actinomyces bovis (false fungi)
Actinomyces israeli
Aspergillus auricularis
Aspergillus barbae
Aspergillus bouffardi
Aspergillus clavatus
Aspergillus concentricus

Aspergillus flavus
Aspergillus fumigatus
Aspergillus giganteus
Aspergillus glaucus
Aspergillus gliocladium
Aspergillus mucoroides
Aspergillus nidulans
Aspergillus niger
Aspergillus ochraceus
Aspergillus pictor
Aspergillus repens

Blastomyces brasiliensis
Blastomyces coccidioides
Blastomyces dermatitidis
Blastomyces farciminosus

FUNGI (continued)

Candida albicans
Candida guilliermondi
Candida krusei
Candida parakrusei
Candida stellatoidea
Candida tropicalis
Coccidioides immitis
Coccidioidomyces
Cryptococcus capsulatus
Cryptococcus gilchristi
Cryptococcus histolyticus
Cryptococcus hominis
Cryptococcus meningitidis
Cryptococcus neoformans

Endomyces albicans
Endomyces capsulatus
Endomyces epidermatidis
Endomyces epidermides
Epidermophyton floccosum
Epidermophyton inguinale
Epidermophyton rubrum

False fungi

Geotrichum candidum

Hemisporo stellata
Histoplasma capsulatum
Hormodendrum compactum
Hormodendrum pedrosoi

Lichtheimia corymbifera

Madurella
Malassezia furfur
Malassezia macfadyani
Malassezia tropica
Microspora furfur
Microsporum audouini
Microsporum canis
Microsporum felineum
Microsporum fulvum
Microsporum furfur
Microsporum gypseum
Microsporum lanosum
Mucor corymbifer

Mucor mucedo
Mucor pusillus
Mucor racemosus
Mucor rhizodiformis
Mycoderma aceti
Mycoderma dermatitis
Mycoderma immite

Nocardia asteroides
Nocardia farcinica
Nocardia madurae
Nocardia minutissima

Paracoccidioides brasiliensis
Penicillium barbae
Penicillium bouffardi
Penicillium crustaceum
Penicillium glaucum
Penicillium minimum
Penicillium montoyai
Penicillium notatum
Penicillium patulum
Penicillium spinulosum
Phialophora verrucosa

Rhinocladium

Saccharomyces albicans
Saccharomyces anginae
Saccharomyces apiculatus
Saccharomyces Busse's
Saccharomyces cantliei
Saccharomyces capillitii
Saccharomyces cerevisiae
Saccharomyces coprogenus
Saccharomyces lipsoideus
Saccharomyces epidermica
Saccharomyces exiguus
Saccharomyces galacticolus
Saccharomyces glutinis
Saccharomyces granulomatosus
Saccharomyces guttulatus
Saccharomyces hansenii
Saccharomyces hominis
Saccharomyces lemonnieri
Saccharomyces lithogenes
Saccharomyces mesentericus

LABORATORY EXAMINATIONS

FUNGI (continued)

Saccharomyces mycoderma
Saccharomyces neoformans
Saccharomyces pastorianus
Saccharomyces rubrum
Saccharomyces subcutaneous tumefaciens
Saccharomyces tumefaciens albus

Torula capsulatus
Torula histolytica
Trichophyton album
Trichophyton acuminatum
Trichophyton asteroides

Trichophyton cerebriforme
Trichophyton concentricum
Trichophyton crateriforme
Trichophyton discoides
Trichophyton ectothrix
Trichophyton endothrix
Trichophyton neoendothrix
Trichophyton ochraceum
Trichophyton radians
Trichophyton rosaceum
Trichophyton violaceum
Trichosporon beigelii
Trichosporon pedrosianum

PROTOZOAN PARASITIC INFECTIONS IN MAN

Protozoa represent the lowest division of the animal kingdom with organisms as small as one cell. They are divided into four classes on the basis of their adaptations for locomotion.

(1) SPOROZOA possesses no means for locomotion and reproduces through spore formation
(2) MASTIGOPHORA (flagellates) possess flagella
(3) SARCODINA (rhizopoda) possess pseudopodia
(4) INFUSORIA (ciliates) possess cilia

Most protozoan diseases are comparatively rare in the United States. Many of the infections seen in this country are developed by travelers and servicemen returning from those areas of the world where the infections are particularly prevalent.

AMEBIASIS, amebic dysentery and hepatic amebiasis are diseases produced by Endamoeba histolytica. Amebiasis is world wide. It is an asymptomatic carrier state in most individuals. Persons so infected pass cysts in their stools which are the most important source of new infections. The cysts are often transmitted on vegetables in countries where human excreta are used as fertilizer, and where food is not properly protected against contamination by flies. The ingested cysts are known to pass through the stomach of man unchanged. At the level of the ileum the cyst wall disintegrates and the eight trophozoites (immature amebas) are produced. These organisms migrate to the colon where they attack the mucosa. In the order of frequency, the sites of involvement are cecum and ascending colon, rectum, sigmoid, appendix, and terminal ileum. Experiments conducted on volunteers produced some interesting observations in that not all subjects fed cysts from the same source, developed the disease. Men were observed to develop the disease more commonly than women. It was also observed that germ free animals in the experimental laboratory cannot be infected with Endamoeba histolytica. However, infection will take place after the intestines are allowed to develop a normal bacterial content. These findings suggest that the bacterial flora of the intestine may be an important factor in the extent to which the disease develops in an individual.

Laboratory examinations for this protozoan form are not usually employed. When the diagnosis is suspected clinically, patients are often treated with antiamebic drugs. Complete cures occur in about 75 to 95% of cases, usually after several courses of treatment. The fatality rate from amebiasis is less than 5%.

MALARIA is another protozoan disease. It is transmitted to man by the bite of Anopheles mosquitoes. The etiologic agents in the disease are protozoa of the genus Plasmodium. Laboratory diagnosis may be made by finding the plasmodium, in one of its stages, in a blood smear.

Man is only an intermediate host for this disease which develops in approximately 200 million persons each year. The mosquito is the actual host for these organisms. Sporozoites are injected into man by the bite of the mosquito. In man they continue to develop outside the red blood cells and then invade the red blood cells where they reproduce asexually. The infected red cells eventually rupture and release them to attack other circulating red blood cells. Some of the red cells become loaded with the gametocytes (sexual forms) which fail to undergo further development until they are again ingested by the appropriate mosquito during a blood meal on the human. Fertilization takes place in the stomach of the mosquito with the release of sporozoites which migrate to the mosquito salivary glands. When they are injected into man through the bite of the mosquito, the cycle begins again.

LEISHMANIASIS is a collective term for three separate diseases caused by protozoa of the genus Leishmania and transmitted to man by the bite of sand flies.

Visceral leishmaniasis, also called kala-azar, is caused by Leishmania donovani. This disease occurs in China, India, East Africa, Egypt, Russia, Sudan, Greece, Crete, and Malta. The disease has also been reported in certain areas of Central and South America.

Cutaneous leishmaniasis, also called oriental sore, is caused by Leishmania tropica. This disease is most prevalent in Southwest Asia, North Africa, Asia Minor and in countries of Europe bordering the eastern Mediterranean.

American leishmaniasis (espundia) has been reported in every country of Central and South America except Chile. It is caused by Leishmania braziliensis. Laboratory diagnosis is possible through skin scrapings or through culture taken from sites of infection. The Montenegro skin test is highly specific for diagnosing this disease.

TOXOPLASMOSIS results from infection by Toxoplasma gondii. Surveys performed on the population of several American cities showed positive results in as high as 33 per cent of the population. The mode of transmission to man has not yet been determined. There is no indication that the disease is contagious. Human infections may be acquired or congenital. Mothers may produce congenitally damaged offspring as a result of this infection without having experienced symptoms of the disease during pregnancy. Chorioretinitis characterized 94% of these infants in a recent survey, with other symptoms including psychomotor retardation, hydro- or microcephaly, convulsive episodes and cerebral calcification. The disease does not plague the newborn of subsequent pregnancies.

The extent and variety of symptoms in acquired toxoplasmosis is considerable. The infection sometimes resembles infectious mononucleosis with lymphocytosis, and atypical lymphocytes. Other symptoms may include enlarged and painful lymph nodes, maculopapular skin rash, muscle and joint pains, encephalitis, pneumonitis, and myocarditis.

Laboratory diagnosis may be made using serologic methods or by demonstrating the organisms in blood smears.

TRICHOMONIASIS is produced by protozoa of the genus Trichomonas. The most important disease produced by this organism is a vaginal and urethral infection produced by Trichomonas vaginalis. Symptoms include itching and burning of the vagina with production of a profuse, frothy, creamy, yellow discharge. In the male, the organisms invade the urethra causing a urethritis. The disease is transmitted through sexual intercourse, use of common toilet articles and other items which might harbor the organisms.

Laboratory diagnosis may be made by examining a fresh sample of the discharge under the microscope for trichomonads.

TRYPANOSOMIASIS, also called sleeping sickness or Chagas' disease, is caused by protozoa of the genus Trypanosoma. The organisms are usually transmitted to man through the bite of an insect.

Laboratory diagnosis may be made by examination of wet blood films and stained smears.

The following table lists protozoa parasitic in man, by name, in alphabetical order. The first letter of the genus name should always be capitalized while the second portion of the name always begins with the lower case, exactly as is shown in this list. Where there are two acceptable versions of a name, one of these will appear in parentheses.

PARASITIC PROTOZOA

Balantidium coli

Chilomastix mesnili

Dientamoeba fragilis

Endolimax nana
Endamoeba (Entamoeba) coli
Endamoeba (Entamoeba) gingivalis
Endamoeba (Entamoeba) histolytica

Giardia lamblia

Iodamoeba bütschlii (williamsi)
Isospora hominis

Leishmania brasiliensis

Leishmania donovani
Leishmania tropica

Plasmodium falciparum
Plasmodium malariae
Plasmodium ovale
Plasmodium vivax

Toxoplasma gondii
Trichomonas hominis
Trichomonas tenax (T. buccalis)
Trichomonas vaginalis
Trypanosoma cruzi
Trypanosoma gambiense
Trypanosoma rhodesiense

PARASITIC DISEASES DUE TO WORMS

Diseases resulting from infestation by parasitic worms are not a common medical problem in the United States except as they occur in some of the southern and southeastern states, and in returning servicemen, travelers as well as immigrants from tropical countries.

ASCARIASIS is an infestation of the bowel by the roundworm Ascaris lumbricoides. Ovum of the worm is transmitted from one host to another by flies, water and food. The incidence of this infection is not common in the United States. Ova may readily be detected in the stool of infested persons. An eosinophilia of 10 to 30 per cent is also frequently seen in these cases.

ENTEROBIASIS (oxyuriasis) also called pinworm infection is caused by Enterobius vermicularis. This parasite is found in all climates all over the world and is probably the most common parasitic infestation of man. The most common symptom is extreme itching in the anal area particularly at night when the female worm migrates to the anal area to deposit her eggs.

The infection is high among children and in households where there are children. It is not uncommon for all of the adults in a family to be likewise infected. The ova may be carried from the anus to the mouth and reinfect the same person. Other modes of transmission include contaminated hands, food and drink. Special care must also be exercised in handling the clothes and bed clothing of infected persons. Shaking of these items results in airborne transmission of the infection.

Diagnosis is made by finding adult forms of the small white pinworms in the stool or on a Scotch tape swab.

FILARIASIS is an infection of the lymphatic system of man by Wuchereria bancrofti or other species such as Wuchereria malaya, Acanthocheilonema perstans, Loa loa, Mansonella ozzardi, and Onchocerca volvulus. Manifestations of the disease include obstruction of the lymphatics with lymphangitis, enlargement of the scrotum and elephantiasis.

The disease is commonly seen in the western Pacific islands such as Samoa and Fiji, as well as in the Philippines, East China, Malaya, and India.

The reproductive cycle of these worms requires a mosquito, man, mosquito host relationship. In the absence of reinfection, man harbors the embryos which may be transmitted to the proper mosquito during a blood meal, for 5 to 10 years. This is the average reproductive life span of the adult worm. Embryos continue to develop only if ingested by the proper mosquito where they can develop further before being reinjected into a human host.

Laboratory diagnosis is sometimes made by demonstration of the motile microfilariae in wet smears.

HOOKWORM is a parasitic infection caused by Ancylostoma duodenale or Necator americanus. Larvae of the worm hatch in warm moist soil where they are picked up by barefoot persons. The larvae penetrate the skin of the host and gain entrance to blood vessels which carry them to the lungs. They migrate from the lungs to the trachea, esophagus, stomach and into the small intestine where they attach themselves and continue to mature.

This infection is still important in southern and southeastern regions of the United States. Improved facilities for sanitation and the wearing of footwear have been factors in reducing the incidence of this disease, in areas where the infection has been reported.

Laboratory examination can be made from hookworm eggs present in direct fecal smears.

SCHISTOSOMIASIS is a term for a group of parasitic diseases caused by blood flukes such as Schistosoma mansoni, S. japonicum, and S. haematobium. This disease must be numbered among the most important parasitic diseases of man. It is estimated that over 150 million persons are infected throughout the world.

The disease is developed by persons swimming, bathing, washing clothes or working in fresh waters contaminated by unsanitary untreated sewage disposal. The worms require a man-snail-man cycle for development. The infective form of the organism called the **cercaria** penetrate the skin and enter the capillary bed, migrating through the venous system, right heart, lungs, mesenteric arteries and portal system. The larvae grow to adult worms in the hepatic portion of the portal system. Manifestations of this infection may include colitis, hepatitis, cirrhosis of the liver, and diarrhea. A high incidence of primary carcinoma of the liver has also been observed in persons infected with this parasite.

The infection is particularly prevalent in Puerto Rico, certain areas of South America, China, the Philippines, Africa, Japan, and the Middle East. Acute schistosomiasis is not found in the United States, except in servicemen who were stationed in the Philippines and in many of the Puerto Ricans who have moved to the United States.

Laboratory diagnosis is made by finding the ova in stool specimens.

STRONGYLOIDIASIS is a parasitic disease caused by the worm Strongyloides stercoralis which is particularly prevalent in tropical countries. The infection is intestinal. The larvae may be ingested through contaminated food and drink; however, the most common mode of transmission is penetration of the skin by larvae present in contaminated soil.

The laboratory diagnosis is made by finding motile larvae in the stool.

TAPEWORMS (Cestodiasis) These infections caused by Taenia saginata (beef tapeworm), Taenia solium (pork tapeworm), and Diphyllobothrium latum (fish tapeworm) may be present without producing clinical symptoms. Diagnosis may be made by identification of ova, proglottids (segments of the worm), or the scolex (head of the worm) in the stool specimen. These infections are developed through the ingestion of poorly cooked infected beef, pork, or fresh water fish.

The most common tapeworm in the United States, particularly in the southern states is Hymenolepis nana (dwarf tapeworm). The infection may be transmitted from man to man without an intermediate host.

TRICHINOSIS is a parasitic infection of the intestines and muscles caused by Trichinella spiralis. The infection is contracted through the ingestion of poorly cooked pork.

Trichinosis is common in the United States and Europe with a much lower incidence in other parts of the world. The incidence in the United States is believed to be between 15 and 20 per cent. There are no methods for detection of trichinosis in pork and for this reason, thorough cooking, freezing, pickling or smoking of all pork is necessary in the prevention of this infection.

Laboratory diagnosis may be made by microscopic examination of laked capillary, arterial or venous blood for larvae. Muscle biopsy as well as examination of the cerebrospinal fluid is sometimes used. A skin test which may be positive as early as the third week after the infection, is also used to diagnose this condition. An immediate and a delayed reading of the skin test are taken. An immediate positive test results in the form of a wheal surrounded by redness. A delayed reaction may be noted after 24 hours or more. Persons may show a positive reaction without any active evidence of the infection. This is believed to be due to the ingestion of nonliving Trichinella in pork.

LABORATORY EXAMINATIONS

The following table lists worms parasitic in man by name. The first letter of the genus name is capitalized while the second portion of the name appears in the lower case, exactly as shown in the table.

WORMS PARASITIC IN MAN

Parasite	Type Worm
Acanthocheulonema perstans	filaria
Ancyclostoma braziliense	hookworm
Ancyclostoma duodenale	hookworm
Ascaris lumbricoides	roundworm
Clonorchis endemicus	liver fluke
Clonorchis sinensis	Chinese liver fluke
Cysticercus cellulosae	larval tapeworms
Dibothriocephalus	fish tapeworm
Diphyllobothrium latum	fish tapeworm
Dipylidium caninum	tapeworm
Dracunculus medinensis	Guinea worm
Echinococcus granulosus	flatworm (hydatid disease)
Enterobius vermicularis	pinworm
Fasciola hepatica	flatworm
Fasciola buski	intestinal fluke
Heterophyes heterophyes	intestinal fluke
Hymenolepis diminuta	tapeworm
Hymenolepsis nana	dwarf tapeworm
Loa loa	filarial eyeworm
Mansonella ozzardi	filaria
Metagonimus ovatus	intestinal fluke
Metagonimus yokogawai	intestinal fluke
Necatur americanus	new world hookworm
Onchocerca volvulus	filaria
Opisthorchis felineus	fluke
Paragonimus westermani	oriental lung fluke
Schistosoma haematobium	blood fluke
Schistosoma japanicum	blood fluke
Schistosoma mansoni	blood fluke
Strongyloides stercoralis	roundworm

WORM PARASITES (continued)

Parasite	Type Worm
Taenia echinococcus	hydatid disease tapeworm
Taenia saginata	beef tapeworm
Taenia solium	pork tapeworm
Trichinella spiralis	porkworm
Trichostrongylus instabilis	roundworm
Trichostrongylus orientalis	roundworm
Trichostrongylus vitrinus	roundworm
Trichuris trichura	whipworm
Wuchereria bancrofti	filaria
Wuchereria malayi	filaria

AUTOMATION IN THE CLINICAL LABORATORY

Within the past fifteen years hospital laboratories have been confronted with an ever increasing workload. An answer to this problem has been sought in automated instrumentation. The first such instrument was the AutoAnalyzer, introduced in 1957, by the Technicon Corporation of Tarrytown, New York. This specialized equipment is a train of interconnected modules that automate the time consuming, step-by-step procedures formerly performed by manual analysis. A variety of biological materials may be tested which include whole blood, plasma, serum, urine and cerebrospinal fluid. With refinement of instrumentation, fast and accurate methods have been developed for reporting a wide variety of laboratory information. It has been found that it is more economical and useful to subject every specimen to a battery of automated tests than to limit the examinations to one or two tests. Through this system of routine total biochemical profiling additional disease screening tests are routinely performed on all admissions. Most large hospitals and many smaller ones today use the SMA 12 or the more current SMA 12/60. All twelve test results obtained on each such profile are reported on an $8\frac{1}{2}$ x 11 sheet of precalibrated chart paper called an SCG (Serum Chemistry Graph). On this report form the normal range of the test is shaded. A graphic line reporting the results on the patient appear in each colume. When the level of the test result appears outside the shaded area in the colume, the physician is alerted to pursue his investigation in this area further.

A sample report form for the SMA 12/60 profile appears on the opposite page.

COPYRIGHT© 1965, 1966 and 1967 by TECHNICON CORPORATION, Ardsley, New York   CHART NO. R01029 A

SMA 12/60

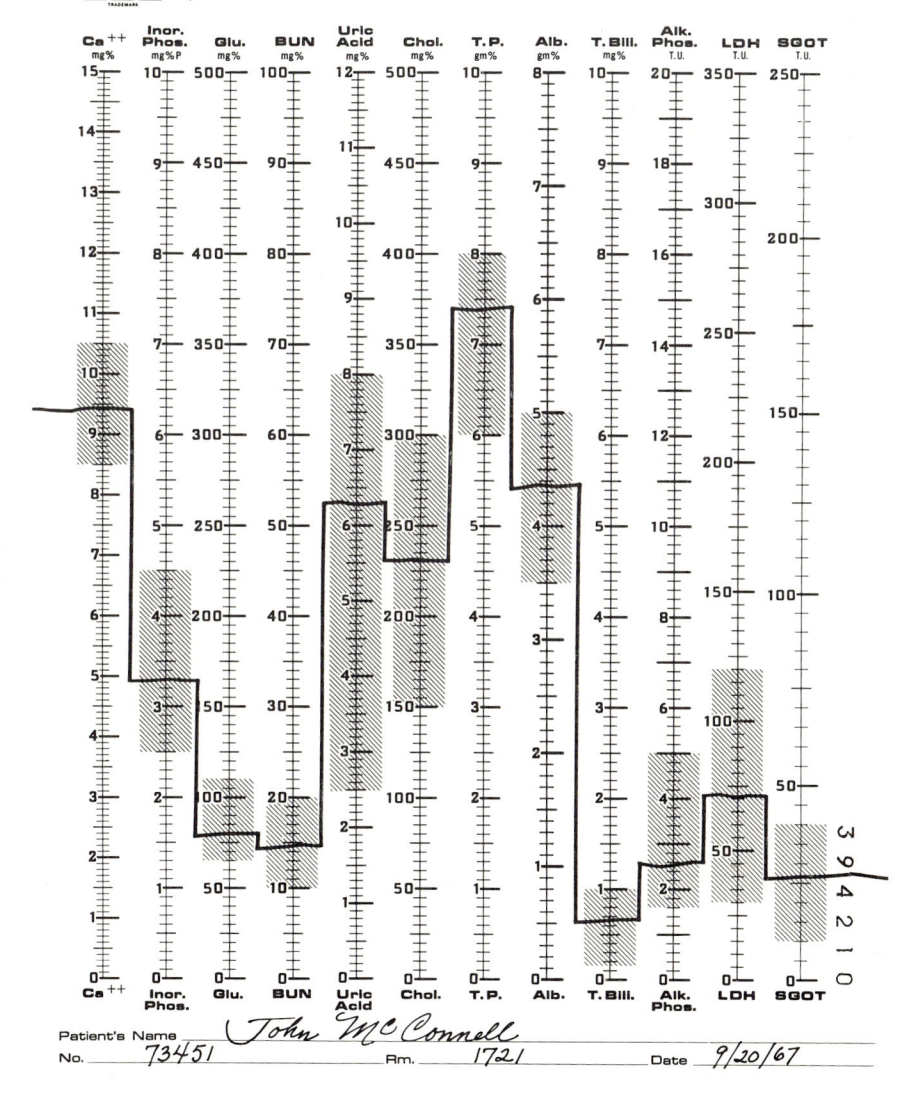

Ca++ mg%	Inor. Phos. mg%P	Glu. mg%	BUN mg%	Uric Acid mg%	Chol. mg%	T.P. gm%	Alb. gm%	T. Bili. mg%	Alk. Phos. T.U.	LDH T.U.	SGOT T.U.

Patient's Name: John McConnell
No. 73451   Rm. 1721   Date 9/20/67

LABORATORY EXAMINATIONS

TEST	PERFORMED ON	NORMAL RANGE	SIGNIFICANCE
Acetone (aceto-acetic acid) (diacetic acid)	Urine	None	Present in metabolic acidosis caused by diabetes, eclampsia, starvation, cachexia, digestive disturbance, febrile disease, vomiting of preg., and sometimes after chloroform or ether anesthesia.
Acid Phosphatase	Blood serum	0.5 to 2 Gutman Units 0 - 1.1 Bodansky u. 0.5 - 3.5 King-Armstrong units	As high as 30 G. units in bone metastases due to CA of prostate, breast, thyroid or colon.
ACTH Test	Patient by injection	In normal persons plasma steroid level up 2 to 4 times	In Addison's disease—no response. In pituitary deficiency ACTH stimulates adrenal cortical activity.
Addis Count	Urine 12 hour	Hyaline casts 0 - 5,000 RBC's 0 - 5,000,000 WBC's 35,000 to 1,000,000	Greatly increased values in nephritis. This test used to differentiate kidney damage.
A/G ratio (albumin-globulin)	Blood serum	1.5:1 to 2.5:1	Reversal of ratio occurs in cirrhosis with ascites, hepatitis, lipoid nephrosis, multiple myeloma and diseases causing loss of albumin and compensatory increase in globulin.

Agglutination tests
See: Bacterial aggl.

LABORATORY EXAMINATIONS

TEST	PERFORMED ON	NORMAL RANGE	SIGNIFICANCE
Albumin	Blood serum	3.5 - 5.5 Gm./100 cc.	Decreased in liver disease, malnutrition and nephrosis.
Albumin (qualitative)	Urine	0 - 15%	Idiopathic albuminuria seen in some persons in the absence of disease. Increase may accompany hypertension, kidney disease or severe heart failure.
Albumin (quantitative)	Urine	None	Test to measure amount of protein being lost in urine.
Aldolase	Blood serum	7.14 units per cc.	Abnormal in values over 10.5 units. Increased in early muscular dystrophy, within 24-48 hours of myocardial infarction and in early acute hepatitis. Also increased in erythroblastosis fetalis, gangrene of extremities, hemolytic anemia, leukemia with high wbc, large pul. infarcts and hemorrhagic pericarditis.
Aldosterone	Urine—24 hr.	2 - 23 microgm. per 24 hours	Increased in primary aldosteronism.
Alkaline phosphatase	Blood serum adults: children:	2 - 4.5 Bodansky units 4 - 13 King-Armstrong u. 5 - 14 Bodansky units 15 - 20 King-Armstrong	Elevated in children, and in women during third trimester of preg. Increased in bone diseases, healing fractures, osteoblastic bone tumors, and hyperparathyroidism.
Alpha amino nitrogen	Plasma	3.0 to 5.5 mg.	Elevated in extensive liver damage.

LABORATORY EXAMINATIONS (continued)

TEST	PERFORMED ON	NORMAL RANGE	SIGNIFICANCE
Amylase	Blood serum	70 - 200 Somogyi u. 8 - 18 Russell units	Increased following abdominal surgery, in perforated peptic ulcer, pancreatic diseases, ruptured ectopic pregnancy, mumps, peritonitis, and other abdominal conditions.
Amlyase	Urine 24 hr.	6 - 30 Wohlgemuth units per cc. or 5,000 Somogyi u. per 24 hours.	
Amlyase	Urine	2 - 50 Wohlgemuth units per cc.	Decreased in severe burns and liver necrosis.
Antistreptolysin O titer (ASO titer)	Blood serum	to 400 units/cc.	Increased in rheumatic fever, and acute glomerulonephritis caused by hemolytic strep.
Ascheim-Zondek	Patient's urine injected into single virgin female rabbit	Negative	Reliable pregnancy test one week after missed period. Positive also in hydatidiform mole, chorioma of placenta, ovary and testicle, and in 50% of ectopic preg, missed and incomplete abortions.
Ascorbic acid	Blood plasma	0.4 - 1.0 mg.%	Lowered in Vit. C deficiency manifested clinically by scurvy.
ASO titer See: Antistreptolysin titer			
Bacterial agglutinations Brucellosis Dysentery Leptospirosis Paratyphoid A & B Typhoid O & H Typhus fever	Blood serum	No agglutination	Certain infections caused by spirochetes, viruses, rickettsiae and bacilli produce antibodies in the patient's serum, which in turn cause agglutination (clumping) of these organisms. Specific organisms are suspended in the patient's serum to determine if they will be agglutinated.

LABORATORY EXAMINATIONS

TEST	PERFORMED ON	NORMAL RANGE	SIGNIFICANCE
Basal metabolic rate (BMR)	Breathing	+ to −15	Elevated in hyperthyroidism. Decreased in hypothyroidism.
BEI (see: Butanol extractable iodine)			
Bence Jones protein	Urine	Negative	Present in 60 to 80% of cases of late mult. myeloma. Also seen in osteogenic sarcoma, osteomalacia and CA of bone.
Bile	Urine Feces	None	Seen in jaundice.
Bilirubin	Urine	Negative	Seen in obstructive jaundice, cholangitis, toxic hepatitis, and partial obstruction of biliary tract.
Bilirubin immediate (Direct)	Blood serum	0.1 - 0.4 mg.%	Increased in obstructive hepatic disease. It is a measure of the free bilirubin in the blood.
Bilirubin, total (Indirect) Also: van den Bergh	Blood serum	0.2 - 0.7 mg.%	Increase indicates elevation in destruction of red blood cells.
Bleeding time	Capillary whole blood	1 to 3 minutes	Bleeding time prolonged in primary thrombocytopenia or secondary thrombocytopenia due to aplastic anemia, pernicious anemia, hemorrhagic disease of newborn, acute leukemias, chronic lymphocytic leukemia, multiple myeloma and Hodgkin's disease of bone marrow.

Blood count
See first seven pages of this chapter

LABORATORY EXAMINATIONS (continued)

TEST	PERFORMED ON	NORMAL RANGE	SIGNIFICANCE
Blood urea nitrogen (BUN)	Blood serum	10 - 20 mg.%	Increased in some kidney diseases. This test preferred to NPN.
BMR See: Basal metabolic rate			
Bromsulphalein (BSP)	Blood serum	Less than 5% retention at 45 min.	Liver function test. Retention of 90% or more indicates severe liver impairment.
BUN See: Blood urea nitrogen			
Butanol extractable iodine (BEI)	Blood serum	3.2 - 6 micrograms %	Used in following patients undergoing iodine therapy for thyroid disease.
Calcium	Blood serum	9.0 to 11.5 mg. per 100 cc.	Increased in hyperparathyroidism, adenoma of parathyroids, bone tumors including metastatic CA of bone, Addison's disease, chronic nephritis with uremia, emphysema, cardiac decompensation.
Calcium (Sulkowitch)	Urine	Positive 1+	Increased in osteitis fibrosa cystica. Decreased in tetany and myxedema.

LABORATORY EXAMINATIONS

TEST	PERFORMED ON	NORMAL RANGE	SIGNIFICANCE
Capillary fragility	Upper arm	Negative	Tourniquet applied to upper arm and pressure pumped to just above diastolic pressure. Test positive if rupture of tiny blood vessels noted. Positive in Vit. K def., chronic nephritis, thrombocytopenic purpura, scurvy, influenza.
Carbon dioxide (CO_2) combining power	Blood serum	56 - 65 Vol.% 25 - 30 mEq/l	Increased in hypoventilation with alkalosis. Decreased in acidosis.
Catecholamines	Urine	Less than 230 microgm/24 hr.	Increased in pheochromocytoma.
Cephalin-Cholesterol flocculation (Hanger's test)	Blood serum	0 to 1+	Liver function test strongly positive in cirrhosis, hepatitis, and catarrhal jaundice. Positive results are also seen in terminal nephritis, infectious mononucleosis, nephrosis, viral or pneumococcic pneumonia, L.E. and bacterial endocarditis.
Chlorides	Blood serum	350 - 390 mg.% 100 - 110 mEq/liter	Decreased in Addison's disease, acidosis and heat prostration. Increased in renal malfunction and Cushing's syndrome.
Cholesterol (total)	Blood serum	110 - 300 mg.%	Increased in liver disease with hepatic impairment, and in hypothyroidism. Decreased in anemias and hyperthyroidism.
Cholesterol esters	Blood serum	75 - 210 mg.%	Decreased in liver damage.
Cholinesterase	Blood serum	0.5 pH units or more	Decreased levels seen in cirrhosis, infectious hepatitis, metastatic carcinoma and extrahepatic biliary obstruction.

LABORATORY EXAMINATIONS (continued)

TEST	PERFORMED ON	NORMAL RANGE	SIGNIFICANCE
Clot retraction time	Venous blood	30 - 60 minutes	Prolonged in primary thrombocytopenia or secondary thrombocytopenia due to Hodgkin's disease, aplastic anemia, pernicious anemia, acute leukemia, multiple myeloma, and hemorrhagic disease of newborn.
Clotting time (Coagulation time)	Blood	6 - 10 min. Lee & White	Measurement of ability of blood to clot properly.
Colloidal gold	Blood serum	1st tube not higher than 4	Complete precipitation seen in first tube in patients with liver damage.
Colloidal gold	Spinal fluid	Negative	Precipitate of colloidal gold may suggest multiple sclerosis, neurosyphilis or other central nervous system diseases.
Congo Red	Blood serum	Less than 40% of dye disappears in one hour.	If over 80% of dye is removed from blood within one hour, amyloidosis suggested. Negative test does not rule out this disease.
Coombs' direct	Blood serum	Negative	Test to determine the globulin coated red cells. Agglutination takes place in positive reactions. Used to test newborn blood for erythroblastosis fetalis. Also used in blood cross matching.
Coombs' indirect	Blood serum	Negative	Test to detect iso-antibodies in serum. Used to detect possible blood incompatibilities in cross matching. Also used to detect Rh incompatibility in maternal blood before delivery by demonstrating anti-Rh antibodies.

LABORATORY EXAMINATIONS

TEST	PERFORMED ON	NORMAL RANGE	SIGNIFICANCE
Coproporphyrin	Urine	50 - 200 micrograms per 24 hours Children: 0 - 80 micrograms/24 hrs.	Increased in coproporphyria, a variant of congenital porphyria.
CPK Creatine phosphokinase; creatine kinase or ATP creatine phospherase	Blood	1 - 10 units 0.2 to 1.42 U. (two methods)	Elevated in myocardial infarction, pul. infarction, pul. edema, muscular dystrophy and D.T.'s
C-reactive protein	Blood serum	None	Found when a variety of inflammatory and necrosis producing diseases.
Creatine	Blood serum	3 - 7 mg.%	Increased in severe muscle damage and malnutrition.
Creatine	Urine	Less than 100 mg. in 24 hours	Increased in pregnancy, fasting, and severe muscle damage.
Creatinine	Blood serum	0.7 - 1.7 mg.	Increased in nephritis and impaired kidney function. Used as a check on BUN for possible renal factor.
Creatinine	Urine	1 - 2 mg.%	Elevated in impaired kidney function.
Cryoglobulin	Blood serum	None	Present in large amounts with multiple myeloma.
Diagnex Blue	Urine	Less than 0.3 mg. standard in color	Color of urine examined for ingested dye. If the blue color in the 2 hour urine compares to or exceeds the 0.6 mg. standard, free hydrochloric acid present in stomach.

LABORATORY EXAMINATIONS (continued)

TEST	PERFORMED ON	NORMAL RANGE	SIGNIFICANCE
Dick Test	Skin inj.	Negative Read 18-24 hrs. after injection	Negative result indicates immunity to scarlet fever. Pink spot or raised area shows a positive result, absence of antitoxin and vulnerability to scarlet fever.
ECG (EKG) Electrocardiogram	Heart function	Read from leads	Used to detect abnormal cardiac function.
EEG Electroencephalogram	Brain waves	Read from graphic record	Used to detect certain brain disorders.
Ellsworth-Howard	Urine	Increase in phosphorus level	Urine studied before and after I.V. injection of parathyroid extract. If phosphorus level in urine does not increase, then pseudohypoparathyroidism must be considered.
Estrogens	Urine 24 hr.	*Female* (nonpreg.) 4 - 60 micrograms per 24 hours *Male* 4 - 25 micrograms per 24 hours	Test of ovarian function.
Erythrocyte uptake of I^{131} (ET_3)	Blood serum	Female: 11 - 17% Male: 12 - 19%	Elevated in hyperthyroidism. Decreased in hypothyroidism.

LABORATORY EXAMINATIONS

TEST	PERFORMED ON	NORMAL RANGE	SIGNIFICANCE
Fertility study male	Semen	Spermatozoa per emission: 400 to 600 million Motility: 85 - 90% active forms Smear for abnormal forms—not over 25% abnormal forms	Male is considered fertile if spermotozoa count is 50 million or more per cc. of semen, there is normal motility and not over 25% abnormal sperm forms.
Fertility studies female (Sims-Huhner Test)	cervical and vaginal secretions	Cervical smear shows about 15 motile spermatozoa per high powered field.	Inactive spermatozoa on cervical smear may indicate nonreceptive cervical secretions.
Fibrinogen	Blood plasma	200 - 600 mg./100 cc.	Increased with infections, inflammations, during pregnancy and menstruation, after X-ray treatment, and in lipoid nephrosis. Decreased in liver diseases, severe malnutrition and anemia, and afibrinogenemia.
Fibrinolysin	Blood plasma	None	Seen in otherwise healthy persons with severe burns or subject to extreme trauma, fear or rigorous exercise.
Fishberg's concentration	Urine	Sp. Gr. 1.022 to 1.032	Decreased values in severe kidney disease.
Fishberg's dilution	Urine	First hour specimen about 400 cc. with Sp. Gr. 1.001 - 1.003	First hour output reduced to less than 200 cc. in persons with impaired renal function.
Fluorescent treponemal antibody (FTA)	Blood serum	Negative	Specific test for primary and secondary syphilis, as well as latent.

LABORATORY EXAMINATIONS (continued)

TEST	PERFORMED ON	NORMAL RANGE	SIGNIFICANCE
Formol gel	Blood serum	Negative	Positive in certain chronic infections, multiple myeloma, and kala-azar.
Frei skin test	Skin	Negative	Injection of diagnostic material read in 48 hours. Positive test shows redness, swelling in cases of lymphogranuloma venereum.
Friedman	Urine	Negative	Pregnancy test performed on rabbit.
Frog test	Urine	Negative	Pregnancy test performed on frog.
Glucose	Blood serum	80 - 120 mgm./100 cc.	Elevated in diabetes mellitus. Decreased in glycogen storage disease (von Gierke's), hypoglycemia and after excessive insulin.
Glucose tolerance intravenous	Blood serum	30 minute blood glucose might rise to 200 mg./100 cc. Level falls to 120 mg. or less in 2 hours	Test positive for diabetes mellitus where blood glucose does not return to normal in 2 hours.
Glucose tolerance Exton-Rose 1 hr.	Blood serum	Normal fasting blood glucose. Response not over 160 mg./100 cc. after ½ hour with drop below ½ hr. level after 1 hour	In diabetes: normal or increased fasting blood glucose with increase of more than 30 mg. after ½ hour and level above 160 mg. after 1 hour.

LABORATORY EXAMINATIONS

TEST	PERFORMED ON	NORMAL RANGE	SIGNIFICANCE
Glucose tolerance standard 3 hour	Blood serum	Fasting blood glucose 80 - 120 mg. per 100 cc. with increase after one hour and return to normal after 2 hrs.	In diabetes, fasting blood sugar 120 mg./100 cc. or higher. Level rises over 180 mg./100 cc. after one hour and does not return to normal in 2 and 3 hour specimens.
Gonadotrophic hormone (pituitary)	Urine	10 to 15 mouse uterine units/24 hr.	Decreased in diseases that reduce anterior pituitary function. Increased in primary deficiencies of the gonads. Used to diagnose panhypopituitarism.
GOT (glutamic oxalacetic transaminase)	Blood serum	10 - 40 units	Increased in myocardial infarction with highest level, which may reach 500 units, 24 hours after attack. Still higher levels seen in liver disease (600 to 2,000 units), such as viral hepatitis. Not consistently elevated in cirrhosis.
GPT (glutamic pyruvic transaminase)	Blood serum	*Colorimetric* 1 to 45 units *Spectrophotometer* 16 ± 9 units	Elevated in liver damage due to drugs and poisons, infectious hepatitis, cirrhosis, and metastatic CA of liver. Increased also in extrahepatic biliary obstruction.
Gravindex	Urine	Negative	Pregnancy test.
Guthrie	Whole blood	Negative	Positive in phenylketonuria.
Hanger's See: Cephalin Cholesterol flocc.			
Hematocrit	Whole blood	Female: 35 - 45% Male: 40 - 50%	Measure of the volume percentage of red cells in whole blood.

LABORATORY EXAMINATIONS (continued)

TEST	PERFORMED ON	NORMAL RANGE	SIGNIFICANCE
Hemoglobin	Whole blood	12 - 18 Gm./100 cc.	Increased in all conditions marked by an increase in red blood cells. Reduced levels seen in all anemias.
Heterophile antibody	Blood serum	Conc. to 1/28	Elevated in serum sickness and infectious mononucleosis.
Hippuric acid (I.V.)	Urine	0.7 - 1.0 Gm./24 hr.	Liver function test seldom used today. Decreased levels indicate liver disease such as cirrhosis or hepatitis.
Hogben	Urine	Negative	Pregnancy test.
Homogentisic acid	Urine	Negative	Presence in urine indicates alkaptonuria.
Howard Test	Urine	Negative	Positive in renal hypertension.
17-Hydroxycorticosteroids (17-OHCS)	Urine	Female: 2 - 8 mg./24 hr. Male: 3 - 10 mg./24 hr.	Adrenal function test.
5-Hydroxyindoleacetic acid (5-HIAA)	Urine	Less than 10 mg./24 hr.	Levels above 25 mg./24 hr. suggest functioning carcinoid tumor.
I^{131} uptake (radioactive iodine)	Thyroid	Uptake of 15 to 45% of administered dose	In hyperthyroidism 50 to 100% uptake; below 15% uptake in hypothyroidism.
Icterus index	Blood serum	3 - 8 units	Used to discover early jaundice.

LABORATORY EXAMINATIONS

TEST	PERFORMED ON	NORMAL RANGE	SIGNIFICANCE
Indican	Urine	4 - 20 mg./24 hr.	May be present in constipated persons, in intestinal putrefaction with obstruction, pernicious anemia, obstructive jaundice, peritonitis, and with conditions causing decomposition of proteins.
Insulin tolerance	Blood serum	Returns to pre-injection level within 2 hours	Diagnostic test for panhypopituitarism where the patient becomes extremely hypoglycemic following insulin injection.
Inulin clearance	Urine	120 - 140 cc./minute per 1.73 sq. meters of body surface	Renal function test.
Iron, inorganic	Blood serum	50 - 200 micrograms per 100 cc.	Increased in acute hepatitis and hemochromatosis. Decreased in chronic infection, uremia and carcinomatosis.
Iron binding capacity	Blood serum	Serum equals 20 to 50% of capacity	Increased in pregnancy and with acute and chronic blood loss. Decreased in malignancy, uremia, pernicious anemia, infections, cirrhosis of liver, and hemolytic anemia.
Isoiodeikon	Blood serum	10 - 15% dye retention in blood 30 minutes after injection	Impaired liver function indicated by retention of more than 20% of injected dye.
Kahn	Blood serum	Negative	Serology test for syphilis.

LABORATORY EXAMINATIONS (continued)

TEST	PERFORMED ON	NORMAL RANGE	SIGNIFICANCE
17-Ketosteroids	Urine	Female: 4 - 15 mg./24 hr. Male: 8 - 21 mg./24 hr.	Increased levels seen in adrenal and testicular hyperfunction such as Cushing's disease and adrenogenital syndromes. Very high values suggest carcinoma of adrenal cortex. Decreased in Addison's disease, myxedema and pituitary deficiency.
Lactic acid	Whole blood	6 - 20 mg./100 cc.	Increased after muscular exercise, and in congestive heart failure, pneumonia, acute hepatitis and terminal cirrhosis of liver.
Lactic dehydrogenase (LDH)	Blood serum	150 - 500 B & B units per cc.	Increased in myocardial infarction, malignant lymphoma, untreated acute leukemia, pulmonary embolism with infarction, CA of kidneys or urinary bladder, sickle cell anemia, megaloblastic anemia.
Latex slide agglutination	Blood serum	1:40 is uppermost serum dilution	Positive in some connective tissue diseases and rheumatoid arthritis.
L.E. Test	Whole blood	Negative	Slide test for antinucleoproteins found in systemic lupus erythematosus.
Leucine aminopeptidase	Blood serum	Female: 80 - 210 u. per 100 cc. Male: 75 - 230 u. per 100 cc.	Increased in carcinoma of pancreas, acute pancreatitis, liver disease, choledocholithiasis, leukemias and lymphoma. Moderately increased in pregnancy and immediately postpartum.
	Urine	Female: 20 - 70 u./24 hr. Male: 50 - 175 u./24 hr.	

LABORATORY EXAMINATIONS

TEST	PERFORMED ON	NORMAL RANGE	SIGNIFICANCE
Levinson	Cerebrospinal fluid	Precip. in mercuric chloride tube 3 X that in sulfosalicylic acid tube.	Test for tuberculous meningitis.
Levulose tolerance	Blood serum	Less than 20 mg. per 100 cc. in 1st hour and less than 8 mg. per 100 cc. after 2 hours.	Test for severe liver damage. Useless if patient has diabetes mellitus.
Lipase	Blood serum	0.2 - 1.5 u.	Increased in pancreatic damage.
Lipids, total	Blood serum	570 - 820 mg.%	Elevated in uncontrolled diabetes mellitus, ketosis and nephrosis.
Magnesium	Blood serum	1.5 - 2.5 mEq/liter	Increased in kidney damage, hypertrophic arthritis, essential hypertension, and arteriosclerosis. Decreased in malignant bone disease with loss of calcium, severe diarrhea.
Malaria film	Whole blood	Negative	Smear study for malarial organisms.
Mallein	Skin test	Negative	Positive for Glanders with reaction at site of injection.
Mastic	Cerebrospinal fluid	Negative	Test for cerebrospinal syphilis.
Melanin	Urine	None	Suggests malignant melanoma.
Mucoproteins	Blood serum	8 - 14 mg./100 cc. in terms of galactose-mannose	Decreased in liver disease, nephrosis and endocrine disorders. Increased in cancer, Tbc, acute and chronic leukemia, pneumonia, myocardial infarction, rheumatic fever, active rheumatoid arthritis, multiple myeloma, Hodgkin's disease, L.E. and lymphosarcoma.

LABORATORY EXAMINATIONS (continued)

TEST	PERFORMED ON	NORMAL RANGE	SIGNIFICANCE
NPN (nonprotein nitrogen)	Blood serum	25 - 40 mg.%	Kidney function test.
PBI (See: protein bound iodine)			
Phenolsulfonphthalien (PSP)	Urine	25% or more/15 min. 40 - 60%/1 hr. 60 - 85%/2 hours	Elevated in some liver diseases. Reduced in chronic nephritis.
Phenylketonuria	Urine of NB	Negative	Used to detect phenylpyruvic acid in the urine of infants after the 4th week. Performed as a diaper test. Ames Co. produces PHENISTIX a test strip which may be dipped in urine or pressed against wet diaper. Mental deficiency results from the child's inability to properly metabolize phenylalanine. A diet deficient in this amino acid must be instituted.
Phosphatase, acid See: Acid phosphatase			
Phosphatase, alkaline See: Alkaline phosphatase			
Phospholipids	Blood serum	220 - 400 mg./100 cc.	Increased in glomerulonephritis, nephrosis, Vit. B def., diabetes with severe malnutrition, secondary anemia with chronic hemorrhage. Decreased in acute infections with fever, anemia and sometimes with hyperthyroidism.

LABORATORY EXAMINATIONS

TEST	PERFORMED ON	NORMAL RANGE	SIGNIFICANCE
Phosphorus Adults	Blood serum	3 - 4.5 mg.% (1.8 - 2.3 mEq/l)	Elevated in hypoparathyroidism, uremia, Bright's disease, and excessive Vit. D intake.
Children		4 - 6.5 mg.% (2.3 - 3.8 mEq/l)	Lowered in hyperparathyroidism, osteomalacia, rickets.
Porphobilinogen	Urine	Negative	Demonstration in urine pathognomonic for acute porphyria.
Porphyrins	Urine	0 - 30 mcg.	Increased in congenital porphyria, pellagra, liver damage and lead poisoning.
Potassium (K)	Blood serum	1.5 - 2.5 Gm./24 hr.	Lowered values in Cushing's disease. Increased in oliguria.
Protein, total Albumin Globulin Electrophoresis	Blood serum	6.3 - 8.0 Gm./100 cc. 4.5 - 5.5 Gm./100 cc. 1.5 - 3.4 Gm./100 cc. Percentage of total protein:	Performed with albumin and globulin. Lowered levels seen in liver disease, malnutrition and chronic kidney disease.
Albumin Globulin: Alpha 1 Alpha 2 Beta Gamma		45 - 55 5 - 8 8 - 13 11 - 17 15 - 25	
Protein bound iodine PBI	Blood serum	4.5 - 8 mcg.	Test for thyroid function.
Prothrombin time	Blood serum	70 - 110% of control 12 - 14 seconds with Difco thromboplastin	When anticoagulation therapy used, prothrombin time kept at from 2 - 2½ times normal.

LABORATORY EXAMINATIONS (continued)

TEST	PERFORMED ON	NORMAL RANGE	SIGNIFICANCE
PSP (See: Phenol-sulfonphthalein)			
Purines	Urine	0.05 gm./24 hr.	Increased by ingestion of foods abundant in nucleins such as liver and sweetbreads. Greatest increase occurs in leukemia, destructive liver disease and during absorption of a pneumonic process. Decreased before onset of gout attack with elevation following onset.
RA Test (Rheumatoid arthritis)	Blood serum	Negative	Visible flocculation in seconds with positive results in about 85-90% of patients with rheumatoid arthritis.
Schick Test	Skin	Negative result indicates immunity to diphtheria	Skin test read 4-6 days after injection to determine immunity to diphtheria. Positive reaction indicates susceptibility to diphtheria.
Sedimentation rate	Whole blood	Westergren: Male 0 - 10 mmph. Female 0 - 20 mmph. Child 0 - 10 mmph.	Values depend upon method used. Lowered values seen in newborn infants, polycythemia, sickle cell anemia and cardiac decompensation.
Sed. rate (continued)	Whole blood	Wintrobe: Male 0 - 9 mmph. Female 0 - 15 mmph. Rourke-Ernstene 0.05 - 0.40 mm./min. Cutler Female 2 - 10 mmph. Male 2 - 8 mmph.	Increased sedimentation rates seen in myocardial infarction, pulmonary infarction, almost all infections, active rheumatoid arthritis, Ca with necrosis, shock, surgical operations, pregnancy and conditions which cause reversal of A/G ratio (hyperglobulinemia).

LABORATORY EXAMINATIONS

TEST	PERFORMED ON	NORMAL RANGE	SIGNIFICANCE
Serology test for syphilis	Blood serum	Negative	Several tests such as Kahn, Kolmer, Wasserman, V.D.R.L. (Venereal Disease Research Lab), Kline, Eagle, Hinton, Mazzini, and R.P.C.F. False positives sometimes obtained. Positive tests confirmed with a complement fixation or TPI (Treponema Pallidium Immobilization). Early syphilis diagnosed by darkfield examination.
Serotonin (See: 5-Hydroxyindoleacetic acid)	Urine		
Serum transaminase (See: Transaminase)			
Sickle Cell Test	Drop of whole blood	Negative for sickle cells	In sickle cell anemia, a red cell is noted which assumes a sickle shape when the oxygen supply is reduced. Sickle cell anemia found in about 8% of American Negroes. These persons are poor OB and surgical risks.
Sims-Huhner Test	Postcoital cervical and vaginal secretions	Active spermatozoa noted	Female fertility study.
Sodium (Na)	Blood serum	136 - 145 mEq/liter Flame photometer	Increased in congestive heart failure, Cushing's disease, after ACTH and cortisone intake, lower nephron nephrosis. Decreased in Addison's disease, vomiting with loss of chloride, excessive perspiration, diabetes with acidosis, glomerulonephritis with uremia, lobar pneumonia and after ether anesthesia.
Sulkowitch See: Calcium			

LABORATORY EXAMINATIONS (continued)

TEST	PERFORMED ON	NORMAL RANGE	SIGNIFICANCE
T-3 uptake (triiodothyronine)	Thyroid function	Depends on lab method	Most frequently used thyroid function test.
TBI (thyroxine binding index)	Blood serum	0.86 to 1.20	Used to evaluate thyroid function.
TGT (thromboplastin generation test)	Blood	Abnormal thromboplastin formation	Test used to differentiate blood coagulation abnormalities.
Takata-Ara Test	Blood serum	Negative	Liver function test which is also positive in some cases of nephritis, pul. tbc, chronic alcoholism and multiple myeloma.
Thorn Test	Blood	50% drop in eosinophil count 4 hr. after injection of ACTH or epinephrine	Test for Addison's disease in which no reduction in eosinophiles occurs.
Thymol turbidity	Blood serum	0 - 5 units	Liver function test with increase indicative of liver damage.
Tourniquet (See: Capillary fragility test)			

LABORATORY EXAMINATIONS

TEST	PERFORMED ON	NORMAL RANGE	SIGNIFICANCE
Transaminase SGOT	Blood serum	10 - 40 units	Serum Glutamic Oxalacetic Transaminase (SGOT) increased 24 hours after myocardial infarction to levels of 500 units. Higher levels seen in liver disease, 600-2000 u., complete biliary obstruction and jaundice with hepatic cirrhosis. Increased to several hundred units in gangrene of extremities, skeletal trauma, muscular dystrophy and with various drugs.
SGPT			Serum Glutamic Pyruvic Transaminase (SGPT) elevated in liver damage.
Trypsin	Blood serum	31 units	Increased in acute pancreatitis, and carcinoma of the pancreas.
Urea	Blood serum	25 - 38 mg. Urea = 2.12 × blood urea nitrogen	Increased in kidney and other diseases causing nitrogen retention. Decreased in toxic hepatitis, eclampsia, celiac disease, lipoid nephrosis.
Urea clearance	Urine	54 cc. - 75 cc.	Decreased in permanent kidney damage, acute nephritis, hypertension with arteriosclerosis, active glomerulonephritis, and congestive heart failure.
Uric acid	Blood serum	2 - 4 mg.%	Increased in gout, leukemia and toxemia.
Urobilinogen	Urine	1 - 4 mg./24 hr.	Increased in hemolytic jaundice, pernicious anemia, liver damage, cardiac decompensation, eclampsia, or infection of the liver.
van den Bergh (See: Bilirubin, total)			

LABORATORY EXAMINATIONS (continued)

TEST	PERFORMED ON	NORMAL RANGE	SIGNIFICANCE
Vanilmandelic acid (VMA Test)	Urine	3 - 10 mg./24 hr.	Screening test for pheochromocytoma with elevated values as high as 250 mg./24 hours. Also elevated in neuroblastomas and related neural tumors.
VDRL (See: Serology test for syphilis)			
d-Xylose tolerance	Urine	5 - 8 Gm. within 5 hours after ingestion of 25 Grams.	Superior to oral glucose tolerance test when there is normal renal function. Decreased in tropical and nontropical sprue. It is one of the best screening tests for intestinal malabsorption.
Zinc flocculation (turbidity)	Blood serum	2 - 12 units	Liver function test.

3 | X-Ray Examinations

Radiology must be counted as one of the fastest growing medical specialties. Its beginning may be traced to the work of the German physicist, Wilhelm Conrad Roentgen, who in 1895 observed a type of radiation which possessed the property of penetrating objects opaque to sunlight. Identification and study of these rays which were called roentgen rays won for him the Nobel prize in physics in 1901.

A year after Roentgen's findings, a French physicist, Henri Becquerel observed radioactive properties occurring from the element uranium. In 1903 he shared the Nobel prize in physics with the Polish physicist, Maria Sklodowska Curie, who discovered the radioactive elements, polonium, named after her homeland, and radium, an element over a million times more active than uranium. She recognized and diagramed three different rays emitted by radium and designated these as alpha, beta and gamma rays. The gamma rays were found to resemble X-rays, but to be more penetrating. She was also awarded the Nobel prize in chemistry in 1911.

The work of these distinguished scientists provided the knowledge from which modern radiology has evolved. Progress in the specialty began slowly. The knowledge was revealed, but man and machine lagged. The new specialty was not without its critics. Prior to 1910, very few hospitals owned X-ray equipment. It was regarded largely as an experimental curiosity which belonged in the laboratory rather than in clinical practice.

Early radiologic examinations were confined to skeletal fractures, foreign bodies and simple chest surveys. Limited as these applications seemed to the hospitals, a great need for these services was generated by World War I (1914-1919). The U.S. Army started the first school of radiology. Industry moved quickly to improve X-ray machinery and photographic materials. The resulting improvement in technology provided better radiologic results. Military surgeons played an influential role in promoting an interest in radiology as they returned to their civilian practices. Hospital demands for radiologic installations provided industry with greater incentive to perfect machinery and supplies. Radiology thus graduated rapidly after the first world war from the obscure status of a scientific oddity, to a valuable medical specialty.

A tour through the radiology department of the modern hospital, particularly in the large teaching centers, makes one acutely aware of the dramatic progress which has been made in this field of medicine. Closed-circuit television screens which permit physicians to monitor radiologic examinations in a viewing room away from the patient represent only one of the recent advances in radiologic equipment. The introduction of contrast media and fluoroscopy for studying hollow organs, anatomic spaces and blood vessels added another dimension to diagnostic radiology. New techniques which include body section radiography, kymography and stereoscopy have greatly enhanced the scope of diagnostic work.

Great strides have also been made in radiation therapy. Modern cobalt teletherapy units are providing valuable support in man's struggle against malignant tumors. Radioactive isotopes are being effectively used in the diagnosis and treatment of a variety of diseases. Even greater achievements are expected as the mysteries of nuclear physics continue to unfold.

X-RAY DIAGNOSTIC TECHNIQUES

X-ray examinations, also referred to as radiographic or roentgenographic examinations, provide an important adjunct to medical and surgical care of the patient. They may consist of a film survey only, or of films obtained in conjunction with fluoroscopic examination.

Fluoroscopy provides the radiologist with a means of observing organs in motion or during function after they are filled with a contrast medium introduced by injection, ingestion or enema. These media serve to differentiate the organ being examined from the surrounding tissues. Contrast media, with the exception of air, are radiopaque (not permitting passage of X-rays). Most of these media used in fluoroscopic examinations represent iodine products.

The following list contains the names of media used in this country as well as abroad. The surgeon as well as the radiologist often specify this important particular in their dictations.

RADIOGRAPHIC CONTRAST MEDIA

Abrodil	Baridol
Acetiodone	Bariform
Acetrizoate	Barium sulfate
Acetrizoic acid	Baropaque A, B, or C.
Air-lipiodol gum tragacanth	Barosperse
Angio-Conray 80	Basolac
Angiopac	BAS 16
Arteray	Biligrafin
Arteriodone	Biliodyl

RADIOGRAPHIC CONTRAST MEDIA (continued)

Biliselektan
Bilitrast
Bilombrine
Bilopaque
Biloptin
Bilospext
Bismuth carbonate

Calcium ipodate
Campiodol
Cardiografin
Cardiotrast
Chloriodized oil
Cholegrafin
Cholepulvis
Choleradiagnost
Cholestim
Cholevic
Cholografin
Cholotrast
Cistobil
Cistopac
Colloidal barium sulfate
Conray 60
Conray 280
Conray 400
Conray 420
Conray 480

Diaginol
Diaginol viscous
Diagnorenol
Diatrast
Diatrizoate sodium
Diatrizoic acid
Dijodin
Dikol
Diodone
Diodrast
Dionosil
Dionosil aqueous
Dionosil oily
Diprotrizoate
Ditriokon
Ditrox

Endografin
Ethiodan
Ethiodol
Ethyl diiodo stearate
Ethyl triiodo stearate

Galisol
Gastrografin
GBD tablets

Hippodin
Hippuran
Hydrombrine
Hypaque 20%
Hypaque 50%
Hypaque—M 75%
Hypaque—M 90%
Hypaque sodium
Hytrast

Intron
Iobenzamic acid
Iodatol
Iod-Cholegnostyl
Iodeikon
Iodipamic acid
Iodipamide
Iodised oil (viscous)
Iodoalphionic acid
Iodochlorol
Iodognost
Iodomethamate sodium
Iodophen
Iodophthalein sodium
Iodopyracet
Iodosol
Iodoxyl
Ioduron
Iopan
Iopanoic acid
Iophendylate
Iophenoxic acid
Iopyracil
Iothalamate
Iothalamic acid
Ipodate

RADIOGRAPHIC CONTRAST MEDIA (continued)

Jodafen
Jodairal
Jodobilan
Jodosol
Jodtetragnost
Joduron

Lipiodol
Lipomul
Lumoxyd

Medopaque
Meglumine diatrizoate
Meglumine iodipamide
Meglumine iothalamate
Methiodal
Metufan
Micropaque
Microtrast
Miokon sodium
Mixobar
Monophen
Morujodol
Mulsopaque
Myodil

Neo-Hydriol fluid (viscous)
Neo-Iodipin
Neo-Iopax
Neo-Methiodal
Neo-Skiodan
Neo-Tenebryl
Nosophen
Nosydrast
Nosylan

Opacin
Opacol
Oparenol
Orabilix (foreign)
Orabilex (U.S.A.)
Oragrafin calcium
Oragrafin sodium
Osbil

Pantopaque
Per-Abrodil
Perjodal
Per-Radiographol
Perurdil
Pheniodol
Phenobutiodil
Phentetiophthalein
Priodax
Propyliodone
Pychokon-R
Pyelectan
Pyelombrine
Pyelosil
Pylumbrin

Radiographol
Raybar
Raybar 75
Renografin
Renovist
Retro-Conray
Rheopac
Rugar

Salpix
Savac
Shadocol
Shadow meal
Sinografin
Skiadin
Skiodan
Skiodan acacia
Sodium buniodyl
Sodium diatrizoate
Sodium diprotrizoate
Sodium methiodal
Sodium metrizoate
Sodium spodate
Sodium tyropanoate
Solu-Biloptin
Sombracol
Sombradil
Steripaque
Steripaque-BR

Steripaque-V
Syntetragnost

Telepaque
Teridax
Thixokon
Thorotrast
Triabrodil
Triiodyl
Triopac
Triosil
Triurol
Trixobar

Umbradil viscous
Umbrathor
Uriodone

Urografin
Urokon sodium
Urombrine
Uropac
Uroselectan B
Urotex
Urotrast
Urumbrine

Vasiodone
Vasoselectan
Veripaque (pre. drug)
Visciodol

X-iodol
Xumbradil

X-RAY EXAMINATIONS

The secretary should be familiar with the purpose and nature of specialized examinations performed in the X-ray department. A description of the commonly obtained film surveys and fluoroscopic examinations follow. It should be noted that the term which describes the technique adds the suffix -graphy. The term for the report adds the suffix -gram.
EXAMPLE: Arteriography (arteriogram)

Abdomen (flat plate; scout film; plain film of abdomen)

When an abnormal condition of the abdomen is suspected a survey film of the abdomen is ordered without use of a contrast medium. Conditions such as abscesses, hematomas or tumors which displace or distort the digestive organs in the abdominal cavity may be diagnosed, in addition to enlarged or perforated organs, intestinal obstruction or ileus.

Examinations limited to one or two roentgenograms are called scout films. Positions for survey of the abdomen vary depending upon the suspected pathology. Films may be taken in the erect or supine position, and be further designated as lateral decubitus, lateral or prone position.

In the plain survey of the abdomen, three films are often taken to include: (1) Bucky anteroposterior film in recumbent (supine) position, (2) erect film, and (3) erect posteroanterior film of the chest.

Aortography (Aortogram)

Examination of the aorta and its branches after the administration of a radiopaque medium. Translumbar aortography is sometimes used by the urologist to evaluate the renal vascular system. This is a useful technique for localizing vascular distribution defects or displacements of the vascular system and can be helpful in assessing their operability.

Arteriography (Arteriogram)

Study of the arterial system after the injection of a contrast medium. The examination may be confined to the brachial, coronary, femoral or renal arteries.

Arthrography (Arthrogram)

Radiographic examination of the interior of a joint into which a gas or fluid dye has been injected. When air is used, the examination is called a pneumoarthrogram.

Autotomography (Autotomogram)

A not too common examination sometimes used with encephalography to demonstrate midline brain structures.

Barium Examinations

Barium sulfate is a thick white solution which provides a contrast medium in radiographic and fluoroscopic surveys of the alimentary tract. Using a fluoroscopic screen, the radiologist is able to observe the course of the barium through the esophagus, stomach and intestines. Intermittent radiographic films are taken at specified intervals for further evaluation of any existing irregularities, filling defects or obstructions.

Barium is administered by mouth or by enema. In some instances of intestinal obstruction, it is injected through a tube to visualize the point of obstruction.

Barium provides the contrast medium in the following examinations:

> *Barium enema*
> Examination of the colon, cecum and terminal ileum with the aid of barium introduced through the rectum by means of an enema.
>
> *Barium meal*
> Barium is swallowed for purposes of radiographic survey of the esophagus, stomach and small bowel.

Barium motor meal
Examination of the terminal ileum and ileocecal region on delayed films after ingestion of barium.

Double contrast
Insufflation of air following barium enema evacuation or concomitant with barium enema for detection of colonic polyps or other small lesions of the colon.

Brachial Arteriography (Brachial arteriogram)

Examination utilizing a contrast medium for evaluation of the brachial artery of the arm and its branches.

Bronchography (Bronchogram)

Fluoroscopic and radiographic examination of the bronchial tree with the aid of a contrast medium which may be administered through a catheter or by needle through the cricothyroid membrane. This examination is used to detect obstruction, bronchial or parenchymal lesions, bronchiectasis and abscesses.

Cardio-angiography (Cardio-angiogram)

Catheterization of the heart is carried out and followed by injection of a contrast medium for evaluation of the heart and great vessels.

Carotid Angiography (Carotid angiogram)

Examination of the brain circulation following the injection of a contrast medium into the common carotid artery, bilaterally or unilaterally. This technique is used to detect space occupying lesions, displaced vessels, defects, aneurysms or obstruction of the vessels, including thrombi and hematomas.

Chest X-ray

Film survey of the chest as a routine measure consists of the large P-A erect film of the chest. Photoroentgens are no longer in common usage because of the associated high exposure to radiation.

Cholangiography (Cholangiogram)
Techniques: I.V., operative, or percutaneous

This examination may be carried out preoperatively, during surgery, or postoperatively.

The *I.V. cholangiogram* utilizes an intravenous dye injection for visualization of the biliary tree, particularly in acute cholecystitis or in patients who have undergone cholecystectomy (gallbladder removal).

The *operative cholangiogram* enables the surgeon to inject contrast medium directly into the common duct. This is particularly useful for detecting stones higher in the biliary tree which might have eluded the surgeon during his digital examination.

In the *percutaneous technique,* injection of dye is performed directly through the abdominal wall into one of the intrahepatic bile ducts for visualization and survey of the biliary tree.

Cholecystography (oral) Graham's Examination (Cholecystogram)

An examination performed to evaluate the structure and function of the gallbladder. An oral dose of dye, usually Telepaque, is administered on the evening prior to X-rays. The dye concentrates in the gallbladder.

A fatty meal which causes the gallbladder to contract is administered after the first set of X-ray films. Post fatty meal films are then taken.

Cystourethrography (Cystourethrogram)

Female—Evaluation of urinary bladder function, particularly in cases of stress incontinence.

Male—Evaluation of the urethra and bladder neck for possible obstruction.

Dacryocystography (Dacryocystogram)

Radiologic evaluation of the lacrimal ducts of the eye.

Discography or Diskography (Discogram or Diskogram)

A roentgenographic technique for visualization of cervical or lumbar intervertebral disk, after direct injection of a dye into the disk. This is not a commonly performed examination.

Encephalography (Encephalogram)

Radiologic study of the ventricular and cisternal systems of the brain through a technique requiring an injection of air or oxygen into the lumbar subarachnoid space or cisterna magna.

Femoral Arteriography (Femoral arteriogram)

Radiologic survey of the femoral artery of the leg and its branches following injection of a radiopaque medium. This examination affords

X-RAY EXAMINATIONS

visualization of the circulation from the inguinal area down the length of the extremity.

Hysterosalpingography also: *Uterosalpingography* (Hysterosalpingogram)

A radiographic examination used particularly in sterility studies to survey the uterus and patency of the fallopian tubes. Contrast medium is introduced through the cervical canal and into the uterine cavity to reveal any defects of the uterus or obstruction in the tubes which might preclude conception.

Kub Film

This is a recumbent film of the abdomen which is used to study the kidneys, psoas shadows, flank area, abdominal wall, bones of the pelvis, gas pattern, unusual masses and opaque shadows.

Lymphangiography (Lymphangiogram)

Roentgenographic survey of the lymphatic system with the use of a contrast medium.

Mastoids

The mastoids are poorly defined divisions of the petrous portion of the temporal bones. They have a honeycomb appearance as a result of air containing cells which develop in this area. The mastoids are a common site of infection. They are usually surveyed with the following projections: (1) Law's projection, (2) Stenvers projection, and (3) occipital projection.

Myelography (Myelogram)

Radiographic evaluation of the spinal cord and canal for possible lesions or disk protrusions, after the injection of a dye.

Paranasal Sinuses

Radiologic survey of the paired, air containing cavities within the maxillary, frontal, ethmoid and sphenoid bones of the face.

Routine X-rays of the paranasal sinuses often include the following projections: (1) submentocervical (axial), (2) frontal (Caldwell), (3) occipital (Granger) and (4) Waters.

Pelvimetry

A roentgenographic determination devised to measure the maternal pelvic outlet. This technique is used when a disproportion is suspected between the head of the fetus and the pelvic opening of the mother. Such an examination is usually performed in the last two weeks of pregnancy and then only when definitely essential because of the radiation hazard to the fetus. See Fig. 19 and 20 for illustration of measurements obtained in this examination.

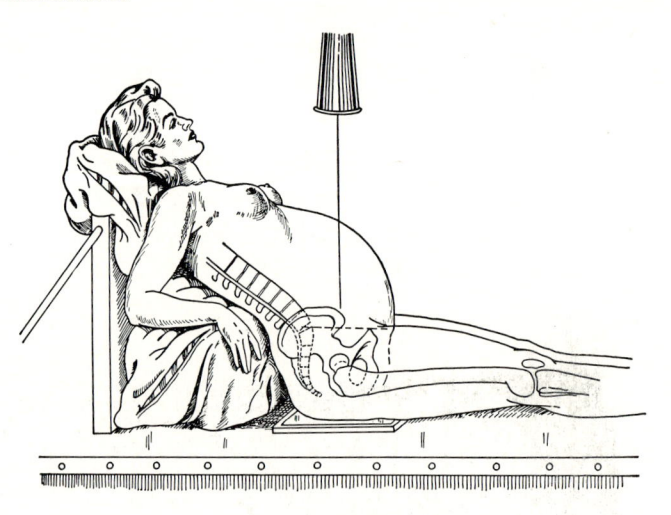

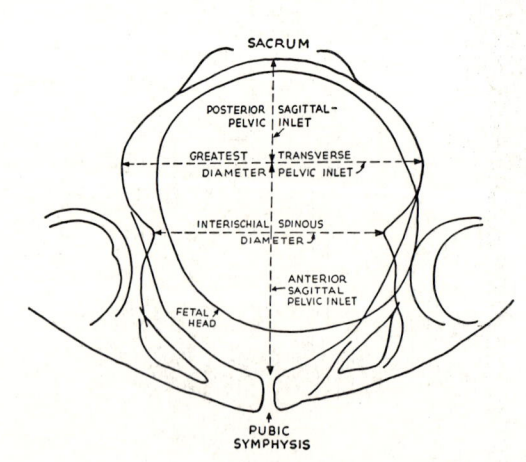

Figure 19 Tracing of radiograph routinely employed in pelvicephalometry for special demonstration of the pelvic inlet and a diagram illustrating the method by which this inlet view is obtained.

By permission. From I. Meschan, Roentgen Signs in Clinical Practice. Philadelphia, W. B. Saunders Co., 1966.

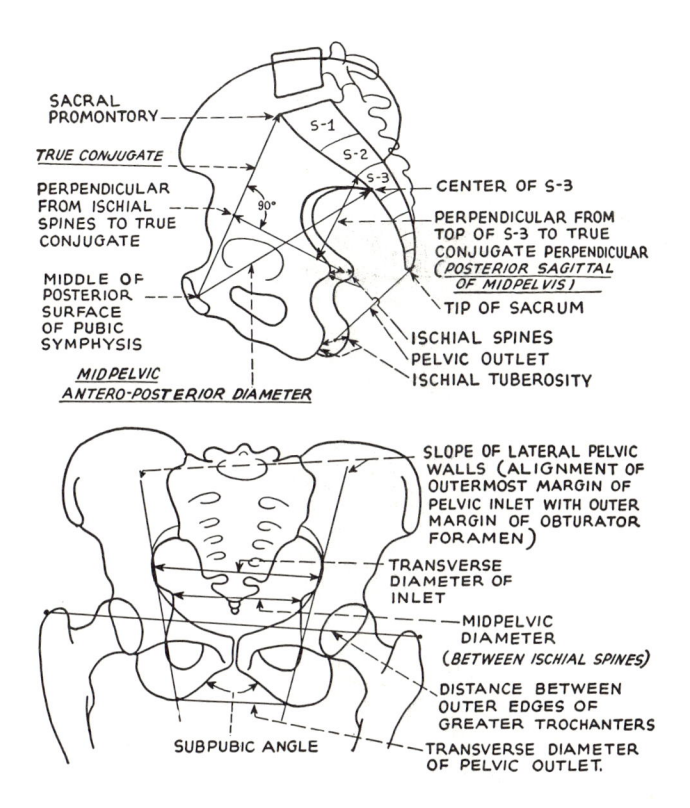

Figure 20 Diagrams illustrating the various measurements which are obtained from routine anteroposterior and lateral teleroentgenograms of the pelvis for pelvic measurement.

By permission. From I. Meschan, *Roentgen Signs in Clinical Practice*. Philadelphia, W. B. Saunders Co., 1966.

Pneumoencephalography (Pneumoencephalogram)

Introduction of air into the subarachnoid space to facilitate study of the ventricular system of the brain.

Portal Venography Also: *Splenoportography* (Splenoportogram)

A technique employing a contrast medium for purposes of outlining the portal vein and its branches. It may be performed in the operating room, under direct vision, or by percutaneous technique, with injection of dye through the abdominal wall into the spleen.

Pyelography Technique: I.V. or retrograde (Pyelogram)

I.V. Pyelography A study of the kidneys, ureters and sometimes of the urinary bladder employing an intravenous injection of radiographic dye which quickly is excreted with the urine.

Retrograde pyelography Study of the kidneys and ureters with the aid of a contrast medium introduced through a catheter, inserted into the ureters. This examination is performed in conjunction with a cystoscopy.

Renal Arteriography (Renal arteriogram)

Radiographic evaluation of the renal arteries, selectively, with the aid of a contrast medium introduced directly into the renal vessels via special catheters.

Sialography (Sialogram)

Radiographic examination of the salivary glands and their ducts where calculi sometimes develop.

Sinography (Sinogram)

Radiographic technique for assessing depth and direction of sinus tracts and their possible connection with internal organs.

Venography (Venogram)

Radiographic evaluation of patency in the communicating and deep veins of the leg.

Ventriculography (Ventriculogram)

Use of air or a contrast medium, introduced directly, for evaluation of the brain ventricles. This procedure is preferred over the pneumoencephalogram when there are signs of increased intracranial pressure.

Vesiculography (Vesiculogram)

Radiographic study of the vas deferens and seminal vesicles of the male genitalia utilizing a contrast medium.

SPECIAL RADIOLOGIC TECHNIQUES

Body Section Radiography

This technique enables the radiologist to study a particular anatomic layer with the blurring out of tissues above and below the layer under survey.

X-RAY EXAMINATIONS

Fluoroscopy

This is a technique used for observing anatomic structures in function or in motion. An X-ray tube is placed under the X-ray table, the patient is placed on the table, and a fluoroscopic screen is placed over the patient in direct line with the X-rays. The radiologist is able to observe from the opposite side of the screen. See Fig. 21.

DIAGRAM OF A FLUOROSCOPE

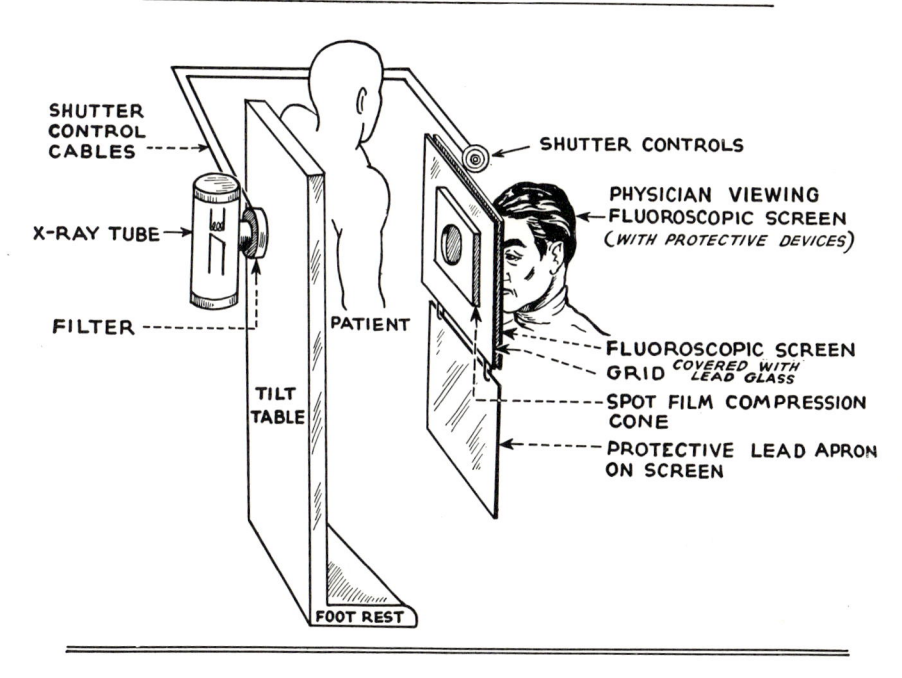

Figure 21 Diagram of a fluoroscope

By permission. From I. Meschan, Roentgen Signs in Clinical Practice. Philadelphia, W. B. Saunders Co., 1966.

Spot film radiography (filming of particular areas for study) is used with fluoroscopy, particularly in gastrointestinal examinations. This technique is also used in surveys of the spine, chest and heart.

The radiologist performing the fluoroscopic examination prepares his eyes for proper accommodation by wearing special goggles at least 20 minutes before the examination. This is done because inadequate accommodation or preparation could result in use of increased milliamperage, kilovoltage or fluoroscopy time with possible dangerous exposure of patient and physician to excessive radiation.

Kymography (Kymogram) Also: Electrokymography

This is a roentgen technique for making a graphic recording of the movements of an organ or structure on a single X-ray film. It is used principally in study of the heart and its component shadows.

Stereoscopy

This is an X-ray examination permitting depth perception and three dimensional reconstruction of an anatomic area. In stereoscopic roentgenograms, a three-dimensional image may be visualized from a two-dimensional film. The films are viewed in a stereoscope consisting of two viewing boxes and a set of mirrors which enables one eye to see one film and the other eye to see the other film. Each eye sees the area at a slightly different angle while the brain registers it as one single composite image with three-dimensional depth.

Stereoscopic radiography is useful in examination of the cranial vault, spine, chest, urinary tract, as well as pelvicephalometry and hysterosalpingography.

THERAPEUTIC RADIOLOGY

Malignancy ranks in second place, after heart disease, as a cause of death in the United States. More than one half million cases of cancer are diagnosed each year in this country where approximately 290,000 persons die of malignancies each year. The American Cancer Society believes that an additional 90,000 Americans could be saved yearly with earlier diagnosis and treatment.

In man's war against disease, it is usual first to recognize the manifestations of a disease, then the cause, and finally the treatment. Not so with cancer. Man has recognized the manifestations of the disease and has devised methods of treatment, but the complete etiologic picture continues to elude him. Until the causative phenomena can be explained, treatment can at best be limited to trial and error. Our knowledge of cancer is still skeletal and our methods of treatment rudimentary. In spite of efforts to develop an effective anti-cancer chemotherapeutic agent, surgery and radiology offer the only successful forms of treatment at this time. Even these methods are not universally successful on all malignant tumors.

Radiation, like surgery, is a local treatment. Once a tumor has metastasized, it is beyond the realm of curative therapy. In such cases, surgery and radiology can only offer palliative benefits.

The problem confronting the radiologist in radiation therapy is the need to preserve the host while destroying the lethal tumor. Despite modern radiologic techniques, we are not yet able to destroy the tumor selectively without damage to the tissues and organs in the irradiated area.

Deep Therapy

Irradiation of deep seated malignant tumors was previously carried out with X-rays produced by 20 kv. (kilovolt) filtered by combinations of copper, tin and aluminum. Modern radiotherapy units currently use 250 kv. constant potential machines. Other modern radiotherapy machines utilize an X-ray beam generated by 2 Mev. (million electron volts), 4-8 Mev., and 15 or more Mev.

With the construction of nuclear reactors it was possible to produce radioactive isotopes by bombarding certain elements with high velocity particles. One such radioactive isotope is radioactive cobalt (Co^{60}) which is being used in teletherapy units to provide radiation comparable to high energy X-ray generators. Only the larger medical centers with comprehensive radiotherapeutic divisions have radioactive cobalt teletherapy units.

Other high energy radiation machines include, (1) linear accelerator for medical radiotherapy, (2) Van de Graaff electrostatic generator, (3) betatron, and (4) resonant transformer X-ray generator. These new supervoltage machines have numerous advantages over the older methods of deep therapy:

1. The maximum tissue dose occurs below the skin and thereby spares the patient disfigurement which often resulted from older modes of deep therapy.
2. Greater depth dose provides more effective radiation of deep seated tumors.
3. The bone absorbs less high energy radiation than it does in the lower energy levels and for this reason there is less danger to the blood supply of the bone.
4. The field may be narrowed with less radiation being dispersed laterally over the patient.

Radium Therapy

Radium therapy was used at a distance from the patient to treat malignant tumors in the past. This method called telecurietherapy is now replaced by high energy radiation such as cobalt-60 teletherapy.

Radium, a naturally occurring radioactive element, is still used to treat malignant tumors seated in body cavities such as the mouth, vagina, uterus, rectum and urinary bladder. The radium salts are permanently enclosed in a small metallic container, usually of platinum, in the form of a needle, seed or tube.

Small radon seeds are sometimes implanted permanently since their radioactivity dies out in about 30 days.

Radioactive Isotopes

Radioactivity is a natural property of all elements with an atomic number above 83. These elements which include radium, uranium, polonium, to mention a few, emit electromagnetic radiations. In 1934, Mme. Irene Joliot, daughter of Marie Sklodowska Curie, and also a nuclear physicist, discovered that radioactivity could be induced in elements which are not otherwise radioactive. Her discovery of induced radioactivity in aluminum by the bombardment of its atoms by swiftly moving alpha particles was followed by further experiments through which several hundred new radioactive isotopes of known elements were produced. Isotopes are different atoms of a single element which have the same chemical and almost the same physical properties, but have different nuclear masses. Radioactive isotopes can be produced through bombardment of an element with fast moving particles such as protons, deuterons, alpha particles or neutrons, in a nuclear reactor. Radioactive elements and isotopes undergo a process of radioactive decay which is expressed in terms of the **half-life** of the element or isotope. The half-life is the time in which the radioactivity originally associated with the radioactive substance is reduced to one half in the process of radioactive decay. The element with the longest half-life period is thorium with 13,400,000,000 years while the shortest half-life period may be assigned to thorium C′ with a hundred millionth of a second. The half-life of radium is 1580 years while the half-life of radon (obtained from radium) is 3.825 days.

Radioactive isotopes have found many valuable applications in industry and in medicine. They are named after the element from which they are produced followed by a number which indicates their atomic mass (a means of distinguishing different atoms of a single element). The following list contains the names and symbols for radioactive isotopes used in modern medicine:

Radioactive isotopes	*Symbol*
Cobalt-60	Co^{60}
Cesium-137	Cs^{137}
Gold-198	Au^{198}
Iridium-192	Ir^{192}
Tantalum-182	Ta^{182}
Strontium-90	Sr^{90}
Phosphorus-32	P^{32}
Iodine-131	I^{131}

X-RAY EXAMINATIONS

Cobalt-60 is being used in teletherapy units in competition with high energy X-ray equipment.

Radioactive gold, in the form of a colloid, is being used in the palliative treatment of abdominal ascites and pleural effusions resulting from malignancy. It has been demonstrated to be effective in controlling fluid formation for various lengths of time. It is also used interstitially with permanent implantation similar to radon seeds.

Iodine-131 is used as a tracer in thyroid testing. It has also been used in the treatment of hyperthyroidism and cancer of the thyroid.

Iridium-192 is being used in the treatment of malignancies where interstitial irradiation is indicated.

Phosphorus-32 has been used in treatment of the leukemias and is also being used in the treatment of polycythemia vera.

Strontium-90 in a sealed applicator is being used in the treatment of corneal and conjunctival ophthalmic conditions.

Tantalum-182 is being used in the treatment of malignancies through interstitial irradiation.

Institutions using radioactive substances are required to take special precautions against contamination and to protect their employees against radiation hazards.

4 ⟩ Pre- and Postoperative Considerations

Anesthesia

Modern surgery has developed with an attending surgical specialty, anesthesiology, without which many of the surgical operations performed today would not be possible.

Neither surgery nor anesthesia are the inventions of modern men. Ancient records, predating Christ by thousands of years, describe primitive surgery and attempts to control and alleviate pain.

Anesthesiology, as we know it today, evolved from the discovery of nitrous oxide (laughing gas) in 1772 by an English chemist, Joseph Priestley, who two years later discovered oxygen. Since that time the list of chemicals with anesthesia inducing properties has grown in refinement and variety.

A listing of the more commonly used anesthetics has been prepared here to assist the secretary in her work. Generic names are used as often as trade names in the profession and for this reason this list purports to be only an alphabetical one. Where an anesthetic is variably known by several names, these will be listed in parentheses.

ANESTHETIC AGENTS

Amethocaine (pontocaine, pantocaine tetracaine)
Amytal
Apothesine hydrochloride
Avertin

Benzocaine
Blockain hydrochloride
Brevital
Butadiene

Carbocaine (mepivacaine)
Chloroform
Chloroprocaine (nesacaine)
Cinchocaine (nupercaine, debucaine, percaine)

Cocaine
Cyclaine (hexylcaine)
Cyclohexane (hexamethylene)
Cyclopentane (C_5H_{10})
Cyclopropane (C_3H_6)

Dibucaine (nupercaine, percaine cinchocaine)
Diethyl ether
Divinyl oxide (vinethene, divinyl ether)
Dyclone

Ethapon (trichloroethanol)
Ether
Ethocaine (procaine, novocain)

ANESTHETIC AGENTS
(continued)

Ethyl chloride
Ethylene
Ethyl ether (ethyl oxide)
Evipan

Fluoromar (trifluoroethyl vinyl ether)
Fluothane (halothane)

Halothane
Hexylcaine (cyclaine)

Lidocaine (xylocaine, lignocaine)
Lignocaine (lidocaine, xylocaine)

Mepivacaine (carbocaine)
Methohexital
Methycaine hydrochloride (piperocaine)
Monocaine

Nesacaine (chloroprocaine)
Nitrous oxide (N_2O)
Novocain (procaine, ethocaine)
Nupercaine crystal
Nupercaine hydrochloride (dibucaine percaine, cinchocaine)

Orthocaine

Pantocaine (pontocaine, amethocaine, tetracaine)
Penthrane
Pentothal (pentothal sodium)
Percaine (nupercaine, dibucaine, cinchocaine)
Piperocaine (metycaine)
Pontocaine hydrochloride (amethocaine, tetracaine, pantocaine)
Procaine hydrochloride (novocain, ethocaine)

Surfacaine
Surital sodium

Tetracaine (pontocaine, pantocaine, amethocaine)
Thiopental
Trichlorethylene (trilene)
Trifluorethyl vinyl ether (fluoromar)
Trimar

Vinamar (vinyl ethyl ether)
Vinethene
Vinyl ethyl ether

Xylocaine (lidocaine, lignocaine)

OPHTHALMIC ANESTHETICS
(eye)

Butyn sulfate & Metaphen ophthalmic ointment

Metycaine hydrochloride and merthiolate

Ophthaine
Ophthetic ophthalmic solution

Tetracaine HCl
Xylocaine hydrochloride 4% solution

PREPARATIONS USED WITH ANESTHESIA

Anectine .... muscle relaxant
Atropine and
  Scopolamine .... twilight sleep
Carbon Dioxide .. CO_2
Chloral .... hypnotic
Codeine .... analgesic
Curare .... muscle relaxant
Ephedrine .... vasopressor (raises blood pressure)
Epinephrine ..... vasopressor and cardiac stimulant

Gallamine .... muscle relaxant
Hydralazine ..... anti-hypertensive agent
Morphine sulfate . analgesic
Oxygen .... symbol = O
Paraldehyde ..... hypnotic
Syncurine .... muscle relaxant
Tolserol .... muscle relaxant
Tuinal .... hypnotic

OPERATIVE CONSIDERATIONS

MODES OF INDUCTION OF ANESTHESIA

Basal narcosis
Block

Caudal
Caudal block
Continuous spinal

Endobronchial
Endotracheal
Epidural block (peridural)

Field block

Infiltration (local)
Inhalation
Insufflation
Intercostal block
Intravenous

Local infiltration

Nerve block:
   brachial plexus
   cervical plexus
   lumbar plexus

Open
Open drop ether
Open endotracheal

Paravertebral block

Rectal
Regional spinal

Sacral block
Saddle block
Segmental block
Spinal block (subarachnoid)
Splanchnic block
Sympathetic block

Topical
Transsacral (sacral & caudal)

SURGICAL SCRUB SOAPS

Derma surgical
Gamophen
Germa-medica
G.S.I.

Hexa-germ
pHisoderm
pHisohex
Septisol

SURGICAL AND EXAMINING POSITIONS

Prior to surgery the chief surgeon decides upon the position in which the patient will be operated. Special positions are also used for certain examinations. Reports of surgery and/or special examinations should always specify the position in which the patient underwent the procedure.

ARM EXTENSION—Patient flat on back with arm extended on an arm board. This position is used for operations on the hand, arm, axilla and breast.

BOYCE—Position for passage of a bronchoscope.

BOZEMAN—Knee elbow genucubital position with patient supported by straps.

CASSELBERRY—Prone position used after intubation.

Sims's position, posterior view

Knee-chest position

Lithotomy position

Trendelenburg position

Surgical position for nephrectomy

Surgical position for spinal fusion

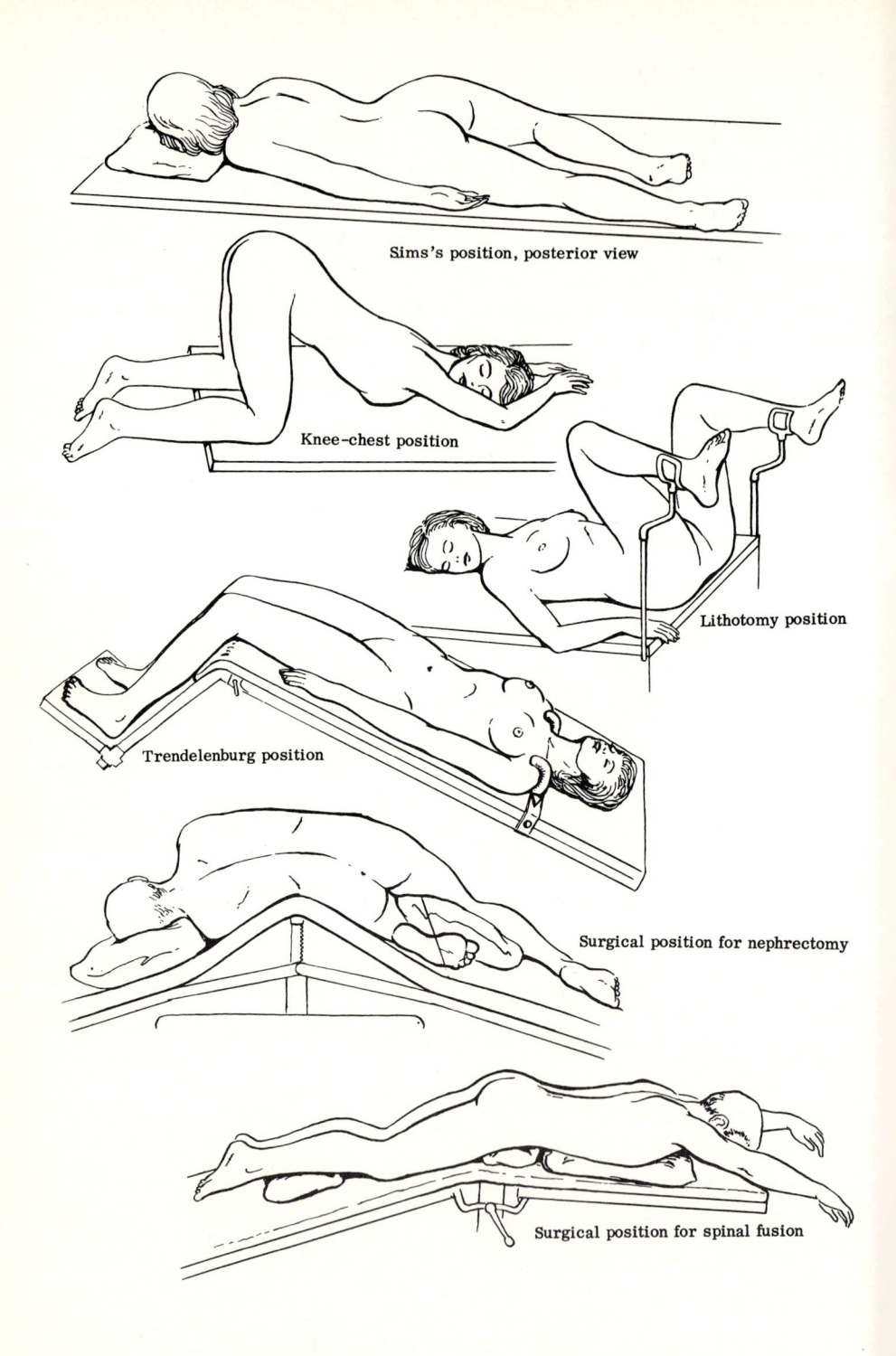

Figure 22 Surgical and Examining Positions

OPERATIVE CONSIDERATIONS 95

CHEST—Patient on side with back to surgeon and shoulder rotated toward surgeon providing access to chest. This position is used in thoracic surgery and is sometimes called the lateral chest position.

DEPAGE—Prone position with pelvis elevated so patient forms an inverted "V."

DORSAL (Supine)—Patient flat on back with legs extended and arms resting at sides. This position is used for abdominal surgery.

DORSAL RECUMBENT—Patient flat on back with knees drawn up and thighs turned outward. This position is used for examinations of the vagina.

EDEBOHLS—Dorsosacral position with patient on back, legs flexed at the knees, thighs flexed onto the abdomen and legs drawn away from the body midline.

ELLIOT—Patient in supine position with back arched over a support facilitating access to gallbladder and bile ducts.

FOWLER—Patient's trunk raised to form a 45 degree angle to the horizontal. The thighs are similarly raised with pelvis forming bottom of the "V."

HEAD DEPENDENT—Patient on back with pillow under neck and head extended over the end of the table. This position is used for removal of tonsils, operations on the mouth and cleft palate repair.

JACKKNIFE—Patient on abdomen with head and foot of table dropped so buttocks are most prominent. This position is used in hemorrhoidectomy operations.

KIDNEY—Patient placed on side and body elevator raised under patient to hyperextend the side to be operated. Head and foot of table are lowered. This position is used for operations on the kidney and its structures.

KNEE-CHEST—Patient kneeling on table, resting on elbows. Also called the genucubital position.

KRASKE—Same as jackknife position and used for sacral excision of rectum.

LATERAL PRONE—Same as kidney position.

LITHOTOMY—Patient on back with legs up in stirrups.

MAYO-ROBSON—Patient supine with back arched over a support facilitating access to gallbladder and bile ducts.

NECK EXTENSION—Dorsal position with support under neck. This position is used for removal of cervical glands and for goiter operations.

PRONE—Patient positioned flat on abdomen with head turned to one side. Used for operations on the back.

REVERSE TRENDELENBURG—The lower end of the table is dropped to a 45 degree angle. This position is sometimes used in abdominal surgery.

ROBSON—Patient placed on back with sandbag under hollow of back.

ROSE—Head lowered for operations on the palate and oropharynx.

SCHULTES (Scultetus)—Body inclined with head downward.

SHOCK—Table inclined with the head lowered.

SIMON'S—Dorsosacral position (Edebohls).

SIMS'—Patient on left side with left arm placed in back of patient causing patient to rest on chest. The right knee is drawn up.

STERN—Patient supine with head lowered over end of table.

TRENDELENBURG—Patient placed on back with table tilted 45 degrees toward the head and broken at the knees. This is a position used in pelvic surgery.

UPRIGHT—Patient seated in an operating chair. This position is sometimes used for submucous resection and for tonsillectomy.

VALENTINE—Urethral access position with patient on back and hips flexed.

WALCHER—Patient on back with hips to the end of the table allowing the legs to hang down.

WOLFENDEN—Prone position with head over the side of the table.

INCISIONS

A properly dictated operative report will contain a reference to the opening incision. The surgeon will specify the site of the incision and its course relative to particular anatomic points.

Some of the more commonly used incisions have been listed here.

Alexander	—Incision above and parallel with the left inguinal ligament.
Auvray	—Splenectomy incision.

INCISIONS (continued)

Bar	—Midline subumbilical cesarean section incision.
Battle	—Vertical appendectomy incision. Same as Battle-Jalaguier-Kammerer incision.
Bergmann	—Kidney exposure incision.
Bevan	—Gallbladder exposure incision.
Brackin	—Incision used in uretero-intestinal anastomosis.
Buttonhole	—A small straight incision into an organ or cavity.
Celiotomy	—Incision through the abdominal wall to permit access to the peritoneal cavity.
Chiene	—Gridiron incision carried medially to open the lateral part of the rectus sheath.
Circumscribing	—Encircling incision.
Codman	—Incision used for removal of subacromial bursa extending 2 inches forward from the acromio-clavicular joint.
Coffey	—Incision used in uretero-intestinal anastomosis.
Confirmatory	—An incision into an organ for purposes of confirming a diagnosis.
Courvoisier	—Same as Kocher incision.
Crescent	—Half-moon shaped incision.
Crosshatch	—An incision consisting of sets of parallel lines crossing parallel lines running crosswise.
Cruciate	—(Crucial) Cross-shaped incision.
Deaver	—Appendectomy incision through the sheath of the right rectus muscle.
Dührssen	—Deep incisions into the cervix uteri to facilitate delivery of an infant.
Edebohls	—Vertical lumbar incision used in nephropexy.
Endaural	—An incision made within the ear.
Exploratory	—An incision for exploratory purposes.
Fergusson	—Incision for excision of the upper jaw.
Fowler	—Angular incision for anterolateral abdominal section.

INCISIONS (continued)

Furniss	—Incision used in uretero-intestinal anastomosis.
Gatellier	—Incision over the lateral malleolus of the fibula.
Gridiron	—An abdominal incision for appendectomy in the line of the fibers of the external oblique muscle.
Halsted	—Inguinal herniorrhaphy incision. A particular radical mastectomy incision.
Harmon	—Incision made on the posterolateral aspect of the leg.
Heerman	—Endaural incision.
Henry	—Shoulder strap incision.
Higgins	—Incision used in uretero-intestinal anatomosis
Hockey-Stick	—J-shaped incision.
Jalaguier	—Same as Battle-Jalaguier-Kammerer incision for appendectomy.
Kammerer	—Vertical appendectomy incision.
Kehr	—An incision for wide opening of the abdomen.
Kocher	—Gallbladder incision.
Küstner	—Semilunar abdominal incision.
Langenbeck	—Abdominal incision through the linea semilunaris parallel to the fibers of the Rectus abdominis muscle.
Lateral Rectus	—An abdominal incision parallel and lateral to the midline of the abdomen.
Lempert	—Endaural incision.
Lilienthal	—A curved parotid incision.
Longuet	—Incision for transplantation of the testicle.
Mackenrodt	—Transverse semilunar abdominal incision.
Mayo-Robson	—Right upper quadrant abdominal incision.
McArthur	—A vertical upper trans rectus incision with transverse division of the peritoneum and posterior sheath.
McBurney	—An appendectomy incision.

OPERATIVE CONSIDERATIONS

INCISIONS (continued)

McLaughlin	—An incision extending forward from the acromion in approach to the subacromial bursa.
Median	—A midline incision in the abdomen.
Meyer	—Hockey stick incision for entering the lower anterior abdomen.
Morison	—(Rutherford Morison) An appendectomy incision.
Ollier	—An ankle incision.
Paramedian	—An incision just lateral to the midline in the upper abdomen.
Parker	—An incision nearly parallel to Poupart's ligament and used for appendiceal abscess operations.
Perthes'	—A gallbladder incision.
Pfannenstiel	—A curved abdominal incision.
Phemister	—An incision along the posterior border of the tibia.
Relief	—An incision made to relieve tension in a region.
Rollet	—Z-flaps for upper eyelid defect repairs.
Saber Cut	—An inverted U incision.
Semilunar	—Half-moon shaped incision.
Stab	—A stab wound usually made for insertion of a drain, etc.
Stellate	—An incision consisting of crossed lines in the shape of a star. This incision is used to drain abscesses, etc.
Visscher	—An incision in the lumbo-iliac region.
Whipple	—Curved incision between the xiphoid process and umbilicus, convex upwards, with division of the recti muscles.
Wilde	—An incision behind the auricle to expose the mastoid region.

SUTURE MATERIALS

Suture materials are described by the surgeon in terms of their size. The U.S.P. surgical ranges, depending upon the particular suture material are: 7-0, 6-0, 5-0, 4-0, 000, 00, 0, 1, 2, 3, 4, and 5.

SUTURE MATERIALS (continued)

Absorbable
Acutrol
Aluminum bronze wire
Ancap silk (braided silk)
Atraumatic
Aureomycin

Babcock suture wire
Barraquer silk
Bed puff
Black braided
Black silk
Black twisted
Blue twisted cotton
Braided
Braided silk
Braided wire
Bronze wire
Bunnell

Cable wire
Cardiovascular
Cargile membrane
Catgut
Catgut celluloid linen
Champion silk
Chinese twisted silk
Chloramine catgut
Chromic catgut
Circumcision
Collagen
Corneo-scleral
Cotton
Cotton, pink, twisted
Cuticular

Dacron
Deknatel surgical silk
Dermal
Dermalene
Dermalon
Dermalon monofilament
D & G Kalmerid catgut
Double armed
Double armed retention
Double stop (glass beads and lead shot)

Equisetene silk
Ethicon (brand name)
Ethicon atroloc
Ethilon nylon
Ethi-pack steel
Extra-chromic

Flaxedil
Flexitone
Flexon stainless steel

Gastrointestinal surgical gut
Gastrointestinal surgical linen
Gastrointestinal surgical silk
General closure
General eye surgery
Gossamer silk
Green braided
Gudebrod
Gut chromic
Gut plain

Horsehair

Iodized surgical gut

Kal-dermic
Kangaroo tendon

Lacidem
Linear polyethylene
Linen
Liver
Luken's iodized catgut

Mayo iron dyed linen
Measuroll
McLean corneoscleral
Medium chromic
Medrafil suture wire
Mersilene
Mesh
Monofilament
Monofilament clear
Monofilament green
Multifilament
Multistrand

Neurological
Non-absorbable

SUTURE MATERIALS (continued)

Nylon
Nylon monofilament

OB double armed
OB-Gyn closure
Oertli silk
Oiled silk
Owens
Oyloidin linen
Oyloidin silk

Pagenstecher linen
Pearsall Chinese twisted silk
Perma-hand surgical silk
Plain gut
Plastic
Polyethylene
Polypropylene button
Pre-op
Pyoktanin catgut

Ramsey County pyoktanin catgut
Reconstructive
Retention
Ribbon gut

Sani-dril
Silicone treated surgical silk
Silk
Silkworm gut
Silver suture wire
Single armed
Stainless steel
Steel

Steel mesh
Supramid-Extra (polyfilament synthetic)
Surgaloy mono-strand stainless steel
Surgaloy multi-strand stainless steel
Surgical gut
Surgical silk
Surgical steel
Surgilon (braided nylon)
Surgilope Sp

Tantalum wire-monofilament
Tension
Tevdek
Thermo-flex
Thoracic
Tiger gut
Tonsil
Twenty day catgut
Twisted cotton
Twisted silk
Tycron

Unabsorbable

Vascular silk
Vienna wire
Viro-Tec

White braided
White nylon
White twisted

Zytor

METHODS OF SUTURING

Primary suture line

The technic of suturing each layer of tissue separately is known as the *primary suture line, the tier plan of suturing, or direct suture approximation.*

Technic for special tissues — The following technics are generally employed when placing sutures in special tissues:

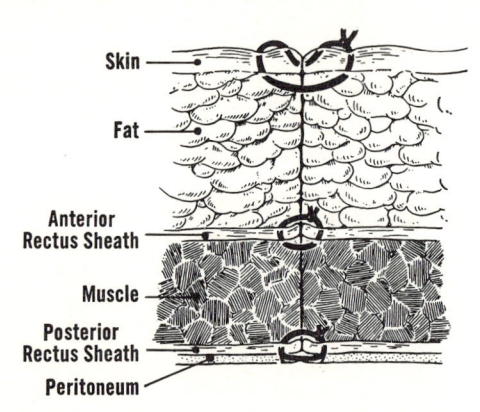

PRIMARY SUTURE LINE
Each layer of tissue is sutured separately.

a. Skin
   Skin is usually closed with nonabsorbable suture material using simple interrupted or vertical mattress stitches. It is essential that accurate, even apposition of the skin be accomplished.

b. Fat
   Fat is seldom sutured because it does not tolerate suture material well, has poor holding power, and adds little to the strength of wound repair.

c. Muscle
   The holding power of muscle is very small and sutures will pull out under moderate tension. Therefore, muscle is seldom sutured except to obliterate dead space. Since the relationship of muscle to fascia is very intimate, many surgeons prefer to approximate muscle by suturing only the fascia.

   During operations where muscles have been split in the direction of their fibers, reapproximation with a few fine sutures will suffice. Muscles divided transversely to their direction of pull require careful repair. It is important in transverse muscle divisions that the stitches include a bite of the over and underlying fascia.

d. Fascia
   Fascia is the tissue most ideally suited to suturing. The strength of its fibrous structure tolerates suture material well. It also possesses great strength when sutured. Generally interrupted stitches are used and so placed that their pull is not parallel to the direction of the fascial tissue fibers.

Courtesy Davis Geck—Division of American Cyanamid

OPERATIVE CONSIDERATIONS

e. Tendons
When suturing tendons it is essential that swelling at the site of repair be kept to a minimum to preserve mobility. The stitching is usually done with very fine interrupted nonabsorbable stitches.

f. Nerves
When suturing divided nerves exact realignment is imperative and only the delicate fibrous perineural sheath is stitched. Very fine interrupted silk stitches are usually used.

g. Blood vessels
Even blood vessels of very fine calibre can be successfully anastomosed when the following basic principles are used:

1. The approximation must be very accurate, preferably everting the innermost lining.

2. Little or no tension should be placed on the suture line.

3. The lining of the vessel must not be traumatized as this favors clotting. The stitches are usually placed with an interrupted or continuous everting stitch employing 5-0, 6-0 or 7-0 silk sutures armed with ATRAUMATIC needles.

h. Gastro-intestinal tract
The strength of repair of a divided gastrointestinal tract lies in the inner or submucosal layer. This layer is sutured with surgical gut employing continuous or interrupted stitches. The outer or sero-muscular layer is usually sutured with interrupted silk or cotton stitches.

Technic for a typical abdominal closure —

a. *Peritoneum*
   Suture size and material: medium chromic surgical gut, size 000 to 1.
   Type of stitching: continuous, with 2-3 interruptions to minimize danger of disruption.

b. *Posterior rectus fascia* (frequently included with the peritoneal layer)
   Suture size and material: medium chromic surgical gut, size 000 to 00 or surgical sik or cotton, size 000 to 00.
   Type of stitching: interrupted mattress

c. *Muscle*
   Suture size and material: plain surgical gut, size 000 to 0.
   Type of stitching: interrupted. A stay or tension suture may be used to obliterate dead space instead of suturing the muscle.

d. *Anterior fascia*
   Suture size and material: medium chromic surgical gut, size 000 to 0 or surgical silk, cotton or wire size 000 to 00.
   Type of stitching: interrupted, placed one centimeter apart and ½ centimeter deep on each edge of the wound.

Courtesy Davis Geck—Division of American Cyanamid

e. *Subcutaneous fat*

Suture size and material: no suture. However, if superficial fascia is well marked 3 or 4 interrupted sutures of plain surgical gut, size 4/0 to 000 may be employed.

f. *Skin*

Suture size and material: silk, cotton, nylon, wire or linear polyethylene, size 4/0 to 00

Type of stitching: interrupted or continuous

Secondary suture line

The secondary suture line is a secondary line of sutures passing through several layers of tissue and placed on each side of the primary suture line. Its purpose is to:

1. Partially relieve the primary suture line of unusual strain
2. To obliterate a dead space which interferes with wound healing
3. Prevent the accumulation of blood and serum

Sutures used for this purpose are commonly called stay sutures, tension sutures or through and through sutures

SECONDARY SUTURE LINE
A line of sutures passing through several layers of tissue and placed on each side of the primary suture line.

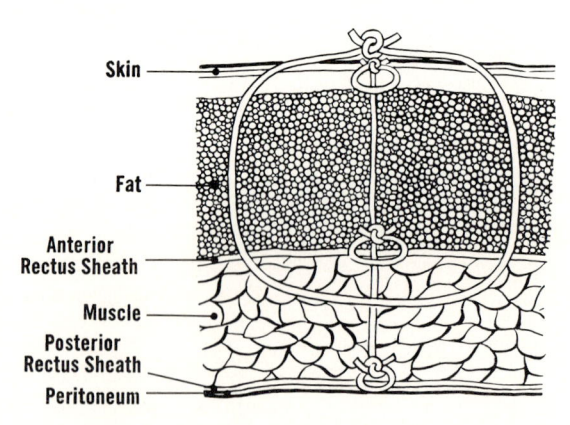

Skin
Fat
Anterior Rectus Sheath
Muscle
Posterior Rectus Sheath
Peritoneum

In long laparotomy wounds the tension sutures are placed with a through and through stitch to include most if not all the layers of tissue of the abdominal wall above the peritoneum. Material, such as nylon, silver or stainless steel wire, or silk may be used. It is advantageous to place the tension sutures at a distance from the wound edges so that the strain is placed on firm issue. After skin closure the exposed portion of the suture is passed through a piece of rubber tubing often called a "boot" or "bumper". The rubber tubing covers the portion of the suture crossing the line of incision

Courtesy Davis Geck—Division of American Cyanamid

and also part of skin. The rubber tubing prevents the tension sutures from cutting into the skin.

Drain fixation

When a drain is to be used it is usually sutured in place to prevent it from slipping in or out of the incision. When the drain is anchored to the skin a nonabsorbable suture (e.g. silk) is used. Enterostomy or gastrostomy tubes may be fixed in place with surgical gut.

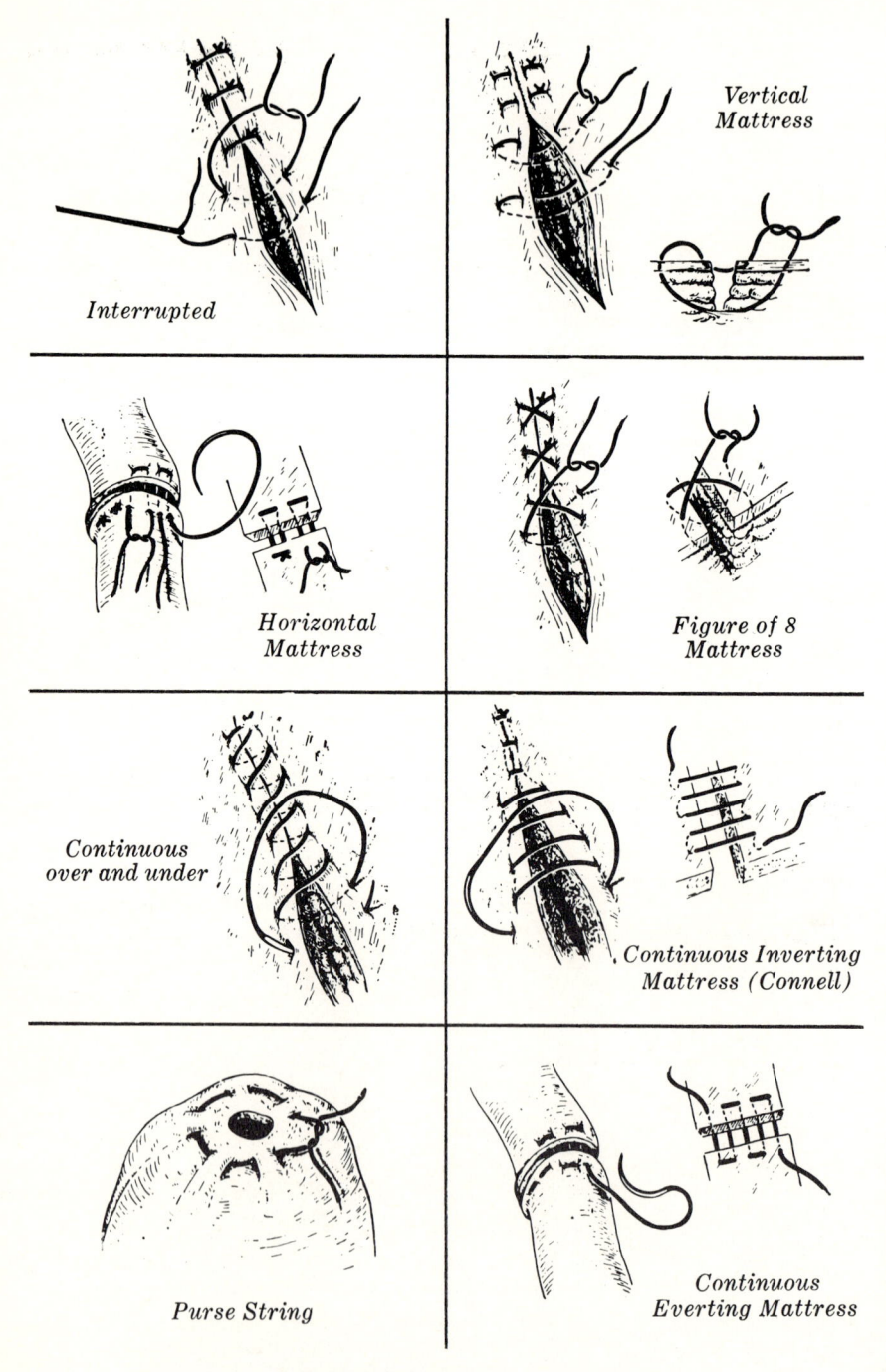

Courtesy Davis Geck, Division of American Cyanamid
Figure 23 Suture techniques

OPERATIVE CONSIDERATIONS

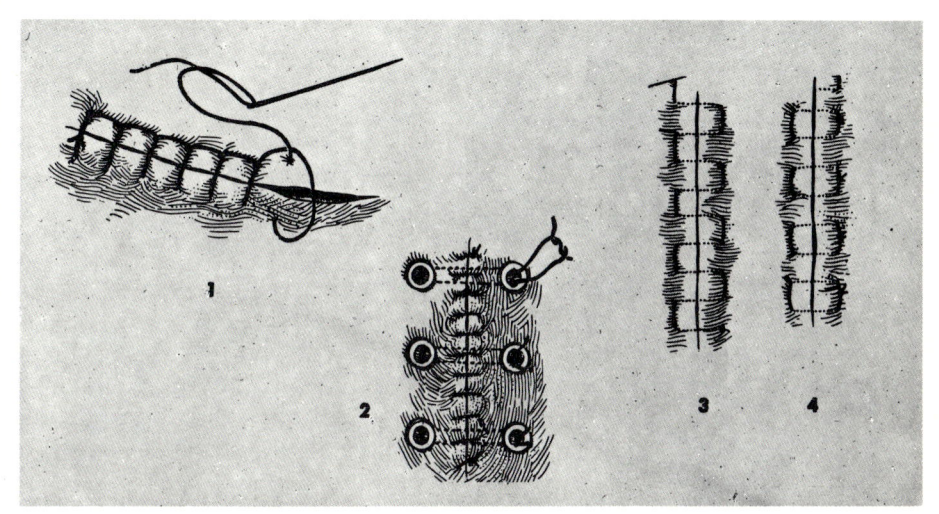

1. The blanket or continuous locked suture. **2.** Continuous suture and method of using perforated buttons to support tension sutures. **3.** Continuous mattress suture. **4.** Interrupted mattress suture.

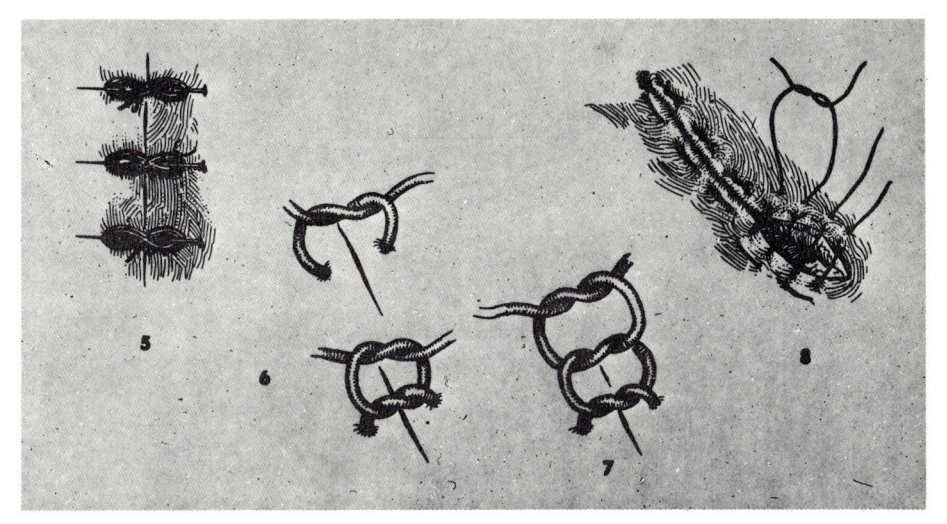

5. Figure-of-eight tension sutures around pins. **6.** Method of placing first and second half-hitches in the square or true knot. **7.** The square knot reinforced by third half-hitch. **8.** The Halsted interrupted mattress suture.

Figure 24   Suture techniques
Courtesy Ethicon, Inc.

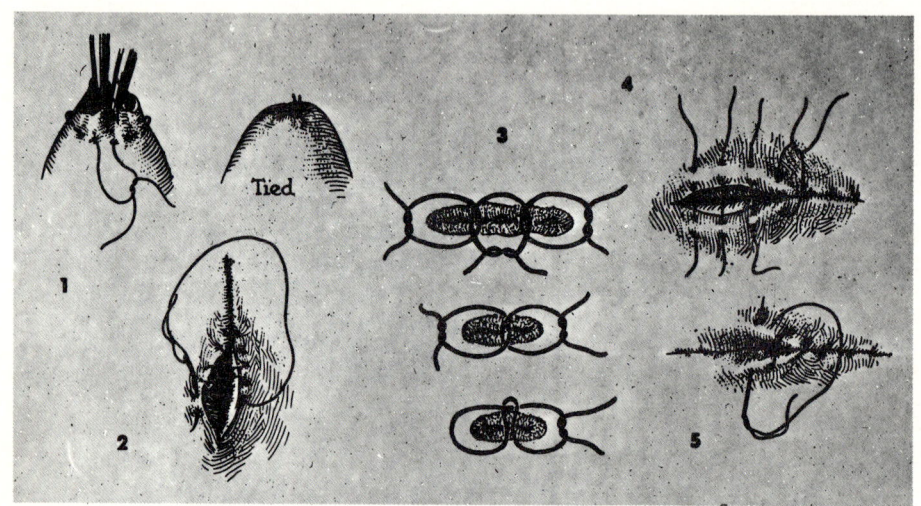

108

1. Purse-string suture around open stump. **2.** Closing stump by Cushing stitch. **3.** Methods for ligation of pedicles with anchored ligatures. **4.** Interrupted Lembert inverting stitch. **5.** Continuous Lembert stitch.

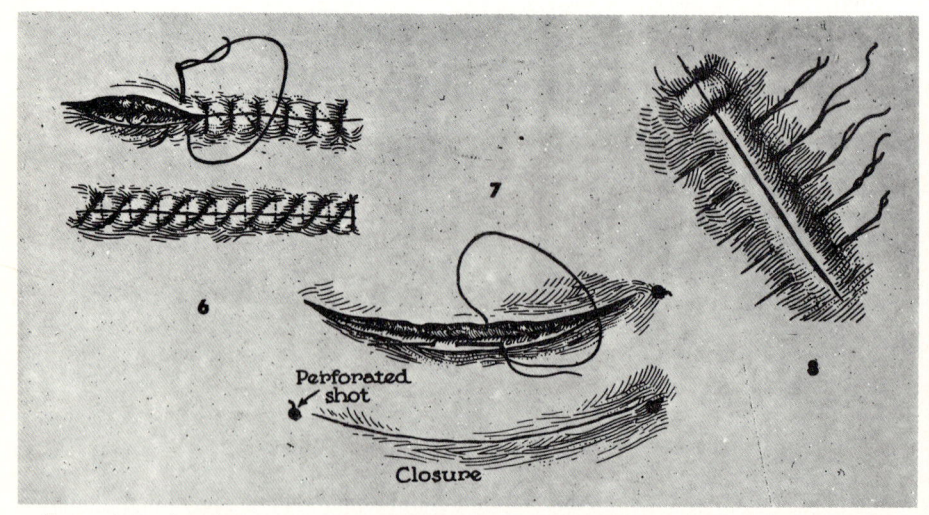

6. Two methods of continuous over-and-over closing sutures. **7.** Subcuticular suture for closure of skin incision. Perforated buck shot used to anchor suture. **8.** Interrupted skin sutures—multiple needle technique.

Figure 25   Suture techniques
Courtesy Ethicon, Inc.

SUTURE TECHNIQUES

Albert	—The first row of stitches passes through the complete thickness of the intestine.
Alternating	—Alternating simple interrupted and mattress sutures used to prevent a depressed scar or improper wound contour.
Appolito	—A continuous cross stitch.
Apposition	—A suture used for closure of cutaneous wound edges.
Approximation	—A suture used for bringing together deep tissues of a wound.
Argyll-Robertson	—Suture for ectropion (turning out of lower eyelid).
Arlt	—Suture for entropion (turning of eyelid inward).
Atraumatic	—Minimizing traumatic or injurious effects.
Axenfeld	—Silk suture for lagophthalmos.
Back and forth	—A continuous suture carried back and forth under the line of incision, thus preventing sutures from lying across the suture line.
Baseball	—A continuous suture carried throughout the length of a wound and placed similar to that with which a baseball is stitched.
Beclard	—Continuous through-and-through using a white and colored thread.
Bell's	—Suture in which the needle is passed from within outward alternately on the two edges of the wound.
Bertrandi	—A back and forth type continuous suture.
Blanket	—A continuous suture.
Bolster	—A suture with ends tied over a segment of rubber tubing or roll of gauze to lessen tension.
Bozeman	—A button suture.
Bridle	—A superior rectus suture (eye muscle).
Bunnell	—Stainless steel suture used in the repair of divided tendons of the hand.

SUTURE TECHNIQUES (continued)

Button	—Suture placed through buttons situated on either side of the line of incision.
Chain	—A continuous suture in which each loop is caught by the next loop.
Circular	—A suture carried through the circumference of an organ.
Coaptation	—Sutures aligning the wound edges.
Cobbler	—Suture with a needle at both ends.
Connell	—A suturing technique used on the intestines in anastomosis procedures where a continuous suture is used on one half of the approximation and the other half of the lumen is closed by a suture carried through the entire wall of the intestine.
Continuous	—A non-interrupted suture.
Corneoscleral	—A suture used in cataract extraction.
Cushing	—A continuous suture traversing the line of incision.
Cutaneous	—A skin suture.
Czerny	—Suturing technique for tenorrhaphy.
Czerny-Lembert	—An intestinal suturing technique.
Double button	—A suture passed across the edges of the wound, deep to the surface, between two buttons, one on each side of the suture line.
Dupuytrens	—A Lembert continuous suture.
Emmet	—Double Lembert suturing technique used in closure of intestinal wounds.
Everting	—The approximated wound edges are turned out.
Figure-of-eight	—Suturing technique in which the thread makes a design resembling the number eight.
Furrier's	—An intestinal suturing technique.
Gaillard-Arlt	—Suture for correction of entropion of the eyelid.
Gely's	—A suture technique consisting of cross stitches made with a suture containing a needle at either end.

SUTURE TECHNIQUES (continued)

Glover's	—A continuous stitch in which the needle after each stitch is passed through the loop of the previous stitch.
Gould	—A mattress intestinal suture technique.
Gussenbauer	—Closure figure-of-eight suture used for instrumentation wounds of the intestine.
Guy	—Sutures inserted in a wound to divide it into small subsections and to support it while further sutures are inserted between the guy sutures.
Halsted	—Intestinal closure technique utilizing mattress sutures, interrupted, each one tieing on the opposite side of the incision line from the previous one.
Harris	—Intestinal anastomosis suture.
Hemostatic	—Two loops of an over and over suture placed at 90 degree angles to each other for control of bleeding, particularly, oozing.
Horizontal mattress	—Stitches made parallel to the wound edges, the suture passing under the wound edges from one side to the other.
Interrupted	—Each stitch is taken with a separate suture on a separate needle.
Intradermic	—A suture placed below the surface of the skin, parallel with the edges of the wound. The needle is inserted at opposite points in the deep layers of the skin.
Inverting	—A suture inverting the approximated wound edges.
Jobert	—Interrupted suture technique for anastomosis of the intestine.
Kalt	—Corneoscleral suture used after section has been completed, in cataract extraction.
Lace	—Fine stitches used for closing a wound or fistula.
LeDentu	—Suture used for repair of a divided tendon.
LeDran	—An intestinal suture technique.
LeFort	—A tenorrhaphy suture technique.

SUTURE TECHNIQUES (continued)

Lembert
—A technique for intestinal repair with interrupted sutures taken through the peritoneum and muscular tunic.

Lespinasse
—Suture technique used in vaso-epididymostomy performed as a sterility procedure, suturing the vas deferens to the epididymis.

Littre
—A suturing method used in creating an artificial anus by ligating the lower end of the bowel and attaching the upper end to the inguinal ring.

Lock stitch
—A hemostatic continuous suture used in surgery of the intestine.

Loffler
—Intestinal repair technique utilizing wire loops in an interrupted fashion.

Loop on mucosa
—A Connell suture.

Mattress
—A stitch carried under the line of incision in the shape of a U and tied to one side of the incisional line where both ends of the stitch can be brought together. These sutures do not cross the line of incision and may be carried as a continuous or interrupted stitch. Also see: horizontal mattress, right angle mattress and vertical mattress suture.

Maunsell
—Suture used in mesenteric layer following the severing of an intestine.

McLean
—Corneoscleral suture used in cataract extraction.

Noose
—An interrupted suture technique.

Over-and-over
—A suture technique by either a continuous or an interrupted method where equal bites are taken in the tissue on each side of the incision with approximation of the edges.

Pagenstecher
—A suture used for correction of ptosis of the eyelid.

Palfyn
—Suture technique for intestinal closure with fixation of the sutures to the skin.

Pancoast
—A suturing technique utilized in plastic surgery where a groove is cut in one wound edge and a tongue in the opposite edge and the two wound edges are sewn together.

OPERATIVE CONSIDERATIONS

SUTURE TECHNIQUES (continued)

Pare	—Closure technique using cloth closure strips on either side of the incision which are sewn together to bring the wound together.
Pin	—A suture technique in which the suture is passed around pins bordering the wound edges to form a figure-of-eight.
Plicating	—A continuous suture pulled tight with folding and puckering of the wound.
Presection	—Stitches placed prior to the incision.
Primary	—The first suture placed in a wound.
Pulley	—A combined relaxation and coaptation suture.
Purse-string	—A suture carried in a continuous in-and-out manner around a gaping opening in such a manner that when the ends of the suture are drawn taut, the wound closes as would a draw string bag.
Quilled	—An interrupted suture technique in which a double suture is passed deep into the wound with a loop emerging on one side of the incisional line and two thread ends on the opposite side. A soft catheter or bougie is placed under the loops which are then tied over it. The free ends are then tied to each other over a second bougie or quill to relieve tension.
Quilted	—Alternating direction continuous mattress sutures.
Ramdohr	—Suture anastomosis technique of the intestine in which the upper portion of the cut intestine is inverted into the lower part and sutured.
Relaxation	—A temporary closure suture which may be loosened to relieve tension.
Retention	—A reinforcement suture for abdominal incisions.
Richter	—Closure technique for intestinal wounds utilizing loops of metal whose ends are brought out of the wound exterior.
Rigal	—Harelip suture using rubber bands.
Right angle mattress	—Same as vertical mattress suture.
Ritisch	—Suture technique for intestinal repair.

SUTURE TECHNIQUES (continued)

Saenger —Closure technique for the uterus in cesarean section utilizing about ten deep silver wire sutures followed by about twenty stitches through the peritoneum.

Secondary —Resuture of a wound after it has once been sutured.

Seroserous —Suturing of two serous surfaces in apposition.

Shotted —A suture of a single strand, each end of which is anchored by a lead shot.

Simon —A method of repair of a lacerated perineum and ruptured sphincter ani by separate suturing of the rectal mucosa, vaginal mucosa and the skin.

Sims's —A shotted suture.

Snellen —Suture technique for ectropion of the eyelid.

Spiroid —Suture technique for enterorrhaphy.

Stallard —Corneoscleral mattress suture placed through the cornea and sclera at 12 o'clock after which section in cataract extraction is performed.

Staple —Wound closure technique using metallic U-shaped wires for approximating the wound edges.

Subcuticular —A continuous buried suture taken in the cutis vera on one side of the incisional line and then on the other side and buried from view by the outer skin layer.

Superficial —A suture which does not include the deeper tissues; a skin closure suture.

Taylor —Suture technique performed on the uterus after amputation of the cervix uteri.

Through-and-through —A suture inserted through the entire thickness of the abdominal wall.

Tongue-and-groove —See pancoast suture.

Track corneoscleral —A suture inserted through the cornea and sclera in cataract extraction.

Transfixion —A suture carried on a needle to transfix the structure around which it is then drawn tight as in the neck of a hernial sac.

SUTURE TECHNIQUES (continued)

Uninterrupted	—A continuous (running) suture.
Verhoeff	—Suture technique for ectropion of the eyelid.
Vertical mattress	—Stitches placed at right angles to the wound taking deep as well as superficial bites of tissue.
Wolfler	—Suture technique for enterorrhaphy. Suture technique for tenorrhaphy.
Wysler	—Suture of the peritoneal surfaces of the intestine.

SUTURE NEEDLES

Surgical needles are classified on the basis of three distinctive features: the eye or lack of eye; the shaft which is straight or curved; and the point which is cutting or noncutting (round). Needles are frequently named after surgeons who popularized them. In addition to the listing of suture needles shown below, a complete listing of surgical needles appears in Chapter 5.

Eyed needles are usually supplied separately from the suture strand with which they are used. These needles may be reused several times, but require examination and resharpening. The exception is prethreaded eyed needles, the most common of which is the straight taper point milliner's needle threaded by the manufacturer with size 000 or 4/0 silk. These needles are discarded after a single use.

The French or split-eye has a split from the end of the needle to the eye through which the suture is drawn to thread it. This type of needle is most commonly used with silk or cotton sutures.

The atraumatic needle is eyeless with the suture permanently swaged to the needle, virtually forming a continuous single strand of material. These needles with their attached suture minimize tissue trauma because the suture strand and needle form a unit of almost uniform diameter. When an eyed needle is threaded, a double suture strand is produced with increased bulk which necessarily causes greater tissue trauma.

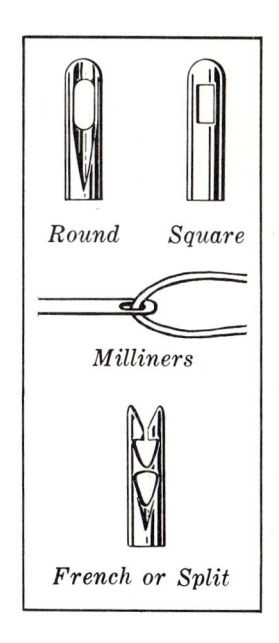

Round   Square

Milliners

French or Split

Eyed needles
Courtesy Davis & Geck

A suture having a needle attached to one end is referred to as a single-armed suture. When needles are attached to both ends of a suture strand, it is referred to as a double-armed suture.

Needle shapes are classified according to the degree of curvature of the shaft, ranging from straight to a 5/8 circle. The principal curvatures are shown below.

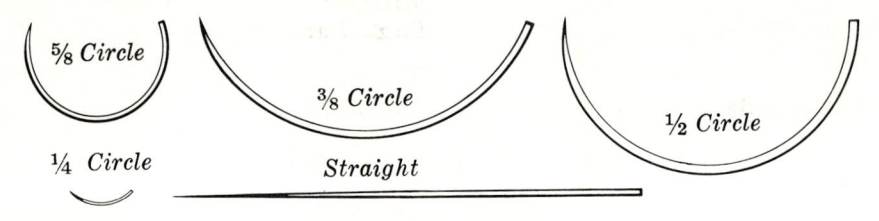

Suture needle shapes
Courtesy Davis & Geck Suture Co.

Points of the atraumatic or eyed needles are classified according to the shape of the point and its extension along the needle shaft, either as cutting or noncutting (round). The taper point needle does not have a cutting edge. It has a round shaft which tapers to a point. The shaft may be curved or straight. This is the most commonly used type of needle point being used primarily on tissues such as the dura mater, viscera and subcutaneous tissues which present little resistance to passage of the needle.

The Spatula (Sulzle diamond point) needle is used in scleral (eye) surgery. The Modified Spatula (Sulzle Diamond Point) needle has been modified for general surgery.

Cutting point needles with a straight shaft have a triangular point with cutting edges extended along the shaft of the needle. These are used primarily for skin closure. Cutting point needles with a curved shaft may be regular cutting needles, having a triangular point with two cutting edges in the horizontal plane and one cutting edge in the vertical plane along the inner curvature of the shaft, or they may be reverse cutting needles, which differ only in that the one cutting edge in the vertical plane is along the outer curvature of the shaft. Cutting needles are used in tough tissues such as fascia or tendon where a taper point needle does not readily penetrate.

SUTURE NEEDLES

Atraumatic
Curved
Cutting
Eyed

Eyeless
Eyeless atraumatic

Flat spatula
French

OPERATIVE CONSIDERATIONS

SUTURE NEEDLES (continued)

Milliner's
Modified spatula

Noncutting

Reverse cutting
Round

Scleral spatula

Spatula
Split
Split eye
Square
Straight
Sulze diamond point

Taper point
Threaded eye

BANDAGES AND DRESSINGS

Ace
Ace adherent
Ace-hesive
Ace longitudinal strips
Ace rubber elastic
Adaptic
Ad-hese-away
Aeroplast
Air pressure
A.R.D. anorectal
Aureomycin gauze

Barrel
Barrier
Barton
Baynton
Belleview surgical wadding
Belleview bridge
Bias cut stockinette
Binocle
Blenderm surgical tape
Bolus
Borsch
Bronson boot
Buller eye

Capeline
Castex rigid
Cilkloid
Cision
Cod liver oil soaked strips
Compound
Compression
Contura medicated
Cotton balls
Cotton elastic

Cotton pledgets
Cotton wadding
Cottonoid
Cravat
Crepe
Crinotene
Cruricast zinc oxide gelatine
Curad plastic

Demigauntlet
Dermicel tape
Desault
Duke spot

Elastic
Elasticfoam pressure
Elastikon wristlet
Elastoplast
Esmarch

Fas-trac traction strip
Felt
Figure-of-eight
Flex-aid knuckle
Flex foam
Foam rubber
Foille
Four tailed
Fricke's scrotal
Furacin
Furacin gauze

Galen
Garretson
Gauntlet
Gauze
Gauztex

BANDAGES AND DRESSINGS (continued)

Gelfilm
Gelocast
Genga
Gibney
Gibson
Gypsonia plaster

Hamilton
Hammock
Heliodorus
Hippocrates
Hueter's perineal

Immobilizing
Ivalon (polyvinyl sponge)

Jelly

Kerlix
Kerlix fluffs
Kerlix roll
Kerlix washed gauze
Kiwisch breast
Kling elastic
Koagamin
Koylon foam rubber

Langier
Larrey
Lister
Livingston

Maisonneuve plaster-of-Paris
Maltese cross
Many tailed
Martin's rubber
Mechanic's waste
Mediplast elastic
Merthiolate
Microdon
Micropore surgical tape
Moleskin traction hitch
Montgomery tapes

No trauma

Oiled silk
Orthoplast
Ostic Plaster

Owens
Oxycel

Peg
Petrolatum gauze
Piedmont all-cotton elastic
Plaster
Plaster-of-Paris
Poly-flex traction
Presso-elastic
Pressoplast compression
Presso-superior
Pressure
Priessnitz
Protective

Quadro

Readiflex elastic
Recurrent
Red cross adhesive
Reversed
Reverse spiral
Ribble
Richet
Rochester pressure
Roller
Rubber

Sayre
Scan spray
Scarlet red gauze
Scultetus binder
Seutin
Sheet wadding
Sof-rol cast wadding
Spica
Spiral
Spiral reverse
Spray
Steri-strip skin closures
Stixon
Stockinette
Superflex elastic
Super-trac adhesive traction
Surgical
Surgicel
Surgipad combine

BANDAGES AND DRESSINGS (continued)

Surgitube
Suspensory

T-bandage
Telfa
Tensoplast elastic adhesive
Tensoplast extension plaster
Tensor elastic
Theden
Thillaye
Tincture of benzoin
Tomac foam rubber traction
Tomac knitted rubber elastic
Trac-a-derm
Trac-grip
Triangular
Tubegauz
Tuffnell

Varick elastic
Vaseline gauze
Vaseline petrolatum gauze
Velpeau
Velroc plaster
Ventfoam traction
Vi-drape surgical film
Vi-hesive

Webril

Xeroform

Y-bandage

Zephyr rubber elastic
Zim-flux
Zimocel
Zoroc resin plaster

SLINGS

Acromioclavicular dislocation harness
Adjustable strap arm
Airplane (Aeroplane)

Banjo

Clavicle strap
Colles'
Cradle arm

Glisson's

Hand cock-up

Lenticular nucleus

Mason-Allen universal
McLeod clavicle

Rauchfuss

Teare arm

Velpeau

Weil pelvic

Zimmer arm
Zimmer clavicular cross

5 Surgical Instruments and Equipment

The following pages contain a comprehensive listing of surgical instruments and equipment which surgeons usually specify in their reports of surgery. More than 2,000 instruments have been added to the listing which appeared in the first edition.

ABRADERS

Dingman otoplasty cartilage
Howard corneal
Iverson dermabrader

Lieberman
Montague

ADENOTOMES

Abelson
Cullom-Mueller
Kelley direct vision
LaForce
LaForce-Grieshaber

LaForce-Stevenson
Mueller-LaForce
Myles guillotine
Shambaugh

AMNIOTOME

Baylor

Beacham

ANASTOMOSIS APPARATUS

Nakayama

ANCHORS

Lemoine-Searcy

Searcy fixation

ANGIOTRIBES

Ferguson

Zweifel

ANOSCOPES

Bacon
Bodenheimer
Boehm
Brinkerhoff
Buie-Hirschman
Fansler
Goldbacher
Hirschman with obturator

Ives
Muer
Otis
Pratt
Pruitt
Rotating speculum
Sims
Welch Allyn

ANTROSCOPE

A.C.M.I.

APPARATUS

Buck's extension
Desault
Fell-O'Dwyer
Kirschner
Nakayama anastomosis
Parham-Martin fracture
Reichert stereotaxic brain

Sayre
Stader extraoral
Tallerman
Taylor spinal support
Tobold laryngoscopic
Zander
Zund-Burguet

APPLICATORS

Allen
Andrew
Brown
Buck
Chaoul
Dean
Ernst radium
Farrell
Gifford corneal
Holinger
Ivan nasopharyngeal
Jackson laryngeal

Kyle
Lathbury
Ludwig
Playfair uterine caustic
Plummer-Vinson radium (esophageal)
Pynchon
Ralks
Roberts
Sawtell
Strontium-90 ophthalmic beta ray
Uebe

ASPIRATORS

Adams
Carabelli
Carmody electric
Clerf
Cook County Hospital
Dieulafoy
Fritz
Gottschalk middle ear

Lukens
Pilling-Negus clamp-on
Potain
Senoran
Stedman suction pump
Thorek gallbladder
Universal

OPERATIVE CONSIDERATIONS

AWLS

Aufranc trochanteric
Carroll
DePuy

Wilson right angled
Zuelzer

BALLOON

Anthony-Fisher antrum

BANDS

Johnson dental
Lukens orthodontic
Magill orthodontic

Matas vessel
Parham-Martin

BARS

Dental arch
Livingston intramedullary

Strut

BASIOTRIBES

Auvard-Zweifel

Tarnier

BLADES

A.S.R.
Balfour center
Bard-Parker
Beaver

Beaver-DeBakey
DeBakey
Dixon
Horgan center

BOLTS

Barr
Cannulated
DePuy
Fenton
Hexhead
Hubbard nylok

Norman tibia
Nylok
Webb
Webb type stove
Wilson
Zimmer

BOUGIES

a-Boule
Acorn tipped
Armed
Bangs
Bellied
Buerger dilating
Bulbous
Chevalier Jackson

Conic
Cylindrical
Dilatable
Dilating
Dourmashkin tunneled
Ear
Elastic
Elbowed

BOUGIES (continued)

Eustachian
Filiform
Fort urethral
Friedman-Otis
Fusiform
Gabriel Tucker
Gruber's
Guyon exploratory
Harold Hayes eustachian
Holinger-Hurst
Holinger infant
Hurst (mercury filled esophageal)
Jackson filiform
Jackson radiopaque
Jackson tracheal
LeFort filiform
Maloney tapered
Mercury filled esophageal

Olive tip
Otis
Phillips urethral whip
Plummer modified
Ravich
Retrograde
Rosary
Ruschelit urethral
Spiral tip
Trousseau esophageal
Tucker retrograde
Urbantschitsch eustachian
Wales rectal
Wax
Whalebone filiform
Whip
Whistler

BOVIE

Clinic
CSV

Liquid conductor
Ritter-Bantam

BRACES

Chairback
Forrester cervical collar
Hudson
Jewett hyperextension
King cervical
Kuhlman cervical
Lyman-Smith toe drop

Milwaukee scoliosis
Murphy
Taylor spine
Taylor-Knight
Teufel cervical
Thomas type cervical collar
Von Lackum transection shift jacket

BROACHES

Barbed
Firtel

Root canal

BRONCHOSCOPES

Albert slotted
Broyles
Bruening
Chevalier Jackson
Davis
Double channel irrigating
Emerson

Foregger
Haslinger
Holinger
Holinger-Jackson
Hook-On
Jackson costophrenic
Jackson full lumen

SURGICAL INSTRUMENTS AND EQUIPMENT

BRONCHOSCOPES (continued)

Jackson standard
Jackson staple
Jesberg
Kernan-Jackson coagulating
Michelson infant
Moersch
Negus
Overholt-Jackson

Pilling
Riecker Respiration
Safar ventilation
Staple
Tucker
Waterman folding
Yankauer

BURS

Adson-Rogers cranial
Allport eustachian
Bailey skull
Ballenger-Lillie mastoid
Burwell corneal
Cavanaugh-Israel
Cavanaugh sphenoid
Cross corneal
Cushing cranial
D'Errico
Diamond
Doyen
Ferris-Smith-Halle sinus
Frey-Freer

Hall mastoid
Halle bone
Hudson
Jordan Day fenestration
Kopetzky sinus
Lempert fenestration
Marin
McKenzie enlarging
Sachs skull
Slotting
Somerset
Wachsberger
Wilkerson choanal
Yazujian cataract

BUTTONS

Boari
Chlumsky
Jaboulay
Lardennois

Murphy
Peritoneal
Todd bur hole
Villard

CALIPERS

Albee bone graft
Burch eye
Castroviejo
Cone ice tong
Green eye

Jameson
Ladd
Thorpe
Townley inside-outside femur
V.M. & Co. ruler

CANNULA (Pl. cannulae)

Abelson curved crico-thyrotomy
Abraham

Adson brain exploring
Adson drainage

CANNULA (Pl. cannulae) (continued)

Bailey
Bellocq
Bishop-Harman irrigating
Bowers
Brodny urethrographic
Bruening
Bucy-Frazier
Calve
Cantlie
Carabelli mirror
Casselberry sphenoid
Castroviejo cyclodialysis
Chilcott
Clagett
Coakley frontal sinus
Colt
Cone biopsy
Cone-Bucy
Cooper chemopallidectomy
Cooper double lumen
Day attic
DeWecker syringe
Dorsey ventricular
Dow Corning
Duke
Dupuis
Elsberg brain exploring
Fischer silicone ventricular
Ford Hospital ventricular
Frazier brain exploring
Goldstein anterior chamber
Goodfellow frontal sinus
Hahn
Haverfield brain
Haynes brain
Hendon venoclysis
Hoen ventricular
Holinger
Holman-Mathieu
Hudgins
Ingals antrum
Ingals rectal injection
Jarcho uterine
Kanavel brain exploring
Killian antrum
Killian-Eicken

Kos attic
Krause
Lacrimal
Lillie attic
Lindemann
Lukens
Luongo
Mandelbaum
Mayo coronary perfusion
Moncrieff anterior chamber
Muller coronary perfusion
Myerson-Moncrieff
Myles sinus
Neal fallopian
New York Eye and Ear
Paterson laryngeal
Penn-Neal
Perfusion
Pierce attic
Pritchard
Pynchon
Randolph cyclodialysis
Robb antrum
Rockey mediastinal
Rolf-Jackson
Roper alpha chymotrypsin
Rubin fallopian tube
Sachs
Scott attic
Scott rubber ventricular
Seletz
Sewall antrum
Silastic coronary artery
Skillern sphenoid
Soresi
Southey
Strauss
Tenner
Topper
Tracheotomy
Trendelenburg
Turnbull
Van Alyea antrum
Von Eicken antrum
Wells
Wolfe return flow

CAPSULOTOMES

Darling

CATHETERS

Acmistat
Alcock return flow hemostatic
Bailey transthoracic
Balloon
Bard
Bardex
Bardex Foley balloon
Bardic cut-down
Bicoude (bicoudate)
Blasucci ureteral
Bozeman
Bozeman-Fritsch
Braasch
Bunts
Campbell
Carlens bronchospirometric
Conical tip
Constantine flexible metal
Coude tip
Councill
Coxeter prostatic
Cummings four wing malecot retention
Cummings nephrostomy
Cummings-Pezzer head
Davol
DeLee tracheal
a demeure
de Pezzer
Devonshire
Elbowed
Eustachian
Faucial eustachian
Filliform
Flexible
Fogarty arterial embolectomy
Fogarty balloon
Foley
Foley-Alcock
Foley bag, inflatable
Four-eye
French
Friend

Friend-Hebert
Fritsch
Furniss female
Garceau ureteral
Gilbert plug self sealing
Gouley
Hagner bag
Hartmann eustachian
Hatch
Higgins
Hryntschak
Indwelling
Itard eustachian
Jaeger-Whiteley
Jelm two-way
Kimball
Lane rectal
LeFort
Lehman aortographic
Lloyd bronchial
Lloyd esophagoscopic
Lobster tail
Malecot
McCaskey antrum
McIver nephrostomy
Mercier
Metras bronchial
Mushroom
Neal
Nelaton urethral
Opaco-Garcea ureteral
Owens
Pezzer
Pharmaseal disposable
Phillips urologic
Pilcher bag
Prostatic
Railway
Retention
Robinson
Rockey-Thompson
Rodriguez-Alvarez
Round tip

CATHETERS (continued)

Ruschelit
Rusch
Rusch-Foley
Schrotters
Self retaining
Shellac covered
Silastic mushroom
Six eye
Skene
Solid tip
Squire
Stitt
Stripseal
Styletted tracheobronchial
Tauber
Thompson bronchial
Tiemann
Tiemann-Coude

Tomac
Touhy
Trattner ureterographic
Two way
Ureteral
Vertebrated
Virden rectal
Walther female
Weber rectal
Whalebone filiform
Whistle tip
Winer
Winged
Wishard tip
Wolf nephrostomy bag
Woodruff ureteropyelographic
Yankauer
Zavod bronchospirometry

CAUTERY

Alkaline battery
Bovie
Burdick
Cold (carbon dioxide)
Corrigan
Downes
Electrocautery
Geiger-Downes
Magielski coagulation
Mueller alkaline battery
Mueller currentrol

National
Paquelin
Prince eye
Rommel Hildreth
Scheie ophthalmic
Souttar
Wadsworth-Todd eye
Wappler
Wappler cold
Wills Hospital eye
Ziegler

CHISELS

Adson laminectomy
Alexander
Andrews
Artmann disarticulation
Ballenger
Ballenger-Hajek
Bishop
Blair
Bowen goose neck
Brittain twin pattern
Brown
Bruening

Brunetti
Brunner
Bruns
Burns guarded
Caltagirone
Cinelli
Cinelli-McIndoe
Clawicz
Cloward spinal fusion
Cloward-Harman
Cloward-Puka
Compere bone

SURGICAL INSTRUMENTS AND EQUIPMENT

CHISELS (continued)

Converse nasal
Costotome
Cottle
Councilman
Crane bone
Derlacki
Derlacki-Shambaugh
D'Errico laminectomy
Eicher tri-fin
Faulkner-Browne
Faulkner trocar
Fomon
Freer
Hajek septum
Halle
Henderson bone
Hibbs
House foot plate
Joseph
Katsch
Keyes splitting
Kezerian
Killian frontal sinus
Killian-Reinhard

Kreischer bone
Lambotte splitting
Lebsche sternum
MacAusland
Magielski stapes
Meyerding
Metzenbaum
Moore hollow
Murphy
Pick
Rish
Roberts hip dissecting
Schuknecht
Sewall ethmoidal
Shambaugh-Derlacki
Sheehan nasal
Silver
Smith-Petersen
Stille pattern bone
Troutman mastoid
Virchow
West
Wilmer wedge
Worth

CLAMPS

Alfred M. Large vena cava
Allen anastomosis
Alyea vas
Ann Arbor double towel
Aorta
Atlee bronchus
Ault intestinal occlusion
Backhaus towel
Bahnson aortic aneurysm
Bailey aortic occlusion
Bailey-Cowley
Bailey-Morse
Bailey duckbill
Bainbridge
Beardsley intestinal
Beck aorta
Beck-Satinsky
Berens muscle
Berke ptosis
Berman

Berry pile
Best right angle
Bigelow calvarium
Black meatus
Blalock stenosis
Blalock-Niedner
Blanchard pile
Böhler os calcis
Boyes muscle
Bradshaw-O'Neill aorta
Brock auricle
Brodny urethrographic
Bronner
Buie pile
Buie-Hirschman pile
Bulldog
C-clamp
Carmalt
Carrel
Castroviejo mosquito lid

CLAMPS (continued)

Charnley bone
Charnley pin
Claiborne lid
Codman cartilage
Collins
Collins umbilical
Cooley anastomosis
Cooley aorta
Cope
Cottle columella
Crafoord coarctation
Crile
Crile appendix
Crile-Crutchfield
Cruickshank entropion
Crutchfield carotid artery
Cunningham incontinence
Daems bronchus
Daniel colostomy
Davidson muscle
Davidson pulmonary vessel
Davis aortic aneurysm
W. Dean McDonald gastric
DeBakey bulldog
DeBakey tangential
DeCourcy goiter
DeMartel-Wolfson intestinal
Dennis anastomosis
Derra anastomosis
Derra vena cava
Derra vestibular
Dieffenbach
Diethrich shunt
Dingman cartilage
Dixon-Thomas-Smith intestinal
Dobbie-Trout bulldog
Doctor Collins fracture
Dogliotti-Guglielmini
Donald
Doyen
Earle pile
Eastman intestinal
Edebohls kidney
Erhardt
Falk vaginal cuff
Farabeuf-Lambotte bone holding
Fehland right angle colon
ferrule (accessory equipment)
Fine-toothed
Finochietto artery
Ford
Forrester
Foss anterior resection
Frahur cartilage
Frazier-Adson osteoplastic flap
Frazier-Sachs
Freeman
Friedrich
Furniss
Furniss-Clute
Furniss intestinal anastomosis
Furniss-McClure-Hinton
Gant
Garland hysterectomy
Gavin-Miller
Glassman non-crushing
Glover auricular appendage
Glover coarctation
Glover patent ductus
Goldblatt
Gomco bloodless circumcision
Goodwin bone
Gray
Green bulldog
Green lid
Gross coarctation
Gross occluding
Gussenbauer
Gutgeman auricular appendage
Guyon-Pean
Guyon vessel
Harken auricle
Harrington-Mixter
Haseltine umbilical
Haverhill
Hayes colon
Heitz-Boyer
Herbert Adams coarctation
Herrick kidney
Hibbs
Hirschman pile
Hopkins aortic occlusion

CLAMPS (continued)

Hudson lung exclusion
Hufnagel valve holding
Hume aortic
Humphries reserve curve aortic
Hunt colostomy
Hurwitz intestinal
Hymes meatus
Jackson bone holding
Jacobs
Jacobson bulldog
Jahnke-Cook-Seeley
Jarvis pile
Javid carotid artery
Jesberg laryngectomy
Johns Hopkins bulldog occluding
Johnston
Jones
Joseph septum
Juevenelle aortic
Julian-Fildes
K-Gar umbilical
Kane umbilical
Kantor circumcision
Kantrowicz thoracic
Kapp-Beck bronchus
Kapp-Beck coarctation
Kapp-Beck colon
Kelsey pile
Kinsella-Buie
Kocher
Ladd lid
Lahey thoracic
Lambert-Lowman
Lane gastroenterostomy
Large
Lees bronchus
Lees right angle
Lees wedge resection
Lem-Blay circumcision
Lewin bone
Lilly rectus tendon
Linnartz stomach
Linton tourniquet
Lockwood
Lowman bone holding
Lowman-Hoglund

MacDonald gastric
Martel
Martin cartilage
Mastin muscle
Mayo
Mayo-Guyon
Mayo-Lovelace spur crushing
McCleery-Miller
McLean pile
McNealy-Glassman-Mixter
McQuigg right angle
Michel
Mikulicz peritoneal
Mikulicz-Radecki
Miles rectal
Mixter thoracic
Mohr pinchcock
Moorehead lid
Moreno gastroenterostomy
Moynihan
Mueller aorta
Mueller bronchus
Muir rectal cautery
Muller-Markham
Nichols aortic
Nicola tendon
Niedner anastomosis
Nunez aortic
Nunez auricular
Nussbaum intestinal
Ochsner
Ockerblad kidney
O'Connor lid
O'Neill
Parham-Martin bone holding
Partipilo
Payr pylorus
Payr resection
Pean hysterectomy
Pean intestinal
Pedicle
Pemberton sigmoid anastomosis
Pennington
Petz
Phillips rectal
Poppen aortic

CLAMPS (continued)

- Poppen-Blalock carotid artery
- Poppen-Blalock-Salibi carotid
- Potts cardiovascular
- Potts coarctation
- Potts-Niedner
- Potts-Smith aorta
- Preshaw
- Price-Thomas bronchus
- Prince
- Pringle
- Ralks thoracic
- Rankin anastomosis
- Rankin intestinal
- Ranzewski intestinal
- Reich-Nechtow artery
- Reynolds dissecting
- Reynolds resection
- Rhinelander
- Richards bone
- Rienhoff arterial
- Rienhoff swan neck
- Rochester sigmoid
- Rockey vascular
- Roeder
- Roosevelt gastroenterostomy
- Rubber dam
- Rubber shod
- Rubin bronchus
- Rubovits
- Rumel myocardial
- Rush bone
- Salibi carotid artery
- Santulli
- Sarnoff aortic
- Sarot bronchus
- Satinsky vena cava
- Schmidt
- Schoemaker intestinal
- Schwartz temporary
- Scudder stomach
- Sellors
- Selman
- Selverstone carotid artery
- Shoemaker aortic
- Smith bone
- Smith cordotomy
- Smith marginal
- Smithwick anastomosis
- Southwick
- Stanton cautery
- Stepita meatus
- Stille kidney
- Stille vessel
- Stockman
- Stone-Holcombe
- Stone intestinal
- Stratte kidney
- Strauss meatus
- Strelinger right angle
- Surgi-Med umbiliclamp
- Swan aortic
- Sztehlo umbilical
- Tatum
- Thomson lung
- Towel
- Trendelenburg-Crafoord coarctation
- Truncus
- Trusler infant vascular
- Vanderbilt vessel
- Umbiliclamp
- Vasconcelos-Barretto
- Verbrugge
- von Petz stomach & intestinal
- Walther-Crenshaw meatus
- Walther kidney pedicle
- Wangensteen gastric crushing
- Wangensteen patent ductus
- Warthen spur crushing
- Watts locking
- Weaver chalazion
- Weck
- Wells pedicle
- Wertheim parametrium
- Wertheim pedicle
- Wertheim-Cullen
- Wertheim-Reverdin
- Wester meniscus
- Whitver penis
- Willett (**OB-Gyn**)
- Wire tightening
- Wolfson intestinal
- Wolfson spur crushing

SURGICAL INSTRUMENTS AND EQUIPMENT

CLAMPS (continued)

Yellen circumcision
Young renal pedicle
Zachary-Cope-DeMartel triple colon
Ziegler-Furniss
Zimmer cartilage
Zipser penis
Zutt

CLIPS

Adson scalp
Ahlquist-Durham vena cava
Autoclips
Callender
Children's Hospital scalp
Cushing
Duane "U"
Edwards parallel jaw spring
Ethicon
Hemoclips
Hesseltine umbiliclips
Hoxworth fashures
Ingraham-Fowler tantalum
Mayfield
McDermott surgiclip
McKenzie brain
Michel
Olivecrona silver
Penfield silver
Pool Pfeiffer self-locking intracranial aneurysm
Raney scalp
Scoville-Lewis aneurysm
Serature
Smith aneurysm
Smithwick silver
Sugar aneurysm
Surgiclip
Tantalum hemostasis
Totco autoclips
von Petz
Wachtenfeldt

COAGULATORS

Ballantine-Drew
Bantam bovie
Birtcher hyfrecator
Codman & Shurtleff neo-coagulator
Electricator
Hyfrecator
Magielski coagulation forceps
Malis bipolar
MPC coagulation forceps
National electricator
Poppen electrosurgical
Ritter
Ritter Bantam bovie

COLLECTORS

Carabelli cancer cell
Clerf cancer cell
Davidson
Hershenson esophageal cytology
Lukens
Pilling
Ware

COMPRESSORS

Anthony orbital enucleator
Berens enucleation
Deschamps'
Devilbiss

CONDUCTORS

Adson
Bailey

Davis
Kanavel

CONTRACTORS

Bailey
Bailey-Gibbon rib

Effenberger
Graham rib

COSTOTOME

Tudor-Edwards

Vehmehren

COUNTERBORES

Curry hip nail

with Lloyd adapter

CRANIOCLASTS

Auvard
Braun

Zweifel-DeLee

CRANIOTOMES

Verbrugghen-Souttar

Williams

CRYOEXTRACTOR

Amoils
Bellows CO_2

Krwawicz cataract
Thomas cryoptor

CRYOPHAKE

Alcon

CRYOPTOR

Thomas

CRYOSTYLET

Kelman

CRYPTOTOME

Blanchard

CULDOSCOPES

Decker fiber optic

Decker photo

SURGICAL INSTRUMENTS AND EQUIPMENT

CURETTES (Also: curet)

Alvis foreign body
Ballenger ethmoid
Barnhill adenoid
Billeau ear
Blake
Bromley uterine
Bronson-Ray pituitary
Brun bone
Brun ear
Buck ear
Buck mastoid
Bumm uterine
Bush intervertebral
Carmack ear
Carroll hook
Carter
Cloward cone ring
Coakley
Cobb
Cone ring
Converse
DeLee
Dench uterine
DePuy bone
Derlacki
Duncan endometrial
Epstein down-biting
Faulkner double ended ring
Faulkner ethmoid
Ferguson bone
Fink
Fox dermal
Franseen rectal
Freimuth ear
Garcia-Rock endometrial suction
Gifford corneal
Goldstein
Govons pituitary
Green corneal
Green uterine
Gross ear
Gusberg endocervical biopsy
Halle ethmoid
Hannon endometrial
Harrison scarifying
Hartmann adenoid
Hayden tonsil
Heaney uterine
Heath chalazion
Hebra corneal
Hibbs bone
Holden uterine
Hotz ear
House ear
Houtz endometrial
Hunter uterine
Ingersoll
Jones
Kelly-Gray uterine
Kezerian
Lempert
Lounsbury placenta
Luer bone
Luongo
Lynch
Magielski
Mayfield
McCaskey antrum
Meigs endometrial
Meyerding saw toothed
Meyhoeffer
Middleton adenoid
Mosher ethmoid
Myles antrum
Nolan-Budd cervical
Novak uterine suction
Piffard dermal with Luer hub
Pratt antrum
Randall endometrial biopsy
Raney spinal fusion
Raney stirrup-loop
Ray pituitary
Recamier uterine
Reich-Nechtow
Reiner
Reverse angle skid
Rheinstaedter uterine
Richards mastoid
Ridpath ethmoid
Rock endometrial suction
Rosenmueller fossa
St. Clair-Thompson adenoid

CURETTES (continued)

Schaeffer mastoid
Schede
Schroeder uterine
Schwartz endocervical
Scoville ruptured disc
Semmes spinal
Shapleigh ear
Sharman
Sheaffer
Simones spinal
Simpson antrum
Sims uterine
Skeele eye
Skene uterine spoon
Skid
Skillern sinus
Smith-Petersen
Spinal fusion
Spratt mastoid
Stirrup loop

Strully ruptured disc
Stubbs adenoid
Tabb ear
Thomas uterine
Thorpe
V.M. & Co. mastoid
Vogel adenoid
Volkmann bone
Voller
Walker ring
Walker ruptured disc
Wallich
Walsh hook type dermal
Walton
Weisman ear
West-Beck spoon
Whiting mastoid
Wullstein
Yankauer salpingeal

CUTTERS

Beaver ring
Cloward-Dowel
Expand-O-Graft (disposable)

Lempert malleus
Porter-O-Surgical

CYSTOMETER

Lewis recording

CYSTOSCOPES

Braasch direct catheterizing
Brown-Buerger convertible
Brown-Buerger fiber optic convertible
Brown-Buerger fiber optic universal
Brown-Buerger 14 French double catheterizing
Brown-Buerger 16 French double catheterizing
Butterfield
Kelly
Kidd

Laidley double catheterizing
Lowsley-Peterson
McCarthy foroblique panendoscope
McCarthy infant cystoscope
McCarthy routine
McCarthy-Campbell miniature
McCarthy-Peterson
National general purpose
Nesbit
Ravich convertible

CYSTOSCOPE ACCESSORIES

A.C.M.I. cystoscopic tip
Ball tip electrode

Bard tip
Bayonet tip electrode

CYSTOSCOPE ACCESSORIES (continued)

Beaked sheath
Biopsy loop electrode
Bridge, three way
Bugbee fulguration electrode
Burns converting bridge
Collings knife electrode
Concave sheath & obturator
Conical tip electrode
Convertible telescope & fin
Convex sheath & obturator
Double catheterizing fin
Double catheterizing sheath and obturator
Double catheterizing telescope
Electrodes
Foroblique telescope
Fulgurating electrode
Hamm fulgurating electrode
Infant telescope
McCarthy coagulation electrode
McCarthy diathermic knife electrode
McCarthy fiber optic foroblique telescope
McCarthy fulguration electrode
McCarthy loop operating electrode
Neil Moore meatotomy electrode
Obturator
Operating telescope
Retrospective telescope
Right angle examining telescope
Ureteral meatotomy electrode

CYSTOTOMES

Beard
Graefe
Holth
Knapp
von Graefe
Wheeler
Wilder

DEBRIDER

Sauer corneal

DERMABRADERS

Iverson
Sand paper

DERMATOMES

Air
Bard-Parker
Barker Vacu-tome
Brown air
Brown electro-dermatome
Hall air
Hood electro-dermatome
Hood manual
Manual
Meek-Wall microdermatome
Padgett
Padgett-Hood electrodermatome
Reese
Stryker
Stryker rolo-dermatome

DILATORS

Arnott
Atlee uterine
Bailey
Bakes common duct
Bakes-Pearce
Bard urethral

DILATORS (continued)

Barnes common duct
Barnes cervical
Beardsley aortic
Berens punctum
Black-Wylie
Bossi cervical
Bowman lacrimal
Bransford-Lewis ureteral
Brock cardiac
Browne-McHardy
Broyles esophageal
Cardiospasm
Castroviejo lacrimal
Clerf
Cooley valve
Creevy urethral
Crump
Crump-Himmelstein
DeBakey-Cooley valve
Delaborde
Derra cardiac valve
DeSeigneux
Dick cardiac valve
Dourmashkin
Einhorn esophageal
Esophagospasm
Feldbausch
Ferris
Frommer
Galezowski lacrimal
Gerbode mitral
Glover modification of Brock aortic
Gohrbrand cardiac
Goodell uterine
Guggenheim-Gergoiye
Guyon
Hank uterine
Hank-Bradley uterine
Harst
Heath punctum
Hegar uterine
Hosford
Jackson bronchial
Jackson esophageal
Jackson-Mosher cardiospasm
Jackson-Plummer

Jackson-Trousseau
Johnston infant
Jolly uterine
Kahn uterine
Kearns bladder
Kelly sphincter
Kollmann
Kron gall duct
LaBorde tracheal
Leader-Kollmann
Mantz rectal
Mixter common duct dilaprobe
Mosher cardiospasm
Muldoon lacrimal
Murphy common duct
Nettleship-Wilder
Norris modified Browne-McHardy
Olive
Ottenheimer common duct
Outerbridge uterine
Palmer uterine
Patton esophageal
Plummer esophageal
Plummer-Vinson esophageal
Pneumatic
Potts expansile
Potts-Riker
Pratt rectal
Pratt uterine
Ramstedt pyloric stenosis
Rapaport
Reich-Nechtow
Ritter meatal
Rolf punctum
Royal Hospital
Ruedemann lacrimal
Russell hydrostatic
Sims uterine
Sinexon
Sippy dilating olives
Starlinger uterine
Steele bronchial
Theobold lacrimal
Trousseau tracheal
Trousseau-Jackson esophageal
Tubbs mitral valve

DILATORS (continued)

Tucker cardiospasm
Turner
Wales rectal
Walther
Wilder lacrimal

Williams lacrimal
Wylie uterine
Young rectal
Ziegler lacrimal

DIRECTORS

Durnin angled
Grooved

Larry rectal
Pratt rectal

DISSECTORS

Allerdyce
Allis
Aufranc
Brunner goiter
Butte
Carpenter
Cheyne dry
Collin pleura
Crabtree attic
Falcao
Hamrick suction
Harris
Heath trephine flap
Herczel
Holinger laryngeal
Hurd tonsil
Hurd-Wieder
Israel
Judet
Kocher goiter
Lane
Lang
Lewin
Logan
Lothrop
Lynch blunt

MacAusland
McWhinnie tonsil
Milligan
Moorehead
Morrison-Hurd
Mulligan
Oldberg
Olivecrona
Penfield
Pierce submucous
Potts
Raney
Rayport dura
Rienhoff
Rogers submucous
Rosen
Shelden-Pudenz hydrostatic
Sloan goiter flap
Smithwick
Stolte tonsil
Walker suction tonsil
Wangensteen
Watson-Cheyne
Yoshida
Young

DRAINS

Angle Pezzer
Bardex
Cigarette
Controlled
Freyer

Henrickson suprapubic
Keith
Latex
Malecot four wing
Malecot two wing

DRAINS (continued)

Marion
Mikulicz
Mikulicz Radecki
Mosher
Penrose
Pezzer
Pharmaseal closed
Quarantine
Ritter suprapubic suction
Rubber dam
Soft rubber
Sovally suprapubic suction cup
Stab wound
T-tube
Whistle tip
Wylie

DRILLS

Adson spiral
Bjork rib
Bosworth crown
Bunnell hand
Bur
Cannulated cortical step
Carmody perforator
Carroll-Bunnell
Cloward cervical
Codman Shurtleff cranial
Collison body
Collison cannulated hand
Collison tap
Crown
Crutchfield
Cushing cranial
Dental
Deyerle
DePuy
D'Errico
Dr. Light-Veley automatic cranial
Hall micro air
Hall step down
Harris-Smith anterior interbody
Hudson cranial
Jacobs chuck
Jordan-Day
Kirschner wire
Loth-Kirschner
Lusskin bone
Magnuson twist
McKenzie cranial
Michelson-Sequoia air
Modny
Moore bone
Neill perforator
Orthopedic universal
Patrick
Pease bone
Ralks bone
Ralks fingernail
Raney cranial
Richter bone
Sherman-Stille
Smedberg
Smith
Stille pattern bone
Stille-Sherman
Thornwald antrum
Twist
Ullrich drill guard
Universal two speed hand
Vitallium
Wolferman
Zimalate
Zimmer Kirschner hand
Zimmer universal

DRIVERS

Ken
Massie
McNutt
McReynolds
Moore
Moore-Blount

SURGICAL INSTRUMENTS AND EQUIPMENT

DRIVERS (continued)

Neufeld
Pugh
Rush
Zimmer

ELECTRICATOR
Also see: Electrosurgical units

National

ELECTRODES

ACMI retrograde
Air spaced
Angular tip
Angulated blade
Arrowsmith
Ball tip
Ballenger follicle
Bard
Baumrucker
Bayonet tip
Beaver tail tip
Berens bident
Biopsy loop
Birtcher
Biterminal
Blade
Bovie conization
Bugbee
Buie fulgurating
Coagulating
Collings fulguration
Collings knife
Conical tip
Conization
Coude
Cuff type inactive
Cup shaped
Cutting loop
Davis coagulation
Disc
Domed angle tip
Fine needle
Flat tip
Flexible radiothermal
Fulgurating
Galloway
Gradle
Grantham lobotomy
Haiman tonsil
Hamm fulgurating
Hubbard
Hurd angular
Hurd bipolar diathermy
Hurd turbinate
Hymes-Timberlake
Iglesias
Inactive
Indifferent
Kronfeld
Lane ureteral meatotomy
Large loop
Loop
Loop ball
Lynch
McCarthy coagulation
McCarthy diathermic knife
McCarthy fulguration
McWhinnie
Moersch
Multipurpose ball
Myerson
National cautery
Needle
Neil Moore meatotomy
Nesbit
New's
Padd
Patient
Pischel
Platinum blade meatotomy
    fulgurating
Pointed tip
Prostatic aluminum
Punctate

ELECTRODES (continued)

Retrograde
Riba electro-urethrotome
Ringenberg
Rod
Roller
Round loop
Rychener-Weve
Semi-flat tip
Shank
Sluder cautery
Small loop
Smith
Stern-McCarthy

Straight blade
Straight point
Straight tip
Timberlake
Tongue plate
Turner cystoscopic fulgurating
Ureteral meatotomy
Vaginal aluminum
Wappler
Weve
Williams tonsil
Wrap around inactive
Zinc ball

ELECTRODIAPHAKE

LaCarrere

ELECTROSCOPE

Bruening

ELECTROSURGICAL UNITS
Dessication—Fulguration—Coagulation

AG bovie
Birtcher hyfrecator
Bovie
Burdick microwave diathermy
Burdick short wave diathermy
CSV bovie

Electricator
L-F uniflex diathermy
Mettler model 50 dia-sonic
Ritter coagulator
Ritter-Bantam bovie
Ultrasonic diathermy

ELECTROSURGICAL UNIT ACCESSORIES

Bovie liquid conductor
Coagulation-aspirator tube
Dessication-fulguration needle
Electrodes:
  angulated blade
  ball
  blade
  conization
  disc
  fine needle
  indifferent
  loop ball
  multipurpose ball

  needle
  patient
  proctological ball
  rod
  round loop
  shank
  straight blade
  straight point
  wrap around inactive
Epilation needle
Indifferent plate
Patient plate
Tissue dessication needle

ELECTROTOMES

McCarthy infant
McCarthy miniature
McCarthy punctuate
Nesbit
Stern-McCarthy
Timberlake obturator

ELEVATORS
Also see: periosteal elevators

Abraham
Adson
Alexander-Farabeuf
Allerdyce
Amerson bone
Apexo
Artmann
Ballenger-Hajek
Ballenger septum
Bennett
Bethune
Blair cleft palate
Boies nasal
Brophy tooth
Brown tooth
Cannon-Rochester lamina
Carter submucous
Chandler
Clinic exolever
Cobb spinal
Cohen
Converse-MacKenty
Cooper spinal fusion
Cordes-New laryngeal punch
Cottle septum
Cottle skin
Coupland's
Crawford dural
Cryer dental
Cushing little joker
Cushing pituitary
Cushing staphylorrhaphy
Davidson-Sauerbruch-Doyen
Dewar
Dingman zygoma
Doyen rib
Dunning
Farabeuf
Fay suction
Ferris-Smith
File
Fomon nostril
Frazier dura
Frazier suction
Freer
Freer double
Freer septum
Friedrich rib
Gillies
Graham scalene
Hajek-Ballenger septum
Halle septum
Hamrick suction
Hatt golf stick
Hayden palate
Hedblom
Henner
Hertzel raspatory
Hibbs costal
Hibbs spinal fusion chisel
House ear
Howorth
Hurd septum
Jackson perichondrial
Joseph-Killian septum
Killian septum
Kinsella
Kirmisson
Kleesattel
Kocher
Ladd
Lamont
Lane
Langenbeck
Lee-Cohen septum
Lempert
Logan
Love-Adson
Luongo septal
Magielski

ELEVATORS (continued)

Matson rib
MacKenty
Moore bone
Moorehead
Overholt
Pennington septum
Phemister raspatory
Pierce
Poppen
Presbyterian Hospital
Proctor mucosa
Ray-Parsons-Sunday staphylorrhaphy
Rochester
Roger septum
Rosen
Sauerbruch-Frey rib
Sayre
Schuknecht
Sedillot
Sewall ethmoidal
Sewall mucoperiosteal
Shambaugh
Shambaugh-Derlacki
Smith-Petersen
Sokolec
Staphylorrhaphy
Sunday staphylorrhaphy
Tabb ear
Tarlov nerve
Tobolsky
Turner cord
Walker submucous
Warwick James
Winter
Woodson

ENTEROSCOPE

Goldberg-MPC operative

ENUCLEATOR

Young prostatic

ERISIPHAKES (also: erysiphake)

Barraquer
Bell
Dimitry
Dimitry-Bell
Dimitry-Thomas
Harrington
Kara
L'Esperance right angled
Maumenee
Nugent-Green-Dimitry
Post-Harrington
Sakler
Searcy
Viers

ESOPHAGOSCOPES

Ballooning
Boros
Bruening
Chevalier Jackson
esophageal bougies (used with)
Haslinger
Holinger
Jackson full lumen
Jesberg
Lell
Moersch
Mosher
Moure
Roberts folding
Roberts oval
Schindler optical
Tucker
Yankauer

EVACUATORS

Creevy
Crigler
Ellik bladder
Hutch
Ice clot
Kennedy-Cornwell bladder

McCarthy bladder
McKenna Tide-Ur-Ator
Snyder hemovac
Thompson
Timberlake
Toomey bladder

EXCAVATOR

Lempert

EXOPHTHALMOMETER

Luedde

EXPRESSOR
Also see: lens expressor

Heath follicle lid
Hess tonsil

Wilmer-Badgley

EXTRACTORS

Cherry
Cloverleaf pin
DePuy
Dolan
Eric Lloyd
Jewett bone
McDermott
McNutt
McReynolds
Massie
Moore-Blount

Moore hooked
Moore nail
Moore-T
Murless head
Rush
Saalfield comedone
Schamberg comedone
Smith-Petersen
Torpin vectis
Unna comedone
Zimmer

EYE IMPLANTS

Acorn shaped
Acrylic ball
Acrylic conformer
Arruga
Berens conical
Berens pyramidal
Berens-Rosa scleral
Berens sphere
Brown-Dohlman design silastic
    corneal
Conventional shell type

Corrected cosmetic contact shell
Curl back shell
Doherty sphere
Forty five degree bend reform
Fox sphere
Frey tunneled
Front build-up
Full dimpled lucite
Glass sphere
Gold sphere
Guist sphere

EYE IMPLANTS (continued)

Haik
Hemisphere
Hook type
Ivalon sponge
Levitt
Lincoff design scleral sponge
Magnetic
Mules sphere
Mullers shield (conformer)
Peanut eye
Plastic sphere
Plexiglas
Reverse shape
Semishell
Shelf type
Shell
Silastic corneal (Brown-Dohlman design)
Silastic scleral buckler
Snellen conventional reform
Tantalum mesh
Vitallium
Wheeler sphere
Wire mesh

FACIAL FRACTURE APPLIANCE

Dental arch bars
Erich

Joseph septum clamp

FASCIA STRIPPER
(See: Stripper)

FASCIATOME

Luck

FIBERSCOPE

Hirschowitz gastroduodenal

FLANGE

Callahan

Scuderi-Callahan

FORCEPS

Abbot-Mayfield
A.C.M.I.
Adair-Allis
Adair uterine
Adson
Adson-Brown
Alderkreutz
Allen uterine
Alligator grasping
Allis
Allis-Adair
Allis-Coakley tonsil
Allis-Duval
Allis-Ochsner tissue
Allis-Willauer
Almeida
Alvis fixation
Amenabar capsule
Andrews tonsil
Anterior
Arruga capsule
Arruga-Gill
Arruga-McCool
Artery
Asch septum straightening
Ashby fluoroscopic foreign body

SURGICAL INSTRUMENTS AND EQUIPMENT

FORCEPS (continued)

Ayer chalazion
Babcock
Babcock intestinal
Babcock lung grasping
Baby Lane bone holding
Backhaus towel
Bacon cranial
Bailey chalazion
Bailey-Williamson OB
Bainbridge thyroid
Baird chalazion
Ballenger tonsil
Ballenger-Forster
Bane
Bane rongeur
Bardeleben bone holding
Barkan iris
Barlow
Barnes-Simpson OB
Barraquer cilia
Barraya
Barrett placenta
Barrett-Allen uterine
Barrett-Murphy
Barrett uterine tenaculum
Barton OB
Bauer dissecting
Bayonet
Bead
Beaupre cilia
Beebe
Beer cilia
Benaron scalp rotating
Bengolea artery
Bennett epilation
Berens corneal transplant
Berens recession
Bergeron pillar
Bergh cilia
Berke ptosis
Berne nasal
Berry uterine elevating
Best stone
Bevan gallbladder
Beyer
Billroth tumor

Bishop-Harman iris
Blake ear
Blake gallstone
Blakesley
Blanchard hemorrhoid
Bland cervical traction
Bland vulsellum
Blum
Boettcher tonsil
Boies
Bolton
Bonaccolto
Bond placenta
Bone
Bonn peripheral iridectomy
Bonney tissue
Boston Lying-In cervical
Botvin iris
Boys-Allis
Bozeman uterine packing
Braasch bladder specimen
Bracken fixation
Bracken iris
Bradford thyroid traction
Braun uterine tenaculum
Bridge deep surgery
Brigham brain tumor
Brophy
Brown-Adson
Brown side grasping
Bruening septum
Brunner tissue
Brunschwig viscera
Buerger-McCarthy bladder
Buie
Bulldog
Bullet
Bumpus
Bunker modified Jackson
    laryngeal cup
Burch biopsy
Burnham biopsy
Burns bone
Cairns dissection
Cairns hemostatic
Callahan

FORCEPS (continued)

Cane bone holding
Cannulated
Capsule
Carmalt
Carmody tissue
Carroll-Adson dura
Carroll tendon pulling
Cassidy-Brophy
Castroviejo transplant grafting
Chamberlen
Champoniere
Chandler iris
Chang bone cutting
Charnley suture
Cheatle
Cheron uterine dressing
Cherry-Adson
Chester
Child
Children's Hospital
Cicherelli rongeur
Citelli
Clark capsule fragment
Clark-Guyton
Clark-Verhoeff
Clerf
Coakley tonsil
Cohen nasal dressing
Coller
Collins
Collins mucous
Collins uterine elevating
Collins-Duvall
Coloviras-Rumel thoracic
Colver tonsil
Colver-Coakley tonsil
Cooley tangential
Coppridge grasping
Corbett bone cutting
Cordes-New laryngeal punch
Corey placenta
Cornet
Corwin tonsil
Cottle
Cottle-Arruga cartilage
Cottle-Jansen

Cottle-Kazanjian nasal
Cottle-Walsham
Cowhorn tooth extracting
Crafoord bronchial-pulmonary
Craig septum
Crawford-Knighton
Crenshaw caruncle
Crile hemostatic
Crossen puncturing tenaculum
Culler fixation
Cullom septum
Curtis tissue
Cushing brain
Cushing I.V. disc
Cushing tissue
Dandy
Dartigues uterine elevating
Davidson pulmonary vessel
Davis bayonet
Davis capsule
Davis diathermy
Dean tonsil
DeBakey thoracic
DeBakey-Bahnson
DeBakey-Bainbridge vascular
DeBakey-Cooley
D'Errico
Defourmental rongeur
DeLee
DeLee shuttle
DeLee-Simpson
Demarest
DeMartel scalp
Demel wire tightening
Dench ear
Dennis intestinal
Desjardin gallstone
Desmarres chalazion
Detakats-McKenzie
Devilbiss
Dewees obstetrical
Dieffenbach
Dieter malleus
Dingman bone holding
Docktor
Dodrill

SURGICAL INSTRUMENTS AND EQUIPMENT 149

FORCEPS (continued)

Donberg iris
Dorsey bayonet
Double concave rat tooth
Douglas eye
Doyen uterine vulsellum
Dunhill
Duplay uterine tenaculum
Duval lung
Duval-Allis
Duval-Crile lung grasping
Eastman
Eber
Elliot gallbladder
Elliott OB
Elschnig fixation
Elschnig-O'Brien fixation
Elschnig-O'Connor
Elschnig secondary membrane
Emmet OB
Endospeculum
English
Epilating
Episcleral
Erhardt eyelid
Erich biopsy
Essrig tissue
Ethridge hysterectomy
Ewald (Hudson)
Ewing
Extracting
Falcao fixation
Falk lion jaw
Farabeuf bone holding
Farabeuf-Lambotte bone holding
Farnham nasal cutting
Farrington septum
Farris tissue
Fauvel laryngeal
Feilchenfeld splinter
Fenestrated blade
Ferguson angiotribe
Ferguson bone holding
Ferguson tenaculum
Ferris-Smith
Ferris-Smith fragment
Ferris-Smith-Kerrison rongeur

Fink fixation
Fink-Jameson
Finochietto lobectomy
Fischmann angiotribe
Fish nasal grasping
Fisher advancement
Fisher-Arlt iris
Fisher capsule
Fitzgerald aortic aneurysm
Fitzwater peanut sponge holding
Fixation
Fletcher-Van Doren
Foley vas isolation
Förster eye
Foss cardiovascular
Foss intestinal clamp
Fraenkel laryngeal (Fränkel)
Francis chalazion
Frankfeldt grasping
Freer-Gruenwald
French pattern
Fry nasal
Fuchs iris
Fulpit tissue
Furniss polyp
Gabriel Tucker
Galea
Garland hysterectomy
Garrigue uterine dressing
Gavin-Miller
Gaylor biopsy
Geissendorfer
Gellhorn biopsy punch
Gelpi hysterectomy
Gelpi-Lowrie hysterectomy
Gerald
Gifford iris
Gilbert
Gill
Gill-Fuchs
Gill-Hess iris
Gill-Safar
Ginsberg
Girrard
Glassman-Allis
Glenner vaginal hysterectomy

FORCEPS (continued)

Gold deep surgery
Goldman-Kazanjian nasal
Gomco
Good OB
Goodyear-Gruenwald
Gordon vulsellum
Gradle cilia
Graefe eye
Graefe fixation
Gray
Gray cystic duct
Grayton
Green fixation
Green suction tube
Green-Armytage
Greenwood coagulation & suction
Gross hyoid cutting
Grotting
Gruenwald-Bryant
Gruenwald nasal
Guggenheim adenoid
Guist fixation
Gunderson recession
Gutgemann auricular appendage
Gutglass cervix hemostatic
Guyton-Noyes
Haig Ferguson
Hajek sphenoid punch
Hajek-Koffler sphenoid punch
Halsted mosquito
Hamby clip applying
Hamilton deep surgery
Hammer
Harken cardiovascular
Harman
Harrington vulsellum
Hartmann alligator
Hartmann-Citelli ear punch
Hartmann-Gruenwald nasal cutting
Hartmann mosquito
Hawkins cervical biopsy
Hawks-Dennen
Hayes-Olivecrona clip
Healy gastrointestinal
Healy uterine biopsy
Heaney-Ballentine

Heaney hysterectomy
Heaney-Kanter hysterectomy
Heaney-Rezek hysterectomy
Heath chalazion
Heath nasal
Hegenbarth
Heise artery
Heise vulsellum
Hemostatic
Hendren cardiovascular
Henke punch
Henrotin uterine vulsellum
Herman bone holding
Herzfeld
Hess-Barraquer
Hess capsule
Hess-Gill eye
Hess-Horwitz
Hibbs bone holding
Hirschman hemorrhoidal
Hirst OB
Hirst-Emmet OB
Hodge
Hoen
Hoffman, W. J.
Hoffmann ear punch
Hodge
Holinger specimen
Holmes fixation
Holth punch
Horsley bone cutting
Hosford-Hicks transfer
House strut
Howard closing
Howard tonsil
Hoxworth fashure
Hoyt deep surgery
Hoytenberger tissue
Hubbard corneoscleral
Hudson cranial
Hufnagel mitral valve holding
Hunt
Hurd septum bone cutting
Hurdner tissue
Hurteau
Imperatori laryngeal

SURGICAL INSTRUMENTS AND EQUIPMENT

FORCEPS (continued)

Iowa membrane puncturing
Jackson approximation
Jackson broad blade staple
Jackson cross action
Jackson cup round punch
Jackson cylindrical object
Jackson double concave rat tooth
Jackson double prong
Jackson down jaw
Jackson dull pointed
Jackson fenestrated meat
Jackson fenestrated peanut grasping
Jackson forward grasping
Jackson hollow object
Jackson laryngeal
Jackson laryngofissure
Jackson papilloma
Jackson rotation
Jackson sharp pointed
Jackson side curved
Jackson sister hook
Jackson square specimen
Jackson triangular punch
Jacob uterine vulsellum
Jameson recession
Jansen bayonet
Jansen ear
Jansen nasal dressing
Jansen-Gruenwald
Jansen-Middleton septum cutting
Jansen-Struycken septum
Jarcho uterine tenaculum
Javerts polyp
Jesberg
Johns Hopkins serrefine
Johnson brain tumor
Johnson thoracic
Jones towel
Joplin bone holding
Judd-Allis
Judd-DeMartel
Juers-Lempert
Juers lingual
Julian thoracic
Jurasz laryngeal
Kadesky

Kahler polyp
Kalt capsule
Katzin-Barraquer
Kazanjian nasal hump cutting
Kelly hemostatic
Kelly-Murphy
Kelly placenta
Kennedy vulsellum
Kent deep surgery
Kern bone holding
Kielland OB (Kjelland)
Kielland-Luikart OB
Killian septum compression
King-Prince
Kingsley grasping
Kirby eye
Kirkpatrick tonsil
Kirschner-Ullrich
Kittner
Knapp trachoma
Knight turbinate
Knight-Sluder nasal
Kocher artery
Koffler septum
Koffler-Lillie septum
Kolb bronchus
Kolodny
Krause punch
Kronfeld micro pin
Kuhnt capsule
Kulvin-Kalt iris
Laborde
Lahey
Lahey goiter
Lahey lock artery
Lahey-Pean
Lahey thyroid traction
Lambert chalazion
Lambotte bone holding
Lane bone holding
Langenbeck bone holding
Laplace
Larsen tendon
Laryngeal sponging
Lauf-Barton OB
Lauf-Barton-Kielland

FORCEPS (continued)

Lauf-Piper OB
Laufman
Laval advancement
Lawrence deep surgery
Lawrence hemostatic
Lawton
Leahey suture
Lebsche sternum punch
Lefferts bone cutting
Lejeune hemostatic
Leland Jones peripheral vascular
Lemmon-Russian
Lempert rongeur
Leo Schwartz multipurpose
Leonard deep surgery
Levenson tissue
Levora fixation
Levret
Lewin bone
Lewin spinal perforating
Lewis septum
Lewkowitz lithotomy
Leyro Diaz thoracic suture
Ligamenta flava
Lillie-Killian septum bone
Linnartz
Lister conjunctival
Lister fixation
Liston bone cutting
Liston-Stille
Litt
Littauer bone cutting
Littauer cilia
Littauer-Liston bone cutting
Livingston
Lobell
Lobenstein-Tarnier
Lockwood
Lockwood-Allis
Lombard-Beyer rongeur
London tissue
Long hysterectomy
Lordan chalazion
Lore subglottic
Lore suction tube holding
Lothrop
Love-Gruenwald alligator
Love-Kerrison
Lovelace bladder
Lovelace lung grasping
Lovelace thyroid traction vulsellum
Low
Lowenberg
Lower gall duct
Lowis I.V. disc rongeur
Lowsley
Luc ethmoid
Lucae ear
Luikart OB
Luikart-McLean
Luikart-Simpson
Lutz septal ridge cutting
Lynch laryngeal
Lyon
MacKenty tissue
Magielski coagulating
Magill
Maier uterine dressing
Mansfield
Marshik tonsil
Martin nasopharyngeal biopsy
Maryan biopsy punch
Mathieu tongue
Mathieu urethral
Matthews
Maumenee
Mayo
Mayo bone cutting
Mayo tissue
Mayo ureter isolation
Mayo-Blake
Mayo-Harrington
Mayo-Pean
Mayo-Robson
Mayo-Russian
McCarthy visual hemostatic
McCarthy-Alcock hemostatic
McCoy septum cutting
McCravey
McCullough
McGannon lens
McGuire marginal chalazion

SURGICAL INSTRUMENTS AND EQUIPMENT

FORCEPS (continued)

McHenry tonsil
McKay ear
McKenzie brain clip cutting
McKenzie grasping
McLean muscle
McLean OB
McLean-Luikart
McLean-Tucker-Luikart
McLearie bone
McNealy-Glassman-Babcock viscera
McNealy-Glassman-Mixter
McPherson micro pin
McQuigg
McQuigg-Mixter
Meacham-Scoville
Meat
Meeker deep surgery
Mendel ligature
Metzenbaum tonsil
Metzenbaum-Tydings
Michel
Michigan intestinal
Mid
Mikulicz tonsil
Miller bayonet
Millin capsule grasping
Millin lobe grasping
Millin T-shaped angled
Mills tissue
Mixter
Mixter-McQuigg
Moehle corneal
Moersch bronchoscopic specimen
Monod punch
Montenovesi cranial rongeur
Moore
Moritz-Schmidt laryngeal
Mosher
Mosher ethmoid punch
Mosquito hemostatic
Mount I.V. disc rongeur
Mount-Mayfield aneurysm
Mount-Olivecrona
Mouse tooth
MPC coagulation
Muck tonsil

Muldoon meibomian
Muller-Markham patent ductus
Munde placenta
Murphy tonsil
Murray
Museholdt nasal dressing
Museux uterine vulsellum
Musial tissue
Myerson bronchoscopic
Myerson laryngeal
Myles
Nelson
Nevins
Newman uterine tenaculum
New Orleans Eye and Ear
New York Eye and Ear
New's tissue and biopsy
Niedner dissecting
Nisbet eye
Nissen's hallux
Noble iris
Norwood
Noyes nasal dressing
Nugent
Nugowski
O'Brien fixation
Obstetrical
Occluding
Ochsner
Ochsner-Dixon
O'Connor U-shaped
O'Dell spicule
Ogura
Oldberg I.V. disc
Olivecrona clip applying
O'Shaughnessy artery
Otto tissue
Overholt
Overstreet
Page tonsil
Pang biopsy
Paton corneal transplant
Paterson laryngeal
Payne-Ochsner artery
Payne-Pean artery
Payne-Rankin artery

FORCEPS (continued)

Pean
Pean G.I.
Peanut fenestrated
Peapod I.V. disc
Peet
Pelkmann uterine dressing
Penfield dissection
Penfield suture
Pennington
Percy intestinal
Perritt
Pfau polypus
Phaneuf uterine artery
Phaneuf vaginal
Phipps
Pin bending
Piper OB
Pischel micro pin
Pitha
Pley capsule
Plondke uterine elevating
Poppen I.V. disc rongeur
Porter duodenal
Potter tonsil
Potts coarctation
Potts patent ductus
Potts-Smith tissue
Poutasse renal artery
Pratt
Pratt-Smith hemostatic
Pratt T-shaped
Preston ligamentum flavum
Price-Thomas bronchus
Prince trachoma
Proctor phrenectomy
Providence Hospital
Quervain cranial rongeur
Quevedo conjunctival
Raaf-Oldberg I.V. disc
Ralks clip removing
Randall kidney stone
Raney rongeur
Rankin
Rankin-Crile
Ratliff-Blake gallstone
Ray kidney stone
Reese advancement
Reich-Nechtow hysterectomy
Reiner-Knight ethmoid cutting
Reisinger lens
Rezek
Riba-Valeira
Rich
Richard tonsil grasping
Richter-Heath
Rienhoff arterial
Ripstein
Robb tonsil
Roberts artery
Roberts bronchial biopsy
Robertson tonsil
Rochester
Rochester-Carmalt
Rochester-Ewald
Rochester-Harrington
Rochester-Ochsner hemostat
Rochester oral
Rochester-Rankin
Roeder
Rolf
Roller
Rongeur
Ronis cutting
Rowe bone drilling
Rowland double action hump
Rugby deep surgery
Rugelski artery
Rumel lobectomy
Ruskin bone cutting
Ruskin-Liston
Ruskin rongeur
Russell hysterectomy
Russian
Russian-Pean
Sachs
St. Clair
St. Clair-Thompson
St. Martin eye
Sam Roberts bronchial biopsy
Santy dissecting
Santy ring-end
Sarot intrathoracic

SURGICAL INSTRUMENTS AND EQUIPMENT

FORCEPS (continued)

Sarot pleurectomy
Sauer
Sawtell
Scheinmann laryngeal
Schlesinger I.V. disc
Schmidt-Rumpler
Schnidt
Schoenberg intestinal
Schoenberg uterine elevating
Schroeder-Braun uterine tenaculum
Schroeder uterine tenaculum
Schubert biopsy punch
Schutz
Schwartz
Schweigger capsule (eye)
Schweizer uterine
Scobee-Allis
Scoville
Scoville-Greenwood
Scoville-Hurteau
Scudder intestinal
Scuderi bipolar coagulating
Searcy capsule
Segond tumor
Seiffert laryngeal grasping
Seletz foramen plugging
Selman
Semb
Semb-Ghazi dissecting
Semken
Semmes dural
Senturia
Sequestrum
Shaaf foreign body
Shallcross gallbladder
Shallcross nasal packing
Shearer chicken bill rongeur
Sheathed flexible gastroscopic
Shuster tonsil
Silcock's dissection
Simons stone removing
Simpson OB
Simpson-Luikart
Singley tissue
Skene uterine tenaculum
Skillman

Smith OB
Smith-Petersen
Smithwick
Smithwick-Hartmann
Snellen entropion
Snyder deep surgery
Somers uterine elevating
Speculum
Spence-Adson
Spence rongeur
Spencer chalazion
Spero meibomian
Spicule
Spurling I.V. disc
Stark vulsellum
Staude-Moore uterine tenaculum
Staude uterine tenaculum
Stevens fixation
Stevens iris
Stevenson grasping
Stille
Stille-Adson
Stille-Bjork
Stille-Horsley bone cutting
Stille-Liston bone cutting
Stille-Luer bone rongeur
Stille-Waugh tissue
Stone tissue
Storey Hillar dissecting
Strabismus
Stratte
Struempel ear
Struyken ear
Struyken turbinate
Suker iris
Suker transplant grafting
Sweet
Szuler
Takahashi nasal
Takahashi neuro
Tarnier OB
Teale uterine vulsellum
Tenaculum
Terson capsule
Thoms
Thoms-Allis

FORCEPS (continued)

Thoms-Gaylor uterine
Thorek-Mixter
Thorpe corneoscleral
Thumb
Tischler cervical biopsy
Tivnen tonsil
Tobold-Fauvel grasping
Tobold laryngeal
Tomac
Torsion
Tower muscle
Townley tissue
Trachoma
Trotter
Trousseau dilating
Trylon hemostatic
Tubular
Tucker
Tucker bead
Tucker hallux
Tucker-McLean
Tucker reach and pin
Tucker tack and pin
Turell biopsy
Turnbull adhesions
Tuttle OB
Tuttle thoracic
Tuttle tissue
Tydings tonsil
Tydings-Lakeside tonsil
Uterine vulsellum
Van Buren sequestrum
Vanderbilt deep vessel
Van Doren uterine biopsy punch
Van Struycken
Varco gallbladder
Vectis (cesarean section)
Verbrugge
Verbrugghen bone holding
Verhoeff
Victor Bonney
Virtus splinter
Von Graefe
Voris-Oldberg I.V. disc rongeur
Vulsellum
Wachtenfeldt

Wainstock eye
Waldeau fixation
Waldron
Walker
Walsham septum straightening
Walter (Carmalt) splinter
Walther tissue
Wangensteen tissue
Watson-Williams nasal
Weil ear
Weil ethmoid
Weingartner ear
Weis chalazion
Wells, T.S.
Wertheim parametrium
Wertheim vaginal
Wertheim-Cullen pedicle
White tonsil
White-Oslay prostatic
White-Lillie tonsil
White-Smith
Wilde ear
Wilde ethmoid
Wilde I.V. disc rongeur
Wilde septum
Wilde-Blakesley
Willauer-Allis
Willett placenta previa
Williams uterine tenaculum
Wills Hospital
Winter placenta
Winter-Nassauer placenta
Wolfe cataract delivery
Worth strabismus
Wound clip
Wrigley
Wullstein ear
Wullstein-House
Wylie uterine tenaculum
Yankauer ethmoid cutting
Yankauer-Little
Yeomans
Young
Young uterine biopsy
Ziegler cilia

SURGICAL INSTRUMENTS AND EQUIPMENT

FRACTURE APPLIANCES

Dental arch bar   Erich facial

FRACTURE FRAMES

Alexian Brothers overhead   Goldthwait
Balkan   Granberry hyperextension
Böhler reducing   Herzmark hyperextension
Bradford   Janes
Charest head   Stryker CircOlectric
Cole hyperextension   Stryker turning
Crawford head   Thomas
DePuy rainbow   Thomson hyperextension
DePuy reducing   Vasocillator
Doctor Plymale lift   Zimmer
Foster turning

GAGS (See: mouth gags)

GASTROSCOPES

ACMI Examining   Hirschowitz gastroduodenal
Benedict operating   fiberscope
Bernstein modification   Housset-Debray
Chevalier Jackson   Janeway
Eder   Kelling
Eder-Chamberlin   Peroral Chevalier Jackson
Eder-Hufford   Schindler
Eder-Palmer   Taylor, H.
Ellsner   Wolf-Schindler
Herman Taylor

GAUZE PACKERS

Allport   Kitchen postpartum
Bernay   Torpin automatic uterine

GONIOMETERS

Conzett   International standard
Finger   Osborne
Frykholm   Tomac

GOUGES

Alexander bone   Aufranc arthroplasty
Andrews mastoid   Ballenger
Army pattern bone   Bowen

GOUGES (continued)

Campbell arthroplasty
Cave scaphoid
Cobb
Cooper spinal fusion
Crane
Derlacki
Dix
Flanagan spinal fusion
Freer nasal
Hibbs bone
Hoen lamina
Holmes cartilage
Kezerian
Kuhnt
Lahey Clinic spinal fusion
Lillie
Martin hip

Meyerding
Moore spinal fusion
Murphy
Nicola
Pilling
Putti arthroplasty
Rowen spinal fusion
Schuknecht
Smith-Petersen arthroplasty
Stille pattern bone
Todd foreign body
Trough
Troutman mastoid
Turner spinal
Walton foreign body
West bone

GUIDES

Adson Gigli saw
Bailey Gigli saw
Blair Gigli saw
Borchard Gigli saw
Caldwell
Cloward
Cone
Cooper basal ganglia
Cottle cartilage
Cushing Gigli saw
Ferciot wire
Harrison forked type strut
House strut
Kendrick Gigli saw

Modny
Morrissey Gigli saw
Mumford Gigli saw
Poppen Gigli saw
Rand-Wells pallidothalmomectomy
Raney Gigli saw
Rhinelander
Scaphoid screw
Schlesinger Gigli saw
Stille Gigli saw
Telescoping
Todd stereotaxic
Todt-Heyer cannula

GUILLOTINES

Lilienthal rib
Sluder tonsil

Sluder-Sauer tonsil
Van Osdel

HALTERS

Cerva crane
DePuy head
Diskard head
Forrester head

Neck wrap
Tracto-halter
Zimfoam head
Zimmer head

SURGICAL INSTRUMENTS AND EQUIPMENT

HAMMERS

Cloward
Epstein

House tapping
Quisling intranasal

HAND PIECES

Chayes
Emesco

Revelation
Wullstein

HEAD HOLDERS

Bayless neurosurgical
Derlacki-Juers

Haslinger
Killian suspension gallows

HEMOSTATS

Boettcher
Broadbill with push fork
Corwin
Crile
Dean
Jackson tracheal

Mathrop
McWhorter
Sawtell-Davis
Schnidt
Shallcross

HEMOSTATIC BAGS

Aberhart disposable urinal
Alcock
Bardex
Brake
Brodny
Coude
Emmet
Foley
Foley-Alcock
Hagner
Hendrickson
Higgins

Nesbit
Owens
Paul Condom
Pearman transurethral
Pear-shaped fluted
Pilcher suprapubic
Severance transurethral
Short tip
Soanes
Thackston retropubic
Two-way
Wolf

HOOKS

Adson brain
Adson knot tier
Allport
Aufranc
Bane
Barr crypt
Berens scleral

Bethune nerve hook
Boettcher tonsil
Bose tracheostomy
Boyes-Goodfellow
Braun decapitation
Braun OB
Brown

HOOKS (continued)

Carroll bone
Chavasse
Cloward cautery
Cloward dura
Colver examining
Converse
Converse hinged skin
Cottle
Cottle-Joseph
Crile nerve
Culler rectus muscle
Cushing dura
Cushing gasserian ganglion
Dailey fixation
Dandy nerve
Davis
Day ear
Double pronged
Dudley rectal
Dudley tenaculum
Edwards rectal
Emmet uterine tenaculum
Fink
Fixation
Frazier cordotomy
Frazier dura
Frazier skin
Freer skin
Gillies bone
Gillies skin
Gillies-Dingman
Goldman universal nerve
Graefe strabismus
Graham nerve
Green strabismus
Gross ear
Guthrie skin
Gwathmey
Haven skin graft
Henton tonsil suture
Hoen nerve
House crura
House foot plate
House incus
House strut
Iris

Jaeger strabismus
Jameson strabismus
Jardine
Jaw
Johnson
Joseph tenaculum
Kelly uterine tenaculum
Kilner skin
Kimball nephrostomy
Kirby double fixation
Kirby intracapsular lens expressor
Klemme dura
Lahey Clinic dura
Lillie attic
Lillie ear
Linton vein
Lordan muscle splitting
Loughnane prostatic
Madden sympathectomy
Magielski
Malgaigne patellar
Martin
Mayo fibroid
McMahon nephrostomy
McReynolds lid retracting
Muelly
Murphy ball end
Neivert
Newhart
Nugent iris
O'Brien rib
O'Connor
Pajot decapitation
Palate
Penn swivel
Pratt rectal
Ramsbotham decapitation
Rolf muscle
Rosser crypt
Russian fixation
Sachs dural
Sadler bone
Schnitman skin
Schuknecht foot plate
Scobee muscle
Scoville curved nerve

HOOKS (continued)

Searcy fixation
Selverstone cordotomy
Shambaugh endaural
Sharpley
Sluder sphenoid
Smellie OB (& crochet)
Smith lid retracting
Smithwick button
Smithwick sympathectomy
Speare dura
Speer suture
Squint
Stevens traction

Stevens tenotomy
Stewart crypt
Strully dura twist
Strut bar
Tauber ligature
Tracheal
Tyrrell iris
Tyrrell skin
von Graefe
Walsh endaural
Weary nerve
Wiener corneal
Zoellner

HYFRECATOR
Also see: Electrosurgical units

Birtcher

IMPLANT MATERIALS
Also see: Eye implants and Prostheses

Acrylic
Adhesive silicone
Bone
Cartilage
Celluloid
Edwards Teflon intracardiac patches
Ethrone
Hollow sphere
Homograft
Ivalon (polyvinyl sponge)
Marlex mesh
Paladon
Paraffin
Plexiglas
Polyether
Polyethylene
Polystan
Polyurethane
Polyvinyl

Shell
Silastic
Silastic Cronin (mammary)
Silastic medical adhesive silicone
Silastic subdermal
Silastic (testicular)
Silicone
Stainless steel
Subdermal
Supramid
Tantalum
Tantalum mesh
Teflon
Teflon mesh
Usher's Marlex mesh
Vitallium
Vivosil
Wire mesh

INSUFFLATORS

Buckstein colonic
Kidde tubal

Weber colonic

INVERTERS

Barrett appendix
Mayo-Boldt

Wangensteen tissue

IRRIGATORS

Baumrucker clamp
Bishop-Harman anterior chamber
Devilbiss eye
Doss automatic percolator
Dougherty anterior chamber
Fox hydrostatic
Gibson anterior chamber

Goldstein anterior chamber
McKenna Tide-Ur-Ator
Moncrieff anterior chamber
Rollet anterior chamber
Sylva anterior chamber
Wells, C.A.

KERATOMES

Agnew
Atkinson
Berens
Castroviejo
Czermak
Daily
Grieshaber
Jaeger

Kirby
Lancaster
Landolt
Lichtenberg
McReynolds pterygium
Rowland
Thomas
Wiener

KNIVES

Abraham
Agnew canaliculus
Allen-Barkan
Atkin tonsil
Austin dental
Ayre cone
Bailey-Glover-O'Neil commissurotomy
Bailey-Morse mitral
Ballenger mucosa & cartilage
Ballenger swivel
Bard-Parker
Barkan goniotomy
Barker vacutome suction
Baron
Barraquer corneal
Barrett uterine
Beard lid
Beck tonsil
Beer's cataract

Berens sclerotomy
Bistoury
Blair-Brown skin graft
Blair cleft palate
Bonta mastectomy
Bosher commissurotomy
Brock mitral valve
Brock pulmonary valve
Brophy bistoury
Brophy cleft palate
Brown cleft palate
Buck ear
Buck myringotome
Bucy cordotomy
Caltagirone skin graft
Canfield tonsil
Carpenter tonsil
Carter septum
Castroviejo ophthalmic
Catling amputating

SURGICAL INSTRUMENTS AND EQUIPMENT

KNIVES (continued)

Cave cartilage
Collings
Colver tonsil
Converse
Cornman dissecting
Cottle nasal
Crescent plaster
Crile cleft palate
Crile ganglion
Crosby
Curdy sclerotome
Cushing dura hook
Davidoff cordotomy
Daviel chalazion
Davis, F.A.
Dean tonsil
DeLee laparotrachelotomy
Dench's ear
DePalma
Derlacki capsule
Derra commissurotomy
Derra guillotine
D'Errico lamina
Desmarres paracentesis
Deutschman cataract
Devonshire
Dintenfass ear
Dintenfass-Chapman
Douglas tonsil
Downing cartilage
Dupuytren
Elschnig cataract
Elschnig pterygium
Equen-Neuffer laryngeal
Ferris-Robb tonsil
Ferris-Smith
Fisher tonsil
Fletcher tonsil
Fomon
Frazier cordotomy
Frazier pituitary capsulectomy
Freer septum
Freer-Ingal submucous
Freiberg cartilage
Friesner ear
Gandhi

Gerzog ear
Gerzog-Ralks
Gill corneal
Goldman guillotine nerve
Goodyear tonsil
Graefe cataract
Graf cervical cordotomy
Green cataract
Groff electrosurgical
Guy tenotomy
Haab
Harris tonsil
Harrison capsule
House ear
House incudostapedial joint
House myringoplasty
Hufnagel commissurotomy
Hundley knee
Humby
Hymes scleral
Jackson tracheal bistoury
Jaeger keratome
Johnson evisceration
Joseph angular
Joseph bistoury
Joseph button end
Joseph cervical
Joseph double edge
Joseph nasal
Joseph-Maltz
Killian tonsil
Kirby cataract
Knapp cataract
Kreissl meatotomy
Krull acetabular
Kyle crypt
Ladd
Lancaster
Lance
Lang eye
Langenbeck flap
Lanigan cartilage
Lebsche sternum
Lee cartilage
Lee Cohen
Leland tonsil

KNIVES (continued)

Lempert
Lillie tonsil
Liston amputating
Lothrop tonsil
Lowe-Breck cartilage
Lowell glaucoma
Lundsgaard-Burch
Lynch obtuse angle laryngeal
MacCallum, P.M.
MacKenty cleft palate
Maltz cartilage
Mandelbaum ear
Marcks
Mayo
McHugh facial nerve
McHugh flap
McKeever cartilage
McMurray tenotomy
McPherson-Wheeler eye
McReynolds pterygium
Mead lancet
Mercer cartilage
Metzenbaum septum
Meyhoeffer eye
Milette tonsil
Milette-Tydings
Miltex ligature
Mitchell cartilage
Moorehead ear
Murphy plaster
Neivert
Newman uterine
Niedner commissurotomy
Nunez-Nunez mitral stenosis
Pace hysterectomy
Page tonsil
Parker serrated discission
Parker tenotomy
Paton corneal
Politzer angular ear
Pope rectal
Potts expansile
Ralks reversible
Rayport dura
Reese ptosis
Reiner
Ridlon plaster
Rish cartilage
Robb
Robertson tonsil
Rochester mitral stenosis
Rosen incision ear
Royce
Scheie goniotomy
Schuknecht roller
Schultze embryotomy
Schwartz cordotomy
Seiler tonsil
Sellor mitral valve
Semilunar cartilage
Sexton ear
Shambaugh
Shambaugh-Lempert
Sheehy canal
Sichel iris
Sluder
Smillie cartilage
Smillie meniscus
Smith cataract
Smith cordotomy
Smith-Fisher cataract
Smith-Green eye
Somer tonsil
Speed-Sprague
Stewart cartilage
Strayer meniscus
Stryker-Scholl meniscus
Suker spatula
Tabb ear
Taylor, C.B.
Tobold laryngeal
Tooke corneal
Tubby tenotomy
Tydings tonsil
Ulrich uterine
Vacutome
Vannas abscess
Vaughan abscess
Virchow skin graft
von Graefe cataract
Walb, P.M.
Walton ear

SURGICAL INSTRUMENTS AND EQUIPMENT

KNIVES (continued)

Weber
Weber canaliculus
Webster skin graft
Weiss pattern
Wheeler discission

Woodruff spatula
Wullstein double edged
Ziegler iris
X-Acto utility

LARYNGOSCOPES

Adult reverse bevel
Albert Andrews modified Jackson
Anterior commissure
Atkins-Tucker shadow free
Bizzarri-Giuffrida
Broyles anterior commissure
Broyles optical
Broyles wasp waist
Chevalier Jackson
Clerf
Dual distal lighted
E.S.I.
Fink
Flagg
Foregger
Guedel
Haslinger
Holinger anterior commissure
Holinger hour glass anterior commissure
Holinger modified Jackson
Holinger slotted anterior commissure
Hook-on folding

Hopp laryngoscope blade
Jackson
Lewy
Lundy
Lynch suspension
MacIntosh
Miller
Multipurpose
Polio
Roberts self retaining
Rotating
Rusch
Sam Roberts self retaining
Sanders intubation
Siker mirror
Standard
Tucker anterior commissure
Welch-Allyn
Wisconsin
Wis-Foregger
Wis-Hipple
Yankauer

LARYNGOSTATS

Jackson

Priest wasp waist

LENS EXPRESSORS

Arruga
Bagley-Wilmer
Berens
Kirby intracapsular with curved zonal separator
Kirby intracapsular with cylindrical separator
Kirby intracapsular with double ball separator

Kirby intracapsular with flat separator
Rizzuti
Smith lid
Verhoeff
Wilmer-Bagley

LENS LOUPES

Amenabar
Arlt
Beebe
Berens
Berger
Daviel

Levis
Lewis
May hook-on
New Orleans
Wilder
Zeiss-Gullstrand

LEUKOTOMES

Bailey
Dorsey transorbital
Freeman transorbital
Lewis

Lours
Love
McKenzie
Nosik transorbital

LID EVERTERS

Berens
Luther Peter
Pess

Siniscal-Smith
Vail
Walker

LIGHTS

Co-Axa lite
Gass neurosurgical

Goodlite super headlight
Overhead

LITHOTRITES

Alcock
Bigelow
Hendrickson
Keyes

Lowenstein
Ravich
Reliquet
Teale gorget

LITHOTRIPTOSCOPE

Ravich with Luer lock

LOOPS (Also see: Lens loupes)

Amenabar
Beck twisted wire
Billeau ear

Cannon endarterectomy
McKenzie leukotomy
Weber-Elschnig

LUMEN FINDERS

Carabelli full view

Tucker vertebrated

MAGNETS

Alnico magneprobe
Berman
Coronet

Equen stomach
Firlene eye
Grafco

SURGICAL INSTRUMENTS AND EQUIPMENT

MAGNETS (continued)

Gruening eye
Haab eye
Hirschberg electromagnet
Holinger bronchoscopic
Holinger endoscopic
Horseshoe
Lancaster

Mellinger
Mueller giant eye
Norris tip
Ralks
Sweet eye
Thomas
Wildgen-Reck metal locator

MALLETS

Bakelite
Boxwood
Carroll aluminum
Chandler
Cottle
Crane
Fibre head
Gerzog
Hajek
Hibbs

Kirk orthopedic
Lucae
MacAusland bone
Meyerding
Nylon head
Ralks
Rush
Smith-Petersen
Standard pattern
White

MASTOID SEARCHER

Allport

MEATOSCOPE

Hubell

MEATOTOMES

Bunge ureteral
Ellik

Riba electric ureteral

MECHANICAL FINGER

Quire

MEDIASTINOSCOPE

Goldberg MPC

MENISCOTOMES

Bowen-Grover

Ruuska

METAL LOCATORS (Also see: Magnets)

Berman

Wildgen-Reck

MICRO-MIKE

Jacobson millimeter

MICROSCOPES

Barraquer-Zeiss movie
Beta ray
Binocular
Capillary
Centrifuge
Comparison
Compound
Corneal
Darkfield
Derlacki-Shambaugh
Electron
Epic
Epimicroscope
Fluorescence
Greenough
Infrared
Integrating
Interference
Ion
Jenoptik surgical
Keeler surgical
Light
Olympus MTX

Opaque
Operating
Oto-microscope
Phase
Phase-contrast
Photon
Polarizing
Rectified
Reflecting
Rheinberg
Schlieren
Shambaugh-Derlacki
Slit lamp & fundus camera
Stereoscopic
Stroboscopic
Trinocular
Ultramicroscope
Ultrasonic
Ultraviolet
X-Ray
Zeiss
Zeiss diploscope

MOBILIZER

Derlacki ear

MOUTH GAGS

Boettcher-Jennings
Boyle Davis
Brophy
Brown-Fillebrown-Whitehead
Brown-Whitehead
Collis
Danns-Jennings
Davis
Davis-Crowe
Denhardt
Denhardt-Dingman
Dott with Kilner modification
Doyen-Jansen

Ferguson-Brophy
Ferguson-Gwathmey
Frohn
Fulton
Green
Green-Sewall
Heister
Hewitt mouth prop
Hibbs
Jennings loktite
Jennings-Skillern
Lane
Lewis

SURGICAL INSTRUMENTS AND EQUIPMENT

MOUTH GAGS (continued)

Maunder oral screw
McIvor
McKesson
Mithoefer-Jansen
Molt
Newkirk
Oral screw
Oral speculum
Proetz
Proetz-Jansen
Pynchon

Ralks-Davis
Roser
Roser-Koenig
Sluder-Ferguson
Sluder-Jansen
Sydenham
Wesson
Whitehead
Wolf
Wolf loktite

MUCOTOME

Norelco

NAILS

Augustine boat nails
Barr bolts
Boat nail
Cannulated
Cloverleaf
Curry hip
Delitala T-nail
Diamond
Dooley
Engel-May
Four flanged
Gissane spike
Hansen-Street self broaching
Hansen-Street solid intramedullary
Hooked intramedullary
Jewett
Ken
Knowles pin
Kuntscher cloverleaf
Kuntscher intramedullary
Lottes
Lottes triflange intramedullary
Massive sliding
McKee tri-fin

Moore adjustable
Neufeld
Noncannulated
Nylok self-locking
Pidcock
Pugh self adjusting
Rush
Schneider intramedullary
Smillie
Smith-Petersen cannulated
Staples type osteotomy
Steinmann
Temple University
Thatcher
Thornton
Tiemann
V-medullary
Venable-Stuck
Vesely-Street split
Vitallium
Watson Jones
Webb bolt
Z-fixation

NASOPHARYNGOSCOPES

Broyles
Holmes

Meltzer
National

NEEDLES

Abscission
Adson aneurysm
Adson-Murphy trocar point
Agnew tattooing
Alexander tonsil
Amsler
Atraumatic
Babcock
Barker, A.E.
Barrett hebosteotomy
Beyer paracentesis
Biegeleisen
Blair-Brown
Bonney
Bowman iris
Brockenbrough
Brophy
Brophy-Deschamps'
Brown staphylorrhaphy
Browne cleft palate
Bunnell
Calhoun
Calhoun-Merz
Campbell ventricular
Carpule
Carroll
Cataract
Charleton antrum
Child-Phillips intestinal plication
Cloquet
Colver tonsil
Cone ventricular
Conrad-Crosby
Cooper chemopallidectomy
Cope pleural biopsy
Cournand
Cournand-Grino
Craig biopsy
Curry cerebral angiography
Cushing ventricular
Dailey cataract
Dandy ventricular
Dattner
Davis
Dean iris knife
Dees renal

Deknatel "K"
Denis Browne cleft palate
Depuy-Weiss tonsil
Deschamps'
Desmarres' paracentesis
Dingman
Discission
Dix
Docktor
Dos Santos lumbar aortography
Duff debridement
Durham
Emmet
Estridge ventricular
Federspiel
Fein
Ferguson
Fischer pneumothorax
Fisher eye
Fish hook
Floyd pneumothorax injection
Flynt aortogram
Frackelton
Francke
Frankfeldt hemorrhoidal
Franklin-Silverman
Frazier ventricular
Frederick pneumothorax
French spring eye
Gallie fascia
Gardner
Goldbacher rectal
Gordh
Gorsch
Grantham lobotomy
Greenfield
Grieshaber 8¾
Haab knife
Hagedorn suture
Halle septum
Harken heart
Hessberg
Hingson-Edwards
Hourin tonsil
House-Barbara
House-Rosen

SURGICAL INSTRUMENTS AND EQUIPMENT

NEEDLES (continued)

Howard-Jones
Hutchins biopsy
Hypospray jet injector
Ingersoll
Jameson strabismus
Kader fish hook
Kalt corneal
Kaplan
Karras
Keith abdominal
Knapp iris knife
Kobak
Koontz
Kronecker aneurysm
Lahey
Lane suture
Lichtwicz antrum
Linton-Blakemore
List
Longdwel catheter
Loopuyt
Lowsley ribbon gut
Luer lock
Lundy fascia
Lundy-Irving caudal
Luongo
Maddox caudal
Magielski
Maltz
Masson fascia
Mayo
McCurdy staphylorrhaphy
McGowan
Menghini liver biopsy
Meyer cyclodiathermy
Mixter ventricular
Murphy intestinal
Nelson
Newman rectal injection
New's
Oldfield
Overholt rib
Pace ventricular
Pannett
Parhad-Poppen arteriogram
Parker knife

Penfield biopsy
Pitkin
Poppen ventricular
Presbyterian Hospital ventricular
P.S. New
Retter aneurysm
Reverdin
Rider-Moeller
Riedel corneal
Riley arterial
Robb
Rochester-Meeker
Rolf lance
Roser
Ross
Ruskin antrum
Sabreloc
Sachs
Salah
Sanders-Brown-Shaw aneurysm
Saunders cataract
Schuknecht
Scoville ventricular
Shambaugh
Sheldon-Spatz vertebral arteriogram
Sheldon-Swann
Shirodkar aneurysm
Silverman biopsy
Singer
Sluder
Smiley-Williams arteriogram
Spring eye
Stocker cyclodiathermy puncture
Strauss
Sturmdorf cervical
Sturmdorf pedicle
Sutton biopsy
Swaged
Swann-Sheldon
Titus venoclysis
Todd eye cautery
Torrington French spring
Trupp ventricular
Tuohy lumbar aortography
Turkel
Univ. of Illinois marrow

NEEDLES (continued)

Updegraff staphylorrhaphy
Veenema-Gusberg prostatic biopsy
Verres
von Graefe iris knife
Walker tonsil
Wangensteen
Ward
Ward French
Watson-Williams
Wolf antrum
Wood type aortography
Yankauer septum
Ziegler knife
Zoellner

NEUROTOME

Bradford enucleation

OBTURATORS

Alcock-Timberlake
Cripps'
Ellik-Shaw
Timberlake
Ureteral catheter

OPHTHALMODYNAMOMETERS

Bailliart
Dial type

OSTEOCLAST

Phelps-Gocht

OSTEOTOMES

Albee
Alexander perforating
Army pattern
Blount scoliosis
Bowen
Campbell
Carroll
Carroll-Legg
Carroll-Smith-Petersen
Cherry
Clayton
Cloward spinal fusion
Converse
Cottle
Crane
Dingman
Epstein
Frazier
Hibbs
Hoke
Howorth
Kezerian
Lahey Clinic thin
Lambotte
Lambotte-Henderson
Leinbach
Legg
Mayfield bayonet
Meyerding
M.G.H.
Miner
Moore
New Lambotte
Rowland
Sheehan
Silver's nasal osteotome
Smith-Petersen
Stille pattern
U.S. Army pattern

SURGICAL INSTRUMENTS AND EQUIPMENT

OTOSCOPES

Bruening pneumatic
Brunton
Politzer air bag
Siegle pneumatic

Toynbee
Welch Allyn dual purpose
Welch Allyn operating

PANENDOSCOPE

McCarthy fiber optic foroblique

PELVIMETERS

Breisky
Collyer
DeLee
DeLee-Breisky

Hanley-McDermott
Martin
Thoms
Williams

PENCILS

Electrosurgery

Weck electrosurgery

PERFORATORS

Bishop antrum
Cushing cranial
DeLee-Perce membrane
Joseph antrum
Lempert
Royce tympanum

Smellie OB
Stein membrane
Thornwald antrum
Wellaminski antrum
Williams

PERIOSTEAL ELEVATOR
(Also see: Elevator)

Adson
Allis
Aufranc
Behrend
Berry-Lambert
Bethune
Bowen
Bristow
Brophy
Cameron
Cameron-Haight
Campbell
Carroll
Carroll-Legg
Cheyne
Cloward

Cobb
Coryllos
Coryllos-Doyen
Costal
Crego
Cushing-Hopkins
Cushion
Davidson
Davidson-Mathieu-Alexander
Davis
D'Errico
Dingman
Doyen
Farabeuf
Federspiel
Fiske

PERIOSTEAL ELEVATORS (continued)

Fomon
Freer
Goodwillie
Harper
Herczel
Hibbs
Hoen
Iowa University
Joseph
Key
Kinsella
Kirmisson
Kocher
Lane
Langenbeck
Love-Adson
Lowis
MacDonald
MacKenty

Massachusetts General Hospital
MGH
Neurological Institute
Norcross
Overholt
Pace
Poppen
Raney
Richardson
Rubin-Lewis
Sayre's double ended
Scott-MacCracken
Sedillot
Sewall mucoperiosteal
Spurling
Steele
Turner
Urquhart
Willauer-Gibbon

PERIOSTEOTOMES

Alexander
Alexander-Farabeuf
Ballenger
Brophy
Brown
Dean
Ferris-Smith-Lyman
Fomon

Freer
Jansen
Joseph
Moorehead
Potts
Speer
Vaughan
West-Beck

PESSARIES

Albert Smith
Chambers intrauterine
Cup
Diaphragm
Doughnut
Emmet-Gellhorn
Findley folding
Gariel
Gehrung
Gellhorn
Globe prolapsus
Gold
Gynefold prolapse
Gynefold retrodisplacement

Hodge style
Hollow lucite
Lever
Menge stem
Plexiglas Gellhorn
Prochownik
Ring
Safety
Smith retroversion
Smith style
Stem
Thomas
Wylie stem
Zwanck (radium)

SURGICAL INSTRUMENTS AND EQUIPMENT

PICKS

Burch ophthalmic
Hoffman scleral fixation
House
Wells scleral suture

PINS

Beaded hip
Böhler
Bohlman
Breck
Compere threaded
Conley
Davis
Depuy
Deyerle
Fahey
Fahey-Compere
Hagie
Hansen-Street
Hatcher
Haynes
Jones
Knowles
Kuntscher
Marble bone
Modny
Moore fixation
Oris
Pidcock
Pischel micro-pins
Rhinelander
Roger Anderson
Rush
Schneider self-broaching
Schweitzer
Shriner
Smith-Petersen fracture
Steinmann
    calibrated
    with Crowe pilot point
    with pin chuck, ball bearing
    with twist drill points
Street
Strut type
Turner
Venable-Stuck fracture
von Saal medullary
Zimmer

PLATES

Anchor
Badgley
Batchelor's
Blade
Blount
    bent blade plate
    double angle blade
    V-blade plate
Bosworth spline
Coaptation
Depuy
Deyerle
Eggers
Elliott femoral condyle
Elliott, R.B. knee plate
Finger
Hansen-Street anchor
Harlow
Hicks lugged
Hoen skull
Hubbard
Jaeger lid
Jewett double angle osteotomy
Jewett slotted
Kessel osteotomy
L-plate
Laing osteotomy
Lane, W.A. fracture
Lundholm
McBride
McLaughlin
Meurig Williams spinal fusion
Milch resection
Moe intertrochanteric
Moore blade
Moore-Blount

PLATES (continued)

Neufeld
Newman toenail
Nicoll
Osborne osteotomy
Plain pattern
Rhinelander
Schweitzer spring
Senn bone
Serpentine bone
Sherman
Slotted
Smith-Petersen
SMO
Temple University
Thornton
Townsend-Gilfillan

Trochanteric
Tupman osteotomy
Venable bone
V-type intertrochanteric
Vitallium
Vitallium Elliot knee
Vitallium Hicks radius
Vitallium Wainwright blade
Vitallium Walldius mechanical knee
Wenger slotted
Wilson spinal fusion
Wright knee plate
Y-bone
Zuelzer hook
Z-plate

PLIERS

Allen's root
Berbecker

Fisherman's
Vice-grip

PLUGS

Counsellor mould
Johnston gastrostomy

Sims vaginal
Reich-Nechtow

PNEUMOTHORAX APPARATUS

McKesson pneumothor
R & B portable
Robinson artificial

Singer portable
Zavod aneroid

PROBES

Amussat
Anel lacrimal
Arbuckle sinus
Barr fistula
Bowman lacrimal
Brackett
Bresgen frontal sinus
Brock
Buck
Buie
Bunnell dissecting
Coakley nasal

Desjardin gallstone
Earle rectal
Emmet uterine
Esmarch tin bullet
Fenger spiral gallstone
Fish antrum
Fluhrer bullet
Fränkel sinus
French pattern lacrimal
Girdner
Gross
Hotz

SURGICAL INSTRUMENTS AND EQUIPMENT

PROBES (continued)

Jansen-Newhart
Kistner
Knapp iris repositor & probe
Kron gall duct
Larry rectal
Lente
Liebreich
Lilienthal
Lillie frontal sinus
Lucae
Mayo common duct
Meerschaum
Mixter dilaprobe
Moynihan
Myrtle leaf
Nelaton
Ochsner
Pratt rectal

Rockey dilating
Rolf lacrimal
Rosen ear
Silver
Sims uterine
Skillern sphenoid
Spencer
Spiesman fistula
Theobald
Uterine vertebrated
Wasko
Welch Allyn
Whale bone eustachian
Williams lacrimal
Wire
Yankauer salpingeal
Ziegler needle

PROCTOSCOPES

ACMI
Boehm
Fansler
Gabriel
Goldbacher
Hirschman
Hirschman-Martin
Kelly
Lieberman

Montague
National
Newman
Pruitt
Turell
Tuttle
Vernon-David
Welch Allyn
Yeomans

PROFILOMETER

Cottle

PROSTHESES
Also see: Eye Implants and Implant Materials

Austin-Moore hip
Bateman finger joint
Bifurcated seamless
Cardona keratoprosthesis
Cartwright heart
Celestin endoesophageal
Clamp stainless steel
Collagen tape
Crimped dacron

Dacron arterial
Dacron bifurcation
Dacron vessel
DeBakey
DePalma hip
DePuy hip with Scuderi head
Ear pinna
Edwards seamless
Edwards Teflon intracardiac patches

PROSTHESES (continued)

Eicher hip
Fascia lata
Fett carpal
Gott low profile
Harrison interlocked mesh
Helanca seamless tube
Hollow sphere
House piston
House stainless steel mesh
House wire
Hufnagel low profile heart valve
Joplin toe
Judet type
Kay-Suzuki disc valve
Lippman hip
Lorenzo SMO
MacIntosh tibial plateau
Mackler intraluminal tube
4-A Magovern valve
Magovern-Cromie sutureless ball valve
Matchett & Brown
McKeever patella cap
Medi-graft vascular
Microcrimped
Minneapolis hip
Modified Moore hip locking
Moore hip
Moseley glenoid rim
Mulberger
Mulligan silastic

Neer shoulder
Orbital floor
Rosi L-type nose bridge
Sampson
Sauerbruch
SCDT heart valve
Schuknecht Teflon wire piston
Scuderi
Sheehy-House incus replacement
Shier's knee
Silastic penile
    Pearman design
    Lash-Loeffler design
Silastic testicular
Smith-Petersen hip cup
Solid silicone orbital
Speed radius cap
Starr-Edwards
Stenzel rod
Teflon mesh
Teflon sheeting
Teflon tri-leaflet
F.R. Thompson hip
Townley
Two prong stem finger
Ushers Marlex mesh
Vitallium Moore self locking
Wada hingeless heart valve
Walldius vitallium mechanical knee
Wesolowski weavenit vascular
Zimaloy femoral head

PUNCHES

Abrams pleural biopsy
Adler attic ear
Ainsworth
Alexander antrostomy
Berens corneoscleral
Beyer atticus
Brock infundibular
Brooks
Bruening cup biting
Castroviejo corneoscleral
Cault
Citelli laminectomy
Citelli-Meltzer atticus

Cloward intervertebral
Cloward-Dowel
Cloward-English
Cloward-Harper cervical
Cone bone
Cordes circular
Cordes semicircular
Cordes sphenoid
Cordes square
Corgill bone
Deyerle
Dorsey cervical foramental
Eppendorfer

PUNCHES (continued)

Faraci
Faraci-Skillern sphenoid
Flateau oval
Gass cervical
Gellhorn uterine biopsy
Goldman cartilage
Graham-Kerrison
Gruenwald
Gundelach
Gusberg endocervical biopsy
Haitz canaliculus
Hajek antrum
Hajek-Koffler sphenoid
Hajek-Skillern sphenoid
Harper cervical laminectomy
Hartmann nasal
Hartmann tonsil
Hoffmann biopsy
Hoffmann ear
Holth corneoscleral
Ingraham skull
Jackson
Jacobson vessel
Johnson-Kerrison
Joseph
Kerrison
Keyes cutaneous
Klause antrum
Klause-Carmody antrum
Knighton-Kerrison
Krause angular oval
Lange antrum
Lebsche sternal
Lempert malleus
Lermoyez nasal
MacKenty sphenoid
McGoey vitallium
Meltzer
MGM glenoid
Mixter brain biopsy
Mosher ethmoid
Mulligan cervical biopsy
Murphy, J.B.
Myerson biting
Myles nasal
Noyes chalazion

Ostrom
Pfau atticus sphenoid
Phemister
Pritikin scleral
Raney laminectomy
Reaves
Ronis adenoid
Rowe glenoid
Rubin-Holth sclerectomy
Sachs cervical
Scheinmann biting
Schlesinger cervical
Schmeden tonsil
Schmithhuisen ethmoid & sphenoid
Schnaudigel sclerotomy
Schubert biopsy
Seiffert grasping
Seletz universal Kerrison
Smillie nail
Sokolowski antrum
Spencer oval
Spencer triangular adenoid
Spies ethmoid
Spurling-Kerrison
Stevenson capsule
Storz antrum
Struyken
Sweet sternal
Takahashi ethmoid
Thompson, G.J.
Thoms-Gaylor biopsy
Tischler cervical biopsy
Turell angular rotating
Turkel prostatic
Van Struycken nasal
Veenema-Gusberg prostatic
Wagner antrum
Walton corneoscleral
Walton-Schubert
Watson-Williams ethmoid
Whitcomb-Kerrison laminectomy
Wilde nasal
Wittner cervical biopsy
Yankauer
Yeomans biopsy

RASPS

Aufricht
Aufricht-Lipsett nasal
Austin-Moore
Berne nasal
Brawley sinus
Brown
Cohen sinus
Converse
Cottle
Dean
Eicher
Epstein
Facet
Fomon
Gallagher antrum
Gleason
Good antrum
Israel
Joseph nasal

Lamont nasal
Lewis nasal
Lundsgaard-Burch corneal
Maliniac nasal
Maltz
Maltz-Lipsett
Moore
Putti bone
Ringenberg
Ritter
Schantz sinus
Schmidt
Spratt
Sullivan
F.R. Thompson
Thompson frontal sinus
Watson-Williams sinus
Wiener universal frontal sinus
Woodward antrum

RASPATORY

Alexander
Artmann
Babcock
Bacon periosteal
Ballenger
Bastow's
Beck pericardial
Berry rib
Bronchocele sound
Brunner
Coryllos rib
Davidson-Mathieu rib
Davidson-Sauerbruch rib
Davis
Dolley
Doyen rib
Farabeuf
Fishtail spatula (Davis)
Friedrich
Hedbloom rib
Hein
Herczel rib
Hoen periosteal
Hopkins Hospital periosteal
Jansen mastoid

Joseph
Kirmisson periosteal
Kleesattel
Kocher
Kokowicz
Ladd
Lambert-Berry Rib
Lane periosteal
Langenbeck-O'Brien
Langenbeck periosteal
Lebsche
Lewis periosteal
Mathieu
Matson
Ollier
Overholt
Phemister
Plenk-Matson
Sauerbruch-Frey
Sayre periosteal
Scheuerlen
Schneider
Sedillot
Semb
Stillenberg

SURGICAL INSTRUMENTS AND EQUIPMENT

RASPATORY (continued)

Trelat
Willauer

Zenker
Zoellner

REAMERS

Aufranc finishing ball
Aufranc finishing cup
Aufranc offset
Cannulated four flute
DePuy cannulated
Duthie
Gruca hip
Jergeson
Kuntscher
Lorenzo
Lottes
MacAusland
MacAusland finishing ball
MacAusland finishing cup
Marin

Medullary canal
Moore bone
Murphy ball
Norton adjustable cup
Norton ball
Phemister
Rowe glenoid
Rush awl
Shaft reamer
Shelf
Smith-Petersen hip
Sovak
Spiral trochanteric
Sturmdorf cervical

RESECTOSCOPES

Bard
Baumrucker
Iglesias
McCarthy miniature
McCarthy multiple
Nesbit

Scott rotating
Stern-McCarthy electrotome
Streak
Thompson direct full vision
Timberlake obturator

RETINOSCOPES

Boilo
Copeland streak
Electric

Welch Allyn May type
Welch Allyn standard
Welch Allyn streak

RETRACTORS

Adson cerebellum
Adson splanchnic
Agricola lacrimal sac
Alden
Alexian Hospital model
Allison lung
Allport mastoid
Allport-Gifford
Alm microsurgery
Alm self-retaining

Alter's lip
Amenabar
Amoils iris
Anderson-Adson self-retaining
Andrews tracheal
Ann Arbor phrenic
Anthony
Apicolysis
Aufranc femoral neck
  (Also: hip, push, psoas)

RETRACTORS (continued)

Aufricht nasal
Austin
Automatic skin
Bacon cranial
Badgley laminectomy
Bahnson sternal
Balfour
Ballantine hemilaminectomy
Bankhart shoulder
Baron
Barr
Barrett-Adson cerebellum
Beatty pillar
Becker
Beckman
Beckman-Adson laminectomy
Beckman-Eaton laminectomy
Beckman-Weitlaner
Bellfield wire
Beneventi self-retaining
Bennett tibia
Berens eye
Berens mastectomy skin flap
Berens thyroid
Bergen
Berna infant abdominal
Bernay tracheal
Bethune phrenic
Bicek vaginal
Blair
Blair-Brown vacuum
Blakesley uvula
Blanco
Bland perineal
Blount knee
Bosworth nerve root
Boyes-Goodfellow hook
Brantley-Turner
Brawley
Breen
Brewster phrenic
Brompton Hospital
Bronson-Turz
Brown uvula
Brunner
Brunschwig visceral

Bucy spinal cord
Buie-Smith anal
Burford-Finochietto
Burford rib retractor
Button hook
Byford
Cairn's scalp
Campbell lacrimal sac
Carroll offset hand
Carroll self-retaining spring
Carroll-Bennett finger
Carter mitral valve
Castallo eyelid
Castroviejo
Cave knee
Chandler laminectomy
Charnley
Cherry S-shaped
Cloward cervical
Cloward self-retaining
Cloward-Hoen laminectomy
Cole duodenal
Colver tonsil
Cone scalp
Contour scalp
Converse nasal
Cook rectal
Cooley atrial
Coryllos
Cottle
Cottle alae
Cottle sharp prong
Cottle-Neivert
Craig-Sheehan
Crawford aorta
Crego
Crile
Crotti
Cushing
Cushing aluminum cortex
Cushing decompression
Cushing "S"
Cushing vein
Danis
Davidoff trigeminal
Davidson erector spinae

SURGICAL INSTRUMENTS AND EQUIPMENT

RETRACTORS (continued)

Davidson scapular
Davis scalp
Deaver
DeBakey-Balfour
DeBakey-Cooley
Decker
Delaney phrenic
DeLee corner
DeLee universal
DeLee vaginal
DeLee vesical
D'Errico nerve
D'Errico-Adson
DeMartel self-retaining brain
Desmarres' lid
Dingman
Dorsey nerve root
Downing
Doyen vaginal
Dumont
Duryea
Eastman vaginal
Effenberger
Elschnig lid
Emmet OB
Falk vaginal
Farabeuf double ended
Farmingdale
Farr wire
Federspiel cheek
Ferguson-Moon rectal
Ferris-Smith orbital retractor
Ferris-Smith-Sewall orbital
Finger rake
Fink lacrimal
Finochietto
Finochietto-Giessendorfer rib
Fisher lid
Fisher tonsil
Fisher-Nugent
Flexsteel ribbon
Fomon
Foss gallbladder
Four prong
Franklin malleable
Franz abdominal

Frater intracardiac
Frazier cerebral
Frazier laminectomy
Frazier lighted
Frazier-Fay
Freer submucous
Freiberg hip
Freiberg nerve root
French S-shaped
Friederich-Ferguson
Friedman perineal
Fritsch
Gelpi perineal
Gelpi self-retaining
Ghazi rib
Gifford mastoid
Glaser laminectomy
Glenner vaginal
Goelet double ended
Goldstein lacrimal sac
Gooch
Goodhill
Goodyear tonsil
Gosset abdominal
Gradle eyelid
Green thyroid
Grieshaber spring wire
Groenholm lid
Gross patent ductus
Gross-Pomeranz-Watkins atrial
Guttmann OB
Guzman-Blanco epiglottis forceps
Haight pulmonary
Haight rib
Hajek antrum
Hamby brain
Hamby-Hibbs
Hand
Harken
Harrington bladder
Harrington-Pemberton
Harrington splanchnic
Harrison chalazion
Haslinger palate
Haslinger uvula
Haverfield hemilaminectomy

RETRACTORS (continued)

Haverfield-Scoville hemilaminectomy
Hays hand
Heaney vaginal
Heaney-Simon
Hedblom rib
Helfrick anal
Henderson self-retaining
Henner endaural
Hertzler baby
Hibbs
Hill-Ferguson rectal
Hillis lid
Himmelstein sternum
Hipps self-retaining
Hoen
Holman lung
Holscher nerve root
House
House-Urban
Howorth toothed
Hudson bone
Hunt bladder
Hupp trachea
Iron interne
Israel
Jackson vaginal
Jacobson bladder
Jaeger lid plate
Jansen
Jansen mastoid
Jansen scalp
Jansen-Gifford
Jansen-Wagner
Jefferson self retaining
Johnson cheek
Johnson ventriculogram
Judd-Masson
Kalamarides dural
Kel
Kellig
Kelly-Sims vaginal
Kerrison
Killian-King goiter
King goiter
Kirkland
Klemme appendectomy
Klemme gasserian ganglion
Knapp
Kocher bladder
Kocher-Crotti goiter
Kozlinski
Krasky
Kretschmer
Kristeller vaginal
Kronfeld eyelid
Lack's tongue
Lahey Clinic nerve root
Lange
Langenbeck
LaPlace liver
Latrobe soft palate
Leatherman trochanteric
Legueu kidney
Lemmon sternal
Lempert
Lempert-Colver
Levinthal surgery
Levy perineal
Lewis
Lilienthal-Sauerbruch
Lillie pillar
Linton splanchnic
Little
Lorie cheek
Lothrop tonsil
Love nasopharyngeal
Love nerve
Love uvula
Lowsley
Luer
Lukens
Lukens epiglottis
Lukens thymus
Luongo hand
Luther, Peter
MacAusland muscle
MacAusland-Kelly
MacKay contour
Maison
Maliniac nasal
Maltz
Markham-Meyerding

RETRACTORS (continued)

Martin abdominal
Martin cheek and lip
Martin nerve root
Masson-Judd bladder
Mathieu
Matson-Mead apicolysis
Mattison-Upshaw
Mayo-Adams
Mayo-Collins
Mayo-Lovelace abdominal
Mayo-Simpson
McBurney
McCullough externo-frontal
McGannon iris
Meller lacrimal sac
Meyer biliary
Meyerding finger
Meyerding laminectomy
Meyerding-Deaver
Middledorpf
Miller
Miller-Senn
Millin-Bacon bladder
Miltex
Miskimon cerebella
Moorehead dental
Moorehead cheek
Morrison-Hurd
Morse modified Finochietto
Morson
Mosher lifesaver
Mott
Mueller lacrimal sac
Mueller-Balfour
Mufson-Cushing
Muldoon lid
Munro self-retaining scalp
Murphy rake
Murtagh self-retaining infant scalp
Myers knee
Neivert
New York Hospital
O'Brien phrenic
O'Brien rib
Ochsner
Oldberg brain
Oliver's scalp
Ollier
O'Sullivan self-retaining abdominal
O'Sullivan-O'Connor vaginal
Otto Barkan bident
Overholt
Parker
Parker-Mott
Paul
Peet lighted splanchnic
Pemberton
Percy amputation
Percy-Wolfson
Phiefer-Young
Picot vaginal
Pierce cheek
Piper lateral wall
Proctor cheek
Pryor-Pean vaginal
Purcell self-retaining abdominal
Quervain-Sauerbruch
Radcliff perineal
Ragnell
Rake
Raney laminectomy
Rankin prostatic
Ribbon
Richardson
Richardson-Eastman
Richter
Rigby bivalve
Rigby rectal
Rigby vaginal
Rizzo
Rizzuti iris
Robinson lung
Rochester atrial
Rochester colonial
Rochester-Ferguson
Rollet eye
Rose tracheal
Rosenbaum-Drews plastic
Ross aortic valve
Roux
Rowe humeral head
Rowe scapular neck spike

RETRACTORS (continued)

Rudolph trowel
Ryerson bone
Sachs
Sachs-Cushing
St. Luke
Sauerbruch
Sauerbruch-Zukschwerdt rib
Sawyer rectal
Schnitker scalp
Schuknecht
Schwartz laminectomy
Scoville hemilaminectomy
Scoville nerve root
Scoville psoas muscle
Seletz-Gelpi self-retaining
Semb
Senn
Senn-Dingman
Senn-Kanavel
Senturia
Serrefine
Sewall orbital
Shambaugh endaural
Shearer lip
Sheehan
Sheldon hemilaminectomy
Sherwood
Shriners Hospital
Shriners interlocking
Shurley tracheal
Simon, G.
Sims vaginal
Sims-Kelly
Sistrunk band
Sloan goiter
Sluder palate
Smillie knee joint
Smith anal
Smith nerve root suction
Smith-Buie anal
Smith-Petersen capsule
Snitman endaural
Sofield
Splanchnic
Stevenson lacrimal sac
Stookey

Strully nerve root
Sweeney posterior vaginal
Sweet amputation
Taylor spinal
Temple-Fay laminectomy
Theis vein
Three prong
Tillary
Tower interchangeable
Tuffier rib
Tuffier-Raney
Tyrer nerve root
Ullrich laminectomy
U.S. Army pattern
Vacher
Vail lid
Valin hemilaminectomy
Veenema retropubic
Verbrugghen
Volkmann-Rake
Walker gallbladder
Walker lid
Walter-Deaver
Webb-Balfour
Weber
Webster abdominal
Weder-Solenberger
Weinberg vagotomy
Weitlaner
Wesson
Wexler
Wexler-Balfour
White-Proud uvula
Wieder pillar
Wieder-Solenberger pillar
Wilder scleral wound
Willauer-Deaver
Wilson hand
Wolfson gallbladder
Wort antrum
Wullstein
Young bifid
Young bulb
Young lateral
Young prostatic
Zalkind

RIB CONTRACTORS

Adams
Bailey
Bailey-Gibbon
Graham
Sellors
Waterman

RIB SHEARS

Bacon
Bethune
Bethune-Coryllos
Bortone
Brunner
Coryllos-Bethune
Coryllos-Moure
Coryllos-Shoemaker
Doyen
Duval-Coryllos
Eccentric lock
Giertz-Shoemaker
Gluck
Horgan-Coryllos-Moure
Horgan-Wells
Lebsche sternum
Lefferts
Moure-Coryllos
Nelson-Bethune
Pott's infant
Roberts
Roberts-Nelson
Sauerbruch
Sauerbruch-Coryllos
Sauerbruch-Frey
Sauerbruch-Lebsche
Semb
Shoemaker
Stille
Stille-Giertz
Stille-Horsley
Thompson
Thomsen rib
Tudor-Edwards
Walton

RIB SPREADERS

Burford-Finochietto
Davis modified Finochietto
DeBakey infant and child
Finochietto
Gerbode modified Burford
Haight
Harken
Hertzler
Lefferts
Lilienthal
Lilienthal-Sauerbruch
McGuire
Miltex
Nelson
Overholt
Overholt-Finochietto
Reinhoff
Reinhoff-Finochietto
Nissen
Sauerbruch-Lilienthal
Sweet
Sweet-Burford
Theis infant
Tuffier
Tudor-Edwards
Wilson

RINGS

Bonaccolto flieringa scleral

ROD

Knodt distraction
Stenzel fracture

ROLLER

Spence cranioplastic

RONGEURS

Adson bone
Andrews-Hartmann
Bacon bone
Bailey aortic valve
Bane
Beyer bone
Beyer endaural (ear)
Blumenthal
Bogle
Bruening-Citelli
Cairns
Campbell laminectomy
Carroll
Cherry-Kerrison laminectomy
Cicherelli
Citelli
Cloward I.V. disc
Cloward pituitary
Colclough laminectomy
Converse nasal
Cranial bone
Cushing bone
Dean bone
Dench
DePuy pituitary
Devilbiss cranial
Duckbill
Dufourmental nasal
Duggan
Echlin duckbill
Falconers
Ferris-Smith pituitary
Ferris-Smith-Gruenwald
Ferris-Smith-Kerrison
Ferris-Smith-Takahashi
Fulton
Glasgow pattern
Glover
Gruenwald pituitary
Hajek antrum
Hakansson
Hartmann bone
Hartmann ear
Hartmann-Herzfeld ear
Hein
Henny laminectomy
Hoen laminectomy
Hoffmann ear
Horsley bone
Houghton
Husks mastoid
Ivy mastoid
Jansen
Jansen bayonet
Jansen-Zaufel
Juers-Lempert endaural
Kerrison
Kerrison-Costen
Kerrison mastoid
Killearn
Lebsche
Leksell laminectomy
Lempert bone
Lempert endaural
Lilly
Littauer
Lombard
Lombard-Beyer
Lombard-Boies mastoid
Love-Gruenwald pituitary
Love-Kerrison
Luer
Luer-Hartmann
Meade bone
Montenovesi double action cranial
Nichols infundibulectomy
Noyes
O'Brien
Oldberg pituitary
Olivecrona endaural
Pennybacker
Pierce
Poppen pituitary
Prince
Raaf-Oldberg
Raney

SURGICAL INSTRUMENTS AND EQUIPMENT

RONGEURS (continued)

Reiner
Rowland nasal
Ruskin bone
Ruskin duckbill
Ruskin mastoid
Ruskin multiple action
St. Luke's double action
Sauerbruch
Sauerbruch-Coryllos rib
Sauerbruch-Lebsche
Scaglietti
Schlesinger
Schwartz-Kerrison
Selverstone I.V. disc
Semb
Semb-Sauerbruch
Shearer chicken bill
Smith-Petersen
Spurling-Kerrison (Colclough)

Spurling laminectomy
Spurling pituitary
Spurling-Love-Gruenwald-Cushing
Stille
Stille-Leksell
Stille-Luer
Stookey
Strully-Kerrison
Strümpel (Struempel)
Taper jaw
Tobey ear
Von Seemen
Voris I.V. disc
Walton
Watson-Williams I.V. disc
Weil pituitary
Weingartner
Whiting mastoid
Zaufel-Jansen

RULERS

Berndt hip
Chernow notched
Joseph measuring
Metal

Millimeter
Pischel scleral
Tabb
Walker scleral

SAFETY PIN CLOSER

Clerf-Arrowsmith

SAWS

Adams, W.
Albee
Bailey-Gigli
Becker-Joseph
Bishop oscillatory electric bone
Bosworth
Brown
Butcher
Chain
Charriere aseptic metacarpal
Clerf laryngeal
Converse
Crego-Gigli
Crown

Electric laryngofissure
Engel plaster
Farabeuf
Gigli
Gigli wire
Gottschalk transverse
Hetherington circular
Hey skull
Hub
Joseph bayonet
Joseph-Maltz angular
Joseph nasal
Lamont nasal
Langenbeck metacarpal

SAWS (continued)

Lell laryngofissure
Luck bone
Magnuson circular twin
Magnuson double counter-rotating
Magnuson single circular
Maltz bayonet
Mueller
Myerson laryngectomy
Rotary hub
Satterlee amputating
Satterlee aseptic
Seltzer
Shrady
Silver
Slaughter nasal
Stille Gigli wire saw
Stryker
Tyler spiral Gigli
V. M. & Co. amputating
Wigmore plaster
Woakes nasal

SCARIFIER

Desmarres'

SCISSORS

Ada
Adson
Aebli
Alligator
American pattern umbilical
Atkinson-Walker
Ball tipped
Baltimore nasal
Bantham wire cutting
Barraquer-DeWecker iris
Baruch circumcision
Beaded tip
Becker septum
Berens iridocapsulotomy
Blanco
Blum arterial
Boettcher tonsil
Bowman strabismus
Boyd dissecting
Braun episiotomy
Brooks gallbladder
Brophy
Brown
Buerger-McCarthy
Buie rectal
Bull dog
Burnham
Busch umbilical
Canalicular
Cannula
Castroviejo corneal
Caylor
Chevalier Jackson
Church pediatric
Classon pediatric
Converse
Cottle bull dog
Cottle dorsal
Cottle nasal
Crafoord lung
Craig
Craniotomy
Crown & collar
Curved-on-flat
Dandy trigeminus
Dean dissecting
Dean tonsil
Deaver
DeBakey endarterectomy
DeBakey stitch
DeBakey-Metzenbaum
DeMartel vascular
deWecker iris
deWecker-Pritikin iris
Doyen abdominal
Dubois decapitation
Duffield
Dumont thoracic
Emmet uterine
Enucleation
Esmarch
Essrig dissecting

SCISSORS (continued)

Federspiel
Ferguson abdominal
Ferguson-Metzenbaum
Finochietto
Fomon saber back
Frahur
Frazier dura
Fulton pediatric
Gauze
Gillies suture
Good tonsil
Graham pediatric
Guggenheim
Guillotine
Guist enucleation
Guyton
Haimovici arteriotomy
Harrington
Heath suture and wire cutting
Heyman nasal
Hoen laminectomy
Holinger curved
Hooper pediatrics
House
Huey
Iris
Irvine
Jackson esophageal
Jackson laryngeal
Jackson turbinate
Jacobson
Jamison-Metzenbaum
Jones dissecting
Jorgenson
Joseph-Maltz
Kahn
Katzeff cartilage
Katzin corneal
Kelly
Knapp iris
Knapp strabismus
Knight nasal
Knowles
Kreuscher semilunar cartilage
LaGrange
Lahey
Lakeside

Lawton corneal
LeJeune laryngofissure
Lexer dissecting
Lillie tonsil
Lincoln pediatric
Lister
Liston plaster-of-Paris
Littauer
MacKenty
Maclay tonsil
Malis neurological
Mancusi-Ungaro
Martin ballpoint
Martin cartilage
Martin throat
Mattis
Maunoir
Mayo dissecting
Mayo round blade
Mayo-Harrington
Mayo-New
Mayo-Noble
Mayo-Potts dissecting
Mayo-Sims
Mayo-Stille
McAllister
McClure iris
McGuire corneal
McLean capsulotomy
McPherson-Castroviejo
McPherson-Vannas
McReynolds eye
Metzenbaum
Metzenbaum-Lipsett
Microscopic
Miller rectal
Mixter operating
Morse backward cutting aortic
Munro brain
Nelson lobectomy
New's
Noble
Northbent suture
Noyes iris
Noyes-Shambaugh
Nugent-Gradle
O'Brien-Mayo

SCISSORS (continued)

Ochsner ball tipped
Ochsner diamond edge
Olivecrona angular
Olivecrona guillotine
O'Neill cardiac
Panzer gallbladder
Poppen sympathectomy
Potts
Potts-Smith
Pratt rectal
Prince dissecting
Prince-Potts
Prince tonsil
Quimby gum
Ragnell
Reinhoff thoracic
Resano
Reynolds dissecting
Rochester-Ferguson
Saber back
Sadler cartilage
Satinsky vena cava
Schmeden
Schroeder operating
Schuknecht
Seiler turbinate
Serrated
Serratex
Shortbent
Sims uterine
Sistrunk dissecting
Smart enucleation
Smellie OB
Southbent

Spencer stitch
Stevens tenotomy
Strabismus
Straight
Strully hook
Sweet esophageal
Sweet delicate pituitary
Taylor dural
Tenotomy
Thorek
Thorek-Feldman gallbladder
Thorpe-Westcott cataract
Toennis
Vannas iridocapsulotomy
Verhoeff dissecting
Vezien abdominal
Waldmann episiotomy
Walker corneal
Walker-Apple
Walker-Atkinson
Walton
Weber tissue
Westcott tenotomy
Westcott-Scheie
Wester meniscectomy
White
Willauer
Wilmer iris
Wincor enucleation
Wullstein
Wutzler
Yankauer
Zoellner

SCLERA MARKER

Gonnin-Amsler

SCLEROTOMES

Alvis-Lancaster
Atkinson
Curdy
Guyton-Lundsgaard

Lancaster
Lundsgaard-Burch
Walker-Lee

SCOOPS

Arlt fenestrated lens
Beck abdominal

Berens common duct
Berens lens

SURGICAL INSTRUMENTS AND EQUIPMENT

SCOOPS (continued)

Daviel lens
Desjardin gall duct
Elschnig
Ferguson gallstone
Ferris common duct
Green lens
Hess lens
Knapp lens
Lang eye
Lewis lens

Luer fenestrated lens
Luer-Korte gallstone
Mayo common duct
Mayo-Robson gallstone
Moore gallstone
Moynihan gallstone
Mule's
Pagenstecher lens
Wells enucleation
Wilder lens

SCREWS

Basile hip
Bosworth coracoclavicular
Buttress thread
Carpal scaphoid
Carrell-Girard
Collison
Cruciate head
Cruciform head bone
Cubbins
Demuth hip
Doyen tumor
Duo-drive cortical
Eggers
Geckeler
Jewett pick-up
Johannsen lag
Kristiansen eyelet lag
Lag
Leinbach olecranon
Lorenzo

Lundholm
Marion
McLaughlin carpal scaphoid
Morris bi-phase
Phillips recessed head
Sherman bone
Sherman molybdenum
Stryker
Stryker type lag
Thatcher
Townley bone graft
Townsend-Gilfillan
Transfixion
Venable
Virgin hip
Vitallium
Wood
Woodruff
Zimmer

SCREW DRIVERS

Automatic
Becker
Children's Hospital
Collison
Cruciform
Cubbins bone
DePuy
Dorsey screw holding
Johnson
Lane
Lever type
Lok-it
Massie
Master

Moore-Blount
Phillips
Plain
Richter bone
Sherman
Sherman-Pierce
Stryker
Trinkle
V. M. & Co.
White
Williams
Woodruff
Zimmer

SEPARATORS

Benson pylorus
Davis nerve
Dorsey
Frazier dura
Grant dura
Harris
Hoen dura
Horsley dura
House ear
Hunter

Kirby:
   curved zonule
   cylindrical zonule
   Double ball
   Flat zonule
Luys, G.
Rosen bayonet (ear)
Sachs dura
Sachs nerve

SEPTUM STRAIGHTENERS

Asch
Cottle-Walsham

Walsham

SHEARS
Also see: Rib shears

Clayton laminectomy
Cooley-Pontius sternum
Diertz
Esmarch plaster
Gluck
Jackson esophageal
Jackson-Moore
Lebsche sternum

Liston
Pilling laryngofissure
Sauerbruch-Frey
Seutin plaster
Semb
Stille plaster
Weck

SHUNTS

Ames ventriculo-peritoneal
Pudenz ventriculo-atrial

Silastic ventriculo-peritoneal

SIGMOIDOSCOPES

Boehm
Buie
Frankfeldt
Kelly
Lieberman with swinging window
Montague

Solow
Turell
Tuttle
Vernon David
Visiline disposable
Welch Allyn

SKIDS

Davis
MacAusland hip
Meyerding
Murphy bone

Murphy-Lane
Ryerson bone
Scudder

SURGICAL INSTRUMENTS AND EQUIPMENT

SNARES

Alfred
Banner enucleation
Beck-Shenk tonsil
Boettcher-Farlow
Bosworth nasal
Brown tonsil
Bruening ear
Bruening nasal
Buerger
Castroviejo enucleation
Crapeau nasal
Douglas nasal
Douglas tonsil
Eves tonsil
Farlow tonsil
Farlow-Boettcher
Foerster enucleation
Frankfeldt rectal
Jarvis
Krause ear
Krause laryngeal
Krause nasal

Laryngeal
Lewis tonsil
Martin
Myles tonsillectome
Neivert-Eves
Nesbit tonsil
Newhart-Casselberry
Norwood
Pynchon ear
Quires mechanical finger
Reiner-Beck tonsil
Robert
Sage tonsil (automatic ratchet)
Stutsman nasal
Storz-Beck tonsil
Tydings automatic ratchet
Tydings tonsil
Weston rectal
Wilde-Bruening ear
Wilde-Bruening nasal
Wright nasal
Wright tonsil

SOUNDS

Bellocq
Benique
Campbell miniature
Davis interlocking
Dittel urethral
Fowler urethral
Gouley tunneled urethral
Guyon urethral
Guyon-Benique urethral
Hunt metal
Jewett urethral
Kocher bronchocele

Lacrimal
LeFort urethral
McCrea infant
Otis
Pratt urethral
Schroeder interlocking
Simpson uterine
Sims uterine
Van Buren urethral
Walther urethral
Woodward

SPATULAS

Castroviejo cyclodialysis
Cave scaphoid
Children's Hospital brain
Culler
Cushing brain
Davis brain
D'Errico brain

Dorsey
Elschnig cyclodialysis
Freer
Garron
Green
Gross brain
Jacobson endarterectomy

SPATULAS (continued)

Kirby iris
Knapp iris
Laird
Lindner cyclodialysis
Mayfield malleable brain
McReynolds
Meller cyclodialysis
O'Brien
Olivecrona brain
Paton
Peyton brain
Raaf flexible lighted
Roux
Sachs
Schuknecht

Scoville flat brain
Segond vaginal
Smith-Fisher cataract
Smith-Fisher iris
Smith-Green double end
Smith-Petersen
Suker cyclodialysis
Tauber vaginal
Thomas
Weary brain
Wecker iris
Wheeler cyclodialysis
Woodson
Wullstein transplant
Wurmuth

SPECULA (Speculum)

Adson
Allen-Heffernan nasal
Allingham rectal
Arruga eye
Aufricht septum
Aural
Auvard weighted vaginal
Auvard-Remine vaginal
Barr anal
Barr rectal
Barr-Shuford
Barraquer-Colibri eye
Beard eye
Beckman
Beckman-Colver nasal
Bedrossian eye
Berens eye
Berlind-Auvard
Bodenheimer
Bosworth nasal
Boucheron ear
Bozeman
Brewer vaginal
Brinkerhoff rectal
Bruner vaginal
Buie-Smith rectal
Carter septum
Castallo eye
Castroviejo eye
Chelsea-Eaton anal

Chevalier Jackson laryngeal
Coakley nasal
Coldlite
Coldlite-Graves vaginal
Collins vaginal
Converse nasal
Cook eye
Cook rectal
Cottle septum
Cusco vaginal
David rectal
DeLee
De Roaldes
Devilbiss vaginal
Devilbiss-Stacey
Douglas mucosa
Doyen vaginal
Duck billed
Dudley-Smith rectal
Duplay nasal
Duplay-Lynch nasal
Eaton nasal
Erhardt ear
Eye
Fansler rectal
Farkas urethral
Farrior ear
Fergusson tubular vaginal
Flannery ear
Flint glass

SURGICAL INSTRUMENTS AND EQUIPMENT

SPECULA (continued)

Forbes esophageal
Foster-Ballenger
Fox eye
Fränkel
Garrigue vaginal
Gerzog nasal
Gilbert-Graves
Gleason
Goldbacher anoscope
Goldstein septum
Graefe eye
Graves vaginal
Gruber ear
Guild-Pratt rectal
Guist eye
Guist-Black eye
Guttmann vaginal
Guyton-Park eye
Halle nasal
Halle-Tieck nasal
Hartmann nasal
Hartmann-Dewaxer
Heffernan nasal
Helmholtz
Helmont
Henrotin vaginal
Higbee vaginal
Hinckle-James rectal
Hood-Graves vaginal
Huffman infant vaginal
Huffman-Graves
Ingals nasal
Ives rectal
Jackson vaginal
Jonas-Graves vaginal
Kahn-Graves vaginal
Kelly rectal
Killian septum
Klaff septum
Kleen-spec disposable
Knapp eye
Kogan endospeculum
Kramer ear
Kristeller vaginal
Kyle nasal
Lancaster eye
Lancaster-O'Connor

Lang eye
Lawford
Lempert-Colver endaural
Lillie nasal
Lister-Burch eye
Luer eye
Macon Hospital
Mason-Auvard weighted vaginal
Mahoney intranasal antrum
Martin rectal
Mathew rectal
McHugh oval
McKinney
McLaughlin
McPherson eye
Mellinger eye
Metcher eye
Miller vaginal
Montgomery vaginal
Montgomery-Bernstine
Mosher nasal
Mosher urethral
Mueller
Murdock eye
Murdock-Wiener eye
Myles nasal
Myles-Ray
National ear
National Graves vaginal
Nott vaginal
Nott-Guttmann vaginal
Noyes
O'Sullivan-O'Connor vaginal
Park eye
Park-Guyton eye
Patton septum
Pederson vaginal
Pennington rectal
Picot
Pilling-Hartmann
Plain wire
Politzer ear
Pratt bivalve
Pratt rectal
Preefer eye
Pynchon nasal
Ray nasal

SPECULA (continued)

Richard Gruber
Roberts esophageal
Rosenthal urethral
Sauer eye
Scott ear
Senturia pharyngeal
Shoe horn
Siegle
Simmonds vaginal
Simrock
Sims rectal
Sims vaginal
Sluder sphenoidal
Smith anal
Smith eye
SMR
Sonnenschein nasal
Stearns
Storz septum
Steiner-Auvard
Stop eye
Sweeney posterior vaginal
Tauber

Taylor vaginal
Terson
Tieck
Tieck-Halle
Toynbee ear
Trelat
Troeltsch ear
Vauban
Vernon-David rectal
Vienna nasal
Voltolini
Von Graefe
Watson
Weeks eye
Weisman-Graves vaginal
Welch-Allyn
Wiener eye
Williams eye
Wire bivalve vaginal
Worchester City Hospital vaginal
Yankauer nasopharyngeal
Ziegler eye
Zower

SPHERE INTRODUCER

Allen

Carter

SPHINCTEROTOME

Doubilet

SPLINES

Bosworth

Rowland-Hughes osteotomy

SPLINTS

Abduction finger
Abduction thumb
Adam & Eve rib belt
Agnew
Airfoam
Airplane (aeroplane)
Alumafoam nasal
Aluminum fence
Aluminum finger cot

Anchor
Anderson, R.
Angle
Anterior acute flexion elbow
Asch nasal
Ashhurst leg
Balkan femoral
Ball-peen
Banjo

SURGICAL INSTRUMENTS AND EQUIPMENT

SPLINTS (continued)

Basswood
Bavarian
Baylor adjustable cross
Baylor metatarsal
Böhler wire
Böhler-Braun (King's traction)
Bond arm
Bowlly arm
Bracketed
Brant aluminum
Browne, Denis
Buck's extension, leg
Bunnell knuckle bender
Bunnell outrigger
Cabot leg
Calibrated clubfoot
Campbell airplane
Campbell traction humerus
Carl P. Jones traction
Carter intranasal
Chandler felt collar
Chatfield-Girdleston
Coaptation
Cock-up hand
Colles
Cramer wire
Culley ulna
Curry walking
Davis metacarpal
Denis Browne clubfoot
Denis Browne hip
DePuy
DePuy aeroplane
DePuy any angle
DePuy coaptation
DePuy open thimble
DePuy-Pott's
DePuy rocking leg
DePuy rolled Colles
Drop foot
Dupuytren's
Dynamic
Easton cock-up
Eggers contact
Engelmann thigh
Erich nasal

Fence
Ferciot tip toe
Fillauer night
Forrester head
Fox clavicle
Frac-Sur
Frejka
Fruehevald
Funsten supination
Gibson
Gilmer dental
Gooch
Gordon's Colle Fracture
Granberry's
Gunning (Jaw)
Hammond
Hand cock-up
Hart extension finger
Haynes-Griffin mandible
Hinged Thomas
Hirschtick utility shoulder
Hodgen hip
Hodgen leg
Infant abduction
Interdental
Jelenko
Jonell countertraction finger
Jonell thumb
Jones arm
Jones forearm & metacarpal
Jones nasal
Joseph septum
Kanavel cock-up
Kazanjian nasal
Keller-Blake half ring leg
Kerr abduction
Keystone
Lambrinudi
Levis arm
Lewin baseball finger
Lewin finger
Lewin-Stern thumb & finger
Liston
Live
Love nasal
Lytle metacarpal

SPLINTS (continued)

Magnuson abduction humerus
Mason
Mason-Allen universal hand
Mayer nasal
McGee
McIntire
Mohr finger
Murray-Jones arm
Murray-Thomas arm
Neubeiser adjustable forearm
O'Donaghue knee
O'Donaghue stirrup
Opponens
Orthopedic strap clavicle
Peabody
Phelps
Plaster
Ponseti
Poroplastic
Porzett
Pott's
Protecto
Putti
Quik splint
Roger Anderson well leg
Rumel aluminum bridge
Safety pin
Sayre
Scott humerus
Simpson sugar tong
Skin
Speed hand
Spigelman baseball finger
Stader
Strampelli eye
Strap clavicle
Stromeyer
Stuart Gordon hand
Sugar tong
Taylor
Teare arm
Therapeutic
Thomas full ring
Thomas hinged
Thomas knee
Thomas leg
Thomas posterior
Thompson modification of
    Denis Browne
T-finger
Tobruk
Toronto
Valentine
Volkmann
Wertheim
Yucca wood
Zimmer
Zimmer airplane
Zimmer clavicular cross
Zim-Zip rib belt
Zucker

SPOONS

Bunge exenteration
Coyne
Culler lens
Cushing pituitary
Cushing spatula
Daviel lens
Elschnig lens
Falk appendectomy
Fisher
Gross ear
Hatt
Hess lens
Hoke
Hoke-Roberts
Kalt eye
Kirby lens
Knapp lens
Kocher brain
Moore gallbladder
Ray brain
Royal
Skene uterine
Volkmann
Wells enucleation

SPREADERS
Also see: Rib spreaders

Blanco valve
Cloward vertebra
Gross ductus
Inge lamina
Kimpton vein
Lemmon sternal

Millin-Bacon bladder neck
Morris mitral valve
Tudor-Edwards
Turek spinous process
Ventura
Wiltberger spinous process

SPUDS

Alvis
Bennett foreign body
Corbett foreign body
Davis foreign body
Dix foreign body
Ellis foreign body
Fisher
Francis knife

Gross ear
Hosford foreign body
LaForce knife
Levine foreign body
Nicati foreign body
O'Brien foreign body
Walter corneal
Whittle

SPUR CRUSHERS

Baby
Berger
DeWitt-Stetten colostomy
Garlock
Gross
Mayo-Lovelace
Mikulicz

Ochsner-DeBakey
Pemberton
Stetten
Warthen
Wolfson
Wurth

STAPLES

Blount type
du Toit shoulder

Zimaloy epiphyseal

STERNAL APPROXIMATOR

Lemmon

Nunez

STONE BASKETS

Councill
Browne
Ferguson

Johnson
Robinson

STONE DISLODGERS

Councill
Creevy calyx
Davis modification of Councill
Dormia

Howard spiral
Howard-Flaherty spiral
Johnson stone
Johnson ureteral basket

STONE DISLODGERS (continued)

Levant
Mitchell ureteral
Morton
Ortved

Robinson
Woven loop
Wullen
Zeiss

STRIPPERS

Babcock jointed vein
Bartlett fascia
Brand tendon
Bunnell tendon
Cannon type
Carroll forearm tendon
Clark vein
Cole polyethylene vein
Crile vagotomy
Doyle vein
Dunlop
Emerson vein
Friedman vein
Joplin tendon
Keeley vein
Kurten vein
Lempka vein
Linton vein
Masson fascia
Matson rib

Matson-Alexander rib
Matson-Mead periosteum
Mayo vein
Mayo-Myers
Myers spiral vein
Nabatoff vein
Nelson rib
Nelson-Roberts
New Orleans
Phelan vein
Price-Thomas rib
Rib edge
Roberts-Nelson rib
Shaw carotid artery clot
Smith posterior cartilage
Trace hydraulic vein
Webb vein
Wilson vein
Wurth vein
Wylie endarterectomy

SUCTION TUBES

Adson brain
Anderson flexible
Andrews-Pynchon
Anthony mastoid
Asepto
Baron
Bel-O-Pak
Buie
Buyes air-vent
Chaffin-Pratt bedside
Cone
Cook County tracheal
Cooley
Coupland
DeBakey
Devilbiss
Fay suction elevator

Fitzpatrick
Frazier brain
Gomco
Gwathmey
Hemovac
Hossli
Hough-Cadogan
House
Humphrey coronary sinus sucker
Immergut
Kay-Cross suction tip
Lezius
Lore
Madoff
Mason
McKesson suction bottle unit
Millin

SUCTION TUBES (continued)

Morse
Morse-Andrews
Morse-Ferguson
Mosher life saving
Mueller-Frazier
Mueller-Pool
Mueller-Pynchon
Mueller tip-trol
Mueller-Yankauer
N.Y. glass
O'Hanlon-Pool
Pleur-evac
Pool abdominal
Pool pediatric
Porto-vac
Pribram
Pynchon
Redi-vacette
Sachs
Samson-Davis infant
Silastic sucker
Snyder hemovac
Stedman continuous
Underwater seal
Weck
Yankauer
Yeder

SUSPENSION APPARATUS

Killian suspension gallows
Lewy
Lynch

TAMP

Kiene bone

TELESCOPES

Atkins esophagoscopic
Best direct forward vision
Burns bridge
Clamp on
Fiber optic right angle examining
Foroblique
Kramer direct vision
McCarthy foroblique operating
McCarthy miniature
Negus
Retrospective
Transilluminating
Tucker direct vision
Vest direct forward vision
Walden

TENACULUMS

Adair breast or uterine
Barrett uterine
Braun uterine
Brophy
Corey
Cottle
Duplay uterine
Emmet
Jackson tracheal
Jacob uterine
Jarcho
Kahn traction
Lahey goiter
Potts
Revots vulsellum
Ritchie cleft palate
Schroeder
Skene uterine
Staude-Moore
Straight's
Thoms
Watts
Weisman

TENOTOME

Ryerson

TENDON PASSERS

Bunnell
Carroll
Gallie

Joplin
Ober
Withers

TENDON STRIPPERS
See: Strippers

TENDON TUCKERS
See: Tuckers

THERMOPORE

Shahan

THERMOSECTOR

Thermosector electrosurgical unit

THORACOTOME

Bettman-Forvash

THORACOSCOPES

Coryllos
Cutler forceps
Jacobaeus

Jacobaeus-Unverricht
Moore
Sarot

TONG (Traction)

Barton traction
Barton-Cone
Böhler

Cherry
Crutchfield skull
Raney-Crutchfield skull

TONGUE DEPRESSORS

Andrews
Andrews-Pynchon
Balmer
Beatty
Blakesley
Boebinger
Bosworth
Chamberlain
Colver-Dawson

Dorsey
Farlow
Granberry
Hamilton
Israel
Jobson-Pynchon
Kellogg
Layman
Lewis

SURGICAL INSTRUMENTS AND EQUIPMENT

TONGUE DEPRESSORS (continued)

Mullins
Oral screw
Pirquet
Proetz
Pynchon
Pynchon-Lillie
Titus
Weder

TONOMETERS

Bailliart
Gartner
Goldman applanation
McLean
Mueller electronic
Musken
Nuvistor electronic
Recklinghausen
Schiotz
Sklar

TONSILLECTOMES

Ballenger-Sluder
Beck-Mueller
Beck-Schenck
Brown
Daniels hemostatic
Hemostatic
LaForce
Mack lingual tonsil
Meding tonsil enucleator
Moltz-Storz
Myles guillotine
Sauer
Sauer-Sluder
Searcy
Sluder
Sluder-Ballenger
Sluder-Demarest
Sluder-Sauer
Tydings
Van Osdel tonsil enucleator
Whiting

TOURNIQUETS

Adams modification of Bethune
Automatic
Bethune lung
Campbell-Boyd
Carr lobectomy
Conn pneumatic
Conn universal
Dupuytren
Esmarch
Field
Fouli
Horseshoe
Ideal
Kidde
Kidde-Robbins
Linton
Momberg
Petit
Pneumatic
Robbins automatic
Roberts-Nelson lobectomy
Rumel cardiovascular
Rumel-Belmont
Samway
Signorini
Truesdale
Universal
Velket Velcro
Weiner

TRACHELOTOME

Spencer

TRACHEOSCOPE

Haslinger
Jackson

TRACHEOTOMES

Salvatore-Maloney
Sierra-Sheldon

TRACTION BOWS

Anderson
Bendixen-Kirschner
Boehler (Böhler)
Crego-McCarroll
Granberry finger
Keys-Kirschner
Logan
Pease-Thomson
Beaded wires
Petersen skeletal

TRACTORS

Anderson
Barton-Cone traction
Blackburn skull traction
Boehler (Böhler)
Buck's extension
Cherry traction
Freiberg traction
Gerster traction bar
Handy-Buck's extension
Hoke-Martin
Kestler ambulatory head
Kirschner wire
Lowsley prostatic
Moleskin traction
Nauth os calcis apparatus
Orr-Buck's extension
Perkins
Pugh
Rankin prostatic
Rocking chair truck
Russell traction
Russell-Buck's extension
Steinmann traction
Syms's
Vinke skull
Watson-Jones
Wells tractor
Young prostatic

TRANSILLUMINATORS

All purpose
Briggs
Finnoff
Hooded
National all-metal
National opal glass
Rotating
Speculum illuminator
Tatum ureteral
Widner

TREPHINES

Arruga eye
Barraquer corneal
Becker skull
Blackburn
Blakesley lacrimal
Boiler septum
Brown-Pusey corneal
Castroviejo corneal
Cross scleral
Damshek sternal
D'Errico skull
Devilbiss skull
Dimitry chalazion
Dimitry dacryocystorhinostomy

TREPHINES (continued)

Elliot corneal
Galt skull
Gradle corneal
Green automatic corneal
Greenwood spinal
Grieshaber corneal
Hand
Harris
Hippel
Horsley
Jentzer
Lahey Clinic skull
Lichtenberg corneal
Lorie antrum
Michele

Mueller electric corneal
Paton corneal
Paufique corneal
Polley-Bickel
Schuknecht temporal
Scoville skull
Searcy chalazion
Sidney Stephenson corneal
Stille
Thornwald antrum
Turkel
Walker corneal
Wilder
Wilkins

TROCARS

Allen cecostomy
Arbuckle-Shea
Babcock empyema
Barnes internal decompression
Beardsley cecostomy
Birch
Boettcher antrum
Campbell suprapubic
Charlton antrum
Coakley antrum
Curschmann
Davidson
Dean antrum
Denker
Diederich empyema
Douglas antrum
Duchenne's
Duke
Durham tracheotomy
Emmet ovarian
Faulkner
Fein antrum
Frazier brain exploring
Gallagher
Hargin antrum
Hunt
Hurwitz
Intercostal

Judd
Kidd
Kolb
Kreutzmann
Lichtwicz antrum
Lillie antrum
Livermore
Morson
Myerson antrum
Neal catheter trocar
Nelson
Nested
Ochsner gallbladder
Paterson
Pierce antrum
Pierce-Kyle
Plain vesical
Potain aspirating
Pool
Rectal
Ruskin
Sewall antrum
Singleton's empyema
Southey anasarca
Southey-Leech
Sweet antrum
Van Alyea
Walther aspirating bladder

TROCARS (continued)

Wangensteen internal decompression
Wiener-Pierce antrum
Wilson amniotic

Wright-Harloe empyema
Yankauer antrum

TUBES
Also see: Suction Tubes

Abbott
Abbott-Rawson
Alesen
Arrow
Ayre
Bardic
Beall, Feldman, Cooley sump
Beardsley empyema
Bellocq
Bettman empyema
Billroth
Blakemore nasogastric
Blakemore-Sengstaken
Bouchut laryngeal
Broyles esophagoscope
Bruecke
Buie
Buyes air-vent suction
Cantor
Carabelli endobronchial
Carman rectal
Carrel
Cattell forked type T-tube
Celestin endoesophageal
Chaussier
Colton empyema
Coolidge
Davol
Deaver T-tube
Debove
Denker
DePaul
Dr. Bruecke aspirating
Dr. Twiss duodenal
Donaldson eustachian
Duke
Duralite
Durham tracheostomy
Einhorn
Ewald

Greiling gastroduodenal
Holinger trachea
Honor-Smathers double lumen
House endolymphatic
Houser
Jackson cone shaped tracheal
Jackson velvet eye
Jackson warning stop
Javid bypass
Johnson intestinal
Jutte
Kaslow
Kelly
Kidd U-tube, bladder
Killian
Kistner plastic tracheostomy
Kozlowski
Kuhn endotracheal
LaRocca nasolacrimal
Lahey Y-tube
Leiter
Lell trachea
Lepley-Ernst
Levin duodenal
Lewis laryngectomy
Lindeman-Silverstein
Linton
Lonnecken
Lord-Blakemore
Lore-Lawrence tracheotomy
Luer speaking
Luer trachea
Lyon
MacKenty laryngectomy
Mackler intraluminal
Magill
Martin tracheotomy
McGowan-Keeley
McMurtry-Schlesinger shunt
Miller, T.G.

SURGICAL INSTRUMENTS AND EQUIPMENT

TUBES (continued)

Miller-Abbott double lumen intestinal
Mixter
Momburg
Morch type swivel tracheostomy
Mosher
Muldoon
Nachlas gastrointestinal
Nephrostomy
Neuber bone
Nunez ventricular ventilation
O'Beirne sphincter
Ochsner gallbladder
O'Dwyer
Paul, F.T. intestinal drainage
Paul-Mixter
Pierce antrum wash
Pilling duralite
Polisar-Lyons adapted trachea
Polyvinyl
Polyethylene
Puestow-Olander G.I.
Rehfuss duodenal
Rochester trachea
Rusch
Ryle duodenal
Sachs
Schall laryngectomy
Sengstaken nasogastric
Sengstaken-Blakemore
Sheehy collar button
Southey capillary drainage
Souttar
T-tube
Toynbee diagnostic
Tucker flexible tip
Tucker tracheal
Turkel
Valentine irrigation
Vernon antrum wash
Voltolini ear
Von Eichen antrum wash
Wangensteen
Webster infusion
Welch Allyn
Wendl
Winsburg-White bladder
Yankauer
Zyler

TUCKERS

Bishop tendon
Bishop-Black tendon
Bishop-DeWitt tendon
Bishop-Peter tendon
Burch-Greenwood tendon
Fink tendon
Green strabismus
Harrison
Smuckler
Wayne

TUNNELER

Crawford-Cooley
DeBakey

TURNBUCKLE

Giannestras

URETHROTOMES

Otis
W.A. Keitzer infant

VAGINOSCOPE

Huffman infant

VALVULOTOMES

Bakst
Brock
Chalnot
Derra
Dogliotti
Gohrbrand
Harken
Himmelstein pulmonary

Longmire
Longmire-Muller curved
Malm-Himmelstein pulmonary
Niedner
Potts expansile
Potts-Riker
Sellor
Universal malleable

VECTIS

Torpin

WHISTLES

Barany noise apparatus

Galton ear

WIRE

Kirschner

WIRE CRIMPER

Gruppe
McGee

McGee-Caparosa

WRENCHES

Hexagonal
Hex socket
Kurlander orthopedic

Petersen fracture
Thomas
Waldon

Section II-Anatomy

6 The Anatomy of Structure, Circulation and Innervation

Regional anatomy is alphabetically listed under the specialty sections in this book to assist the secretary with transcription of anatomic terms. The anatomy of the musculoskeletal system, circulatory system and peripheral nervous system cannot be limited to any one specialty exclusively. In order to obviate duplication, alphabetically arranged tables of ARTERIES, VEINS, BONES, JOINTS, LIGAMENTS, MUSCLES AND NERVES are listed in this chapter. These tables are designed to provide a ready reference for transcription purposes.

NB: Although the tables listing anatomic structures in the following pages show the first letter of each item capitalized, in context the English version of anatomic terms is used with the lower-case. Structures named after individuals in these tables are used with the upper-case as are the proper (B.N.A.) names of muscles.

CIRCULATION

A survey of the circulatory system in the body provides an appreciation of the role of the arteries and veins in this circuit. Venous blood enters the right atrium (auricle) of the heart, passes to the right ventricle, is pumped to the lungs by way of the pulmonary artery and into the pulmonary capillaries. In the capillaries of the lung, carbon dioxide is given off and oxygen is absorbed. The oxygenated blood is returned to the left atrium of the heart by the pulmonary veins. The blood then passes into the left ventricle from which it is pumped out into the aorta, arteries and capillaries. In the arterial capillaries, oxygen is given up to the tissues and carbon dioxide is absorbed. The blood then passes into the venous system and with its collection of carbon dioxide and metabolic wastes, is returned by the veins to the venae cavae. It is then carried back into the heart through the right atrium.

Blood Circuit:

right atrium — right ventricle — pulmonary artery — pulmonary capillaries — pulmonary veins — left atrium — left ventricle — aorta — arteries — capillaries throughout the body and into the venous system — venae cavae — right atrium of heart.

The circuit from the heart, through the lungs and back to the heart is called the pulmonary (lesser) circulation. The course of the blood from the left ventricle out into the tissues and back to the right atrium of the heart is termed the systemic (greater) circulation. The systemic circulation time in an adult is about 23 seconds.

The volume of blood in the body is related to body weight. The blood volume, in pints, may be approximated by dividing the body weight in pounds by 14.

Blood pressure is a measure of the pressure of the blood on the walls of the arteries and is expressed as the systolic (maximum) pressure over the diastolic (minimum) pressure. The systolic arterial blood pressure rises during excitement or activity and falls during sleep. In a normal relaxed adult it is between 110 and 145 mm. of mercury.

ARTERIES

Acetabular
Acromial
Acromiothoracic
Alar (nose)
Alveolar
Angular
Anterior, superior, dental
Aorta, arch
Aorta, ascending
Aorta, thoracic
Appendicular
Arciform
Arcuate, of foot
Arcuate, of kidney
Auditory
Auricular, anterior
Auricular, posterior
Axillary
Azygos, of vagina
Basilar
Brachial
Bronchial
Buccal
Buccinator

Calcaneal
Calcarine
Caroticotympanic
Carotid, common
Carotid external
Carotid, internal
Carpal
Cavernous
Cecal
Celiac
Central, of retina
Cerebellar, inferior, anterior
Cerebellar, superior
Cerebral, anterior
Cerebral, middle
Cerebral, posterior
Cervical, ascending
Cervical, deep
Cervical, transverse
Charcot's
Choroid
Ciliary
Circumflex, of fibula
Circumflex, of humerus

ARTERIES (Continued)

Circumflex, iliac
Circumflex, lateral of thigh
Circumflex, medial of thigh
Circumflex, of scapula
Clitoral
Colic
Collateral
Common carotid
Communicating
Conjunctival
Coronary
Cortical
Costocervical
Cricothyroid
Crural
Cystic
Deferential
Dental
Digital, of fingers
Digital, of toes
Diploic
Dorsal, of clitoris
Dorsal, of feet
Dorsal, of nose
Dorsal, of penis
Epigastric
Episcleral
Esophageal
Ethmoidal
External carotid
Femoral
Frontal
Gastric
Gastroduodenal
Gastroepiploic
Genicular
Glaserian
Gluteal
Hemorrhoidal
Hepatic
Hepatic, proper
Humeral
Hypophyseal
Ileal
Ileocolic
Iliac, common

Iliac, external
Iliac, internal
Iliolumbar
Inferior dental
Inferior hemorrhoidal
Inferior mesenteric
Inferior pancreatic
Infraorbital
Infrascapular
Innominate
Intercostal
Interlobar, of kidney
Interlobular, of kidney
Internal carotid
Interosseous, common
Interosseous, dorsal
Interosseous, recurrent
Interosseous, volar
Interventricular
Intestinal
Jejunal
Labial
Lacrimal
Laryngeal
Lateral nasal
Lateral striate
Lenticular
Lenticulostriate
Lienal
Lingual
Lumbar
Macular
Malleolar
Mammary, internal
Mandibular
Marginal
Masseteric
Mastoid
Maxillary
Medial striate
Median
Mediastinal
Medullary
Meningeal
Mental
Mesenteric

ARTERIES (Continued)

Metacarpal, dorsal
Metacarpal, volar
Metatarsal, dorsal
Metatarsal, plantar
Musculophrenic
Neubauer's
Nutrient, of femur
Nutrient, of fibula
Nutrient, of humerus
Nutrient, of tibia
Obturator
Occipital
Omphalomesenteric
Ophthalmic
Ovarian
Palatine, ascending
Palatine, descending
Palmar
Palpebral, lateral
Palpebral, medial
Pancreatic
Pancreaticoduodenal
Perforating, of thigh
Pericardiacophrenic
Perineal
Peroneal, of tibia
Pharyngeal
Phrenic, inferior
Phrenic, superior
Plantar
Pontine
Popliteal
Posterior dental
Posterior pancreaticoduodenal
Principal, of thumb
Principal, of pterygoid canal
Pubic
Pudendal
Pulmonary
Pyloric
Quadriceps
Radial
Radicular
Ranine
Recurrent, radial
Recurrent, tibial
Recurrent, ulnar
Renal
Sacral
Scapular
Scrotal
Septal, of nose
Sigmoid
Somatic
Spermatic
Sphenopalatine
Spinal
Spiral
Splanchnic
Splenic
Stapedial
Sternal
Sternocleidomastoid
Sternomastoid
Striate
Stylomastoid
Subclavian
Subcostal
Sublingual
Submental
Subscapular
Sulcal
Supraorbital
Suprarenal
Sural
Tarsal
Temporal
Terminal
Testicular
Thoracic, long
Thoracoacromial
Thoracodorsal
Thymic
Thyrocervical
Thyroid
Tibial
Tonsillar
Transverse, scapular
Transverse, of face
Transverse, of neck
Tympanic
Ulnar

STRUCTURE, CIRCULATION AND INNERVATION

ARTERIES (Continued)

Umbilical
Urethral
Uterine
Vaginal
Vertebral
Vesical
Volar, digital, common

Volar, digital, proper
Volar, radial, index finger
Wilkie's
Willis
Zinn's
Zygomatico-orbital

VEINS

Accessory, cephalic
Accessory, hemiazygos
Accessory, saphenous
Angular
Anterior auricular
Anterior bronchiole
Anterior coronary
Anterior facial
Anterior jugular
Anterior mediastinal
Anterior parotid
Anterior tibial
Anterior vertebral
Articular, of knee
Articular, of mandible
Ascending lumbar
Axillary
Azygos
Basilic
Basivertebral
Brachial
Bronchial
Cephalic
Cerebellar
Cerebral
Choroid
Colic
Comitans lateralis
Comitans medialis
Common digital
Common facial
Common iliac
Coronary
Coronary, of the stomach
Costoaxillary
Cystic
Deep

Deep cervical
Deep circumflex iliac
Deep femoral
Deep iliac circumflex
Deferentiales
Dental
Digital
Diploic
Dorsal digital of hand
Dorsal digital of foot
Dorsal metacarpal
Dorsal metatarsal
Dorsal, of penis
Ductus venosus
Duodenal
Emissary
Esophageal
External iliac
External jugular
External nasal
External pudic
Femoral
Femoropopliteal
Frontal
Galen
Gastroepiploic
Gluteal
Great cardiac
Great saphenous
Hemiazygos
Hepatic
Hypogastric
Ileocolic
Iliolumbar
Inferior epigastric
Inferior gluteal
Inferior mesenteric

VEINS (Continued)

Inferior ophthalmic
Inferior palpebral
Inferior petrosal sinus
Inferior phrenic
Inferior thyroid
Inferior vena cava
Innominate
Intercapitular
Intercostal
Internal auditory
Internal circumflex
Internal iliac
Internal jugular
Internal mammary
Internal maxillary
Internal pudendal
Internal pudic
Internal vertebral
Intervertebral
Jugular, external
Labial
Lateral circumflex femoral
Lateral plantar
Lateral sacral
Left coronary
Lienal (splenic)
Lingual
Long thoracic
Lumbar
Marginal, right
Medial plantar
Median
Median antebrachial
Median temporal
Mediana cubiti
Meningeal
Metacarpal
Middle cardiac
Middle colic
Middle hemorrhoidal
Middle sacral
Musculophrenic
Nasofrontal
Obturator
Occipital
Ophthalmic, inferior

Ophthalmic, superior
Orbital
Ovarian
Palatine
Palmar digital
Palmar metacarpal
Pancreatic
Pancreaticoduodenal
Paraumbilical
Pericardial
Peroneal
Pharyngeal
Plantar digital
Plantar metatarsal
Popliteal
Portal
Posterior auricular
Posterior bronchiole
Posterior external jugular
Posterior facial
Posterior mediastinal
Posterior parotid
Posterior scrotal
Posterior tibial
Prostatic
Pubic
Pudendal
Pyloric
Radial
Renal
Short gastric
Short saphenous
Sigmoid
Small cardiac
Small saphenous
Spermatic
Sphenopalatine
Sphenoparietal
Splenic
Stylomastoid
Subclavian
Subcutaneous abdominal
Subcutaneous thoracic
Superficial circumflex iliac
Superficial epigastric
Superficial, of penis

STRUCTURE, CIRCULATION AND INNERVATION

VEINS (Continued)

Superficial temporal
Superior epigastric
Superior gluteal
Superior hemorrhoidal
Superior mesenteric
Superior ophthalmic
Superior palpebral
Superior phrenic
Superior thyroid
Superior vena cava
Supraorbital
Suprarenal
Testicular
Thoracoepigastric

Transverse cervical
Transverse facial
Transverse scapular
Ulnar
Urethral
Uterine
Uterovaginal
Vaginal
Vein of cochlear canal
Vertebral
Vesical
Vesicular
Volar digital
Volar metacarpal

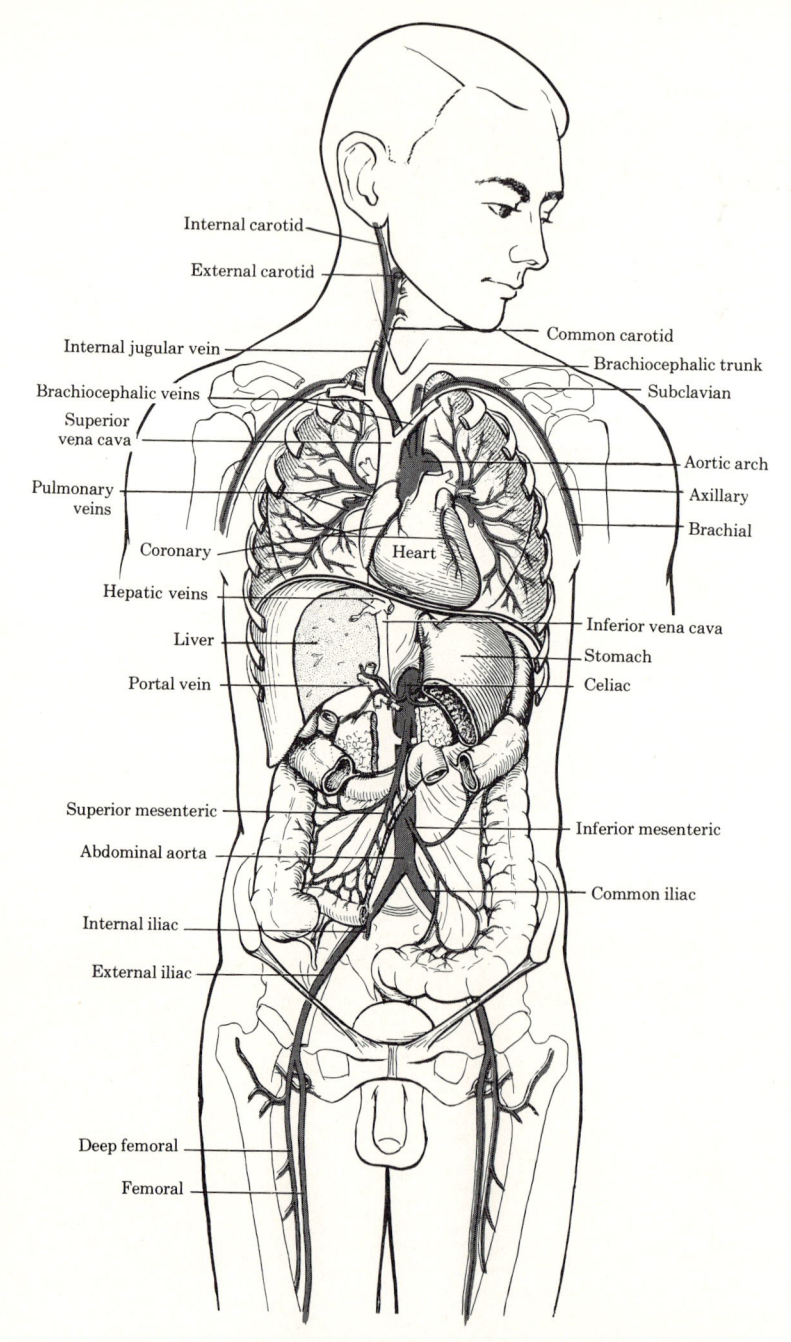

Figure 26 Principal Arteries of the Body and Pulmonary Veins
(From Dorland's Illustrated Medical Dictionary Courtesy W. B. Saunders Co.)

STRUCTURE, CIRCULATION AND INNERVATION 221

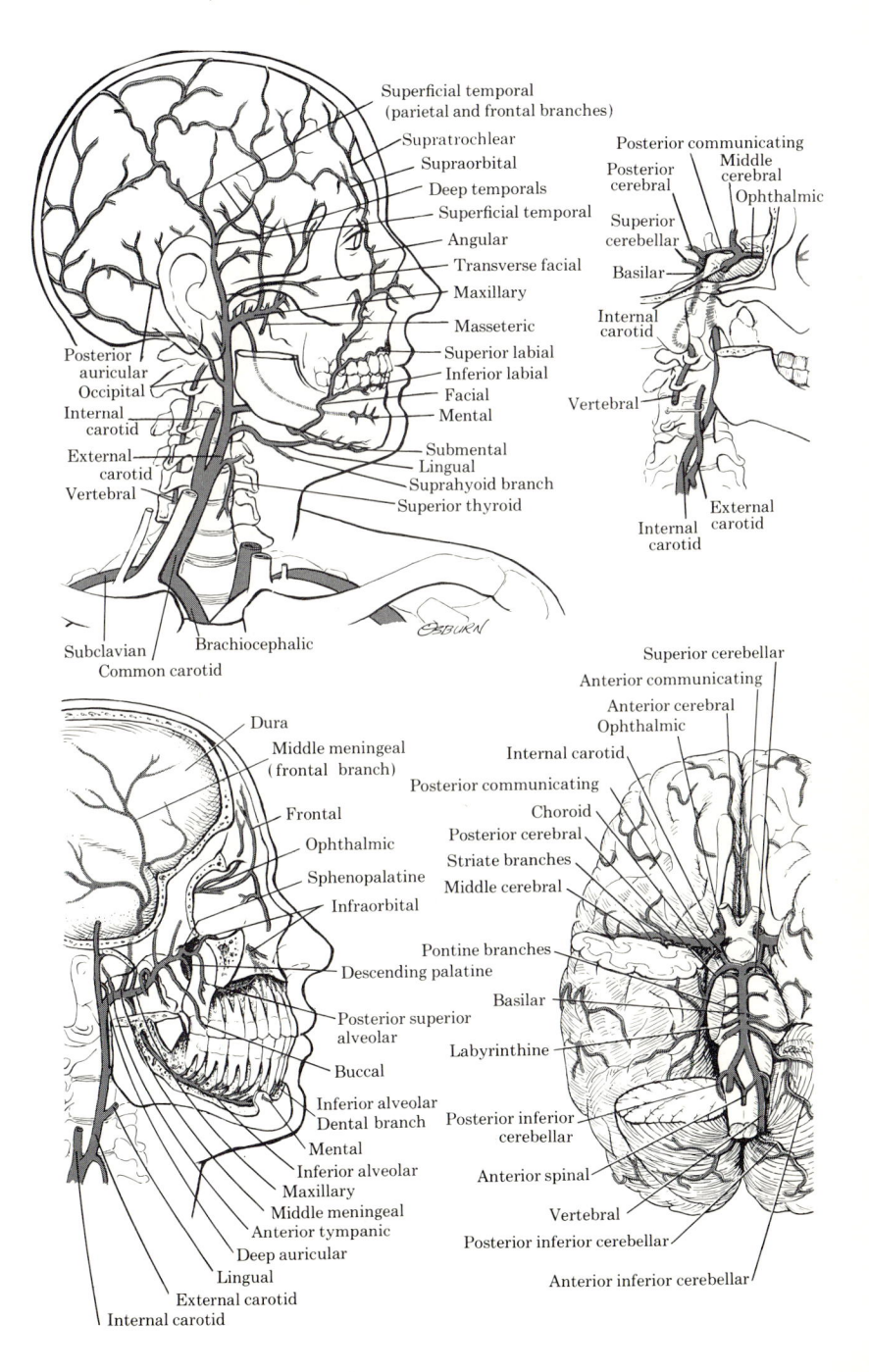

Figure 27 Arteries of the Head, Neck, and Base of the Brain
(From Dorland's Illustrated Medical Dictionary Courtesy W. B. Saunders Company)

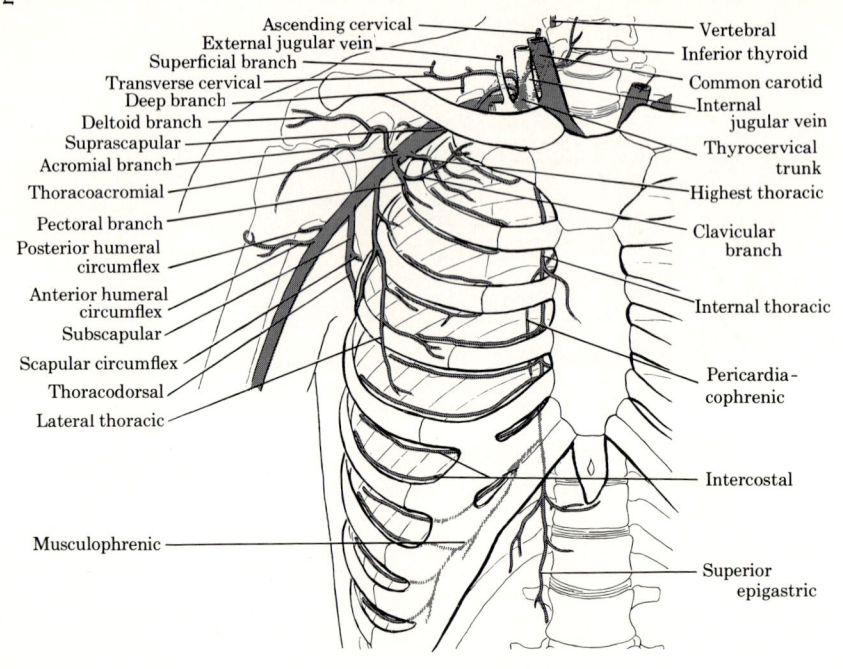

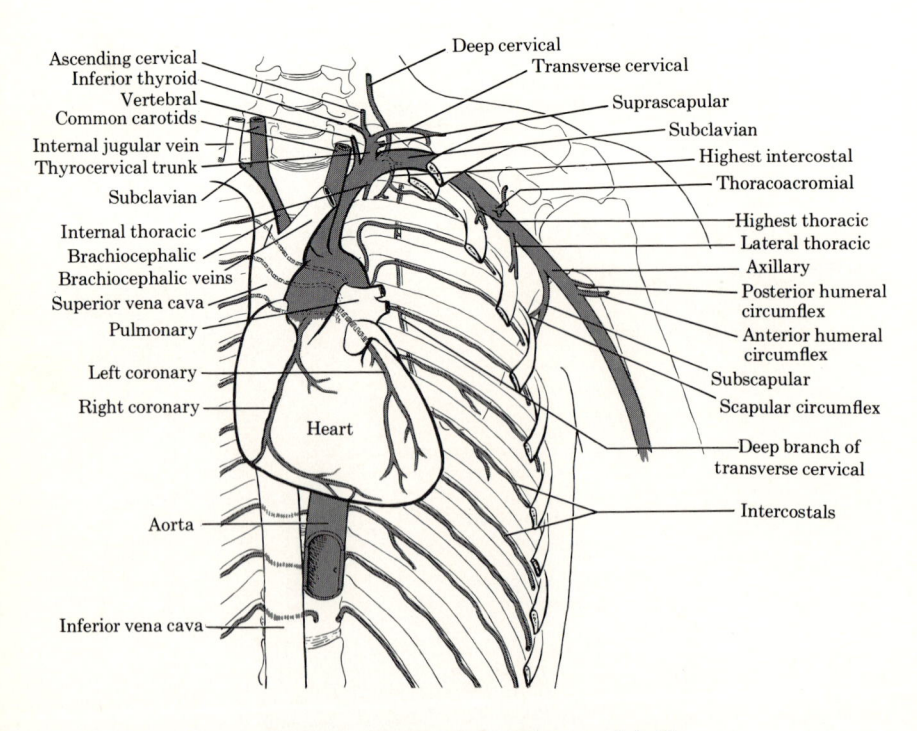

Figure 28   Arteries of the Thorax and Axilla
(From Dorland's Illustrated Medical Dictionary Courtesy W. B. Saunders Company)

STRUCTURE, CIRCULATION AND INNERVATION

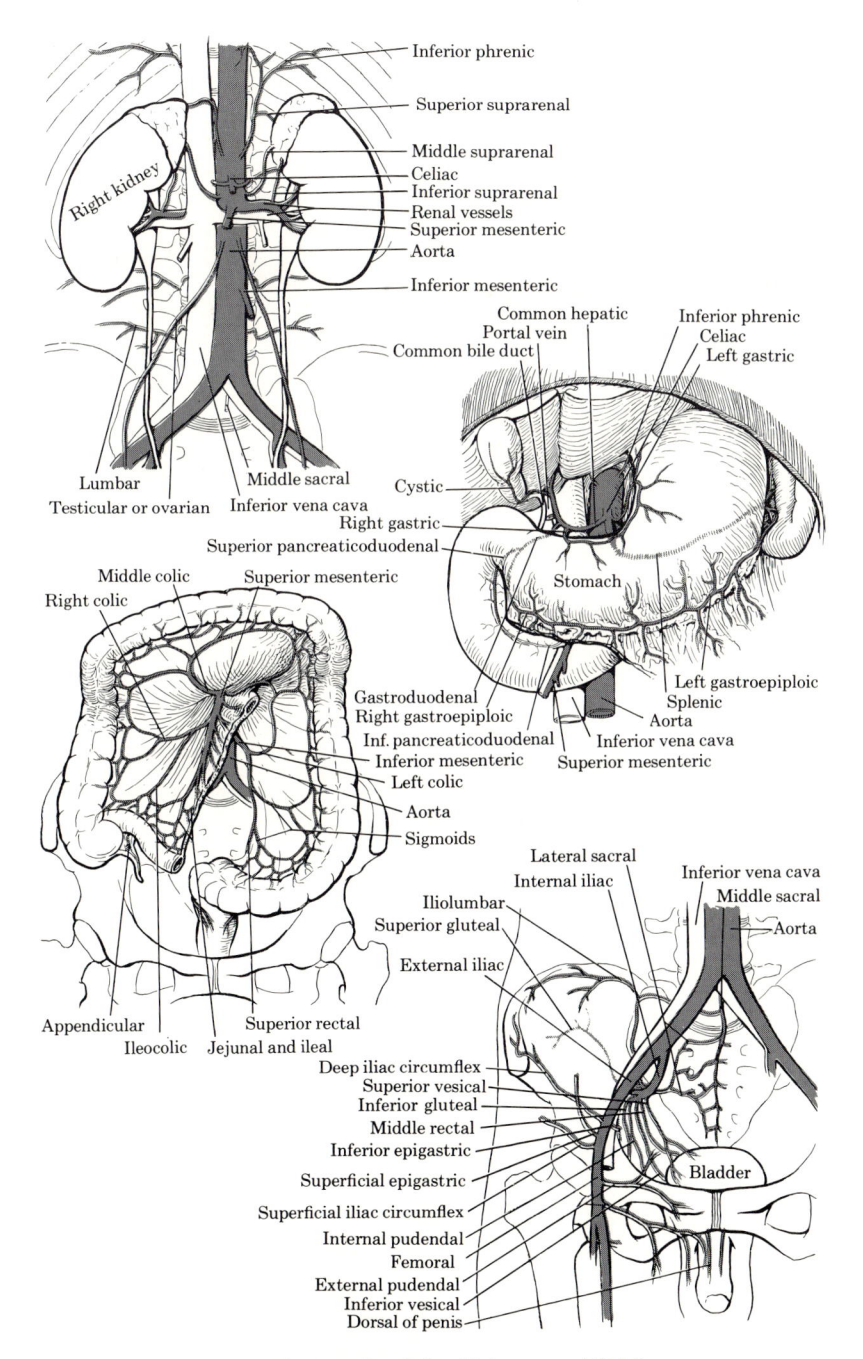

Figure 29 Arteries of the Abdomen and Pelvis
(From Dorland's Illustrated Medical Dictionary Courtesy W. B. Saunders Company)

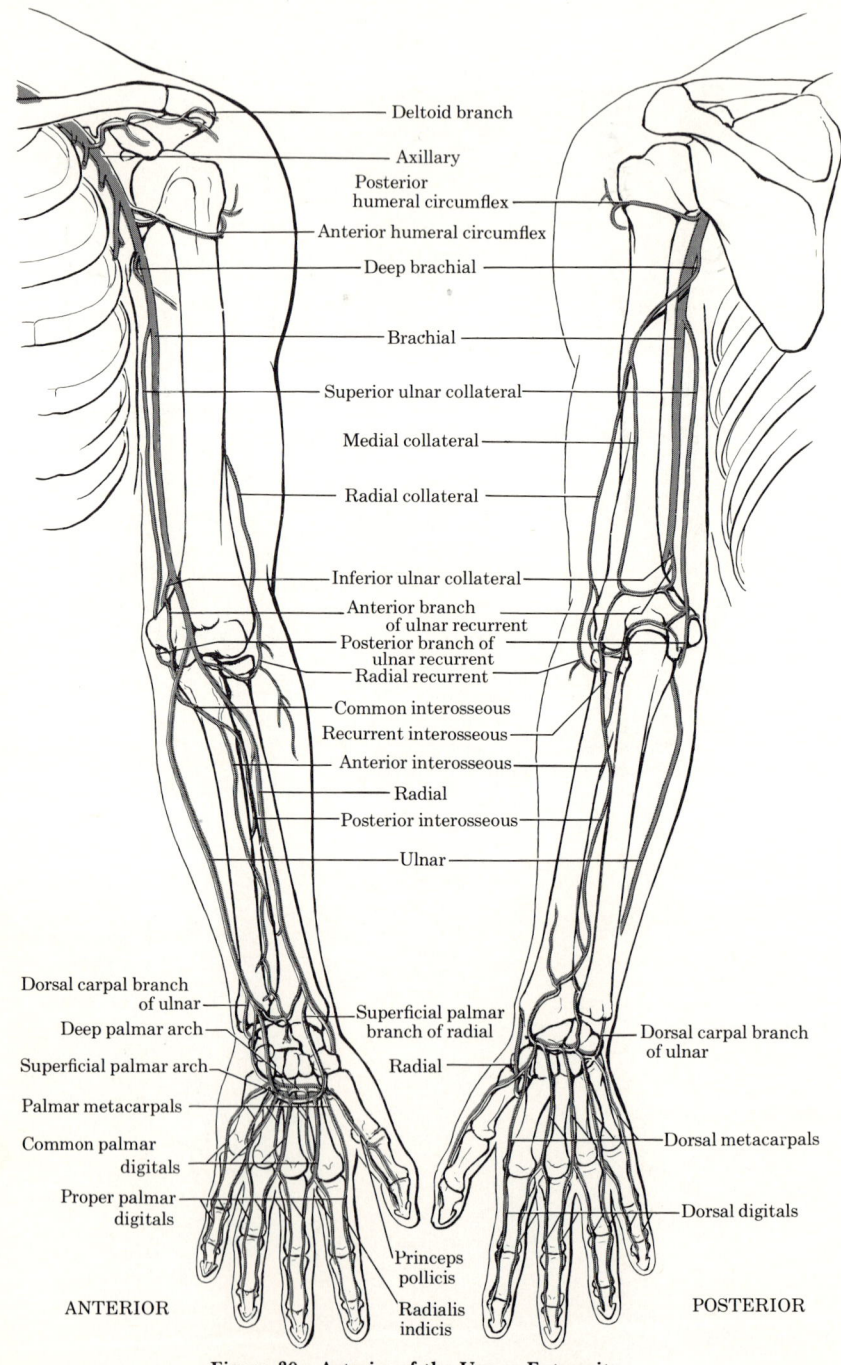

Figure 30 Arteries of the Upper Extremity
(From Dorland's Illustrated Medical Dictionary Courtesy W. B. Saunders Company)

STRUCTURE, CIRCULATION AND INNERVATION 225

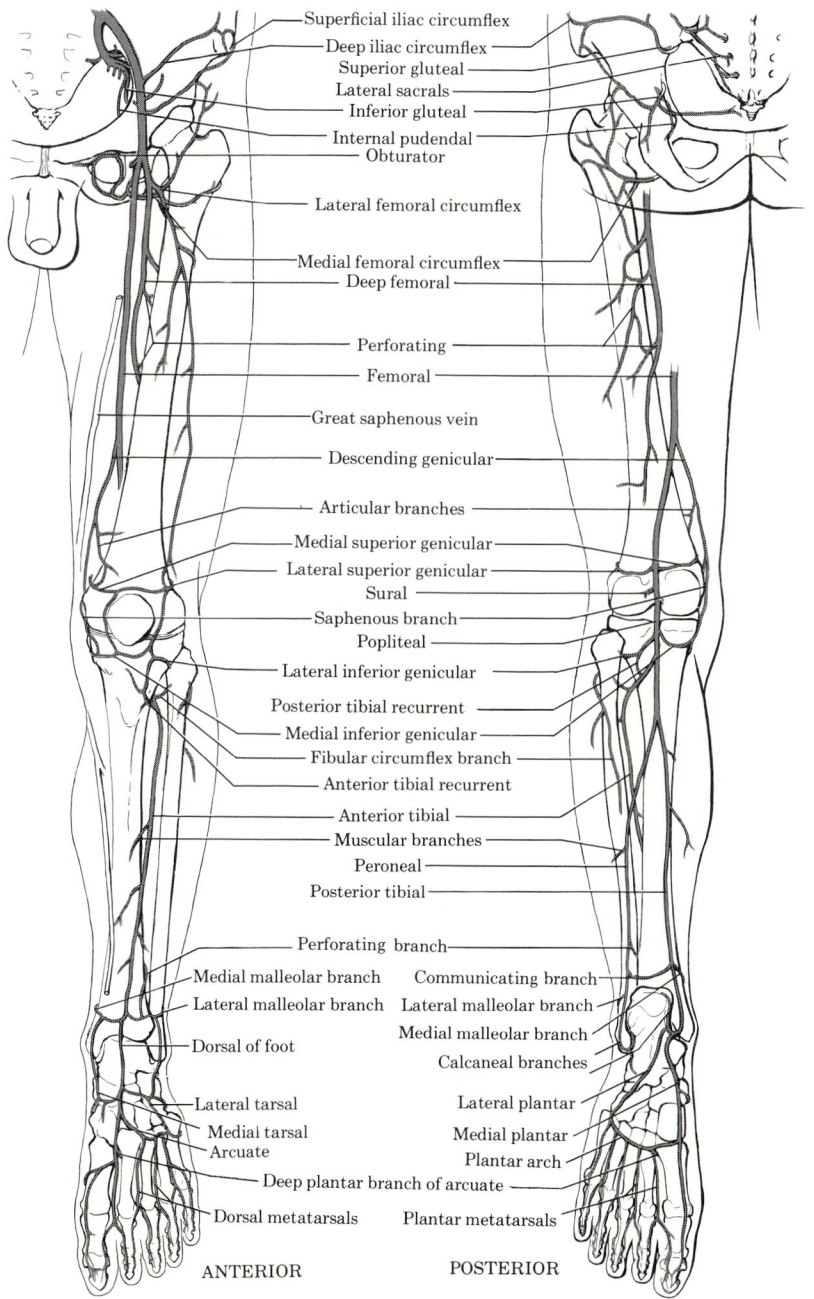

Figure 31 Arteries of the Lower Extremity
(From Dorland's Illustrated Medical Dictionary Courtesy W. B. Saunders Company)

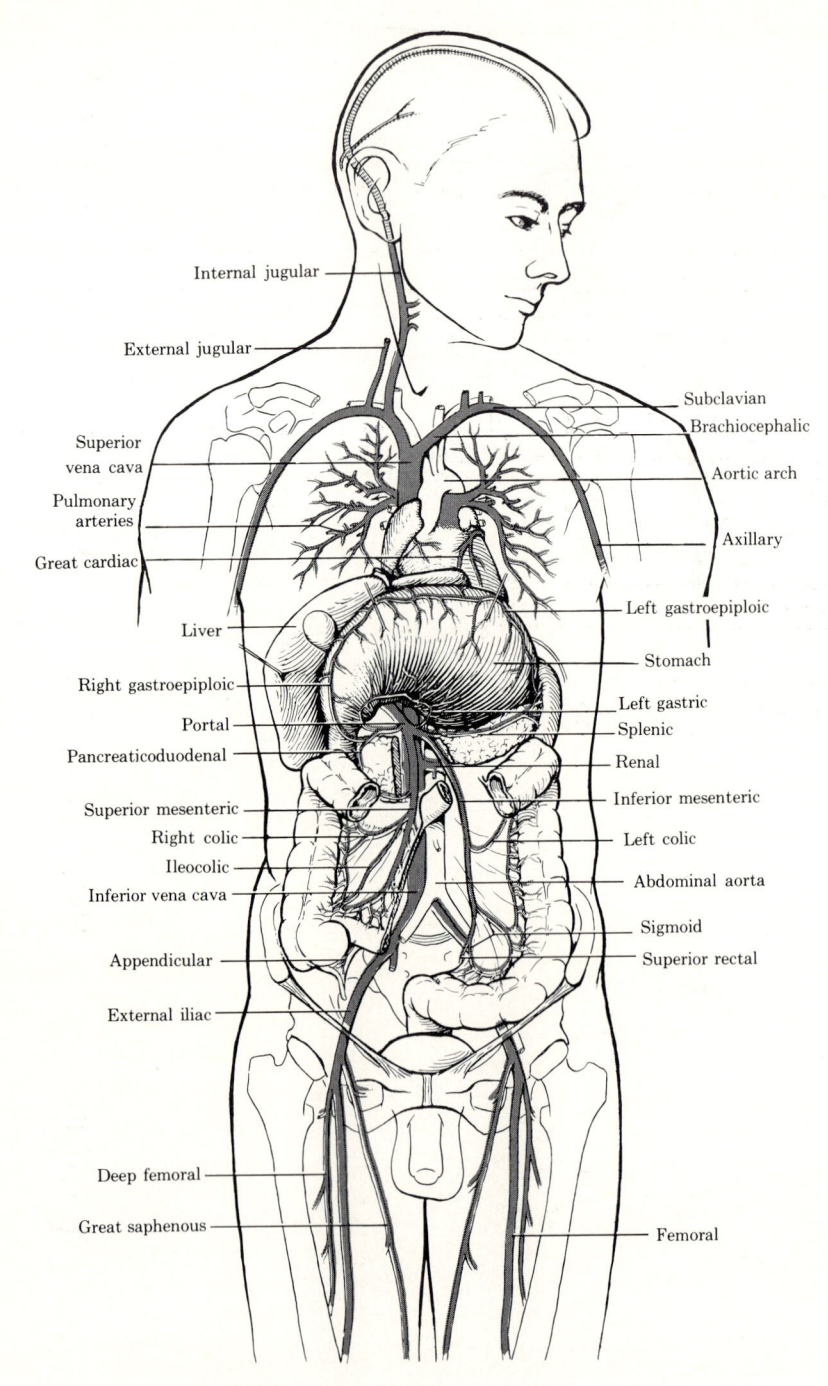

Figure 32 Principal Veins of the Body
(From Dorland's Illustrated Medical Dictionary Courtesy W. B. Saunders Company)

STRUCTURE, CIRCULATION AND INNERVATION 227

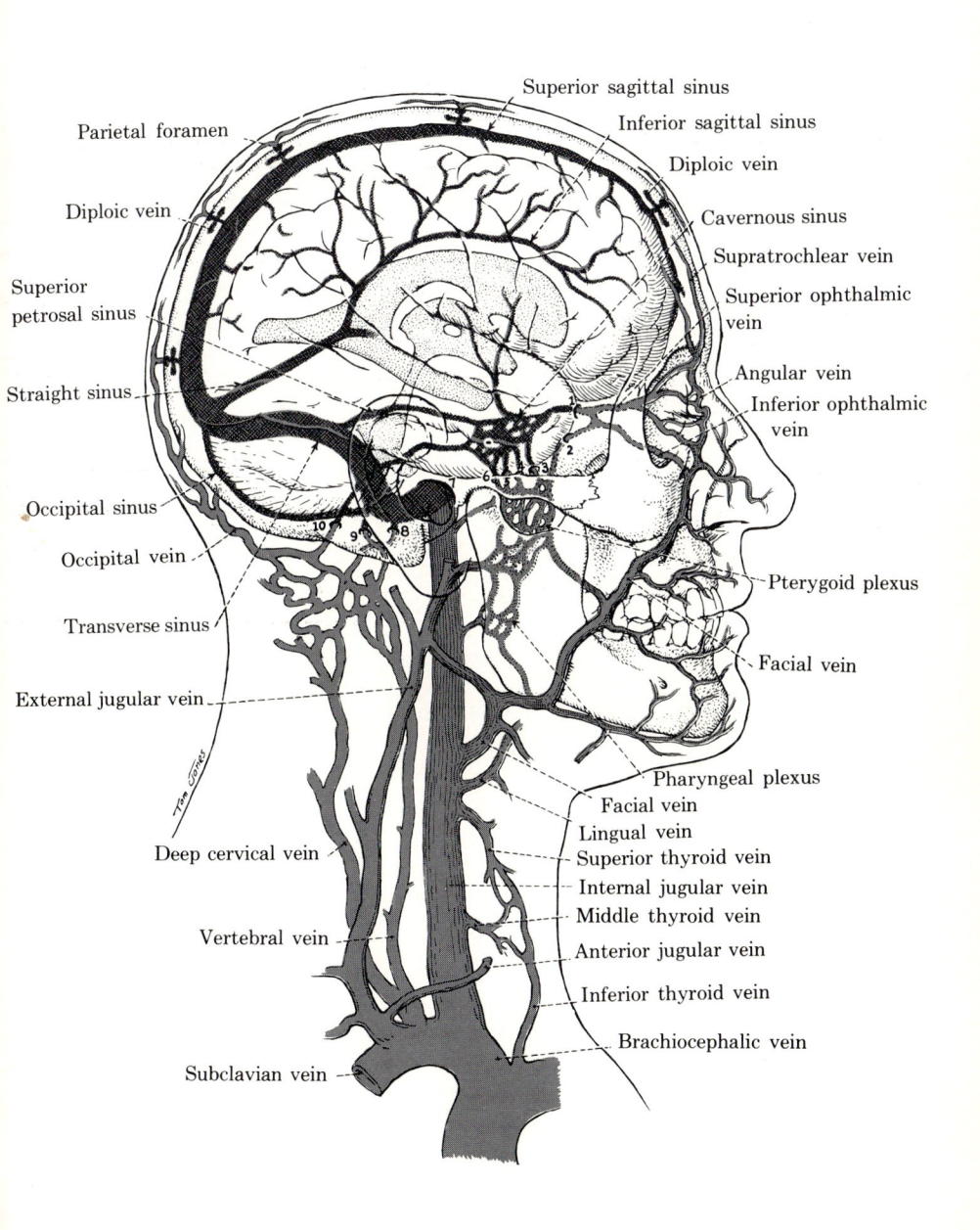

Figure 33 Veins of the Head and Neck
(From Dorland's Illustrated Medical Dictionary Courtesy W. B. Saunders Company)

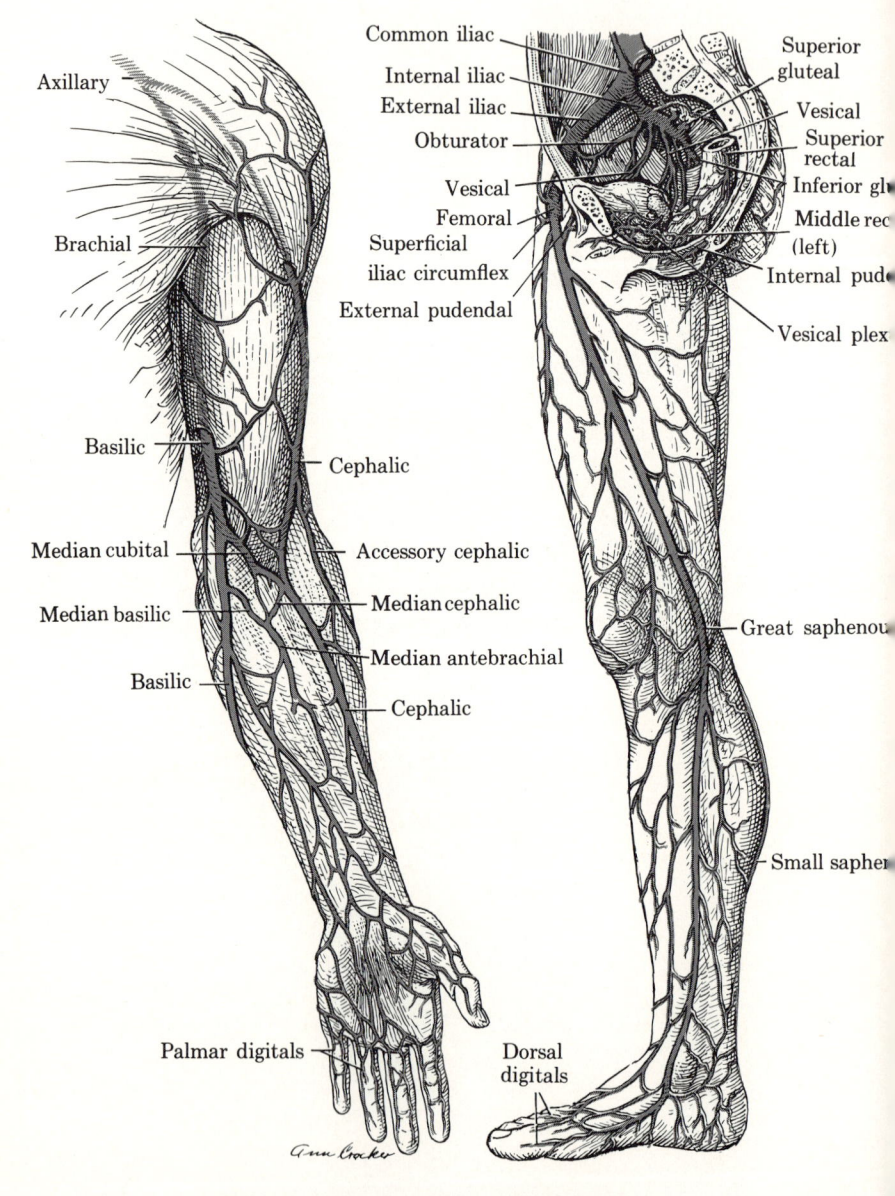

Figure 34 Superficial Veins of the Extremities
(From Dorland's Illustrated Medical Dictionary Courtesy W. B. Saunders Company)

STRUCTURE, CIRCULATION AND INNERVATION 229

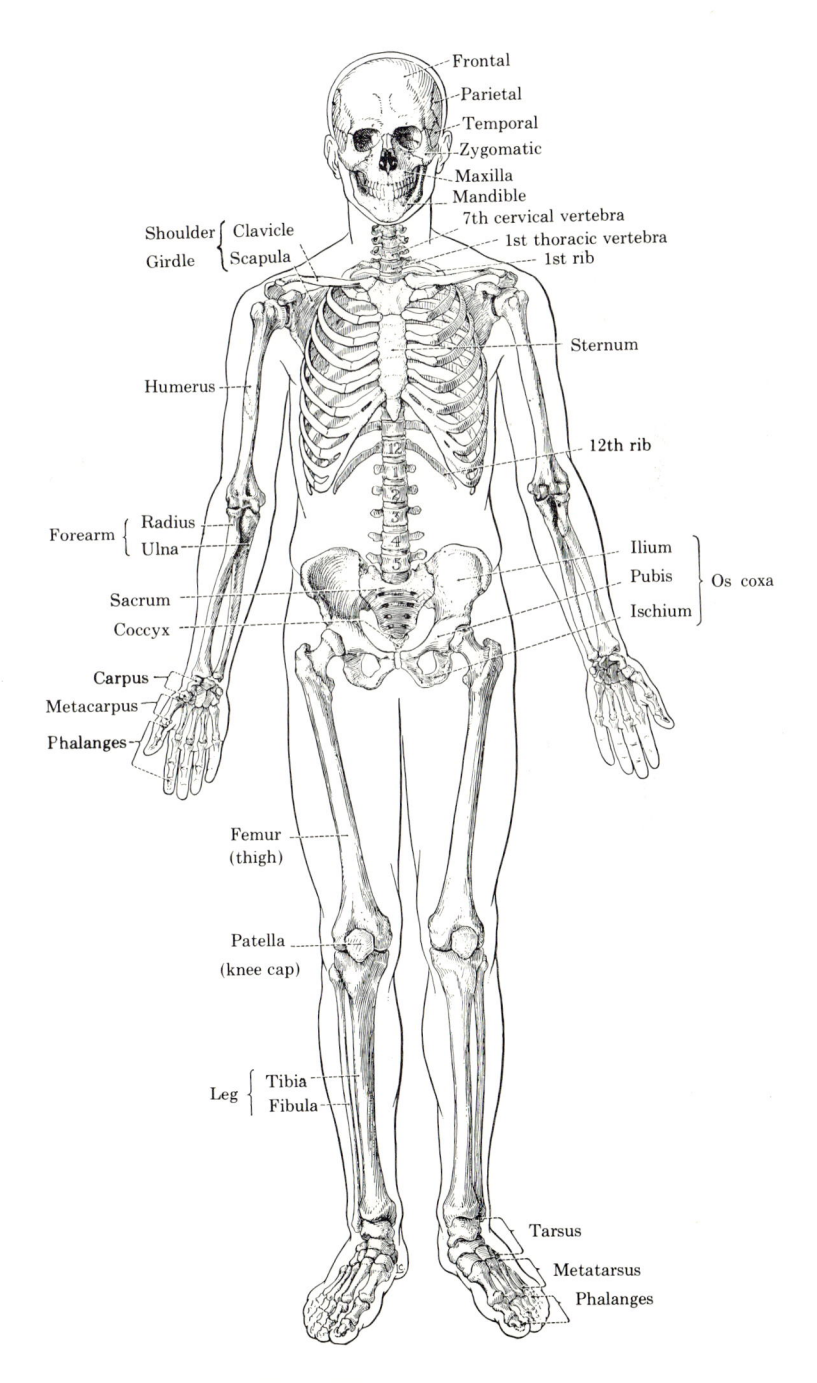

Figure 35 Anterior View of the Human Skeleton
From Human Anatomy and Physiology by King and Showers by permission

THE MUSCULOSKELETAL SYSTEM

The bony skeleton with its attachments consisting of muscles, ligaments, tendons, tendon sheaths, fasciae, bursae and cartilages are collectively called the musculoskeletal system.

The skeletal portion of this system provides the framework and general shape of the body. Other functions of the skeleton include protection of the internal organs (viscera), reaction with the muscles to produce movement, storage for calcium and phosphorus, and sites of blood cell formation.

Bony tissue consists of dense compact exterior bone and an inner spongy cancellous bone. The outside covering of bones is called *periosteum* which if saved during surgery and replaced, gives rise to new bone growth.

SKELETAL ANATOMY

The skeletal framework of the body is made up of 206 separate bones which are distributed as follows:

Skull	22
Hyoid bone	1
Vertebral column	26
Ribs and sternum	25
Auditory ossicles (ear)	6
Lower extremities	62
Upper extremities	64
	206

The bones are joined at articulating points called joints. The articular ends of the bones are connected by bands of flexible connective tissue called ligaments. With the aid of muscles, the various parts of the body can be moved voluntarily. The muscles are attached to the bones by tendons. The ends of the muscles are further secured by aponeuroses and fasciae which also exert an influence on the direction of pull.

The bones, joints, ligaments and muscles are presented here to assist the secretary with the nomenclature of these structures.

BONES

CRANIAL BONES

Ethmoid	Occipital
Frontal	Parietal

CRANIAL BONES (Continued)

Sphenoid
Temporal
  mastoid
  petrous
  squamous
  styloid process
  subperiosteal
  tympanic

NECK

Hyoid

FACIAL BONES

Inferior turbinates
Lacrimal
Malar (zygomatic)
  zygomatic arch
Mandible (jaw bone)
  alveolar process
  condyloid process
  coronoid process
  ramus
Maxilla
  alveolar process
  frontal process
  palatine process
Nasal
  ethmoid
  septum
    perpendicular plate
    cribriform process
Vomer

EAR BONES

Incus
Malleus
Stapes

BONES OF THE TRUNK

Ribs
Sternum
  manubrium
  gladiolus
  xiphoid (ensiform)
Vertebrae
  cervical
  thoracic
  lumbar
  sacral (sacrum)
  coccygeal (coccyx)

SHOULDER GIRDLE

Clavicle (collar bone)   Scapula (shoulder blade)

UPPER LIMBS

Humerus
Radius & Ulna
Carpal Bones (wrist)
  capitate (os magnum)
  greater multangular (trapezium)
  lesser multangular (trapezoid)
  hamate (unciform)
  lunate (semilunar)
  navicular (scaphoid)
  pisiform
  triangular (cuneiform)
Metacarpals
Phalanges

PELVIC GIRDLE

Pelvis
  ilium

ischium
os pubis

LOWER LIMBS

Femur (thigh bone)
  condyle, lateral
  condyle, medial
  head
  neck
  shaft
  trochanter, greater
  trochanter, lesser
Tibia & Fibula
Patella (knee bone)
  medial meniscus

lateral meniscus
Tarsal Bones (ankle)
  calcaneus (os calcis)
  cuboid
  cuneiform, inner
  cuneiform, middle
  cuneiform, outer
  navicular (scaphoid)
  talus (astragalus)
Metatarsals (foot bones)
Phalanges (toe bones)

JOINTS AND LIGAMENTS

Joints are points at which the bones of the skeleton are joined to one another. They may be classified into three groups: the immovable, the slightly movable and the freely movable. An example of the immovable joint may be found in the articulations of the bones of the skull. Slightly movable joints may be found between the vertebral bodies. The joints most often referred to in orthopedic surgery are the freely movable, such as the elbow, wrist, hip, knee, etc. These bones are completely separated from one another permitting a wide range of motion. Their articular surfaces are covered with cartilage and a joint capsule and they are attached to one another by strong fibrous bands called ligaments. The ligaments actually form the joint.

The nomenclature for the ligaments and joints constitutes an important phase of surgical terminology and should be familiar to the secretary. Alphabetically arranged tables of these structures are presented in this section for reference and review purposes.

THE JOINTS

The movable joints and some of the slightly movable ones which are important to the surgeon are listed here.

Acromioclavicular .... shoulder
Atlantooccipital .... vertebral colume with **cranium**
Carpometacarpal .... wrist

HEMODIALYSIS UNIT

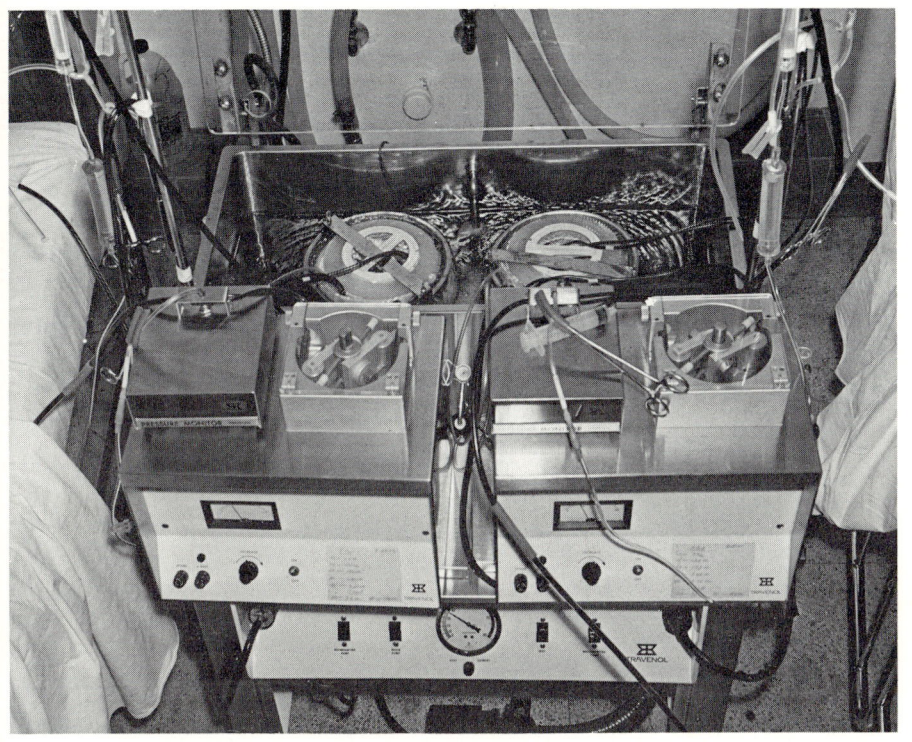

Hemodialysis unit (artificial kidney machine) capable of servicing two patients at a time at the Detroit General Hospital—City of Detroit. Patients who have undergone bilateral nephrectomy (removal of both kidneys) or whose kidneys are nonfunctioning are kept alive by a six hour treatment on this machine twice weekly. Prior to placing patients on hemodialysis, a Scribner or Cimino arteriovenous shunt is performed under the skin in the arm or the foot. In the Scribner procedure, a segment of Silastic tubing is left projecting from the patient's arm to facilitate hook-up to the machine. Blood is circulated from the patient, to the machine for cleansing and then back to the patient. Many patients undergoing such treatment are awaiting kidney transplants.

234

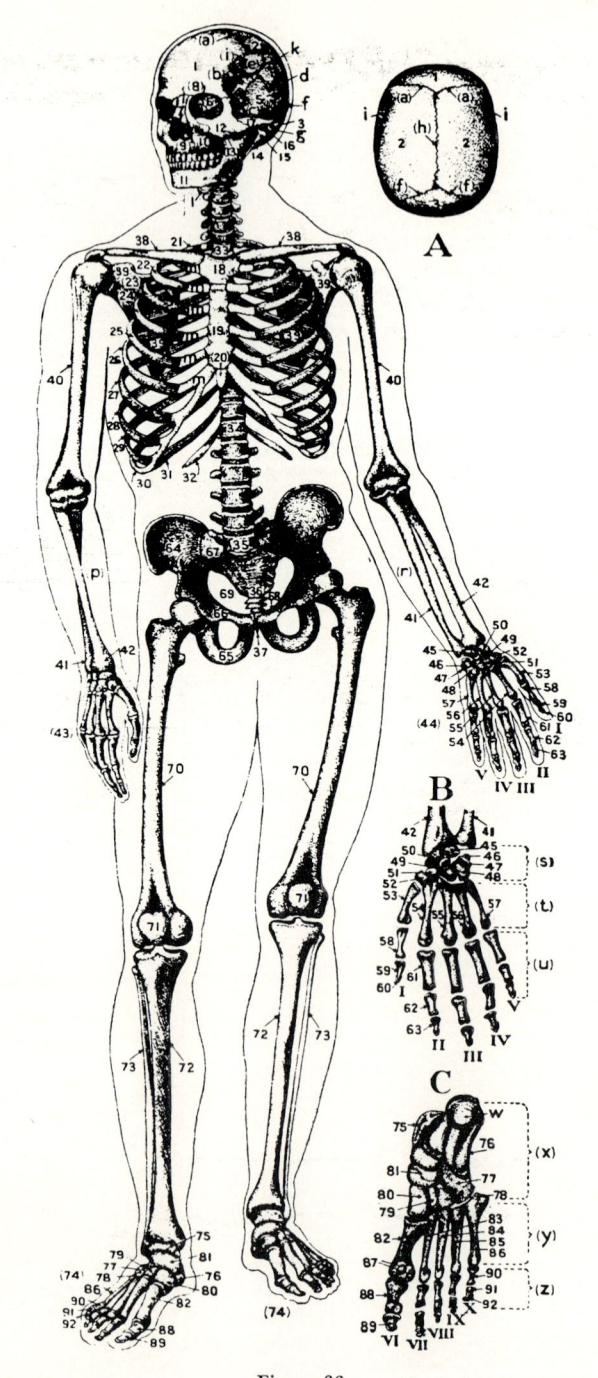

Figure 36

By permission. From Webster's Third New International Dictionary, copyright 1961 by G. & C. Merriam Co., Publishers of the Merriam-Webster Dictionaries.

SKELETON OF ADULT MAN

HEAD OR SKULL
Bones of the Cranium
A Top of Skull showing Sutures
1 Frontal
2 Parietal (two in number)
3 Squamous Portion of Occipital
4 Greater Wing of Sphenoid
5 Squamous Portion of Temporal (two)
6 Ethmoid

Bones of the Face
7 Nasal (two)
8 Lachrymal (two)
9 Vomer
10 Maxilla or Superior Maxillary; (two)
11 Mandible or Inferior Maxillary
12 Zygomatic (two)
(The Palatine Bones (two), the Inferior Conchae or Inferior Turbinated Bones (two), the Ethmoid (two), the Lachrymal (two), the Vomer (one), and the Bones of the Ear — Malleus, Incus, Stapes in each ear — are not indicated)

Principal Features of the Bones of the Head
13 Coronoid Process of Mandible
14 Condyloid Process of Mandible
15 Styloid Process of Temporal
16 Mastoid Process
17 Zygomatic Arch
a Coronal Suture
b Sphenofrontal Suture
c Sphenosquamosal Suture
d Squamous Suture
e Sphenoparietal Suture
f Lambdoid Suture
g Occipitomastoid Suture
h Sagittal Suture
i Superior Temporal Line
k Inferior Temporal Line
l Hyoid Bone

THORAX OR CHEST
Bones of the Breast
18 First Bone of the Sternum, called also Manubrium, Presternum
19 Second Bone of the Sternum, called also Mesosternum
20 Xiphoid process

Sternal or True Ribs
21 to 27 First to Seventh Ribs inclusive (two of each)

Asternal or False Ribs
28 to 32 Eighth to Twelfth Ribs inclusive
(31 and 32 are the Floating Ribs) (two pairs)
m. m. m. etc. Costal Cartilages

TRUNK
Spinal Column
33 First Thoracic Vertebra
34 Twelfth Thoracic Vertebra
35 Fifth Lumbar Vertebra
36 Fifth Sacral Vertebra (last bone of the Sacrum)
37 Coccyx

UPPER EXTREMITY
Shoulder
38 Clavicle or Collar Bone (two)
39 Scapula or Shoulder Blade (two)

Arm
40 Humerus (two)
41 Ulna (two)
42 Radius (two)
(p) Bones of Forearm in Prone Position
(r) Same in Supine Position

Bones of the Hand
(43) Bones of Right Hand (Dorsal, or Back, Surface)
(44) Bones of Left Hand (Volar, or Palm, Surface)
Diagram B Bones of the Left Hand (Dorsal Surface)
(s) Carpus, or Wrist
(t) Metacarpus, or Palm
(u) Phalanges of Thumb and Fingers

Bones of the Carpus
45 Lunatum (two)
46 Pisiform (two)
47 Triquetrum (two)
48 Hamatum (two)
49 Capitatum (two)
50 Navicular (two)
51 Multangulum minus (two)
52 Multangulum majus (two)

Bones of the Metacarpus
53 to 57 First to Fifth Metacarpal Bones (two of each)

Phalanges (28 in all)
58 and 59 First and Second Phalanx of Thumb (two of each)

60 Ungual Tuberosity
61 Proximal, or First, Phalanx of Index
62 Middle, or Second, Phalanx of Index
63 Distal, Terminal, Ungual, or Third, Phalanx of Index

LOWER EXTREMITY
Bones and Principal Parts of Pelvic Girdle
64 Ilium (two)
65 Ischium (two)
66 Pubis (two)
67 Sacrum
68 Brim of Pelvis
69 True Pelvis

Bones of Leg
70 Femur, or Thigh Bone (two)
71 Patella, or Kneepan (two)
72 Tibia, or Shin Bone (two)
73 Fibula (two)

Bones of the Feet
(74) View from Dorsal Surface
Diagram C Bones of Right Foot (Plantar, or Sole, Surface)
(x) Tarsus, or Ankle
(y) Metatarsus
(z) Phalanges of Toes

Bones of the Tarsus
75 Talus, Astragalus, or Ankle Bone (two)
76 Calcaneus, or Heel Bone (two)
w Tuberosity of Calcaneus
77 Cuboid (two)
78, 79, 80 Cuneiform Bones (six in all)
81 Navicular, or Scaphoid, Bone (two)

Bones of the Metatarsus
82 to 86 First to Fifth Metatarsal Bones (ten in all)
87 Sesamoid Bones
VI First Digit, Hallux, or Great Toe
VII to IX Second to Fourth Digits, or Toes
X Fifth Digit, or Little Toe

Phalanges (28 in all)
88 and 89 First and Second Phalanx of Hallux
90 to 92 First, Second, and Third Phalanx of Fifth Digit

By permission. From Webster's Third New International Dictionary, copyright 1961 by G. & C. Merriam Co., Publishers of the Merriam-Webster Dictionaries.

JOINTS (Continued)

Costochondral	ribs and cartilage
Costosternal	ribs and sternum
Costotransverse	ribs and transverse processes
Costovertebral	ribs and vertebrae
Coxal	hip
Cuboideonavicular	ankle-foot
Cuneocuboid	foot
Cuneonavicular	foot
Hip	trunk and leg
Humeral	shoulder
Intercarpal	wrist
Interchondral	cartilages of ribs
Intercuneiform	foot
Intermetacarpal	hand
Intermetatarsal	foot
Interphalangeal	toes or fingers
Intertarsal	ankle
Knee	upper and lower leg
Lumbosacral	trunk
Metacarpophalangeal	hand and fingers
Metatarsophalangeal	foot and toes
Midcarpal	wrist
Midtarsal	ankle
Radiocarpal	wrist
Radioulnar	wrist
Sacrococcygeal	lower trunk
Sacroiliac	lower trunk
Scapuloclavicular	shoulder
Shoulder	upper arm and trunk
Sternal	upper trunk (sternum)
Sternoclavicular	sternum and clavicle
Sternocostal	sternum and ribs
Symphysis pubis	lower trunk
Talocalcaneal	intertarsal (ankle)
Talocalcaneonavicular	intertarsal (ankle)
Talocrural	ankle
Tarsal	ankle
Tarsometatarsal	ankle-foot
Temporomandibular	mandible-temporal bone
Tibiofibular, distal	ankle
Tibiofibular, superior	knee
Tibiotarsal	ankle

THE LIGAMENTS

In addition to connecting the articular ends of bones at the joint, the ligaments also serve to support viscera, muscles and fasciae. These structures are encountered in the surgery of almost all of the specialties. They have been listed here alphabetically to provide an expedient source of reference.

LIGAMENTS

Accessory
Acromioclavicular
Alar
Annular
Anococcygeal
Apical odontoid
Arantius'
Arcuate, lateral
Arcuate, medial
Auricularis
Axis (of malleus)
Bardinet's
Barkow's
Bellini's
Berry's
Bertin's
Bichat's
Bifurcated
Bigelow's
Botallo's
Bourgery's
Broad
Brodie's
Burns's
Calcaneocuboid
Calcaneofibular
Calcaneonavicular, external
Calcaneonavicular, lateral
Calcaneonavicular, plantar
Calcaneotibial
Caldani's
Campbell's suspensory
Camper's
Capsular
Cardinal
Caroticoclinoid
Carpal dorsal
Carpal palmar

Carpometacarpal, dorsal
Carpometacarpal, palmar
Caudal
Cervical
Check, lateral
Check, medial
Ciliary
Civinini's
Clado's
Collateral, fibular
Collateral, metatarsophalangeal
Collateral, radial
Collateral, tibial
Collateral, ulnar
Colles'
Conoid
Cooper's
Coraco-acromial
Coracoclavicular
Coracohumeral
Corniculopharyngeal
Coronary (of knee)
Coronary (of liver)
Costoclavicular
Costocolic
Costotransverse, anterior
Costotransverse, middle
Costotransverse, posterior
Costoxiphoid
Cotyloid
Cricoarytenoid posterior
Cricopharyngeal
Cricosantorinian
Cricothyroid
Cricotracheal
Crucial
Cruciate, of atlas of spine
Cruciate, of knee

LIGAMENTS (Continued)

Cruciate, of the leg
Cruciform
Cruveilhier's
Cubonavicular
Cuneocuboid
Cystoduodenal
Deltoid
Denonvillier's
Dental
Denticulate
Denuce's
Diaphragmatic (kidney)
Epihyal
External lateral (wrist)
Falciform
Falciform, of the liver
Fallopian
Ferrein's
Flood's
Fundiform (penis)
Gastrolienal
Gastrophrenic
Gastrosplenic
Gerdy's
Gillette's suspensory
Gimbernat's
Gingivodental
Glenoid
Glossoepiglottic
Gunz's
Helmholtz'
Henle's
Hensing's
Hepatocolic
Hepatoduodenal
Hepatogastric
Hepatorenal
Hesselbach's
Hey's
Holl's
Heuck's
Humphry's
Hunter's
Hyoepiglottic
Hypsiloid
Iliofemoral

Iliolumbar
Iliopectineal
Iliotrochanteric
Infundibulo-ovarian
Infundibulopelvic
Inguinal
Inguinal reflex
Intercarpal
Interchondral
Interclavicular
Interclinoid
Intercornual
Intercostal
Intercuneiform
Interfoveolar
Intermetacarpal
Intermetatarsal
Internal lateral (wrist)
Interspinous
Intertransverse
Intra-articular
Ischiofemoral
Jarjavay's
Jugal
Krause's median **puboprostatic**
Laciniate
Lacunar
Lannelongue's
Lateral (bladder)
Lauth's
Lienophrenic
Ligament teres of liver
Ligamenta flava (spine)
Ligamentum nuchae
Lisfranc's
Lockwood's
Longitudinal
Lumbocostal
Luschka's
Mackenrodt's
Malleolar
Mauchart's
Meckel's
Nuchal
Occipito-axial (Membrana tectoria)
Odontoid

LIGAMENTS (Continued)

Orbicular (radius)
Ovarian
Palpebral, lateral
Palpebral, medial
Pectinate (iris)
Pectineal
Perineal
Petit's
Phrenicocolic
Phrenicosplenic
Phrenogastric
Phrenosplenic
Pisiunciform
Pisohamate
Pisometacarpal
Plantar
Popliteal arcuate
Popliteal oblique
Poupart's
Pterygospinous
Pterygomandibular
Pubic
Pubocapsular
Pubofemoral
Puboprostatic
Pubovesical
Pulmonary
Quadrate
Radiate
Radiocarpal
Retzius'
Rhomboid
Robert's
Round
Sacrococcygeal
Sacroiliac, anterior
Sacroiliac, interosseous
Sacroiliac, posterior
Sacrosciatic
Sacrospinous
Sacrotuberous
Sappey's
Sheath
Soemmering's
Sphenomandibular
Spinoglenoid

Spiral of cochlea
Spring
Stanley's cervical
Stellate
Sternoclavicular
Sternocostal
Sternopericardial
Stylohyoid
Stylomandibular
Suprascapular
Supraspinous
Suspensory
Sutural
Synovial
Talocalcanean
Talofibular
Talonavicular
Talotibial
Tarsal
Tarsometatarsal
Tarsotibial
Temporomandibular
Teutleben's
Thyroepiglottic
Thyroepiglottidean
Thyrohyoid
Tibiofibular
Tibionavicular
Transverse
Trapezoid
Treitz's
Triangular
Umbilical
Uterosacral
Vaginal
Valsalva's
Ventricular
Vertebropelvic
Vesalius
Vesicouterine
Vesicoumbilical
Vestibular
Vocal
Von Helmholtz'
Weitbrecht's
Winslow's

LIGAMENTS (Continued)

Wrisberg's
Y-shaped
Yellow

Zaglas'
Zinn's

MUSCLES, FASCIA, APONEUROSES AND TENDONS

The muscles are organs of voluntary motion which, through contraction, effect movement of the various parts of the body. Muscle tissue is either smooth or striated (striped). It is either voluntary or involuntary. Smooth muscle, such as that of the intestine and the striated muscle of the heart are involuntary. The striated muscles, except for that of the heart, are voluntary because they can be controlled with conscious effort. When we refer to the muscles, we usually refer to the skeletal, striated, voluntary variety.

Other important musculoskeletal tissues include the fasciae, aponeuroses and tendons which take their names from the muscle with which they are identified.

The fasciae consist of fibrous connective tissues whose function it is to cover, separate and support the muscles, as well as other organs throughout the body. The entire fascial system is divided into three categories: the deep fascia, the subserous fascia, and the superficial fascia. The most extensive of the three types is the deep fascia, binding and enveloping the muscles. The subserous fascia lies within the body cavities. It covers and supports the viscera. It forms the fibrous layer of the serous membranes, such as the peritoneum, pericardium and pleura, and serves as an attachment for the parietal aspect of the serous membranes to the deep fascia situated on the inner surface of the body wall. The superficial fascia permits free movement of the skin by intervening between the deep fascia and the skin.

Another structure of the muscles is the aponeurosis which extends from the muscle as a flattened tendon. These tissues assist in the contraction of the muscle. The tendons also function in this capacity. They are strong flexible cords which connect the muscle to the bone or other structures. With the exception of their point of attachment, they are enveloped in a sheath of fine fibro-elastic connective tissue. These structures are often partially or completely severed in lacerations of the extremities.

An alphabetical table of the muscles and a listing by regions follows.

NB: Although the tables listing anatomic structures throughout these pages show the first letter capitalized in every item listed, in context these terms would appear in the lower-case. Only the Latin B.N.A. names of muscles and those named after an individual are capitalized. The English versions of anatomic titles are used with the lower-case.

STRUCTURE, CIRCULATION AND INNERVATION

MUSCLES

NB: Capitalize first letter in names listed in this table. For authority see Gray's Anatomy.

Abductor digiti minimi manus
Abductor digiti minimi pedis
Abductor hallucis
Abductor pollicis brevis
Abductor pollicis longus
Accelerator urinae
Adductor brevis
Adductor hallucis
Adductor longus
Adductor magnus
Adductor minimus
Adductor obliquus hallucis
Adductor obliquus pollicis
Adductor pollicis
Adductor transversus hallucis
Anconaeus
Antitragicus
Arrectores pilorum
Articularis genu
Aryepiglotticus
Arytenoideus obliquus
Arytenoideus transversus
Aryvocalis
Attollens aurem
Attrahens aurem
Auricularis anterior
Auricularis posterior
Auricularis superior
Azygos uvulae
Biceps brachii
Biceps femoris
Biceps flexor cruris
Biventer mandibulae
Brachialis
Brachioradialis
Bronchooesophageus
Buccinator
Buccopharyngeus
Bulbocavernosus
Caninus
Cephalopharyngeus
Ceratocricoideus
Ceratopharyngeus
Cervicalis ascendens
Chondroglossus
Chondropharyngeus

Ciliaris
Cleidoepitrochlearis
Cleidomastoideus
Cleidooccipitalis
Coccygeus
Complexus
Complexus minor
Compressor naris
Compressor urethrae
Constrictor pharyngis inferior
Constrictor pharyngis medius
Constrictor pharyngis superior
Constrictor urethrae
Coracobrachialis
Corrugator cutis ani
Corrugator supercilii
Cremaster
Cricoarytenoideus lateralis
Cricoarytenoideus posterior
Cricopharyngeus
Cricothyreoideus
Crureus
Cucullarius
Deltoideus
Depressor angulioris
Depressor labii inferioris
Depressor septi
Depressor supercilii
Depressor urethrae
Detrusor urinae
Diaphragma
Digastricus (digastric)
Dilator naris
Dilatator pupillae
Ejaculator seminis
Epicranius
Epitrochleoanconeus
Erector clitoridis
Erector penis
Erector spinae
Extensor brevis digitorum
Extensor brevis pollicis
Extensor carpi radialis brevis
Extensor carpi radialis longus
Extensor carpi ulnaris
Extensor coccygis

MUSCLES (Continued)

Extensor communis digitorum
Extensor digiti minimi
Extensor digitorum
Extensor digitorum brevis
Extensor digitorum brevis manus
Extensor digitorum longus
Extensor hallucis brevis
Extensor hallucis longus
Extensor indicis
Extensor longus digitorum
Extensor longus pollicis
Extensor minimi digiti
Extensor ossis metacarpi pollicis
Extensor pollicis brevis
Extensor pollicis longus
Flexor accessorius digitorum
Flexor brevis digitorum
Flexor brevis hallucis
Flexor brevis minimi digiti
Flexor carpi radialis
Flexor carpi ulnaris
Flexor digiti minimi brevis
Flexor digiti minimi brevis
Flexor digitorum brevis
Flexor digitorum longus
Flexor digitorum profundus
Flexor digitorum superficialis
Flexor hallucis brevis
Flexor hallucis longus
Flexor longus digitorum
Flexor longus hallucis
Flexor longus pollicis
Flexor pollicis brevis
Flexor pollicis longus
Flexor profundus digitorum
Flexor sublimis digitorum
Frontalis
Gastrocnemius
Gemellus inferior
Gemellus superior
Genioglossus
Geniohyoideus
Glossopalatinus
Glossopharyngeus
Gluteus maximus
Gluteus medius

Gluteus minimus
Gracilis
Helicis major
Helicis minor
Hyoglossus
Hyopharyngeus
Iliacus
Iliacus minor
Iliocapsularis
Iliocostalis
Iliocostalis cervicis
Iliocostalis dorsi
Iliocostalis lumborum
Iliocostalis thoracis
Iliopsoas
Incisivus labii inferioris
Incisivus labii superioris
Incisurae helicis
Infracostalis
Infraspinatus
Intercostalis externus
Intercostalis internus
Intercostalis intimus
Interosseus dorsalis manus
Interosseus dorsalis pedis
Interosseus palmaris
Interosseus plantaris
Interosseus volaris
Interspinalis
Intertransversarius
Ischiocavernosus
Ischiococcygeus
Keratopharyngeus
Laryngopharyngeus
Latissimus dorsi
Levator alae nasi
Levator anguli oris
Levator anguli scapulae
Levator ani
Levator costae
Levator glandulae thyreoideae
Levator labii inferioris
Levator labii superioris
Levator labii superioris alaeque nasi
Levator palati
Levator palpebrae superioris

STRUCTURE, CIRCULATION AND INNERVATION

MUSCLES (Continued)

Levator prostatae
Levator scapulae
Levator veli palatini
Longissimus capitis
Longissimus cervicis
Longissimus thoracis
Longitudinalis dorsi
Longitudinalis inferior
Longitudinalis superior
Longus capitis
Longus colli
Lumbricalis manus
Lumbricalis pedis
Masseter
Mentalis
Multifidus
Mylohyoideus
Mylopharyngeus
Nasalis
Obliquus auriculae
Obliquus capitis inferior
Obliquus capitis superior
Obliquus externus abdominis
Obliquus inferior
Obliquus internus abdominis
Obliquus superior
Obturatorius externus
Obturatorius internus
Occipitalis
Occipitofrontalis
Omohyoideus
Opponens digiti minimi
Opponens digiti quinti
Opponens minimi digiti
Opponens pollicis
Orbicularis oculi
Orbicularis oris
Orbicularis palpebrarum
Orbitalis
Orbitopalpebralis
Palatoglossus
Palatopharyngeus
Palatosalpingeus
Palatostaphylinus
Palmaris brevis
Palmaris longus
Papillaris
Pectinatus
Pectineus
Pectoralis major
Pectoralis minor
Peroneocalcaneus
Peroneus brevis
Peroneus longus
Peroneus tertius
Petropharyngeus
Petrostaphylinus
Pharyngopalatinus
Piriformis
Plantaris
Platysma
Pleurooesophageus
Popliteus
Procerus
Pronator pedis
Pronator quadratus
Pronator teres
Prostaticus
Psoas major
Psoas minor
Pterygoideus externus
Pterygoideus internus
Pterygoideus lateralis
Pterygoideus medialis
Pterygopharyngeus
Pterygospinosus
Pubococcygeus
Puboprostaticus
Puborectalis
Pubovesicalis
Pyramidalis
Pyramidalis auriculae
Pyramidalis nasi
Pyriformis
Quadratus femoris
Quadratus labii inferioris
Quadratus labii superioris
Quadratus lumborum
Quadratus menti
Quadratus plantae
Quadriceps femoris
Rectococcygeus

MUSCLES (Continued)

Rectourethralis
Rectouterinus
Rectovesicalis
Rectus abdominis
Rectus capitis anterior
Rectus capitis anticus major
Rectus capitis lateralis
Rectus capitis posterior major
Rectus capitis posterior minor
Rectus externus
Rectus femoris
Rectus inferior
Rectus internus
Rectus lateralis
Rectus medialis
Rectus superior
Rectus thoracis
Retrahens aurem
Rhomboatloideus
Rhomboideus major
Rhomboideus minor
Risorius
Rotatores
Rotatores cervicis
Rotatores lumborum
Rotatores thoracis
Sacrococcygeus anterior
Sacrococcygeus dorsalis
Sacrococcygeus posterior
Sacrococcygeus ventralis
Sacrolumbalis
Sacrospinalis
Salpingopharyngeus
Sartorius
Scalenus anterior
Scalenus medius
Scalenus minimus
Scalenus posterior
Scansorius
Semimembranosus
Semispinalis capitis
Semispinalis cervicis
Semispinalis colli
Semispinalis dorsi
Semispinalis thoracis
Semitendinosus

Serratus anterior
Serratus magnus
Serratus inferior posterior
Serratus posterior superior
Soleus
Sphenosalpingostaphylinus
Sphincter ampullae
  hepatopancreaticae
Sphincter ani externus
Sphincter ani internus
Sphincter oris
Sphincter pupillae
Sphincter pylori
Sphincter urethrae
Sphincter urethrae membranaceae
Sphincter vaginae
Sphincter vesicae
Spinalis capitis
Spinalis cervicis
Spinalis colli
Spinalis dorsi
Spinalis thoracis
Splenius capitis
Splenius cervicis
Splenius colli
Stapedius
Staphylinus externus
Staphylinus internus
Staphylinus medius
Sternalis
Sternochondroscapularis
Sternoclavicularis
Sternocleidomastoideus
Sternofascialis
Sternohyoideus
Sternothyreoideus
Styloauricularis
Styloglossus
Stylohyoideus
Stylolaryngeus
Stylopharyngeus
Subclavius
Subcostalis
Subcrureus
Subscapularis
Supinator

MUSCLES (Continued)

Supinator longus
Supraclavicularis
Supraspinalis
Supraspinatus
Suspensorius duodeni
Tarsalis inferior
Tarsalis superior
Temporalis
Tensor fasciae latae
Tensor palati
Tensor tarsi
Tensor tympani
Tensor veli palatini
Teres major
Teres minor
Thyreoarytenoideus
Thyreoarytenoideus externus
 and internus
Thyreoepiglotticus
Thyreohyoideus
Thyreopharyngeus
Tibialis anterior
Tibialis gracilis
Tibialis posterior
Tibialis secundus
Tibiofascialis anterior
Trachealis
Tracheloclavicularis
Trachelomastoideus
Tragicus
Transversalis abdominis

Transversalis capitis
Transversalis cervicis
Transversalis nasi
Transversospinalis
Transversus abdominis
Transversus auriculae
Transversus linguae
Transversus menti
Transversus nuchae
Transversus perinei profundus
Transversus perinei superficialis
Transversus thoracis
Trapezius
Triangularis
Triangularis labii inferioris
Triangularis labii superioris
Triangularis sterni
Triceps brachii
Triceps surae
Triticeoglossus
Uvulae
Vastus externus
Vastus intermedius
Vastus internus
Vastus lateralis
Vastus medialis
Ventricularis
Verticalis linguae
Vocalis
Zygomaticus (major & minor)

MUSCLES OF THE FACE AND HEAD

Auricularis anterior
Auricularis posterior
Auricularis superior
Buccinator
Caninus
Caput zygomaticum
Depressor septi nasi
Epicranius
Levator palpebrae superioris

Masseter
Mentalis
Nasalis, pars alaris
Nasalis, pars transversa
Obliquus inferior oculi
Obliquus superior oculi
Orbicularis oculi
Orbicularis oris
Platysma

FIGS. 1 AND 2. MUSCULAR SYSTEM OF MAN

FIG. 1, FRONTAL VIEW. FIG. 2, DORSAL VIEW.

Frontal View

Dorsal View

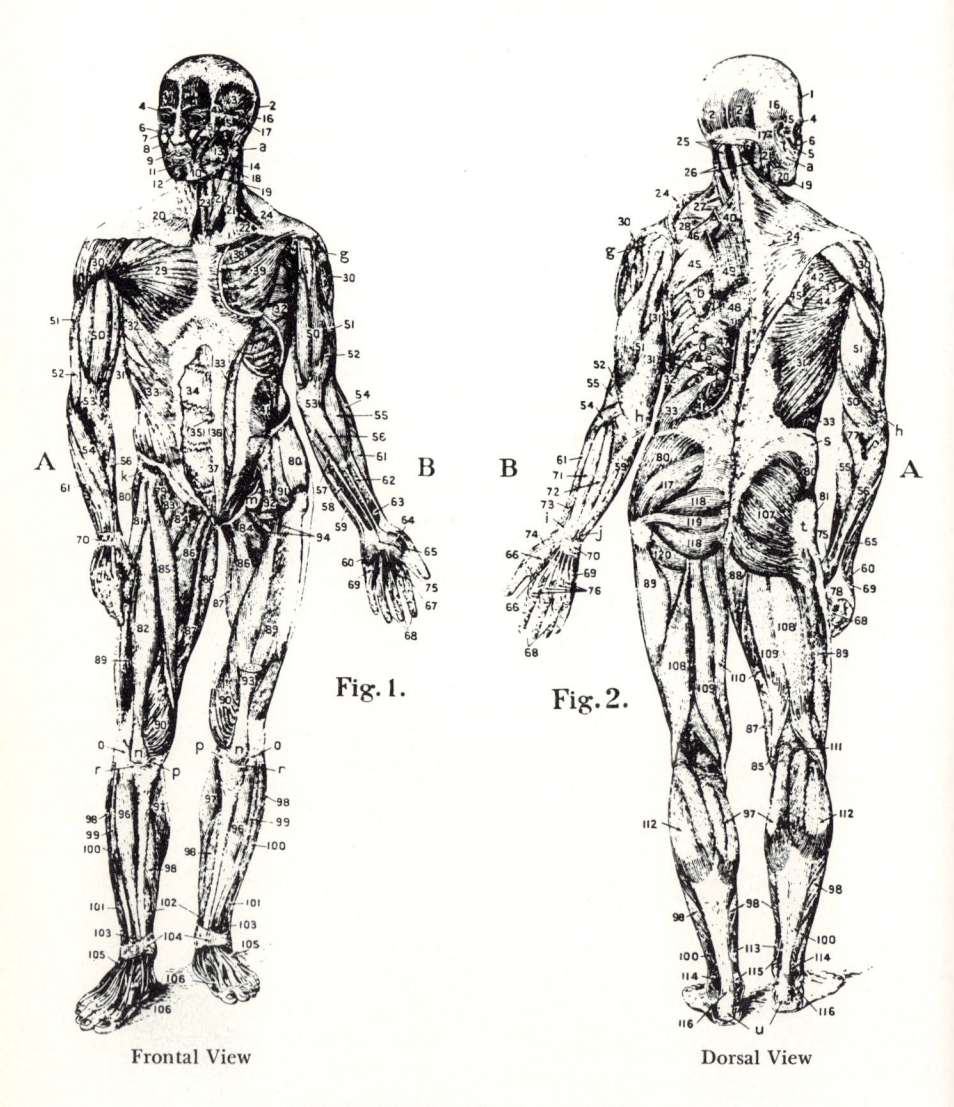

Figure 37 Muscular System of Man

By permission. From Webster's Third New International Dictionary, copyright 1961 by G. & C. Merriam Co., Publishers of the Merriam-Webster Dictionaries.

STRUCTURE, CIRCULATION AND INNERVATION

Figs. 1 and 2. MUSCULAR SYSTEM OF MAN

Fig. 1, FRONTAL VIEW.   Fig. 2, DORSAL VIEW.

HEAD AND NECK

1 Frontalis (2)
2 Occipitalis (2)
3 Temporal (1)
4 Orbicularis Oculi
5 Zygomaticus
6 Zygomatic Head of the Quadratus Labii Superioris, or Zygomaticus Minor
7 Angular Head of the Quadratus Labii Superioris (1)
8 Nasalis (1)
9 Orbicularis Oris (1)
10 Triangularis Menti (1)
11 Quadratus Labii Inferioris (1)
12 Mentalis (1)
13 Masseter (1)
14 Buccinator (1)
15 Auricularis Anterior
16 Auricularis Superior
17 Auricularis Posterior
a Parotid Gland
18 Mylohyoid
19 Digastric
20 Platysma or Platysma Myoides
21 Sternocleidomastoid
22 Omohyoid (1)
23 Sternohyoid (1)
24 Trapezius (1)
25 Splenius Capitis (2)
26 Splenius Cervicis (2)
27 Levator Scapulae (2)
28 Supraspinatus (2)

TRUNK

29 Pectoralis Major (1)
30 Deltoid
31 Latissimus Dorsi
32 Serratus Anterior
33 External Oblique
34 Rectus Abdominis (1)
35 Umbilicus (1)
36 Abdominal Aponeurosis (1)
37 Linea Alba (1)
38 Subclavius (1)
39 Pectoralis Minor (1)
40 Serratus Posterior Superior (1)
41 Internal Oblique
42 Infraspinatus (2)
43 Teres Minor (2)
44 Teres Major (2)
45 Rhomboideus Major (2)
46 Rhomboideus Minor (2)
b Scapula (2)
c 9th Rib (2)
d 10th Rib (2)
e 11th Rib (2)
f 12th Rib (2)
47 Serratus Posterior Inferior (2)
48 Lumbodorsal Fascia (2)
49 Sacrospinalis (2)

UPPER EXTREMITY

50 Biceps Brachii
51 Triceps Brachii
52 Branchialis
53 Lacertus Fibrosus
54 Extensor Carpi Radialis Longus
55 Brachiorodialis
56 Flexor Carpi Radialis
57 Palmaris Longus (1)
58 Flexor Digitorum Sublimis (1)
59 Flexor Carpi Ulnaris
60 Palmaris Brevis
61 Extensor Carpi Radialis Brevis
62 Flexor Pollicis Longus (1)
63 Pronator Quadratus (1)
64 Flexor Pollicis Brevis (1)
65 Palmaris Longus (cut across in Fig. 1)
66 First Dorsal Interosseus
67 First Lumbricalis (1)
68 Fibrous Sheaths of the Tendons
69 Adductor of the Little Finger
70 Annular Ligament of the Carpus
g Head of Humerus (showing Bicipital Groove)
71 Extensor Digitorum Communis (1)
72 Extensor Carpi Ulnaris (2)
73 Extensor Pollicis Longus
h Medial Epicondyle of Humerus (2)
i Lower End of Radius (2)
j Lower End of Ulna (2)
74 Tendons of Extensor Pollicis Longus and Brevis (2)
75 Adductor Pollicis (2)
76 Tendons of the Extensors (2)
77 Pronator Teres (2)
78 Palmar Aponeurosis (2)

LOWER EXTREMITY

k Anterior Superior Spine of Ilium (1)
79 Iliacus (1)
80 Gluteus Medius
81 Tensor Fasciae Latae
82 Rectus Femoris (1)
83 Psoas Major (1)
84 Pectineus (1)
85 Sartorius
86 Adductor Longus (1)
87 Adductor Magnus
88 Gracilis
89 Vastus Lateralis
90 Vastus Medialis
91 Gluteus Minimus (1)
92 Superior Extremity of Rectus Femoris (1)
93 Inferior Extremity of Rectus Femoris (1)
m Head of Femur (1)
94 Inferior Extremities of Psoas and Iliacus (1)
95 Adductor Brevis (not shown)
n Patella (1)
o Head of Fibula (1)
p Medial Condyle of Femur (1)
r Tuberosity of Tibia (1)
96 Tibialis Anterior
97 Gastrocnemius, Medial Head (1)
98 Soleus
99 Extensor Digitorum Longus (1)
100 Peroneus Longus
101 Peroneus Brevis (1)
102 Flexor Digitorum Longus (1)
103 Extensor Hallucis Longus (1)
104 Ligamentum Cruciatum Cruris (1)
105 Extensor Digitorum Brevis (1)
106 Abductor Hallucis (1)
s Ilium
t Greater Trochanter
107 Gluteus Maximus (2)
108 Biceps Femoris (2)
109 Semitendinosus (2)
110 Semimembranosus (2)
111 Plantaris (2)
112 Gastrocnemius, Lateral Head (1)
113 Flexor Digitorum Longus (2)
114 Peroneus Tertius (2)
115 Tendon of Tibialis Posterior (2)
116 Achilles' Tendon (2)
117 Pyriformis (2)
118 Gemellus Superior and Gemellus Inferior (2)
119 Obturator Internus (2)
120 Quadratus Femoris (2)

By permission. From Webster's Third New International Dictionary, copyright 1961 by G. & C. Merriam Co., Publishers of the Merriam-Webster Dictionaries.

MUSCLES OF THE FACE AND HEAD (Continued)

Procerus
Pterygoideus externus
Pterygoideus internus
Quadratus labii inferioris
Quadratus labii superioris
Rectus inferior oculi
Rectus lateralis oculi

Rectus medialis oculi
Rectus superior oculi
Risorius
Temporalis
Triangularis
Zygomaticus

MUSCLES OF THE NECK

Constrictor pharyngis inferior
Constrictor pharyngis medius
Constrictor pharyngis superior
Digastricus
Genioglossus
Geniohyoideus
Glossopalatinus
Hyoglossus
Intrinsic tongue muscles
Levator veli palatini
Longus capitis
Longus colli
Musculus uvulae
Mylohyoideus
Omohyoideus

Pharyngopalatine
Rectus capitis anterior
Rectus capitis lateralis
Scalenus anterior
Scalenus medius
Scalenus posterior
Sternocleidomastoideus
Sternohyoideus
Sternothyroideus
Styloglossus
Stylohyoideus
Stylopharyngeus
Tensor veli palatini
Thyrohyoideus

MUSCLES OF THE TRUNK

Cremaster
Iliocostalis
Intercostales externi
Intercostales interni
Interspinalis
Latissimus dorsi
Levatores costarum
Longissimus
Multifidus
Obliquus capitis inferior
Obliquus capitis superior
Obliquus externus abdominis
Obliquus internus abdominis
Pyramidalis

Quadratus lumborum
Rectus abdominis
Rectus capitis posterior **major**
Rectus capitis posterior **minor**
Rotatores
Sacrospinalis
Semispinalis
Serrati posteriores
Spinalis dorsi
Splenius
Transversus abdominis
Transversus thoracis
Trapezius

MUSCLES OF THE FOREARM AND HAND

Abductor digiti quinti manus
Abductor pollicis brevis
Abductor pollicis longus
Abductor pollicis
Brachioradialis
Extensor carpi radialis brevis
Extensor carpi radialis longus
Extensor carpi ulnaris
Extensor digitorum communis
Extensor digiti quinti proprius
Extensor indicis proprius
Extensor pollicis brevis
Flexor carpi radialis
Flexor carpi ulnaris

Flexor digiti quinti brevis manus
Flexor digitorum profundus
Flexor digitorum sublimis
Flexor pollicis longus
Interossei dorsales manus
Interossei volares
Lumbricales manus
Opponens digiti quinti manus
Opponens pollicis
Palmaris brevis
Palmaris longus
Pronator quadratus
Pronator teres
Supinator

MUSCLES OF THE HIP AND KNEE

Adductor brevis
Adductor longus
Adductor magnus
Biceps femoris
Gemellus inferior
Gemellus superior
Gluteus maximus
Gluteus medius
Gluteus minimus
Gracilis
Iliacus
Obturator externus
Obturator internus

Pectineus
Piriformis
Psoas major
Rectus femoris
Quadratus femoris
Sartorius
Semimembranosus
Semitendinosus
Tensor fasciae lata
Vastus intermedius
Vastus lateralis
Vastus medialis

MUSCLES OF THE PERINEUM AND PELVIS

Bulbocavernosus
Coccygeus
Iliacus
Iliococcygeus
Ischiocavernosus
Levator ani
Obturator internus

Piriformis
Pubococcygeus
Sphincter ani, externus
Sphincter urethrae membranaceae
Transverse perinei superficialis
Transversus perinei profundus

MUSCLES OF THE ARM AND SHOULDER

Anconeus
Biceps brachii
Brachialis
Deltoideus
Infraspinatus
Latissimus dorsi
Levator scapulae
Pectoralis major
Pectoralis minor
Rhomboideus major
Rhomboideus minor
Serratus anterior
Subscapularis
Supraspinatus
Teres major
Teres minor
Trapezius
Triceps brachii

MUSCLES OF THE LEG AND FOOT

Abductor digiti quinti pedis
Abductor hallucis
Dorsal interossei dorsales pedis
Extensor digitorum longus pedis
Extensor hallucis longus
Flexor digiti quinti brevis pedis
Flexor digitorum brevis
Flexor digitorum longus
Flexor hallucis brevis
Flexor hallucis longus
Gastrocnemius
Interossei plantares
Lumbricales pedis
Peroneus brevis
Peroneus longus
Peroneus tertius
Plantaris
Popliteus
Quadratus plantae
Soleus
Tibialis anterior
Tibialis posterior

THE PERIPHERAL NERVOUS SYSTEM

Terminology referable to the peripheral nervous system is used more frequently in surgical dictations than is that of the central nervous system; however, in addition to developing a familiarity with the names of the nerves, the secretary should have an intelligent concept of the divisions of the nervous system as a whole.

Grossly, the nervous system is divided into the central nervous system (brain and spinal cord), and the peripheral nervous system (cranial and spinal nerves and end organs). The peripheral nervous system may be further divided into the cerebrospinal (voluntary) system and the visceral (autonomic or splanchnic) system.

The cerebrospinal system connects the central nervous system with the body wall, controls skeletal muscles and includes those parts of the brain governing consciousness and mental activities. The autonomic system innervates the viscera and involuntary tissues such as the heart, the glands and plain muscle tissue which cannot be consciously controlled.

The autonomic system may be further subdivided into the parasympathetic (craniosacral) and sympathetic (thoracolumbar) systems.

STRUCTURE, CIRCULATION AND INNERVATION

The fibers of the parasympathetic arise from the midbrain, the medulla oblongata and the sacral segment of the spinal cord. Stimulation of the parasympathetic system causes contraction of the smooth muscle of the stomach and intestine, constriction of the arterioles, bronchioles and pupils of the eyes. It also causes a slowing of the heart.

The sympathetic division runs parallel on either side of the vertebral column and is connected to the spinal cord by thoracic and lumbar fibers. Its functions are opposite and antagonistic to those of the parasympathetic system. A balance exists between the two systems to maintain proper body function.

Some of the more important peripheral nerves are the cranial which are referred to by number (based on the order in which they emerge from the brain) as often as by name. Medical students use a rhyme to assist them in recalling the nerves in their proper order, where the first letter of each word coincides with the first letter in the name of each nerve—ON OLD OLYMPUS TOWERING TOPS, A FINN AND GERMAN VIEWED A HOPS.

The Cranial Nerves Are: (12 pairs)

I.	Olfactory		VI.	Abducent
II.	Optic		VII.	Facial
III.	Oculomotor		VIII.	Acoustic
IV.	Trochlear		IX.	Glossopharyngeal
V.	Trigeminal		X.	Vagus
	ophthalmic branch		XI.	Accessory
	maxillary branch		XII.	Hypoglossal
	mandibular branch			

The numbers are just as important as the names in identifying these nerves. The surgeon will often refer to the 5th nerve rather than to specify it as the trigeminal. He is just as apt to refer to a nerve branch by name and the nerve proper by number, as for example, the ophthalmic branch of the 5th nerve.

THE NERVES

The names in this table may be used in the lower case except where they are named after an individual.

Abdominal	**Alveolar, superior**
Abducens	**Anococcygeal**
Accessory	**Aortic plexus**
Acoustic	**Auditory**
Adrenal plexus	**Auricular**
Alveolar, inferior	**Auricular, great**

THE NERVES (Continued)

Auricular, posterior
Auriculotemporal
Axillary
Brachial, cutaneous
Bronchial
Buccal, of facial
Buccinator
Calcaneal, medial
Cardiac
Caroticotympanic
Carotid, of glossopharyngeal
Cavernous, of penis
Celiac, of vagus
Cervical
Chorda tympani
Ciliary, long
Ciliary, short
Circumflex, of clitoris
Clunical
Coccygeal
Cochlear
Crural, anterior
Cutaneous
Cutaneous surae lateralis
Deep branch of radial
Dental
Descending ramus of hypoglossal
Digastric
Digital
Dorsal, of penis
Dorsal scapular
Dural
Erigentes
Esophageal
Esophageal plexus
Ethmoidal, anterior
Ethmoidal, posterior
External nasal
Facial
Femoral
Frontal
Gastric
Gastroduodenal plexus
Genitofemoral
Glossopharyngeal

Gluteal, inferior
Gluteal, superior
Great auricular
Greater occipital
Hemorrhoidal
Hepatic branches of vagus
Hypogastric
Hypoglossal
Iliohypogastric
Ilioinguinal
Incisive
Inferior dental to infrahyoid
Infraorbital
Infrapatellar
Infratrochlear
Intercostal
Intercostobrachial
Intermedius, of Wrisberg
Intermesenteric plexus
Internal calcaneal
Interosseous, anterior
Interosseous, posterior
Jacobson's
Jugular
Labial, inferior
Lacrimal of Lancisi
Laryngeal, inferior
Laryngeal, recurrent
Laryngeal, superior
Laryngopharyngeal
Lesser splanchnic
Lingual
Long ciliary
Lowest splanchnic
Lumbar
Lumbo-inguinal
Mandibular
Masseteric
Maxillary
Median
Meningeal
Mental
Mesenteric plexus
Middle superior alveolar
Motor

THE NERVES (Continued)

Musculocutaneous
Mylohyoid
Nasal
Nasociliary
Nasopalatine
Obturator
Occipital
Oculomotor
Olfactory
Ophthalmic
Optic
Orbital
Ovarian
Palatine
Palpebral, inferior
Pelvic
Perineal
Peroneal, common
Peroneal, deep
Peroneal, superficial
Petrosal, greater superficial
Petrosal, lesser
Petrosal, lesser superficial
Pharyngeal
Phrenic
Phrenic plexus
Plantar
Popliteal
Posterior scrotal
Presacral
Pterygoid
Pterygopalatine
Pudendal
Pudendal plexus
Pudic, internal
Pulmonary
Pyloric
Radial
Recurrent laryngeal
Renal
Respiratory, of Bell
Saphenous
Scapular

Sciatic
Solar plexus
Spermatic
Sphenopalatine
Spinal accessory
Spinosus
Splanchnic
Splenic plexus
Stapedial
Stylohyoid
Stylopharyngeal
Subscapular
Supraclavicular
Supraorbital
Suprascapular
Supratrochlear
Sural
Temporal
Tensor tympani
Tensor veli palatini
Tentorial
Testicular
Thoracic, anterior
Thoracic, long
Thoracodorsal
Thyrohyoid
Tibial
Tibial, anterior
Tibial, posterior
Tonsillar
Trigeminal
Trochlear
Tympanic
Ulnar
Ureteric
Uterovaginal plexus
Vagus to vertebral artery
Vestibular
Vidian (of pterygoid canal)
Volar digital of Wrisberg
Zygomatic
Zygomaticofacial
Zygomaticotemporal

Section III - Regional Surgery

General Surgery	Chapter 7
Gynecology	Chapter 8
Neurosurgery	Chapter 9
Obstetrics	Chapter 10
Ophthalmology (Eye)	Chapter 11
Orthopedics	Chapter 12
Otolaryngology (ENT)	Chapter 13
Plastic Surgery	Chapter 14
Thoracic	Chapter 15
Urology	Chapter 16
Vascular surgery	Chapter 17

INTRODUCTION TO REGIONAL SURGERY

Modern surgery reaching for new goals and pyramiding its knowledge on what has already been learned, continues to open new vistas of thought and imagination in man's struggle to unveil the medical mysteries which surround him. The surgeon does not work alone. His daring achievements have been made possible through the efforts of biologists, biochemists, physiologists, bacteriologists, pharmacologists and other researchers whose work is allied to clinical medicine. Through their research there has evolved a new understanding of cardiovascular dynamics, blood clotting phenomena, system monitoring, tissue transplant, immunologic response and homograft, use of cold in surgery, use of the extraordinary energy of the laser, extracorporeal perfusion, in addition to many other important pharmacologic, physiologic, biochemical and bioelectric relationships in medicine. The modern surgeon is a member of this scientific team, applying what has been learned for the direct benefit of man.

The mysteries in medicine are many. The quest for answers will be an eternal one. New knowledge is always attended by new mysteries, but through knowledge we continue to grow. As the horizons of surgery expand so must those of all persons allied to this field. Modern medicine needs trained workers who perform intelligently rather than mechanically. It is only through the development of such personnel that the physician will be genuinely unburdened of duties which he is able to delegate. Toward this end we have developed the following chapters. The material, gathered in extensive research and consultation with numerous medical specialists, is designed to promote a greater interest, appreciation and understanding of surgery for persons whose work is related to this specialized field of medical endeavor.

CRYOSURGERY

Cryosurgery, a new surgical technique utilizing intense cold and fine instruments, is having a revolutionary impact on almost all surgical specialties. The technique employs the use of a fine instrument known as a cryoprobe which is insulated throughout its length by either silk or Teflon. Tip temperatures drop to a temperature of $-65°$ C. in simple cryoprobes. A cryogenic agent such as Freon 12 or liquid nitrogen is pumped through the evacuated insulated cryoprobe, the latter producing temperatures in the range of $-180°$ C. to $-190°$ C.

This technique is being used where limited necrosis or destruction to a small specific area is required as opposed to a technique which might focus on a more general local target and destroy healthy surrounding tissue.

Some diseases and tumors of the pituitary gland causing acromegaly, Cushing's disease and Nelson's syndrome (a hyperpigmentation seen after adrenalectomy due to the development of a pituitary adenoma), as well as basal ganglia disorders causing dystonia musculorum deformans, and Parkinson's disease are treated successfully by cryogenic destruction of responsible tissue.

Other advantages of this technique are being recognized in the palliative treatment of metastatic breast cancer and prostatic cancer through destruction of the pituitary and thereby, elimination of hormone stimulation to the tumor. Visual losses in some cases which are secondary to hemorrhagic type progressive diabetic retinal disease are also helped by cryohypophysectomy.

Another valuable application which is gaining widespread acceptance is use of this technique in cataract and other fine eye surgery.

With the development of finer instruments, cryosurgery will become increasingly important in all of the specialties, and particularly in those cases where fine selective tissue destruction is necessary.

THE LASER

The laser is a new device for the generation of a beam of light which is more coherent, more monochromatic and capable of greater intensity than any previous light source. It is a unique form of energy which also produces a thermal effect.

The theory of laser action was outlined in 1958, by Townes and Schawlow. In May, 1960, T. H. Maimian built the first operational model which was a solid state laser utilizing ruby. In 1961, Javan, Bennett and Herriott built the first gas laser which utilized a mixture of helium and neon in a glass tube. Its major advantage was its continuous wave emission.

The laser, although employed by some surgeons, is still a quasi-experimental instrument. Its coherently intense beam may be further concentrated and accurately focused by means of lenses and mirrors. The effect of the laser light ray is to set up an inflammation much in the same manner as diathermy coagulation. It actually produces a light coagulation. The high energy source provided by the intense beam appears to be differentially absorbed by pigmented areas. It has been used in experimental treatment of melanomas. It triggers some response within the tumor that appears initially to be a minimal one and yet, in the days which follow, a continuous regression in the tumor takes place. The laser possesses an almost surgical selectivity for pigmented areas with almost no damage to surrounding tissues. Retinal angiomas and retinal melanomas are some of the lesions which have been treated with the laser. It is still too early to assess these results.

In ophthalmology the laser photocoagulator is used for the prevention of retinal detachments. It is not used in the treatment of retinal detachment, but is used to wall off and seal off holes and small tears in the retina which are predisposing factors in the development of retinal detachment. The laser beam is also used to treat abnormal blood vessels on the retinal surface. Such vessels, if not destroyed, produce bleeding into the vitreous which leads to irreparable visual loss.

Dental surgeons have found that colored or discolored materials such as dental caries absorb more laser energy than uncolored materials. The effect of the laser on carious areas has varied from small 2 mm. deep holes to complete disappearance of the caries with some whitening of the rim around. It has been concluded that extensive destruction of carious areas of teeth by focused beams of a high energy pulsed ruby laser is possible. Added advantages in use of the laser for such procedures are the fact that laser light sterilizes the area and the laser burst is so short (1 to 3 milliseconds) that anesthesia is usually unnecessary. Stained tooth enamel is bleached by low laser energies, but cratered by high energies. Lasers can also be used to provide transillumination of teeth more effectively than current X-ray methods. Laser light has also proved effective in tooth cutting.

Other uses for the laser include hemostasis by coagulation, arterial anastomosis and use of the laser as a cutting instrument. Refinement in instrument development along with further experimentation should open many new applications for this valuable concept.

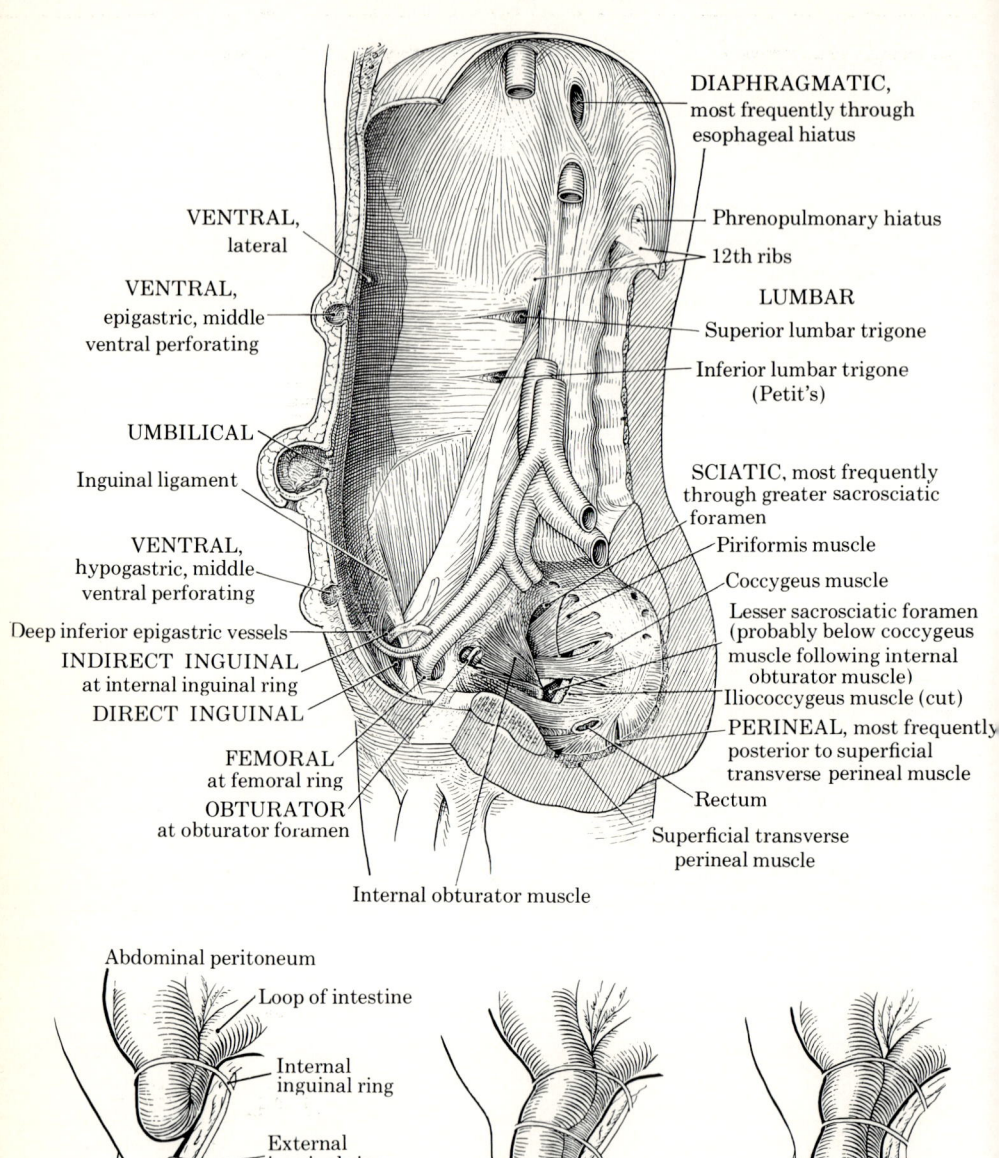

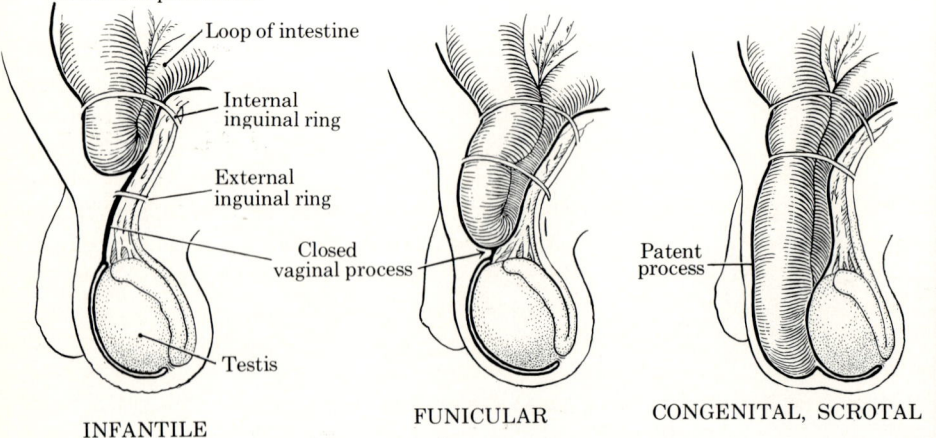

TYPES OF INDIRECT INGUINAL HERNIA.

7 | General Surgery

The field of general surgery encompasses a wide variety of operations and is not confined to particular organs or systems as are the surgical specialties. The modern, well trained general surgeon is qualified to perform many of the operations which we usually think of as specialty surgery with the exception of those procedures which require highly specialized knowledge and training. For example, the general surgeon might perform major ENT surgery such as a laryngectomy and yet not venture into delicate ear operations as, for instance, a stapedectomy or tympanoplasty.

We will confine our considerations of general surgery to those cases which do not encroach on the specialties presented elsewhere in this book. Representative cases, performed most frequently in the general hospital, have been selected to exemplify the work of the general surgeon. Other technical information has been included with these case presentations which should be of value to the secretary.

HERNIA (pl. herniae or hernias)

An abdominal hernia may be congenital or acquired, the latter often developing after a fall, heavy lifting or compression of the abdomen. Transmitted pressure caused by coughing, sneezing or straining at stool or urination may also result in a hernia. Other causes include increased abdominal pressure caused by ascites, pregnancy or tumor. A recent survey conducted in a VA hospital demonstrated that 17 per cent of patients with an intra-abdominal malignancy first presented themselves to the hospital for repair of an inguinal hernia.

The three component parts of a hernia are: (1) an opening in the abdominal wall (hernial ring), (2) a sac, and (3) the sac contents which usually consist of bowel or omentum. The diagnosis of hernia usually takes into account special circumstances prevailing in any of the component parts and indicates the anatomic location of the protrusion. Common hernial sites are illustrated in Fig. 38.

The list below contains qualifying terms frequently used in the diagnosis of hernia to describe special circumstances which prevail.

Complete —An inguinal hernia which passes into the scrotum.

Congenital —A hernia due to a developmental defect.

Direct —An internal inguinal hernia which emerges between the edge of the rectus muscle and deep epigastric artery.

Incarcerated —A hernia in which the contents have become adherent to the sac making the hernia irreducible, but where neither obstruction or circulatory interruption has developed.

Incomplete —An inguinal hernia which has descended through the external ring or inguinal canal but has not entered the scrotum.

Indirect —An external or oblique inguinal hernia which descends out of the abdomen through the internal ring, down through the inguinal canal, external to the deep epigastric artery. It often passes out the external ring into the scrotum. The sac of an indirect inguinal hernia lies in the spermatic cord, while a direct inguinal hernia is unrelated to the spermatic cord.

Interstitial —A hernia in which a knuckle of intestine lies between two layers of the abdominal wall.

Irreducible —A hernia which cannot be returned to the abdomen by manipulation (taxis).

Pantaloon —A combined hernia consisting of an indirect and direct inguinal hernia.

Recurrent —A hernia which reappears after a previous reduction.

Reducible —A hernia in which the contents of the sac may be returned to the peritoneal cavity.

Sliding —A hernia in which a part of the hernial sac is formed by a retroperitoneal organ, most commonly the bladder, cecum, descending colon or sigmoid.

Strangulated —A hernia with interference to the vascular supply of the hernial sac contents, usually the bowel.

TYPES OF HERNIA

Abdominal
Acquired
Adiposa
Amniotic
Barth's
Beclard's (femoral)
Birkett's
Bladder
Cecal
Cloquet's (pectineal)
Complete
Concealed
Congenital
Cooper's (retroperitoneal)
Crural
Diaphragmatic
Direct inguinal
Dry
Duodenojejunal
Encysted
Epigastric
External
Extrasaccular
Fat
Femoral
Foraminal
Funicular
Gastroesophageal
Gibbon's (hydrocele & hernia)
Gluteal
Goyrand's (inguinal)
Gruber's (int. mesogastric)
Grynfelt (superior lumbar)
Hesselbach's
Hey's (encysted)
Hiatal
Hiatus
Holthouse's (inguinal)
Incarcerated
Incisional (ventral)
Incomplete
Indirect inguinal
Infantile
Inguinal
  congenital
  direct

incarcerated
indirect (oblique)
interstitial
recurrent
sliding
strangulated
Inguinocrural
Inguinofemoral
Inguinoproperitoneal
Inguinosuperficial
In recto
Intermuscular
Internal
Interparietal
Intersigmoid
Interstitial
  inguinosuperficial (Küster)
  interparietal
  properitoneal (Krönlein)
Irreducible
Ischiatic
Ischiorectal
Krönlein (inguinoproperitoneal)
Küster (inguinosuperficial)
Labial
Laugier's (femoral)
Levator
Linea alba
Littre
Littre-Richter's
Lumbar
Maydl's (W hernia)
Mesenteric
Mesocolic
Mucosal
Oblique
Obturator
  anterior iliac
  hernia foraminis ovalis
  opeocele
  thyroidal
Omental
Ovarian
Pantaloon
Paraduodenal
Paraesophageal

TYPES OF HERNIA (continued)

Paraperitoneal
Parasaccular
Par glissement
Parietal
Paraumbilical
Pectineal
Perineal
Petit's
Properitoneal
Pudendal
Pulsion
Rectal
Reducible
Retrocecal
Retrograde
Retroperitoneal
Richter's
Rieux's (retrocecal)
Rokitansky's
Sciatic
Scrotal
Sliding (hernia en glissade)
 intraperitoneal—sliding
hernia with complete sac
 paraperitoneal—sliding
hernia with incomplete sac
 extraperitoneal—sliding
hernia without a sac
Slip
Slipped
Spigelian (abdominal)
Strangulated
Subpubic
Thyroidal (obturator)
Treitz's
Tunicary
Umbilical
Uterine
Vaginal
Vaginolabial
Velpeau (femoral)
Ventral
Vesical (urinary bladder)
Voluminous
Von Bergmann (hiatus)
W hernia

TECHNIQUES FOR REPAIR OF INGUINAL HERNIA
(Herniorrhaphy)

Andrews Modification of **Bassini**
Anson-McVay
Babcock
Bassini
Bevans Right-Sliding
Bloodgood
Ferguson
Ferguson-Coley
Gallies
Graham Roscie Sliding Sigmoidal
Halsted Rectus Sheath Flap
Handley Darn & Staylace
Hey Grooves
Hopkins
Hotchkiss
Houget (Pantaloon Hernia)
Hunt's
Inlay
Keel
Lotheissen
Mackid's (sliding)
Mair's Whole Skin **Graft**
Mayo
McArthur
McVay
Mermingas
Nuttall
Ogilvie
Tanner Slide Operation
Turner
Wangensteen
Wise's Method
Wyllys Andrews **Imbrication**
Zieman Indirect **Repair**
Zimmerman (sliding)

ANATOMIC FEATURES INVOLVED IN INGUINAL REPAIRS

Aponeurosis of ext. oblique
Areolar tissues
Circumflex iliac superficial fascia
Conjoined tendon
Cooper's ligament
Cremaster fascia
Cremaster muscle
Deep epigastric vessels
Direct component
External oblique
External pudic vessels
Funiculus spermaticus
Gimbernat's ligament
Hesselbach's triangle
Hypogastric branch of iliohypogastric nerve
Iliohypogastric nerve
Ilioinguinal nerve
Infundibuloform fascia
Inguinal ligament
Inguinal ring
Lacunar ligament
Leaf (leaves) of muscle
Ligamentum inguinale
Os pubis spine
Pampiniform plexus
Pillars, external and internal
Plexus pampiniformis
Poupart's ligament
Processus vaginalis
Properitoneal fat
Pubic bone
Pubic crest
Pudendal vessels
Rectus sheath
Sac
Scarpa's fascia
Shelving edge of Poupart's
Spermatic cord
Transversalis fascia
Vas deferens

McVay Inguinal Herniorrhaphy

After satisfactory general anesthesia, the patient's abdomen was prepared and draped in the usual manner.

A right groin incision was made and carried through the skin and subcutaneous tissues. Hemostasis was secured with clamps and individual ligatures. Sharp and blunt dissection was employed to free the entire inguinal ligament inferiorly and medially. The aponeurosis of the external oblique was sharply incised, opening the external ring. Sharp and blunt dissection was employed to free the round ligament and its contents. Prior to this, the ilioinguinal nerve was visualized, identified, isolated and retracted out of the way.

Rather extensive dissection in the operative area failed to reveal the presence of any hernial sac, even though the indirect area was dilated and loose in character. The round ligament was transected. A high ligation with transfixing suture was done. The internal ring was undisturbed. There was a mild weakness in the direct component. The inferior epigastric artery was identified, visualized and retracted inferiorly. Palpatation along the femoral canal revealed the presence of a defect about 1½ fingerbreadths in diameter. It was elected, therefore, to perform a herniorrhaphy of the McVay (Cooper's ligament) type repair.

Interrupted 00 dacron sutures were employed to coapt Cooper's ligament to the internal oblique aponeurosis and this was accomplished down to the level of the femoral artery and vein, where a transitional suture of the same material was placed, from the inguinal ligament, to Cooper's ligament, to the femoral sheath. This completely closed the defect. The aponeurosis of the external oblique was closed with a running suture of 000 chromic. Subcuticular closure with interrupted sutures of 000 chromic was done and a pull-out suture of 00 nylon was used to close the skin. Blood loss was negligible and none was replaced. Sponge count was correct on two occasions.

Bassini Operation for Inguinal Herniorrhaphy

Under general anesthesia, the patient was sterilely prepared and draped in the supine position.

An oblique incision was made about ½ inch above and parallel to Poupart's ligament, from a point opposite the anterior superior spinous process of the ilium, to the spine of the os pubis. The incision was deepened to expose the fascia of the external abdominal oblique muscle. The incision severed the superficial epigastric vessels, running at right angles to them. These were carefully ligated. The superficial external pudic vessels and the superficial circumflex vessels were also encountered.

Exposure and identification of the components of the external abdominal ring was accomplished. A Kocher was introduced through the external ring. The aponeurosis of the external abdominal oblique muscle was divided from the external ring, along the line of incision, for 2 or 3 inches. The edges of the aponeurotic flaps were retracted and the upper flap was separated inward. The lower flap was separated from Poupart's ligament. The index finger, covered with gauze, was used to strip and expose the lower leaf of the divided external oblique muscle from the underlying structures. The contents of the inguinal canal were exposed. The ilio-inguinal nerve was identified and avoided.

The conjoined tendon was identified. Full exposure was accomplished by retraction. The hernial sac and cord were raised en masse. By stripping and dissection, the sac was completely isolated from the spermatic cord as high as possible in relation to the internal ring. The sac was opened and its contents examined. The contents were returned to the abdominal cavity.

The conjoined tendon was retracted. The hernial sac was transfixed at its base, as high as possible, with chromic catgut. The deep epigastric vessels were avoided. The ligature was tied. The neck of the sac was encircled and the ligature tied once more. The redundant sac was removed. The stump of the sac retracted beyond the internal ring. A strip of tape was insinuated under the cord and it was retracted out of the way. Six # 2 catgut sutures were introduced beneath the cord, from before, backward and from within, outward. This united the conjoined tendon with the transversalis fascia, muscles and the lower fibers of the internal oblique muscle with Poupart's ligament. Sutures were tied and tissues approximated.

The cord was replaced on its new floor. The aponeurosis of the external oblique muscle was approximated with interrupted sutures of # 2 catgut. There was no constriction of the cord at its exit from the newly constructed external ring. This was verified by introduction of the little finger into the external opening. The skin was closed with interrupted silkworm-gut.

FEMORAL HERNIA

A femoral hernia consists of the descending of intestines through the femoral ring, an area in the lower lateral abdomen just above the crease of the thigh. The femoral ring is bounded in front by the inguinal ligament, behind by the Pectineus muscle covered by the pectineal fascia, laterally by the fibrous septum on the medial aspect of the femoral vein, and medially by the base of the lacunar ligament. The ring is closed by extraperitoneal fatty tissue called the septum femorale or crural septum. The round ligament of the uterus in the female lies immediately above the anterior margin of the ring as does the spermatic cord in the male.

Femoral hernias constitute about four per cent of all hernias and appear to be more common in women. The incidence in children is comparatively rare.

TYPES OF FEMORAL HERNIORRHAPHY

Anson-McVay
Combined femoral-inguinal approach
Extra-peritoneal approach
Gallie's
Henry
High Operation (inguinal approach)
Lotheissen (high operation)
Lower Operation (femoral approach)
Marcy Purse-String Method
McEvedy
Ogilvie
Wyllys Andrews

FEMORAL ANATOMIC STRUCTURES

Aponeurosis (pl. aponeuroses)
Conjoined tendon
Cooper's ligament
Cribriform fascia
Crural canal
External iliac vessels
Falciform process of fascia lata
Fascia lata of thigh
Femoral canal
Femoral sheath
Gimbernat's ligament
Hesselbach's triangle
Iliopectineal line
Lacunar ligament
Leaf (leaves) of aponeurosis
Pectineal fascia
Pectineal ligament
Pectineal line
Pectineus fascia
Peritoneum
Poupart's ligament
Properitoneal fat
Scarpa's triangle
Transversalis fascia

Femoral Herniorrhaphy

Under general anesthesia, the patient was placed in the supine position. An incision was made between the left corner of the pubic bone and the left anterior superior iliac spine. It was carried down to the fascia. The bleeders were clamped with Kelly clamps and tied with 000 chromic sutures.

The large hernial sac was visualized. It was opened and found to contain a large piece of omentum. The omentum was partially necrotic and was therefore excised. It was clamped with several hemostats, divided and the hemostats replaced with sutures of 000 chromic catgut. The sac was freed. The remaining omentum was replaced into the abdomen. The base of the sac was sutured with a 00 intestinal catgut, tied and the sac removed. The femoral vessels could easily be palpated.

Poupart's ligament was sutured to the fascia with interrupted 00 cotton sutures. A second layer of suture was placed approximating the aponeurosis of the external oblique to Cooper's ligament with 00 interrupted cotton sutures.

A small catheter drain was inserted into the wound because of oozing. It was brought out below the incision, through a small stab wound. The skin edges along with the subcutaneous tissues were approximated with interrupted mattress sutures of 00 cotton. Pressure dressing was applied to the wound.

GENERAL SURGERY

DIAPHRAGMATIC HERNIA

The diaphragm is a musculomembranous structure which serves as a partition between the chest (thoracic) cavity and the abdominal cavity. An opening called a hiatus exists in this partition through which the esophagus passes to connect with the stomach. It is at this hiatus that herniation most commonly occurs. These are called hiatal hernias.

Defects in the diaphragm may be congenital or may be acquired from injuries to the chest or abdomen. They sometimes develop following subphrenic abscess.

The principal types of diaphragmatic hernia are:
(1) Short esophagus
(2) Sliding (stomach enters thorax)
(3) Paraesophageal (esophagus remains attached to the diaphragm while the gastric cardia moves upward into the thorax, alongside the esophagus)

Diaphragmatic herniorrhaphy may be accomplished either through a transabdominal approach or a transthoracic approach.

Diaphragmatic Herniorrhaphy—Transthoracic approach for hiatal hernia

The patient was prepared and draped after being positioned on his right side. It was decided to enter the thoracic cavity through the 7th intercostal space. A skin incision was made coursing from the spine to the midaxillary line. The skin incision was deepened into the musculature for its entire length. A small section of the 7th and 8th ribs was removed to facilitate entry into the pleural cavity. The left phrenic nerve was crushed.

The abdominal contents were carefully examined and no incarceration was noted. There was no other pathology nor were there any marked adhesions. A few small adhesions were lysed and hemostasis secured. The intestinal contents were replaced in the abdomen after a gastrotomy had been performed and the stomach lining found to be normal. No ulcerations were noted. Adhesions were found binding the fundus of the stomach to the liver. These were freed by blunt and sharp dissection. The gastroesophageal junction was visualized and freed from adhesions. The defect was found and measured approximately 7 cm. in diameter and easily admitted three fingers.

By blunt and sharp dissection, the right and left crus of the diaphragm were freed and reapproximated with interrupted 00 silk. The hiatal hernia was then further diminished by approximating the crus anterior to the esophagus with one interrupted 0 silk stitch. The defect at the termination of the procedure measured approximately 2 cm. in diameter and admitted two fingers.

The peritoneum was then closed with interrupted 00 chromic and the fascia was reapproximated with interrupted figure-of-eight #30 wire. The subcutaneous tissue was closed with chromic and the skin edges brought together with interrupted cotton.

UMBILICAL HERNIA

Umbilical hernia consists of a protrusion at the umbilicus. It may consist of a congenital hernia into the cord (omphalocele) or a hernia through the umbilical ring, the latter being the most common.

Omphalocele is a birth defect in the abdominal wall consisting of a thin walled protrusion through which the abdominal viscera may be seen. It might more accurately be described as an eventration of the abdominal wall than a hernia. Such defects are usually covered with shifting skin flaps shortly after birth to prevent rupture of the hernia with evisceration and peritonitis. A later repair is carried out after the abdominal cavity has developed to the extent where it may contain the displaced organs.

UMBILICAL HERNIA REPAIR TECHNIQUES

Imbrication technic
Repair with omphalectomy

Repair with umbilectomy
Vest-over-pants technic

Umbilical Herniorrhaphy

Under general anesthesia the patient was placed in the supine position. A curved elliptical incision was made inferior to the umbilicus extending laterally for a distance of approximately $1\frac{1}{4}$ inches. The incision was made down through the subcutaneous tissues and down to the fascia proper. The underlying sac was freed from its entire circumference and carefully opened. Upon opening the sac, a small piece of omentum was found to be incarcerated. The omentum was then handled by division between curved Kelly clamps. The sac was freed. The peritoneal contents were in place. The peritoneum, itself, was freed from the surrounding edges.

An attempt was made to explore the abdominal cavity, but because of the fact that there were so many abdominal adhesions from previous surgery, the exploration was quite inadequate. After having excised the redundant peritoneum, the peritoneum was closed with a continuous atraumatic suture.

The rectus sheath had already been freed from the subcutaneous tissue. It was also freed from the underlying peritoneum to permit correction of the midline defect. Following this, an overlapping type of repair was performed by placing a series of mattress sutures which would imbricate the upper flap over the lower flap. The closure was further reinforced by again approximating the upper flap to the distal flap, to the lower flap with interrupted 000 cotton sutures.

After adequate bleeding control was achieved, closure was accomplished by first approximating the subcutaneous tissue with interrupted 000000 cotton sutures. The umbilicus was then sutured to the underlying fascia with one interrupted 000000 cotton suture. Closure of the skin was accomplished with interrupted 00000 dermalon sutures.

500 cc. of 5% glucose in water was used during the operation.

Left Radical Groin Dissection

An incision was made just above a previous hernial incision for the removal of a carcinomatous testicle. The incision was carried through the subcutaneous tissue, to the aponeurosis of the external oblique. It was then carried to the internal oblique muscle, following the extension of the incision through the internal oblique. A portion of the internal oblique muscle and transversalis were incised. Bleeders were clamped, cut and ligated with 000 chromic suture. Following incision through the muscles, the extraperitoneal tissue and preperitoneal fascia were encountered. The peritoneum was reflected medially. The cord, which had been ligated previously, was encountered. This was isolated between the muscle layers and was dissected further towards its origin. Clamps were applied and the vessels were ligated. Following the excision of the spermatic cord, dissection was carried out exposing the ureter. This was reflected medially. The iliac vessels and hypogastric vessels were all isolated and were entered. The internal and external iliacs were exposed. The peri-iliac glands were dissected out carefully. There were several pudendal glands. The nerve was oriented at this point and the obturator palpated. Dissection was carried along the common iliac to the aorta and this was palpated high towards the region of the kidney. All of the perivascular fatty tissue as well as the glands between the aorta, at the bifurcation of the iliac, and at the common, internal and external iliacs were exposed and dissected out. There were no unusual tumor masses palpable anywhere in the extraperitoneal area.

A drain was inserted into the pelvic cavity and brought out through the superior portion of the wound.

Repair was carried out using interrupted 000 and 00 dacron sutures for the various fascial and muscle layers. Partial covering of the internal oblique was accomplished with interrupted 000 dacron. The fascia of the external oblique was approximated with interrupted 00 dacron and the subcutaneous tissue with interrupted chromic. The skin was closed with subcuticular nylon.

A separate longitudinal incision was then made commencing just inferior to Poupart's ligament and extending down along the greater saphenous vein, exposing the femoral artery. There were several small glands encountered here. The artery and vein were carefully dissected out. Several branches of the greater saphenous were clamped, cut and ligated. The perivascular fatty tissue and glands were removed for a distance of about 5 inches. The tissues were approximated with 000 interrupted chromic suture and the skin with subcuticular nylon.

THE NAILS

Traumatic injuries to the fingernails or toenails and ingrown nails of the large toes constitute the principal reasons for surgery of these structures. These conditions often require radical excision of the nail rather than simple excision, and in such instances, the patient is admitted to surgery.

Some of the conditions which may be listed as the pre- or postoperative diagnosis have been listed here with structures commonly referred to in operative dictations of nail excisions.

NAIL STRUCTURES

Body	Lunula
Cuticle	Matrix
Cuticular fold	Nail bed
Dorsal plate	Nail fold
Eponychium	Root

DISEASES OF THE NAILS

Eggshell nails	Onychomycosis
Koilonychia	Onychorrhexis
Leukonychia	Paronychia
Onychauxis	Polyunguia
Onychia	Unguis incarnatus (ingrown)

Radical Excision of Toenails

The patient was admitted with recurrent ingrown toenails for which radical excision of the toenails was proposed.

Under general anesthesia, the patient was prepared and draped in the supine position.

Beginning with the right great toe, a tourniquet was applied to the base of the toe to create a bloodless field. A small incision was made in the soft tissue of the nail fold and eponychium, on a line with the incision, and extended back to the matrix. The nail was raised from its bed with scissors for its entire length. A loose piece of nail was grasped with forceps and by gradual traction and separation from the nail bed, it was removed in one piece.

Using a small curet, the matrix and nail bed were curetted to prevent recurrent nail growth. The same procedure was carried out on the left great toe.

INCISION AND DRAINAGE OF ABSCESS (EXTERNAL)
INSTRUMENTS

Backhaus towel clamp	Mayo Hegar needle holder
Crile forceps	Mayo Pean forceps
Grooved director	Mayo scissors
Kelly forceps	Thumb forceps

Incision and Drainage of Abscess on Buttocks

Under spinal anesthesia the patient was sterilely prepared and draped in the usual manner.

There was an abscess about the size of a small egg on the left buttocks which was incised and drained. The area of the abscess was dissected free and loculations were broken up.

The incision was cross-hatched over the surface of the abscess. A small Penrose drain was inserted. Culture was taken for bacteriologic identification and sensitivity studies.

Incision and Drainage, Dorsum of Hand

With the patient under general anesthesia, the hand was prepared and draped in the usual manner.

The abscess which presented on the dorsum of the hand, over the hypothenar surface, was incised in a stellate fashion and probed. It was then drained and cleaned of all purulent material.

The abscess cavity was packed with Iodoform gauze and the hand bandaged over a gauze compress and wad of mechanic's waste.

The patient tolerated the procedure well and was returned to the room in good condition.

Excision of Pilonidal Cyst

After satisfactory spinal anesthesia was obtained, the patient was placed in the prone flexed position. Sterile preparation and draping was carried out.

An elliptical incision was made after methylene blue injection of the sinus and it was excised en bloc. Hemostasis was secured with clamps and individual ligatures.

Interrupted 000 chromic catgut sutures were employed to coapt the deeper layers employing the fascia of the coccyx also. A maneuver of vertical mattress sutures of 00 cotton was done to coapt the edges entirely. A running subcuticular pull-out type 00 nylon suture was employed to close the skin. Sponge and needle counts on two occasions were correct.

THE BREASTS

The breasts, otherwise known as the mammae or mammary glands, give rise to a variety of surgical lesions which are usually treated by the general surgeon. It is argued in some quarters that surgery of the breasts belongs in the specialty of gynecology; however, this classification is not universally accepted. For this reason, we will consider the breasts in the category of general surgery. Operations designed to augment or reduce the size of the breasts belong in the category of plastic surgery.

One of the most common conditions involving the breast in the male is gynecomastia (excessive enlargement of the male breasts). Frequently seen surgical lesions in the female breast include abscesses, fibrocystic disease, blue dome cysts, cystic mastitis, fibroadenomas and other benign neoplasms.

The most important disease of the female breasts is carcinoma (cancer). In the U.S.A. each year approximately 50,000 new cases are diagnosed and at least 25,000 women succumb to the disease. It is the most common female malignancy. The probability of a woman developing breast cancer, based on American Cancer Society statistics, is one in 20, or about 5 per cent. It does not occur in prepubertal breasts and only rarely before the age of 25 years. The highest incidence is found between the ages of 40 and 70, with the mean age of onset being 57 years. It is interesting to note that there is a very low incidence of this disease among Japanese women. Breast cancer is also rare in the male, the ratio being one male for every 100 females with the disease.

The etiology of breast cancer remains obscure. The belief that it is more common in women who have never been pregnant or have never lactated has not been supported by recent surveys. Also, local injury to the breast is no longer considered a causative factor. Etiology is believed to be related to hormonal, genetic and viral influences with a hereditary tendency suggested by the higher frequency in patients with a family history of this malignancy.

Breast cancer may arise in any part of the breast; however, 50 per cent of these tumors are found in an area which includes the areola and the upper outer breast quadrant. Statistics suggest that these tumors of the outer aspect of the breast have a somewhat better prognosis for cure than tumors of the medial half, the latter often being associated with metastases to the internal mammary chain of lymph nodes adjacent to the sternum, and beneath the ribs.

Common sites of metastases from a primary breast tumor include the axilla, supraclavicular area, mediastinum, lungs and liver. Skeletal metastases develop more commonly in the spine, pelvis, upper end of the femur, ribs, shoulder girdle and skull. The tumor spreads by embolization through lymph channels to regional and distant lymph nodes, by embolization through the veins, and by direct extension.

The surgeon's examination of the breast takes note of such clinical signs as nipple retraction or dimpling, edema of the skin over the tumor causing an orange peel appearance, abnormal nipple discharge (seen more often in benign breast lesions), eruption of the skin of the areola and nipple and enlarged axillary (armpit) lymph nodes. On the basis of these findings the physician determines whether the lesion is operable or inoperable. When there is clinical evidence that the tumor has passed to the incurable stage, only palliative treatment is offered in the form of irradiation therapy.

Lesions which are deemed operable are biopsied first. While the patient is still on the operating table, the removed tissue is examined by the pathologist using a technique called frozen section. The results are reported back to the surgeon in about 10 minutes. When malignancy is diagnosed, the biopsy wound is closed and sealed off with a plastic material. The patient is redraped and a fresh surgical set-up is used to prevent implantation of viable cancer cells into the mastectomy wound. The usual operation for operable breast cancer is radical mastectomy, an operation in which the entire breast, the attached pectoral muscles, axillary lymph nodes and fat are removed as one specimen. When the cancer occurs in the medial (inner) portion of the breast some surgeons remove the internal mammary chain of lymph nodes as well.

If axillary lymph node metastases are found at the time of surgery, or if the tumor is located in the medial portion of the breast, postoperative radiotherapy is often given.

Postmastectomy patients frequently develop edema of the arm as a result of blockage in the venous system or in the deep and superficial lymphatics of the axilla. This condition is sometimes treated by the Kondoleon or Beck operation designed to promote lymphatic drainage.

Inoperable breast cancer in premenopausal patients is often treated by oophorectomy (removal of the ovaries). There is a current prevailing belief that breast tumors may be hormone dependent and therefore estrogen stimulation of the tumor must be removed. In some cases adrenalectomy is employed since this is another source of estrogen production. When it is deemed advisable to eliminate all estrogen production in the body, hypophysectomy (removal or destruction of the pituitary gland at the base of the brain) is performed. The latter two operations are the more radical and are performed less frequently than a bilateral oophorectomy. Patients who undergo adrenalectomy must be maintained thereafter on daily supplements of cortisone and salt, while patients who undergo hypophysectomy must be managed on cortisone, pituitary extract and thyroid extract. Although these three hormones are secreted by different glands, their production is dependent upon the hormones of the anterior pituitary.

The Axillary Region

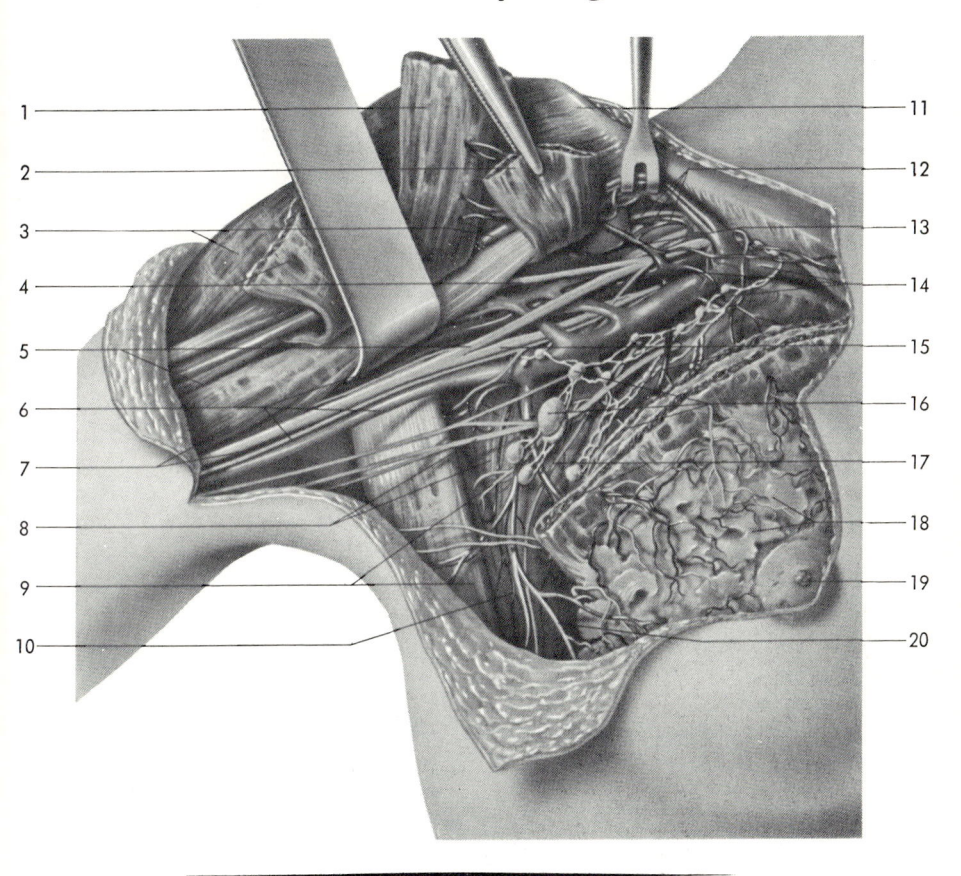

1 Pectoralis major muscle
2 Pectoralis minor muscle
3 Deltoid muscle; cephalic vein
4 Pectoralis major muscle; musculocutaneous nerve
5 Long head of biceps brachii muscle; lateral branch of median nerve
6 Brachial artery and vein; ulnar nerve
7 Short head of biceps brachii muscle; median nerve
8 Intercostobrachial nerve; subscapularis muscle
9 Thoracodorsal nerve; latissimus dorsi muscle
10 Branch of thoracodorsal artery
11 Acromial extremity of clavicle
12 Suprascapular artery, vein and nerve
13 Thoracoacromial artery
14 Axillary artery and vein; subclavian lymphatic trunk
15 Median branch of median nerve; lateral thoracic artery
16 Axillary lymph nodes; pectoralis minor muscle
17 Long thoracic nerve; pectoralis major muscle
18 Lobes of breast
19 Papilla of breast
20 Thoracoepigastric vein

Figure 39 The axillary region
Courtesy of Lederle Laboratories

Premenopausal patients are sometimes treated with testosterone, a male sex hormone which suppresses estrogen formation. It is believed that tumor stimulation by estrogen may continue in a woman for as many as 10 years after her menopause. For this reason, these patients are usually treated as premenopausal patients. In the older (more than 10 years postmenopause) incurable patient with breast cancer, palliative hormonal therapy is employed using male hormones as well as female hormones.

Scientists currently suspect that a biological balance exists between the patient and the tumor, and that this is the factor which predetermines the outcome of a case more so than does time or mode of therapy. This element of balance is believed to determine the growth and spread of the disease before the diagnosis is made (Macdonald). The theoretical curability rate proposed by Macdonald is 45 per cent of any series, a figure which corresponds to the over-all salvage rate for this disease. He suggests that some patients are incurable by any means, that some are curable by simple surgery, while others may be saved only by radical surgery. Much remains to be learned about the tumor-host relationship and the factors which may influence this association in favor of or against the host.

DISEASES OF THE BREASTS

Aberrant breast
Abscess
  retromammary
Absence of one breast
Actinomycosis
Adenocarcinoma
Adenofibroma
Adenomatosis
Agalactia
Chemical burn
Comedo mastitis
Cyst
  retention
Cysticercosis
Cystosarcoma phyllodes
Ductal carcinoma
  in situ
Echinococcosis
Fat necrosis
Fibrosis
Filarial elephantiasis
Fissure of nipple
Fistula
  puerperal

Galactocele
Galactorrhea
Gynecomastia (male)
Hemangiosarcoma
Hematoma
Hypertrophy of female breasts
Hypoplasia of areola
Infarction
Intracystic papillary carcinoma
Inversion of nipple
Involution cyst
Lobular carcinoma
Lymphosarcoma
Mastitis
  acute
  chronic
  cystic
  interstitial
  puerperal with mumps
  suppurative
Mastopathy
Medullary carcinoma
Occlusion of duct
Papilloma of breast

DISEASES OF THE BREASTS (continued)

Plasma cell mastitis
Sarcoma
Supernumerary breast
Supernumerary nipple
Sweat gland carcinoma

Syphilis of breast
Thelitis
Thrush of breast
Tuberculosis of breast
Varicose veins of breast

OPERATIONS ON THE BREASTS

Biopsy
Excision of lesion
Excision of nipple
Incision and drainage
Mammilliplasty (plastic operation of nipple)
  with free graft of nipple
  with position change of nipple
Mammoplasty (also: mammaplasty)
  augmentation with prostheses
  reductive
Mastectomy
  simple complete
  partial
  radical (breast, axillary lymph nodes and pectoral muscles)
Mastopexy
Mastoplasty
Mastotomy
  with drainage
  with exploration
  with removal of foreign body
Suture of breast

ANATOMIC FEATURES OF THE BREAST and AXILLA

Acromiothoracic artery
Alar thoracic artery
Alar thoracic vein
Areola
Areolar glands
Cooper's ligament
Ducts
Fascia of recti muscles
Glands of Montgomery
Internal mammary artery

Lactating breasts
Mammary gland
Nerve of Bell
Nipple
Papilla
Parenchyma
Pectoralis major
Pectoralis minor
Space of Mohrenheim
Sulcus

ARTERIAL SUPPLY

Acromial
Acromiothoracic
Alar thoracic
Intercostals

Internal mammary
Long thoracic
Subscapular artery
Thoracic branch of **axillary**

MASTECTOMY INCISIONS

Elsberg
Halsted
Handley
Jackson
Meyer
Rodman
Stewart
Thomas-Warren

Right Breast Biopsy—Frozen Section—Right Radical Mastectomy

After satisfactory general endotracheal anesthesia, the patient's right breast was prepared and draped in the usual manner.

An areolar incision was made and, by sharp dissection, an excisional biopsy of the right breast was carried out. This mass was approximately 4 cm. in diameter and was immediately sent to the pathologist for frozen section examination. The wound in the areolar area was closed over a gauze pack with a continuous 000 nylon suture. Frozen section report of the excisional biopsy was malignant. A radical mastectomy was elected.

An elliptical incision was made from the middle of the clavicle down to about the end of the thoracic cage and the skin flaps developed. Sharp dissection was employed to develop fairly thin flaps on the medial aspect. These tapered out to relatively thick flaps at the base of the flap, per se. Hemostasis was secured with clamps and electrocautery. Sharp dissection was employed to find the distal attachment of the Pectoralis major. This was doubly cross clamped, divided and then suture ligated. Continuous sharp and blunt dissection was employed to identify the head of the Pectoralis minor. This was also transected between clamps and suture ligated. The entire axillary vein was then cleaned of all its inferior branches and surrounding fat. The axilla was likewise cleaned of its fat and lymphatic node content. The long thoracic nerve was visualized.

By sharp dissection, the Pectoralis major, Pectoralis minor and overlying breast were removed. Hemostasis was secured with clamps and individual ligatures or electrocautery. The Serratus anterior was left intact.

The entire operative area was then inspected for hemostasis and it was found to be secure. Large Penrose drains were placed for drainage purposes and a French catheter for irrigation-suction purposes. The wound was irrigated with Clorpactin solution.

The skin was closed in one layer with vertical mattress type sutures. There was no area of discoloration of the skin and the flaps appeared to be viable. Blood loss sustained during the course of the operation was replaced in the operating room. Sponge counts taken on several occasions were found to be correct. The patient tolerated the operation well and was returned to the recovery room in satisfactory condition.

THE TONGUE

The tongue is a movable muscular organ on the floor of the mouth which assists in the articulation of sound, acts of mastication and swallowing. It has a midline fold of mucous membrane on its undersurface called the frenulum, which serves to attach the tongue to the floor of the mouth. Anatomic relationships of the tongue and its adjacent structures are best exemplified in Fig. 40.

Diseases of the tongue are not commonly encountered except possibly syphilitic and neoplastic lesions. Cancer of the tongue occurs with higher frequency in males over fifty years of age. Lymphatic extension is to the submaxillary, submental and upper deep cervical lymph nodes. Surgical treatment of this condition usually involves radical removal of the areas of lymphatic drainage as well as the primary lesion.

DISEASES OF THE TONGUE

Abscess of tongue
Acanthosis of tongue
Adenocarcinoma
Adhesion of tongue to gum
Adhesion of tongue to roof of mouth
Aglossia (congenital absence)
Ankyloglossia (tongue-tie)
Atrophy of mucous membrane
Atrophy of tongue
Bifid tongue
Bifurcation of tongue
Black hairy tongue
Chemical burn
Chondroma
Cleft tongue
Cyst of tongue
Displacement downward
Double tongue
Elongated frenulum linguae
Epidermoid carcinoma
Fissured tongue
Geographic tongue
Glossitis
Granular cell myoblastoma
Hemangioma
Leukoplakia
Lipoma
Lymphangioma
Macroglossia (congenital hypertrophy)
Median rhomboidal glossitis
Microglossia (hypoplasia)
Monilial infection
Mucous cyst
Papilloma
Senile atrophy
Shortening of frenulum linguae
Syphilis
Thrush
Trichinosis
Tuberculosis
Ulcer of tongue
Vincent's infection

OPERATIONS ON THE TONGUE

Biopsy of the tongue
Clipping of frenum linguae
Glossectomy
    complete
    partial (hemiglossectomy)
Glossoplasty
Glossorrhaphy (suture repair)
Glossotomy
    with drainage of abscess
    with removal of foreign body

Region of the Mouth

LATERAL VIEW OF THE LINGUAL REGION

INNERVATION AND BLOOD SUPPLY OF THE TEETH

LINGUAL BLOOD SUPPLY

GLANDS OF THE MOUTH

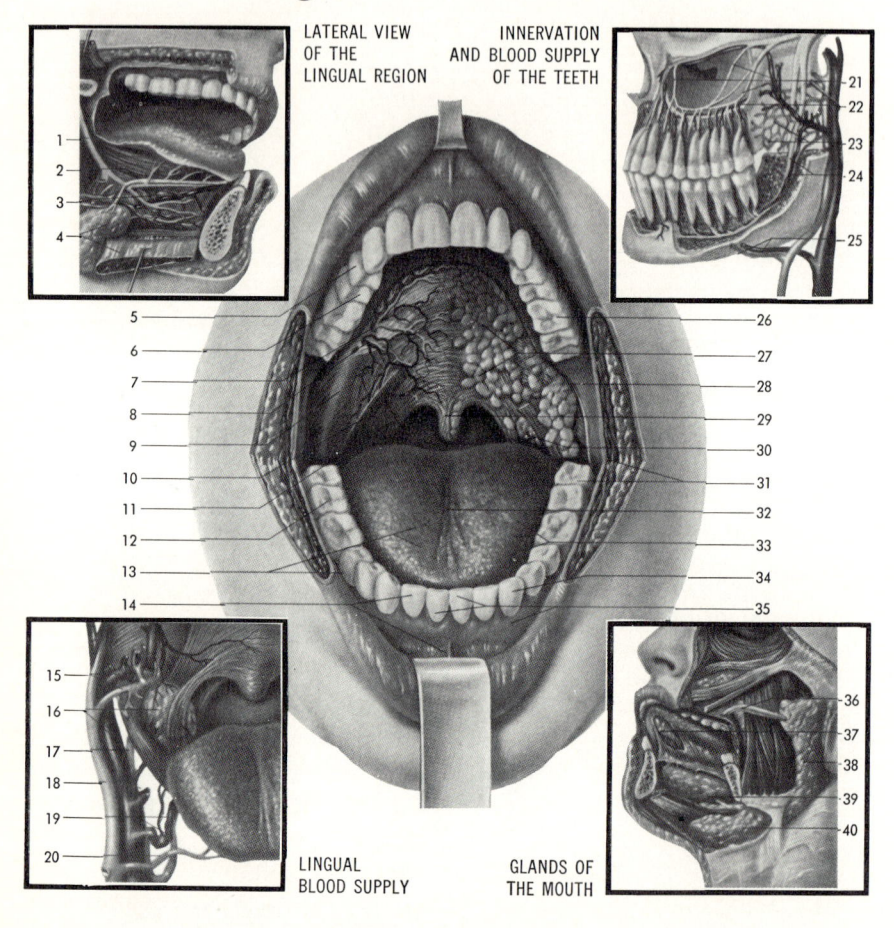

1 Lingual nerve
2 Submaxillary duct
3 Sublingual branches of lingual artery and vein
4 Submaxillary gland; mylohyoid muscle
5 First premolar
6 Second premolar
7 Greater palatine artery and nerve
8 Lesser palatine artery and nerve
9 Pterygomandibular raphe
10 Glossopalatine muscle
11 Pharyngopalatinus muscle
12 Second molar
13 Filiform papillae; second premolar
14 Lateral incisor; frenulum of lower lip
15 Internal maxillary artery and vein
16 External carotid artery; palatine tonsil
17 Internal jugular vein
18 Posterior facial vein
19 Lingual artery and vein
20 Ranine vein
21 Anterior, middle and posterior superior alveolar nerves
22 Posterior superior alveolar artery
23 Pterygoid venous plexus
24 Inferior alveolar nerve and artery
25 External maxillary artery; anterior facial vein
26 First molar
27 Palatine glands
28 Cut edge of mucous membrane
29 Uvula
30 Palatine tonsils
31 Third molar; buccinator muscle
32 Median sulcus of tongue
33 Fungiform papillae
34 Canine
35 Central incisors; gingiva
36 Parotid duct
37 Anterior lingual gland
38 Parotid gland
39 Sublingual gland
40 Submaxillary gland

Figure 40   Region of the mouth and salivary glands
Courtesy Lederle Laboratories

THE SALIVARY GLANDS

There are three pairs of salivary glands which communicate with the mouth, and pour their secretions into its cavity. They are the *parotid, submaxillary,* and *sublingual.* The secretions of these glands combine with those of the small buccal glands of the mouth to form saliva. See Fig. 40.

Parotid Gland

The parotid gland is the largest of the three, situated at the side of the face, below and in front of the external ear. The parotid duct (Stensen's duct) opens upon the inner surface of the cheek opposite the second upper molar tooth. The gland is invested in a capsule continuous with the deep cervical fascia. A portion of the fascia, attached to the styloid process and the angle of the mandible, is somewhat thickened and forms the stylomandibular ligament which courses between the parotid and submaxillary glands.

Structures adjacent to the parotid and other salivary glands are important considerations in surgery of this area and therefore will be reviewed here to provide the secretary with an anatomic reference.

The main body of the parotid is situated between the mastoid process and Sternocleidomastoideus posteriorly and the ramus of the mandible anteriorly. The anterior surface is covered by the Pterygoideus internus and the Masseter. It slopes for a short distance between the two Pterygoid muscles. The outer lip of the gland extends over the superficial surface of the Masseter. There is a detached portion just below the zygomatic arch called the accessory part. The superficial surface of the gland is covered by superficial fascia containing the facial branches of the great auricular nerve. The posterior surface of the gland borders against the external acoustic meatus, the mastoid process, and the anterior edge of the Sternocleidomastoideus muscle. The deep surface of the parotid extends into the deep tissues with two processes, one of which is located in front of the styloid process, contacting the internal jugular vein, internal and external carotid arteries, and the glossopharyngeal and vagus nerves; the other is situated on the styloid group of muscles, styloid process and Digastricus muscle. It projects under the mastoid process and Sternocleidomastoideus.

The parotid duct (Stensen's duct) emerges in several branches from the anterior aspect of the gland, crosses the Masseter muscle, where it receives the duct of the accessory part of the parotid gland, continues through the corpus adiposum of the cheek and Buccinator muscle and finally opens upon the inside of the cheek, just opposite the second upper molar tooth.

STRUCTURES OF THE PAROTID GLAND

Accessory duct
Accessory part of gland
Apophysis
Auriculotemporal nerve
Deep cervical fascia
Facial nerve

Great auricular nerve
Masseter muscle
Parotid duct
Spinal accessory nerve
Stensen's duct
Stylomandibular ligament

VESSELS OF THE PAROTID GLAND

Common facial vein
External carotid artery
   int. maxillary branch
   posterior auricular branch
   superficial temporal branch
External jugular vein

Internal maxillary vein
Posterior auricular vein
Posterior facial vein
Superficial temporal vein
Temporal artery
Transverse facial artery

Parotidectomy (Aveline Gutierrez Technic—preservation of lower maxilla)

Using 0.5% Novocain, the auriculotemporal, auricular and anterior branches of the facial nerve were blocked. The facial nerve was likewise blocked.

Beginning at the malar arch, an incision was made parallel to the zygomatic arch, toward the tragus, under the anterior portion of the ear lobe, following the contour of the ear. The incision was carried further along the auriculomastoid line, toward the base of the mastoid apophysis. It was then carried downward toward the vertex, proceeding toward the anterior border of the sternocleidomastoid muscle, and then curving in the direction of the hyoid bone. The skin and underlying tissues were reflected.

The external jugular vein was ligated and divided at the level of the border of the maxilla. The sternocleidomastoid along with the mastoid apophysis were identified after deep dissection. The digastric muscle was further identified at the point where it meets the sternocleidomastoid. Further identification of structures was carried out to include the external branch of the spinal accessory nerve which courses in front of the transverse apophysis to the atlas. This was isolated. We also identified the great hypoglossal nerve, the internal jugular vein and the external

GENERAL SURGERY 285

Anatomy of the Neck

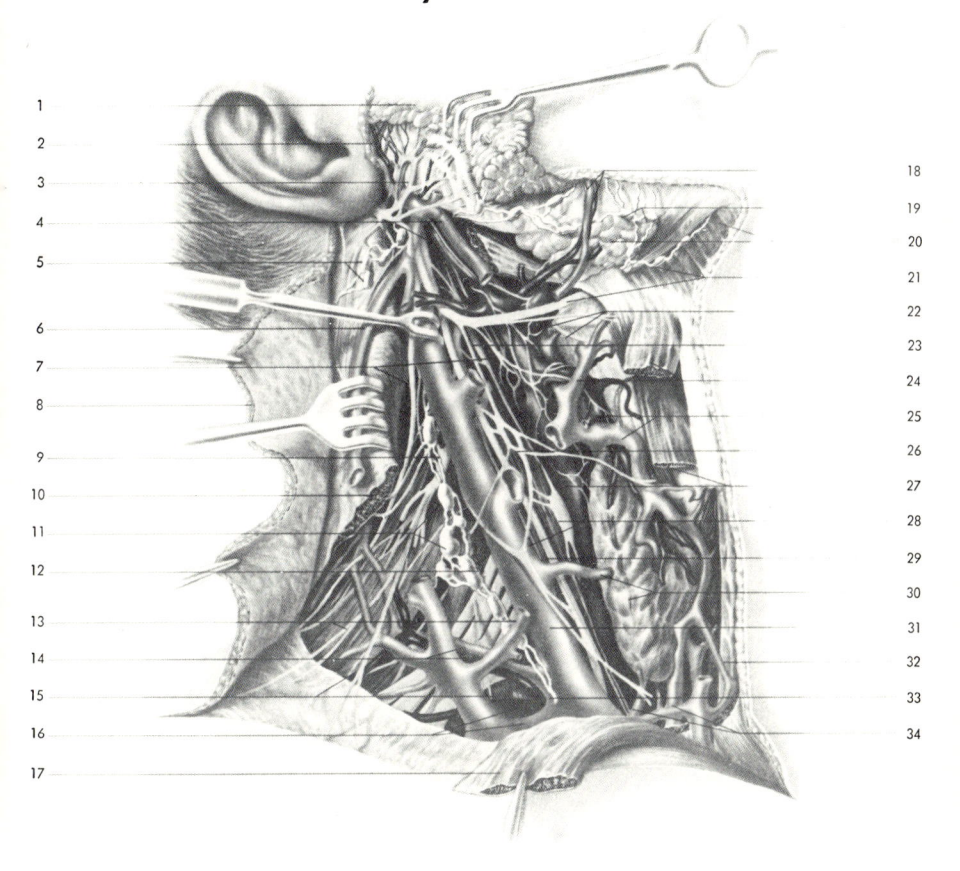

1 Parotid gland
2 Superficial temporal artery and vein
3 Temporal branch of facial nerve
4 External carotid artery and posterior facial vein
5 Superficial cervical lymph nodes
6 External jugular vein
7 Accessory nerve and internal carotid artery
8 Platysma muscle
9 Fourth cervical nerve
10 Superior position of sternocleidomastoid muscle
11 Deep cervical lymph nodes
12 Fifth cervical nerve
13 Posterior supraclavicular nerve and anterior jugular vein
14 Superficial cervical artery and vein
15 Middle supraclavicular nerve and sub·lavian artery
16 Transverse scapular artery and vein
17 Inferior position of sternocleidomastoid muscle
18 External maxillary artery and anterior facial vein
19 Submaxillary lymph nodes and digastric muscle
20 Submaxillary gland and mylohyoid muscle
21 Submental lymph nodes and hypoglossal nerve
22 Superior laryngeal artery and nerve
23 Superior cervical ganglion
24 Superior laryngeal vein and omohyoid muscle
25 Superior thyroid artery and vein
26 Ansa hypoglossi
27 Common carotid artery and sternothyroid muscle
28 Middle cervical ganglion and phrenic nerve
29 Vagus nerve
30 Thyroid gland and middle thyroid vein
31 Internal jugular vein
32 Sternohyoid muscle
33 Jugular lymphatic trunk
34 Inferior thyroid veins

Figure 41 Anatomy of the neck

carotid artery. The external carotid was dissected free and ligated with silk, the ligature passing from within, outward. The artery was divided between these ligatures.

By careful dissection, the parotid gland was divided from the pavilion of the ear and auditory canal. The temporal artery and sternocleidomastoid artery, coursing in front of the tragus, were ligated and divided. By placing forward traction on the parotid, we were able to expose the facial nerve.

An incision was then made for the purpose of removing the skin overlying the lesion of the parotid which extends, from the mid-portion of the zygomatic arch, toward the angle of the mandible. By mobilizing the anterior flap we were able to expose the anterior border of the parotid. This maneuver exposed the transverse facial artery and Stensen's duct. These structures were ligated and divided. The gland was then freed from the Masseter muscle. Bleeding was controlled.

By backward traction on the gland, we were able to expose the internal maxillary veins which were ligated and divided. The pharyngeal portion of the gland was isolated with a Kocher director. The dead space remaining after removal of the gland was obliterated by use of contiguous skin flaps which were mobilized and sutured in place. Horsehair sutures were used to approximate the skin edges. A drain was left in the lower portion of the wound. The specimen was sent to the pathologist for histopathologic examination.

Radical Neck Dissection, left

With the patient in the supine position and the head turned to the right, the left cheek, neck and upper chest were prepared and draped.

A routine double "Y" incision was made in the usual manner. Marked bleeding was encountered due to Cobalt therapy and old surgery in the area. Bleeders were controlled by clamping and ligating and/or electrocoagulation. After the flaps had been adequately elevated in all directions, the sternomastoid muscle was isolated anteriorly and its two heads of attachment sharply divided. The carotid sheath was entered. The internal jugular vein was isolated and doubly ligated, one of which was a suture ligature. The dissection was carried posteriorly to the scalene fat pad which was included in the specimen and carried down to the level of the fascia overlying the brachial plexus and scalene muscles. The phrenic nerve was tentatively identified and preserved. The dissection was carried posteriorly to the anterior border of the Trapezius and upward, including the spinal accessory nerve and its accompanying nodes. The sternomastoid was divided superiorly from the mastoid process. Beneath this, the digastric muscle was identified and retracted anteriorly to expose the upper end of the internal jugular vein. Anterior to this, a portion of the tail of the parotid gland was included as was the submaxillary gland. One additional involved node was noted just anterior to the bifurcation of the common carotid artery and was included with its surrounding fat and nodes in the specimen.

Considerable time was expended in controlling the bleeding. This was accomplished as stated above and the neck flaps reapproximated with a few interrupted 000 chromic catgut sutures.

Hemovac drainage tubes were inserted through two stab wounds and attached to the Hemovac units. The skin was then closed with interrupted simple and vertical mattress 00000 nylon sutures. A light dressing was applied.

Blood loss was approximated at about 1800 cc. During the operative procedure, the patient received 1000 cc. of whole blood and an additional 500 cc. in the recovery room.

Submaxillary Gland

The submaxillary gland is situated under the posterior tongue, largely in the submaxillary triangle, extending backward to the stylomandibular ligament and forward to the anterior belly of the Digastricus. Below, it usually overlaps the intermediate tendon of the Digastricus and the insertion of the Stylohyoideus.

The submaxillary duct (Wharton's duct) extends in branches from the deep surface of the gland and courses between the Genioglossus, Hypoglossus, Mylohyoideus and sublingual gland and opens at the side of the frenulum linguae.

SUBMAXILLARY GLAND STRUCTURES

Deep cervical fascia	Platysma muscle
Deep process	Submaxillary ganglion
Facial nerve	**Submaxillary lymph nodes**
Hypoglossal nerve	Superficial fascia
Lingual nerve	Wharton's duct
Mylohyoid nerve	

SUBMAXILLARY GLAND CIRCULATION

Anterior facial vein
External carotid artery
External maxillary artery
Facial artery
Facial vein
Glandular br. of ext. maxillary

Hypoglossal vein
Jugular vein
Lingual artery
Mylohyoid vessels
Submental vessels

Sublingual Gland

The sublingual gland is the smallest of the salivary glands. It is located under the tongue, in the floor of the mouth, at the side of the frenulum linguae.

SUBLINGUAL GLAND STRUCTURES

Duct of Bartholin
Ducts of Rivinus
Plica sublingualis

Sublingual depression
Sublingual ducts
Submaxillary duct

SUBLINGUAL CIRCULATION

Sublingual arteries

Submental arteries

DISEASES OF THE SALIVARY GLANDS AND DUCTS

Abscess of the salivary gland or duct
Absence of the salivary gland
Accessory parotid glands and ducts
Adenocarcinoma
Adenolymphoma
Adenoma
Atresia of sublingual duct
Atresia of submaxillary gland
Calculus of salivary gland
Cyst of salivary gland
Cyst of sublingual gland (ranula)
Cyst of submaxillary gland
Dilatation of Wharton's duct

Fistula of salivary gland
Fistula of sublingual gland
Fistula of submaxillary gland
Hypertrophy of salivary gland
Mixed tumor of salivary gland
Myoepithelial tumor
Parotitis (mumps)
Ranula
Sialadenitis
Stenosis of salivary duct
Stensen's duct opening in neck
Stone in sublingual duct

OPERATIONS ON THE SALIVARY GLANDS AND DUCTS

Biopsy of the salivary gland
Closure of salivary fistula
Dilation of salivary duct
Excision of lesion
Exploration of salivary gland or duct
Incision and drainage of salivary gland
Incision and removal of calculus
Parotidectomy
Radical excision of salivary glands
Removal of salivary calculus
Sialoadenectomy
Sialodochoplasty (repair of duct)
Sialolithotomy

THE THYROID GLAND

The thyroid is one of the ductless endocrine glands which pour their secretions (hormones) into the blood stream. The hormone secreted by the thyroid is **thyroxine** whose production is controlled primarily by the thyroid stimulating hormone (TSH) of the anterior pituitary.

Thyroid function is important in growth, cellular oxidation and regulation of the basal metabolic rate. Disturbances in function are common. When function is normal the patient is said to be in a **euthyroid** state. Secretion of too little thyroid hormone is termed **hypothyroidism,** a condition which in childhood leads to cretinism, and in adulthood, to myxedema. Excessive thyroid secretion is called **hyperthyroidism** and is the basis for thyrotoxicosis (toxic goiters).

A lack of iodine produces an enlargement of this gland called a goiter, four types of which are recognized clinically: (1) diffuse toxic goiter, (2) nodular toxic goiter, (3) diffuse nontoxic goiter, and, (4) nodular nontoxic goiter.

Nodular goiters are surgical problems. The nodules cannot be distinguished clinically as adenomatous or carcinomatous. Benign adenomas are the most common lesions. The small soft nodules seen in nontoxic nodular goiter are not always removed; however, firm and enlarging nodules, particularly in men and children, are usually excised because of the frequency of neoplastic change in such lesions. The exact etiology of malignant lesions remains obscure. There is convincing evidence that early radiotherapy, even in very low dosage, administered to children for an "enlarged thymus" or for skin conditions contributes to the occurrence of this cancer.

Papillary cancer of the thyroid is a slow growing tumor which is readily removed at surgery. Even when total excision is not successful, patients may live for 15 or more years with very few symptoms. Metastases develop in adjacent lymph nodes. Often the first sign of cancer of the thyroid is a firm solitary nodule in the gland.

Surgical conditions of the thyroid consist primarily of nodular goiters (adenomas or carcinomas) and hyperthyroidism. In patients with malignant lesions, lobectomy or total thyroidectomy is performed with removal of adjacent lymph nodes, often by an en bloc dissection. Such lesions are also treated by radioactive iodine (I^{131}) or external radiotherapy. In cases of hyperthyroidism, a small segment of each lobe is preserved.

Surgeons will often indicate in their operative report that special care was exercised to avoid injury to the recurrent laryngeal nerve and the parathyroid glands. Injury to the recurrent laryngeal nerve is a serious postoperative complication in thyroidectomy which results in partial or complete loss of the voice. When voice changes are noted immediately after surgery, nerve damage is probable which may be permanent. Voice changes which develop later are usually caused by edema and will return to normal.

The parathyroids usually number four, being arranged in pairs on the posterior surface of the thyroid. Their exact location and number varies. They are regarded as essential to life, their function being to regulate calcium metabolism. Operative injury to these organs results in P.O. parathyroid tetany due to hypocalcemia.

Thyroid storm or P.O. toxic crisis is another post-thyroidectomy complication. It is not seen in patients who have been properly prepared and brought to surgery in a euthyroid state. It represents a serious and often fatal accentuation of hyperthyroidism with death occurring due to hepatic failure or cardiovascular collapse.

Patients who undergo radical removal of the thyroid gland or even excessive partial excision develop hypothyroidism and therefore must be managed with replacement therapy of the hormone.

DISEASES OF THE THYROID GLAND

Abscess
Accessory thyroid gland
Adenocarcinoma
Adenoma
Atrophy
Cyst of lateral aberrant thyroid
Cyst of thyroid gland
Fibrosarcoma
Giant cell carcinoma
Goiter
Hashimoto's disease (chronic lymphomatous thyroiditis)
Hürthle cell adenoma
Hürthle cell carcinoma
Hyperthyroidism
Hypothyroidism
Injury of thyroid gland
Lymphosarcoma
Nontoxic diffuse goiter
Nontoxic nodular goiter
Papillary adenoma
Papillary carcinoma
Small cell carcinoma
Solitary adenoma
Syphilis, congenital, thyroid
Thyroglossal cyst
Thyroglossal duct, persistent

Thyroiditis
  acute
  chronic
  chronic lymphomatous

Toxic diffuse goiter
Toxic nodular goiter
Tuberculosis of thyroid gland

OPERATIONS ON THE THYROID GLAND

Biopsy
Excision of aberrant thyroid
Excision of thyroglossal duct, cyst or sinus
Incision and drainage
Ligation of inferior thyroid artery
Ligation of superior thyroid artery
Thyroidectomy
  complete
  partial (hemithyroidectomy)
  isthmectomy
Thyroidotomy
  with drainage
  with exploration
  with transection of isthmus

THYROID AND ASSOCIATED STRUCTURES

Accessory thyroid glands
Carotid sheath
Colloid goiter
Cricothyroid
Deep fascia
Hyoid bone
Isthmus
Larynx
Levator glandulae thyreoideae
Omohyoid muscle
Paratracheal nodes
Parathyroids
Platysma muscle
Pretracheal fascia
Pyramidal lobe

Recurrent laryngeal nerves
Recurrent nerves
Ribbon muscles of the neck
Sternal notch
Sternocleidomastoid muscle
Sternohyoid muscle
Sternothyroid muscle
Strap muscles of the neck
Superficial fascia
Thyroid capsule
Thyroid cartilage
Thyroidea ima
Thyroid notch
Trachea

THYROID CIRCULATION

Anastomotic branch of artery
Brachiocephalic vein
Common carotid artery
Inferior thyroid artery
Inferior thyroid vein

Internal jugular vein
Middle thyroid vein
Subclavian artery
Superior thyroid artery
Superior thyroid vein

THYROID UPTAKE
(Radioisotopes)

Medotopes
Radiocaps

Sodium Radio-Iodide (I^{131})

Subtotal Thyroidectomy—with resection of pyramidal lobe

Under general endotracheal anesthesia, the patient was sterilely prepared and draped in the usual fashion.

An orbicular incision, two fingerbreadths above the sternoclavicular notch, was made. The skin was incised as was the Platysma which was dissected free to the thyroid notch. Dissection was carried inferiorly to the retrosternal space of Burns with sharp dissection. Bleeders encountered were clamped and ligated with 000 intestinal suture. Upon completion of this procedure, a vertical incision was made in the midline between the two prethyroid muscle bundles. This incision was extended from the thyroid notch to the level of the sternal notch. The incision was carried to the sternothyroid and sternohyoid muscles. These were retracted and the surgical capsule of the thyroid gland was incised.

On inspection, the thyroid was noted to be approximately 2 to 3 times larger than normal size and there were diffuse, nodular areas throughout the entire thyroid substance.

Dissection was continued by grasping the superior lobe of the thyroid and using blunt and sharp dissection, the superior thyroid vessels were dissected free. These were clamped and ligated with 00 cotton suture. The middle thyroid vein and inferior thyroid vessels were similarly treated. In the area of the inferior thyroid, blunt and sharp dissection were used to dissect free the recurrent laryngeal nerve. After identification and under good visualization, the inferior thyroid vessels were cut, ligated with 000 cotton suture and checked for hemostasis. At this time, the hemostats were used to transect the base of the thyroid in subcapsular fashion, leaving some thyroid tissue present. Upon completion of the transection to the isthmus of the thyroid, the thyroid was dissected from the trachea using both sharp and blunt dissection. The pyramidal lobe was noted superiorly. This was dissected using blunt and sharp dissection. Bleeders were clamped and ligated with 000 cotton suture. Upon removal of the right lobe, the left lobe was similarly removed. Persistent bleeders were clamped and ligated with 000 cotton suture or 000000 cotton.

Two drains were placed into the thyroid fossa and brought out laterally through the sternocleidomastoid muscle. The midline was closed with interrupted # 60 cotton and the subcutaneous tissue and Platysma with 0000 chromic. The skin was closed with a mattress cotton suture.

The patient tolerated the procedure well and was transferred to the recovery room in good condition.

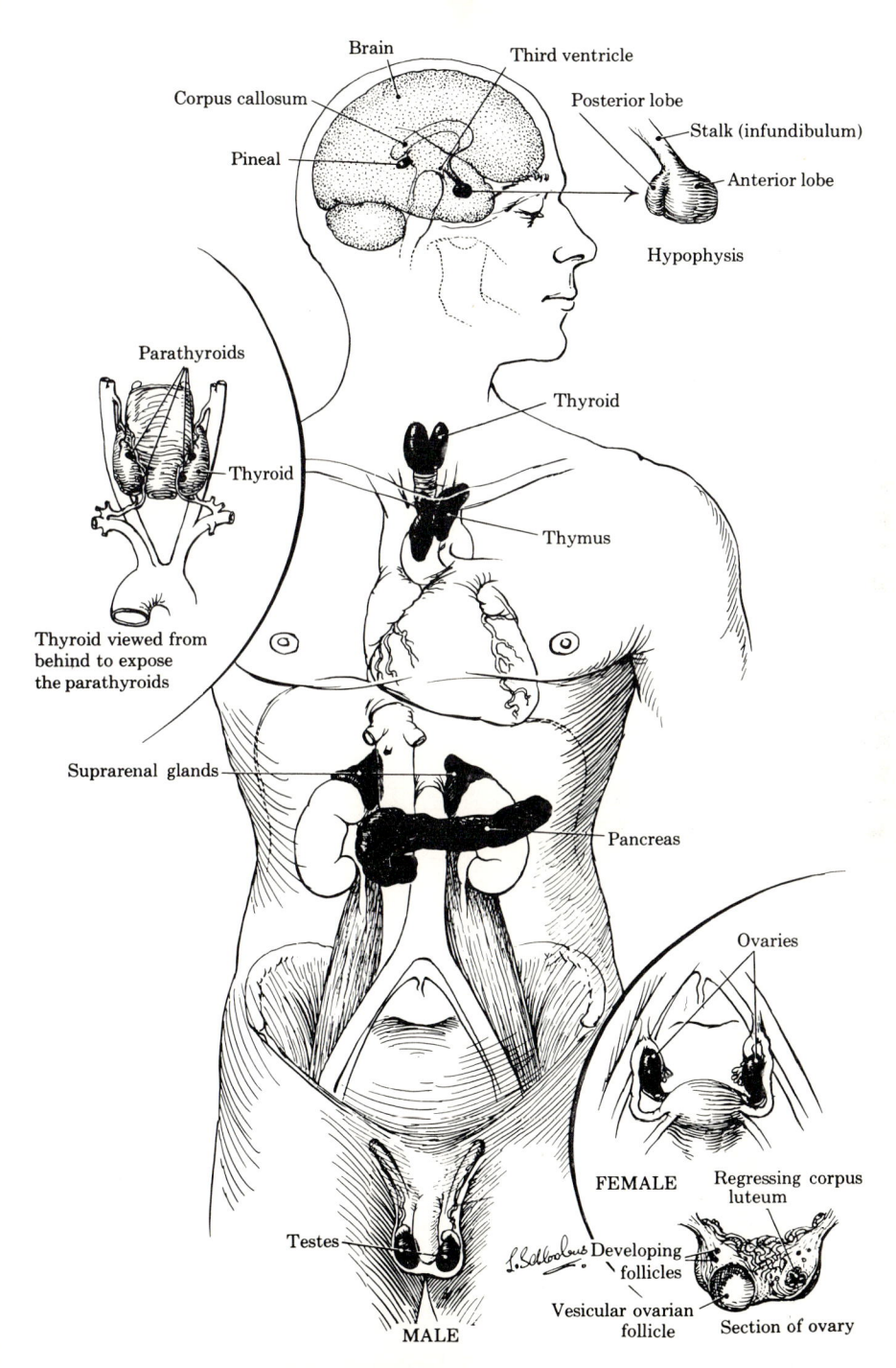

Figure 42   **THE ENDOCRINE GLANDS**

THE ADRENAL GLANDS

The adrenal glands (suprarenals) are two small bodies above and in front of the upper end of each kidney, situated at the back of the abdomen, behind the peritoneum. Their average weight is 3.5 to 5.0 grams each. Small accessory adrenals are sometimes found in the adrenal area. Studies have demonstrated that the adrenals are not necessary to maintain life; however, the secretions of the adrenal cortex are considered essential. It is for this reason that persons who have undergone total adrenalectomy must be maintained on replacement therapy for the remainder of their lives. The effectiveness of such therapy enables these patients to live an almost completely normal life.

Bilateral adrenalectomy (removal of the adrenals), was first performed in 1945, as a palliative procedure for advanced carcinoma of the prostate and is still used in these cases. Its purpose is removal of the secondary source of male hormone after the primary source has been eliminated by removal of the testes. The operation is employed for the same purpose in breast cancer, removing the secondary source of estrogen after the primary source has been eliminated by removal of the ovaries (oophorectomy).

Structurally and functionally, the adrenals consist of two portions, the external surface (cortex) and the internal area (medulla).

The adrenal cortex secretes hormones considered essential to life. These secretions are involved in the intermediary metabolism of organic substances, the regulation of sodium and potassium metabolism as well as estrogenic and androgenic activity. Chronic adrenal cortical deficiency is known as **Addison's disease,** a condition characterized by debility, weakness and a peculiar bronzing of the skin. It is treated by hormone replacement therapy.

Hyperfunction of the adrenal cortex may result in one of several clinical syndromes, namely, Cushing's disease, Conn's syndrome (aldosteronism), virilization or feminization. These conditions are treated surgically when they are caused by carcinoma, adenoma or hyperplasia of the adrenal cortex.

Cushing's disease occurring in childhood is usually caused by an adrenal carcinoma. In adults only about 35 per cent have an adrenal tumor of which only one-half are malignant. About 60 per cent of these patients demonstrate adrenal cortical hyperplasia. Cushing's disease is treated surgically by adrenalectomy with hormone replacement thereafter. Of interest is the finding that one-sixth of postadrenalectomy patients exhibit chromophobe adenomas of the pituitary, a tumor associated with hypopituitarism. These neoplasms are treated by irradiation.

Aldosteronism usually results from an aldosterone-producing adenoma or carcinoma of the adrenal cortex. Some of these patients, however, have normal appearing adrenals or demonstrate only adrenal hyperplasia. Treatment consists of excision of the hyperfunctioning tissue.

Adrenal virilism, like the other diseases of cortical hyperfunction, may result from carcinoma, adenoma or hyperplasia. This condition is characterized by production of excessive amounts of adrenal hormones with androgenic (male hormone) activity. The most common form of noncongenital adrenal virilization is that seen with bilateral adrenocortical hyperplasia. Children with this condition are successfully treated with suppressive doses of glucocorticoid. True virilism in adults is uncommon. The symptoms which simulate virilism are more likely to be associated with Cushing's syndrome due to bilateral hyperplasia.

Adrenal feminization is extremely rare and usually due to adrenal carcinoma.

The medulla of the adrenals produces epinephrine, an internal secretion which prepares the organism for "fight or flight" situations. Although the medulla is not necessary to maintain life, it augments the function of the adrenal cortex in helping the organism cope with stress. Diseases of the medullary portion of the adrenals are usually caused by neoplasms. One such tumor is pheochromocytoma, a disease associated with paroxysmal or sustained hypertension. This condition is treated by excision of the tumor. Nonfunctioning tumors of the adrenal medulla include: sympathogonioma, a rare highly malignant tumor which develops during intrauterine life or infancy with early metastases and a poor prognosis; ganglioneuroma, a slow growing tumor of adults; and neuroblastoma, one of the most common malignancies of early childhood.

DISEASES OF THE ADRENAL GLANDS

Absence of adrenal gland
Accessory adrenal gland
Adenocarcinoma
Adenoma
Adrenal cortical hyperfunction
   with premature puberty
   with Cushing's syndrome
   with virilism
Adrenal cortical hypofunction
   secondary to hypopituitarism
Adrenalitis
Atrophy of adrenal cortex
Cyst of adrenal gland
Degeneration

Displacement
Ganglioneuroma of medulla
Hemorrhage into adrenal gland
Hyperplasia
Hypoplasia
Injury to
Necrosis of adrenal gland
Pheochromocytoma
Sympathicoblastoma of medulla
Syphilis of adrenal gland
Tuberculosis of adrenals
Virilizing adenocarcinoma
Virilizing adenoma

OPERATIONS ON THE ADRENAL GLANDS

Adrenalectomy
Biopsy

Excision of lesion
Exploration of adrenals

THE PITUITARY GLAND

The pituitary (hypophysis cerebri) is an endocrine gland attached to the base of the brain by a pituitary stalk. It is situated within a bony depression in the sphenoid bone of the skull called the sella turcica because of its resemblance to a Turk's saddle. The gland, consisting of an anterior and posterior lobe, produces many hormones with widespread direct effect on many body tissues.

The principal functions of the posterior lobe hormones are to promote the reabsorption of water by the renal tubes through an antidiuretic effect, enhance the secretion of milk from the lactating breast, and stimulate uterine contraction.

The anterior lobe is involved in most of the endocrine activity of the body. The ovaries and testes are completely dependent on hormones of the anterior pituitary for production of their respective hormones. The thyroid is also activated by a hormone of the anterior lobe of the pituitary. Secretions of both these glands influence normal body growth. Other functions of the anterior lobe hormones include maintenance of adequacy of the adrenal cortex, induction of lactation and influence over various metabolic processes.

Hormones produced by the anterior pituitary include: ACTH (adrenocorticotropic hormone), TSH (thyroid-stimulating hormone), FSH (follicle-stimulating hormone), LH (luteinizing hormone) in the female with its analogue in the male of ICSH (interstitial cell-stimulating hormone), LTH (luteotropic hormone) and MSH (melanocyte-stimulating hormone). Because of these many secretions with their far reaching influences throughout the body, it is unusual for only one body system to be effected by a destructive disease process in the gland.

Hypopituitarism, interestingly, is manifested by a general loss of anterior pituitary hormones. In hyperpituitarism a general increase in all hormones does not develop. It is exceedingly rare for more than one pituitary hormone to be produced in excess in any single individual.

Hypophysectomy (excision of the pituitary gland) was first performed in 1951, for metastatic breast cancer. It is used today as a palliative measure designed to diminish hormonal activity and production. Studies have shown remissions following such surgery to exceed 15 months and average survival to surpass 21 months. Removal of the pituitary necessitates management of the patient thereafter on replacement hormonal therapy consisting of pituitary extract, cortisone and thyroid extract.

Surgery of the pituitary gland is generally performed by the neurosurgeon. One of the newest methods at his disposal is cryosurgery, a technique which utilizes intense cold and a fine instrument called a cryoprobe. This modern surgical application of cold enables the surgeon to destroy fine areas of disease producing tissue without undue damage to surrounding healthy tissues.

Diseases of the pituitary are thought of in terms of hypofunction or hyperfunction of the gland. Hypofunction, when it occurs in childhood, results in dwarfism, and sometimes, mental retardation. When it develops in the adult, it results in reduced sexual prowess and impotence. In complete pituitary failure there follows premature senility.

Tumors are common causes of pituitary disease resulting in either hypo- or hyperfunction of the gland. The anterior lobe is most commonly involved. The tumors are either nonsecretory or they secrete large amounts of a specific hormone. The eosinophilic tumors produce excess growth hormone while the basophilic and chromophobic tumors produce excess ACTH.

Chromophil adenoma is associated with hyperfunction and is more prevalent in males. When it develops in young persons who are still growing and in whom the epiphyses have not yet closed, gigantism results. When the tumor manifests itself later in life, it results in acromegaly, a condition marked by enlargement of the facial features, jaw, hands and feet. Resection of the tumor relieves the symptom of the disease, but there is no improvement in the bone changes which have distorted the patient's appearance.

Basophilic adenoma (pituitary basophilism) is a tumor of the adrenal cortex producing hyperadrenocortism. Chromophobe adenoma is more common than the chromophil adenoma. Its size produces symptoms which often include impaired vision as a result of pressure on the optic chiasm of the brain. This tumor has a feminizing influence on males. The disease is primarily one of glandular hypofunction and for this reason surgery is not generally employed except to relieve pressure symptoms on the brain.

There are a variety of cysts which develop about the pituitary. They usually manifest themselves in childhood, resulting in dwarfism and other evidences of hypofunction. When they obstruct the foramen of Monro they can produce hydrocephalus. Although benign in nature, they may be fatal when they encroach on vital centers of the brain. Treatment is surgical when they become symptomatic.

DISEASES OF THE PITUITARY GLAND

Abscess
Adenocarcinoma
Adenoma
Anterior pituitary hyperfunction
　with:
　　acromegaly
　　hypophysial gigantism
　　pituitary basophilism
　　premature puberty
Anterior pituitary hypofunction
　with:
　　adiposogenital dystrophy
　　dwarfism and infantilism
　　hypopituitary cachexia
　　juvenile hypopituitarism
　　sex infantilism
Basophilic adenoma
Calculus
Chromophobe adenoma
Chromophobe carcinoma
Craniopharyngioma
Cyst of Ratke's pouch

Cyst of pituitary stalk (vestigial)
Degeneration
Dyspituitarism
Eosinophilic adenoma

Infarction due to embolism
Injury to
Syphilis of
Tuberculosis of

THE PARATHYROIDS

The parathyroid glands are usually four in number, although occasionally three or five are found. The upper two glands are generally situated close to the lateral thyroid lobes. The lower two have a wider distribution, being situated anywhere from the upper pole of the thyroid to the anterior mediastinum or the pericardium. These glands control calcium metabolism and strongly influence phosphorus metabolism. Excision of all parathyroid tissue is followed by death or severe tetany.

The most common pathology of these glands is adenoma, a benign tumor. Single adenomas account for about 90 per cent of hyperparathyroidism. This disease causes renal stones and demineralization of bone as seen in osteitis fibrosa cystica.

Hyperparathyroidism and hypoparathyroidism (parathyroid tetany) are conditions associated with elevation and decrease of calcium blood levels. Hypoparathyroidism of spontaneous occurrence is rare. It is most frequently seen as a complication of thyroidectomy where the parathyroids have been inadvertently traumatized or removed. Tetany develops in from 24 hours to three weeks after such accident. Function returns to the glands if they were only bruised. Parathyroid tissue also possesses marked regenerative faculty in which remaining tissue undergoes hyperplasia with reduction in the severity of the hypoparathyroidism.

Treatment of hyperparathyroidism consists of excision of the adenoma or subtotal resection of the hyperplastic tissue.

DISEASES OF THE PARATHYROID GLANDS

Adenocarcinoma
Adenoma
Hyperparathyroidism

Hyperplasia
Hypoparathyroidism
Injury due to operation

OPERATIONS ON PARATHYROIDS

Biopsy
Excision of lesion

Exploration
Parathyroidectomy

THE PINEAL GLAND

The pineal gland (pineal body or epiphysis) develops as an outgrowth from the third ventricle of the brain near the midbrain. Following puberty the glandular tissue is gradually replaced by connective tissue. Tumors of this gland are sometimes associated with enlarged genitals and precocious sexual development in boys.

DISEASES OF THE PINEAL GLAND

Calcification
Glioma
Injury to
Pinealoma

Premature puberty due to pineal tumor
Teratoma of the pineal gland

OPERATIONS ON THE PINEAL GLAND

Biopsy
Excision of lesion of

Exploration of
Pinealectomy

SURGERY OF THE SPLEEN

The spleen is a lymph gland with many functions, all of which are not completely known. It is regarded as an organ which is not essential to life. Its removal (splenectomy) is not followed by any significant or permanent dysfunction.

Functions of the spleen include blood production. During embryonic life the spleen is an important blood forming organ, but later it forms only lymphocytes. In a disease like myeloid leukemia, the spleen reverts to its former role of complete hemopoiesis producing red cells, white cells and megakaryocytes (the giant cell of bone marrow). It is known to exert a restraining influence on the bone marrow and to be the site of destruction of red blood corpuscles. It is also involved in bacterial and particle fixation, antibody production, hemoglobin degradation and iron storage.

Location of this organ in the left hypochondriac region, just beneath the diaphragm and behind the stomach, predisposes it to rupture in cases of severe trauma to the abdominal wall. This often proves fatal because the spleen is such a vascular organ being supplied by the splenic (lienal) artery, a branch of the celiac.

The most common indications for surgery are: (1) traumatic rupture of the spleen, (2) hypersplenic syndromes which include hematologic disorders, and (3) congestive splenomegaly. At splenectomy a search is always made for accessory spleens, particularly when the operation is performed in order to cure a hematologic disease. Accessory spleens are actually ectopic functional organs which are found in about 10 per cent of all patients.

Blood disorders where splenectomy is sometimes effective in bringing about a cure include idiopathic thrombocytopenic purpura (platelet deficiency), congenital hemolytic anemia (red cell deficiency), primary neutropenia (neutrophil deficiency), and primary pancytopenia (deficiency of the myeloid cells)

IMPORTANT ANATOMIC FEATURES OF THE SPLEEN

Accessory spleens (supernumerary)
Capsule
Celiac axis
Colic surface
Diaphragm
Ectopic tissue
Gastric surface
Gastroepiploic branch of lienal artery
Gastrolienal ligament
Gastrosplenic omentum
Greater omentum
Hilum
Lienal artery
Lienal vein
Lienorenal ligament
Malpighian bodies
Mesogastrium
Pancreaticosplenic ligament
Pedicle of spleen

Phrenic surface
Phrenicocolic ligament
Phrenicolienal ligament
Phrenicosplenic ligament
Portal vein
Posterior parietal peritoneum
Presplenic fold
Renal surface
Short gastric br.-lienal artery
Splenic artery
Splenic pulp
Splenic vein
Splenocolic ligament
Splenomegaly
Splenunculi
Tunica albuginea
Tunica serosa
Visceral surface

TECHNIQUES OF SPLENECTOMY

Carter thoracicoabdominal
Three clamp method of Federoff

Henry
Rives

Splenectomy

Under general anesthesia, after the patient had been sterilely prepared and draped, a left Kocher incision was made and the rectus muscle was divided and ligated. The peritoneal cavity was entered. There was splenomegaly which descended to the costal margins.

By means of sharp dissection, the short gastric vessels in the gastrosplenic ligaments were isolated, clamped, divided and ligated with cotton. The splenic artery was identified running over the superior border of the pancreas. By means of a ligature carrier, the artery was isolated at a short segment and tied with 00 chromic just distally and proximally and then divided between ligatures. A second suture of 000 cotton was used to transfix the artery proximally; it was ligated for further safety. The artery and veins of the pedicle were clamped, divided and ligated close to the spleen, avoiding the pancreas. The colon and stomach were retracted out of the way to avoid injury. The splenocolic and splenorenal ligaments were clamped, divided and ligated. There were firm adhesions of the diaphragmatic attachments onto the posterior aspect of the spleen. These were lysed by blunt dissection. The spleen was removed. Further hemostasis was achieved with interrupted cotton stitches until the field was entirely dry. A medium size Penrose drain was placed beneath the diaphragm in the left side and brought out through a separate stab wound in the flank.

There were no accessory spleens palpable and the pelvic organs were felt to be entirely normal as was the remaining G.I. tract. The appendix could not be reached through this incision.

The peritoneum and posterior sheath were closed with a continuous locking 00 chromic suture. The fascia was approximated in layers with interrupted figure-of-eight 000 cotton. The subcutaneous tissue was closed with chromic sutures. The skin edges were approximated with a sliding dermalon. The drain was transfixed to the skin with a suture and safety pin. Dressing applied.

DISEASES OF THE SPLEEN

Absence
Accessory
Amyloid disease
Amyloid disease
Aneurysm of splenic artery
Arteriosclerosis of splenic artery
Atrophy
Cysticercosis
Displacement
Echinococcosis of spleen
Embolism of splenic artery
Fibroma
Floating spleen

Hemangioma
Hernia of spleen
Hodgkin's disease of spleen
Infarction
   due to embolism
   due to thrombosis

Injury of spleen
Lobulation of spleen
Lymphosarcoma
Myeloid metaplasia
Passive congestion
Phlebolith of splenic vein
Phlebosclerosis of splenic vein

Reticulum cell sarcoma
Rupture of spleen
Sarcoidosis
Schistosomiasis
Splenitis
Splenomegaly

Splenoptosis
Syphilis of spleen
Thrombosis of splenic vein
Torsion of spleen
Tuberculosis of spleen
Varix of splenic vein

OPERATIONS ON THE SPLEEN

Biopsy of the spleen
Splenectomy (removal of spleen)
Splenic puncture
Splenopexy

Splenorrhaphy (suture repair)
Splenotomy
  with drainage
  with exploration

UPPER ALIMENTARY CANAL

The upper alimentary canal extends from the oral cavity to the duodenal papilla (end of the first portion of the duodenum), including the esophagus, stomach and first portion of the duodenum. It also includes the liver, bile passages and pancreas. Its function is the elaboration and secretion of digestive juices, mixing these with ingested food and conduction of this mixture through the digestive tract.

The Esophagus

The esophagus begins at the lower end of the pharynx and extends downward to become continuous with the stomach at the cardioesophageal junction. It lies in close relationship to the trachea, thyroid glands, aorta, root of the lungs, heart, thoracic duct, diaphragm, spinal column and vagus nerves. These surrounding structures make surgical approach to it difficult. Early spread of infection and neoplasms to inaccessible areas occur commonly. Traumatic and operative wounds are more disposed to leakage because the esophagus has no outer serous covering which could act as a self-sealing membrane.

Surgical conditions of the esophagus are not common. Those which do arise include congenital atresia (narrowing or closure of the passage), tracheo-esophageal fistula, esophageal varices, traumatic injuries and diverticula of the esophagus.

Benign tumors of the esophagus are rare; malignant tumors are common. Carcinoma of the esophagus accounts for two per cent of the total cancer deaths in this country. The incidence of this malignancy in China is several times that of the U.S.A., a difference which some physiologists believe to be due to variations in eating habits and diets.

GENERAL SURGERY 303

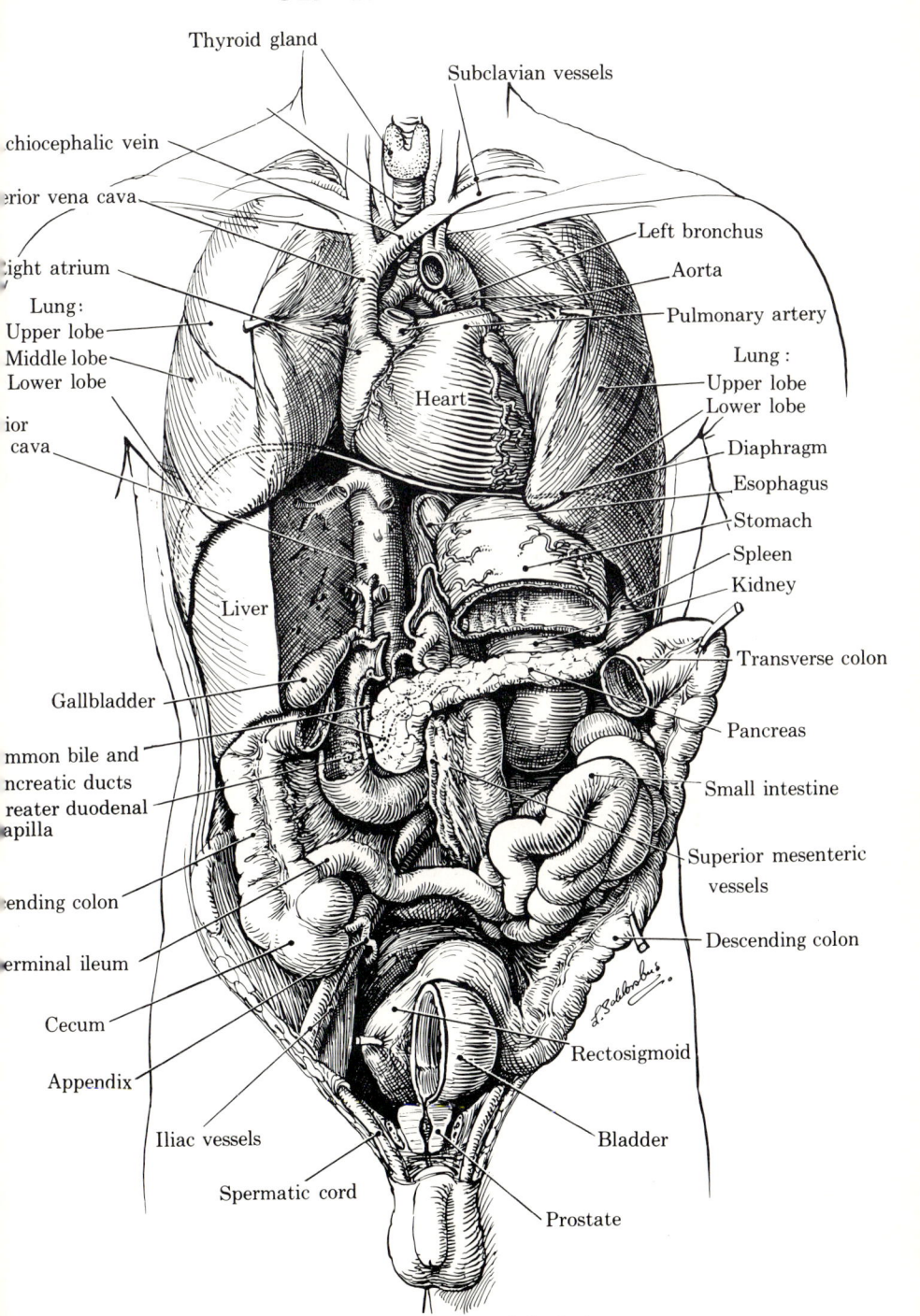

Figure 43   Internal organs of the body
Courtesy W. B. Saunders Co.

Of interest is the statistical evidence that approximately 80 per cent of esophageal cancers occur in males, beyond middle age. It has also been noted that the area between the midportion and the lower third of the esophagus is the more common site of the cancer.

Carcinoma of the esophagus spreads locally invading neighboring structures such as the trachea, bronchi, lymph nodes and also spreads within the wall of the esophagus.

When the lesion involves the lower esophagus it is resected and the stomach is brought up into the thoracic cavity for anastomosis with the shortened esophagus.

When the tumor involves the upper or midesophagus, the right large or small bowel must be brought into the thoracic cavity to replace the diseased portion of the esophagus. Sometimes incisions are required in the abdomen, thorax and neck. For these reasons irradiation is often considered the treatment of choice when carcinoma involves the upper and middle third of the esophagus.

Operative mortality for esophageal cancer is about 20 per cent and five year survival is low, representing about three out of 100 patients.

Inoperable lesions are offered palliative therapy with irradiation provided by rotation and supervoltage therapy. Other palliative measures involve insertion of a tube into the narrowed esophageal passage and gastrostomy for feeding purposes.

DISEASES OF THE ESOPHAGUS

Abscess
Absence, congenital
Achalasia with dilatation
Adenocarcinoma
Atresia
Cysts
Dilatation
Displacement of gastric mucosa
Diverticulum (pulsion or traction)
Duplication, congenital
Epidermoid carcinoma
Esophagitis
Fistula
    esophagobronchial
    esophagocutaneous
Foreign body

Giant esophagus
Leukoplakia
Peptic ulcer
Perforation
Polyp
Rupture
Short esophagus
Spasm
Squamous cell papilloma
Stricture
Syphilis
Thrush
Tuberculosis
Ulcer
Varix (pl. varices)

GENERAL SURGERY

OPERATIONS PERFORMED ON THE ESOPHAGUS

Esophageal anastomosis
Esophageal biopsy
Esophageal dilatation
Esophageal diverticulectomy
    pharyngoesophageal
Esophageal fistula closure
    tracheoesophageal
Esophageal repair or suture
Esophagectomy
Esophagoduodenostomy
Esophagoesophagostomy

Esophagogastrectomy
Esophagogastroplasty
Esophagogastrostomy
Esophagojejunostomy
Esophagoplasty (plastic repair)
Esophagoscopy
    with biopsy
    with excision
    with dilation
Esophagostomy
Esophagotomy

ESOPHAGOSCOPES

Ballooning
Boros

Holinger
Jackson full lumen
Jesberg
Lell
Mosher
Moure

Chevalier Jackson
Haslinger

Roberts folding
Sam Roberts
Schindler optical
Tucker
Yankauer

Esophagogastroscopy

The patient was given Sodium amytal grains 2 prior to coming to the operating room and atropine grains 1/100 on call to the OR. In the operating room, the buccal, oral and pharyngeal mucosa were sprayed with 1% Xylocaine and epinephrine. The patient was given 50 mgm. of Demerol and turned on his left side.

A flexible Eder-Hufford esophagoscope was introduced without difficulty. The epiglottis was visualized as was the pyriform sinus. The lumen of the esophagus was kept in constant view. The scope was gently urged through the Cricopharyngeus muscle as the patient swallowed. A definite hiatal hernia was noted measuring about 2-3 cm. The mucosa of the stomach and distal esophagus were markedly edematous. No true varices were seen. No evidence of esophagitis was noted. The scope was gently withdrawn.

An Eder-Chamberlin gastroscope was introduced to depth I. The pylorus was readily seen, unusually so, in all quadrants and appeared normal throughout. The scope was then withdrawn and reinserted into the body of the stomach and greater curvature. At the junction of the posterior wall there was a large fold, abnormal in color, with two pinpoint ulcerations on its surface measuring about 1-2 cm. and very highly suspicious of malignancy. The mucosa proximal to this area was markedly atrophic with a definite venous pattern. The scope was removed.

Esophagoscopy

The patient was given Sodium amytal grs. 2 I.M. and atropine grains 1/100 on the ward. In the OR, the buccal, oral and pharyngeal mucosa were sprayed with 1% Xylocaine and epinephrine with no untoward results. The patient was given 75 mgm. of Demerol intravenously. He was turned on his left side. The esophagoscope obturator was passed without difficulty. The cardioesophageal junction was identified.

There was no evidence of hiatal hernia, varicosities, ulcerations, tumefactions or areas of inflammation. As the scope was slowly removed, the mucosa was inspected. There were no lesions noted. No hyperemia of the mucosa was seen. The scope was removed and the patient returned to the ward in good condition.

THE STOMACH

The stomach is a J-shaped pouch situated between the esophagus and the duodenum. The upper portion of the stomach where the esophagus enters is called the cardiac portion. The uppermost portion of the stomach which rises above this level is the fundus, the lowermost portion is the pyloric end and the portion between is the body of the organ. The lesser curvature is the shorter curve on the inner surface of the stomach as opposed to the greater curvature on the outer border.

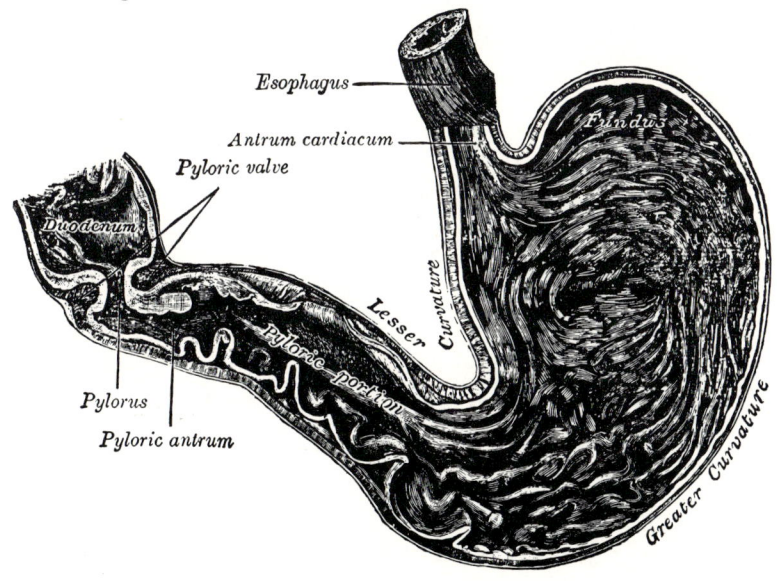

Figure 44   Interior view of the stomach
From Gray's Anatomy 28th edition edited by Dr. Charles M. Goss. Courtesy Lea & Febiger Publishers.

The stomach is covered by peritoneum on all sides and usually is found in the abdominal cavity. It may be introduced into the thoracic cavity through herniation or surgery. Its function is the temporary holding of ingested food until digestion has taken place to the point where the contents may pass through the pyloric sphincter into the duodenum.

The stomach is not essential to life. Surgical lesions sometimes require resection of large portions of the organ or total removal.

DISEASES OF THE STOMACH

Abscess of stomach wall
Achalasia (cardiospasm)
Achlorhydria
Adenocarcinoma

Atony
Atrophic gastritis
Cardiospasm
Diffuse scirrhous carcinoma

DISEASES OF THE STOMACH (continued)

Dilatation
Displacement of esophageal
   mucosa into cardia
Diverticulum (traction or pulsion)
Erosion
Fibroma
Fistula
Foreign body
Gastritis
  acute
  chronic
  atrophic
  hypertrophic
  phlegmonous
Gastroptosis
Gastrostomy opening
Gunshot wound
Hair ball
Hemorrhage
Hernia into thorax
Herniation of gastric mucosa
Hourglass stomach
Leiomyoma (pl. leiomyomata)
Linitis plastica (Brinton's disease;
   leather bottle stomach, cirrhotic
   gastritis)
Lipoma
Lymphosarcoma
Megalogastria
Microgastria
Neurofibroma
Pancreatic tissue in wall of stomach
Perforation
Perigastritis
Perigastric adhesions
Phytobezoar
Polyp
Prolapse of gastric mucosa
Redundancy of gastric mucosa
Scirrhous carcinoma
Stenosis of cardia
Strangulation due to hernia
Syphilis
Transposition
Tuberculosis
Ulcer (with or without perforation)
Varix (pl. varices)
Volvulus

OPERATIONS ON THE STOMACH
(For definitions see glossary at back of book)

Anastomosis of bile duct to
Biopsy
Excision of gastroduodenal, marginal
  or stomal ulcer
Excision of gastrojejunal, jejunal,
  marginal or stomal ulcer
Fistula closure
  cholecystogastric
  gastrocolic
  gastrojejunocolic
Gastrectomy
  complete (total)
  partial
  radical

Gastroduodenostomy
Gastrogastrostomy
Gastrojejunostomy
Gastromyotomy
Gastroplasty
Gastrorrhaphy (repair)
Gastroscopy
Gastrostomy
  closure of
Gastrotomy
Implantation of biliary
  fistulous tract into

OPERATIONS ON THE STOMACH AND INTESTINES

The most frequently performed operation on the stomach is probably the gastrectomy (excision of all or a portion of the stomach), indicated in certain cases of gastric and duodenal ulcer and other surgical lesions of the stomach and duodenum. A partial or subtotal resection is performed more often than a complete or total excision. These resections are usually followed by either a gastroduodenostomy (anastomosis of the stomach and duodenum) or a gastrojejunostomy (anastomosis between the stomach and jejunum).

A number of techniques have been proposed for gastrectomy, all based upon the principles of the Billroth methods. They are, in essence, modifications of the Billroth I and II operations.

BILLROTH I   Resection of a portion of the stomach with an end-to-end anastomosis between the stomach and the duodenum.

BILLROTH II   An anastomosis following gastric resection, closing the end of the stomach and duodenum and attaching a loop of jejunum to a new opening in the stomach.

Other popular gastrectomy techniques include:

Schoemaker Modification of Billroth I

Billroth I except that the cut end of the stomach on the lesser curvature side is closed with a row of continuous chromic catgut and a row of interrupted silk resulting in a stoma of about 2 inches for anastomosis with the duodenum.

Anterior Polya

Resection of a portion of the stomach with end-to-end anastomosis between the stomach and jejunum, anterior to the transverse colon.

Posterior Polya

Removal of a portion of the stomach with end-to-end anastomosis between the stomach and jejunum, posterior to the transverse colon.

Hofmeister Modification of Polya

The stomach is partially resected and the lesser curvature of the remaining stomach is closed leaving a 2 inch opening on the side of the greater curvature. The stoma is anastomosed to the jejunum.

GASTRECTOMY TECHNIQUES

Aquirre
Balfour
Bancroft-Plenk
Billroth I
Billroth II
Braun and Jaboulay
Connell's Tube Operation
  (partial fundusectomy)
Deloyers reverse gastrectomy
Finsterer
Finochietto-Billroth I
Hofmeister
Hofmeister-Billroth II antecolic
Horsley
Krönlein
Lahey
Mayo

McKittricks two stage partial
Mikulicz
Moore
Moynihan
Nissen
Pauchet
Polya, anterior
Polya, posterior
Reichel
Roux-Y (Also: Roux-en-Y)
Schoemaker
Schoemaker-Billroth II
Stevenson
von Eiselsberg
von Haberer
von Haberer-Finney
Warren

GASTRECTOMY INSTRUMENTS

Allis forceps
Babcock forceps
Balfour retractor
Deaver retractor
Doyen clamps
Doyen cross-action forceps
Dunhill hemostats
Eastman clamp
Friedrich-Petz clamp
Furniss clamp
Halsted hemostats
Harrington forceps
Kelly clamps
Kocher clamps
Kocher forceps
Lane clamps
Lockwood clamps

Maingot hemostats
Martin needle
Mayo needle
Mayo scissors
Mayo-Ochsner box-joint forceps
Mosquito clamps
Moynihan clamps
Ochsner clamp
O'Sullivan-O'Connor retractor
Parker-Kerr forceps
Payr clamp
Rankin clamp
Roosevelt clamp
Spencer Wells forceps
Stevenson clamps
von Petz clamp

ANATOMIC STRUCTURES ENCOUNTERED IN GASTRECTOMY

Anterior rectus sheath
Azygos vein
Cardiac orifice
Celiac axis
Crus of diaphragm
Duodenum
Fundus of stomach
Gastric artery
Gastrocolic ligament
Gastroepiploic artery
Gastrohepatic ligament
Gastrohepatic omentum
Gastrolienal ligament
Gastrophrenic ligament
Greater curvature
Greater omentum
Hepatic artery
Hepatogastric ligament
Incisura angularis
Incisura cardiaca
Jejunum
Leaf of mesocolon
Lesser curvature
Ligament of Treitz
Muscularis
Posterior rectus sheath
Pyloric antrum
Pyloric orifice
Pyloric valve
Pyloric vestibule
Pylorus
Recti muscles
Rugae of stomach
Rugal folds
Seromuscular layer
Serosa
Stoma
Suspensory ligament of liver
Transverse colon
Vasa brevia

Gastrectomy and Gastroduodenostomy (Billroth I)

Under spinal anesthesia an incision was made approximately 1½ inches above the umbilicus to approximately 1 inch below the xiphoid. The incision extended through the superficial tissues, down to the linea alba. The linea alba was opened and the peritoneum incised.

Exploration revealed the liver, kidneys and gallbladder to be normal. There was no evidence of duodenal ulcer. Examination of the stomach did not reveal any gross evidence of an ulcer. In view of the difficulty in palpation for an ulcer, a longitudinal incision was made in an avascular area in the anterior wall of the stomach. 000 chromic intestinal sutures were placed. The stomach wall was incised. Upon examining the lumen of the stomach, a posterior penetrating ulcer measuring approximately 1½ cm. in diameter was found. Grossly, it appeared to be benign. In view of this, the opening in the anterior wall of the stomach was closed with continuous running 00 chromic suture.

The gastrocolic omentum was freed by ligating and clamping the vessels. The duodenum, along its inferior border, was freed for a distance of about 1½ inches. The right gastric artery and vein were doubly clamped, cut and ligated with dacron and chromic 0 sutures. The superior portion of the duodenum was freed. The left gastric vessels were doubly clamped, cut and ligated. Following this, the clamp was placed on the duodenum and the prepyloric area, and the stomach was divided. Approximately 65-70% of the stomach was resected.

The lesser curvature of the stomach was closed with three layers. First, the layer beneath the clamp was closed with an overlying 00 chromic suture and a running 000 cotton suture. The stoma of the opening in the stomach was then brought to the duodenum and approximated with it using interrupted 000 dacron sutures for the posterior seromuscular layer. Following the approximation of the posterior layer, through-and-through 00 chromic sutures were used for a posterior approximation of the mucous membrane. This was utilized as a Connell suture anteriorly with a reinforcing row of 000 dacron. Several sutures were placed along the inferior superior border of the duodenum and the stomach to remove any tension between the stomach and duodenal anastomosis. Following the anastomosis, inspection revealed no evidence of any further bleeding anywhere.

The peritoneum was closed with a continuous 00 chromic closure suture. The fascia was approximated with figure-of-eight 00 dacron suture and the skin with 00 nylon suture.

Subtotal Gastrectomy and Gastrojejunostomy (Billroth II)

Under spinal anesthesia the patient was placed in the supine position, prepared and draped in routine fashion.

A midline supraumbilical incision measuring 3 inches in length was made. The incision was carried down to the subcutaneous tissues and down through the anterior rectus sheath. This was incised vertically. The right and left recti muscles were retracted laterally. The posterior rectus sheath and peritoneum were grasped and opened.

Upon entering the abdominal cavity, palpatory exploration of the abdominal organs and contents was carried out. The examination was within normal limits except for the duodenum which contained both an anterior and posterior duodenal scar. On the anterior wall there was a very definite area of erythema and dimpling as well as an extensive area of scarring. By palpation with a finger in the foramen of Winslow, it was felt that the ulcer did not involve the common duct. It was decided that a resection would be the procedure of choice.

Attention was then turned to the stomach, where, under adequate visualization, the gastrocolic and gastrolienal ligaments were divided between curved Kelly clamps and ligated with sutures of 0 chromic catgut. After adequate mobilization of the duodenum and greater curvature, the index finger was placed through the gastrohepatic ligament in an avascular plane and the vessels and ligaments to the lesser curvature of the stomach were divided between curved Kelly clamps and ligated in a similar manner. The duodenum was then ready for division. The clamp was placed just proximal to the pylorus and the duodenum was divided just below this clamp. With the stump of the duodenum open, one could see that there was some posterior scarring. Bile was seen to flow freely from the duodenal stump.

The duodenal stump was closed with a three layer closure using 00 chromic catgut suture which was reinforced with interrupted 000 dacron sutures. The body of the stump was further mobilized by clamping and dividing further the gastrocolic and gastrohepatic ligaments for a distance involving approximately 70% of the stomach. The stomach was then ready for division.

Two long intestinal clamps were placed across two-thirds of the stomach in a transverse manner. The stomach was partially divided. A second set of clamps was placed across the lesser curvature portion of the stomach in 45 degree angles and the stomach divided. A continuous atraumatic chromic catgut suture was placed upon the lesser curvature clamp which was removed and the suture drawn taut. An additional chromic catgut suture was then run back and tied. A third layer of a continuous 000 cotton suture completed the closure of the lesser curvature aspect of the stomach.

The ligament of Treitz was found by grasping the transverse colon, maintaining general traction and bringing up a loop of jejunum, 14 to 18 cm. from the ligament of Treitz, to be anastomosed to the stomach in an antecolic fashion. The anastomosis was closed with a two layer closure using continuous 000 chromic catgut suture which was reinforced with interrupted 000 dacron sutures.

After adequate hemostasis had been attained, the anastomotic site and duodenal stump were checked for bleeding and leakage. None were found and therefore closure of the wound was begun by approximating the peritoneum with 00 general closure suture. The fascia was closed with interrupted 00 dacron figure-of-eight sutures. A medium size Penrose drain was inserted into the subcutaneous tissues and brought out through a separate stab wound incision, inferior to the primary incision. Subcutaneous tissues were then approximated with interrupted 000 chromic catgut sutures and the skin with 00 dermalon in a continuous subcuticular suture.

GASTROSCOPY

The interior of the esophagus and stomach can be examined without recourse to surgery by means of endoscopic procedures called esophagoscopy and gastroscopy. A scope is introduced by way of the mouth and passed into the esophagus and stomach. With the aid of a light and a lens system, the interior of these organs may be visualized and even biopsied. Aspirations can also be collected by this method for Papanicolaou smears and cytologic studies.

Gastroscopy is an adjunct to roentgenologic studies. Any instrumentation is usually preceded by x-ray examinations of the esophagus, stomach and mediastinum to rule out the presence of conditions which would contraindicate such a procedure.

These examinations are performed by specially trained endoscopists who may be internists or surgeons. The otolaryngologist performs endoscopic examinations of the esophagus but does not, as a rule, carry his examination into the stomach.

GASTROSCOPES

ACMI
Benedict Operating
Bernstein modification
Chevalier Jackson
Eder
Eder-Chamberlin
Eder-Hufford
Eder-Palmer

Ellsner
Herman Taylor
Housset-Debray
Janeway
Kelling
Peroral Chevalier Jackson
Schindler
Wolf-Schindler

Gastroscopy

Sodium amytal I.M. and atropine grains 1/150 were administered while the patient was on call to the OR. In the operating room, the buccal, oral and pharyngeal mucosa were sprayed with 1% Xylocaine with epinephrine. There were no untoward results. 100 mgm. of Demerol was given intravenously and the patient turned on her left side.

An Eder-Hufford gastroscope was introduced with minimal difficulty. The scope was passed to depth I. The incisura was readily identified. On the anterior and greater curvature wall of the stomach, just proximal to the incisura, there were noted six separate 3 to 5 mm. polyps, none of which were ulcerative. There was no evidence of surrounding infiltration.

On the anterior wall, proximal to the polyps described, there was a linear fold which was a pseudopolyp. This was hemorrhagic, but without ulceration. The venous pattern could be readily seen throughout the stomach indicating an atrophic gastritis. The lesser curvature was normal.

The scope was gently withdrawn and the patient returned to the ward in satisfactory condition.

GASTROSTOMY

The purpose of all gastrostomy procedures is to establish a fistulous communication between the stomach and the surface of the abdominal wall in order that the patient might be fed. A permanent fistula is formed in cases of inoperable stricture of the larynx, pharynx or esophagus. A temporary and palliative gastrostomy is formed in those cases where the disease process is obstructing and the patient does not have much longer to live or as an expedient measure in conditions which are being corrected.

GASTROSTOMY TECHNIQUES

Beck-Jianu
DePage-Janeway
Kader
Marwedel

Spivack
Stamm
Witzel

Gastrostomy

The patient's abdomen was sterilely prepared and draped. Using ½% Xylocaine as a local anesthetic, an area in the left upper quadrant of the abdomen was infiltrated through the skin and muscle.

A transverse incision was made midway between the umbilicus and xiphoid. The lateral fibers of the rectus muscle were clamped, divided and ligated. The posterior sheath was then infiltrated with Xylocaine and it was entered. The stomach was reached and brought out through the wound with gentle traction. A purse-string of 00 chromic was then used on the greater curvature near the vascular supply.

A stab wound was made in the stomach and a #30 mushroom catheter was inserted. The purse-string was then tied and the catheter was reinserted into the stomach with two other circumferential purse-strings of chromic. This provided a secure gastrostomy. The stomach serosa was then tacked to the anterior peritoneal wall circumferentially with interrupted chromic stitches. The wound was closed in layers.

PYLOROPLASTY AND GASTRODUODENOSTOMY

The pylorus is the distal aperture of the stomach which opens into the duodenum. It is the site of frequent obstructing stenosis necessitating pyloroplasty. Surgery on the pylorus is also indicated to relieve gastric stasis and promote emptying of the stomach which loses its tone following vagotomy. The Heinecke-Mikulicz pyloroplasty is the most widely practiced technique today for facilitating gastric drainage by enlarging the gastric opening.

PYLOROPLASTY TECHNIQUES

Finney
Fredet-Ramstedt pyloromyotomy
Heinecke-Mikulicz
Horsley
Jaboulay

Judd
Ramstedt
Weinberg's Modification
  of Heinecke-Mikulicz

ANATOMIC FEATURES

Duodenum (duodenal)
Gastrocolic omentum
Gastrohepatic omentum
Gastrolienal ligament
Greater and lesser curvature
Greater omentum

Pyloric antrum
Pyloric sphincter
Pyloric valve
Pyloric vestibule
Sulcus intermedius

Ramstedt Pyloromyotomy

Using ether anesthesia administered by drop and open mask method, a vertical 1½ inch rectus muscle splitting incision was made high in the epigastrium. It was carried through the posterior sheath to the peritoneum which was carefully picked up and incised.

The liver was carefully retracted upwards and the pyloric region of the stomach was brought into the wound. A longitudinal incision was then made in the hypertrophied area. A 1 inch incision was begun just proximal to the pyloric vein of Mayo at the gastroduodenal junction. It was carried through the peritoneal and superficial muscular layers over the pyloric lesion and then slightly beyond into the antrum of the stomach. The muscle fibers were bluntly separated with a knife handle for the length of the incision. The dissection continued until the mucous membrane gaped widely in the incision. Constricting fibers were released and patency of the pylorus assured. The duodenum was checked and found to be intact.

The stomach was replaced in the abdomen and the wound closed in layers with two continuous sutures of 000 chromic catgut. The skin edges were approximated with interrupted vertical mattress sutures of fine Deknatel.

Abdominal Vagotomy

In certain cases of duodenal ulcer, where the nervous phase of gastric secretion is found to be abnormally great, complete division of the vagus nerves to the stomach is indicated. This operation is called a gastric vagotomy and is usually performed in conjunction with a gastrojejunostomy or pyloroplasty.

Technique: (using transabdominal approach)

Under general anesthesia the patient was prepared and sterilely draped in the supine position.

A left paramedian incision was made extending from the xiphoid to 2 cm. below the umbilicus. The incision was carried through the anatomic layers of the abdomen. The peritoneum was picked up and incised.

The abdominal viscera were carefully examined and palpated. There was no pathology noted. The left lobe of the liver was pulled down into the operative field disclosed the coronary ligament which was divided with scissors. The left lobe of the liver was retracted to the right, exposing the lower esophagus and upper stomach. A 1 cm. transverse incision was then made about 1 cm. above the esophageal hiatus. This aperture was enlarged by blunt finger dissection. Using gentle finger dissection, the lower portion of the esophagus was separated from its areolar tissue. The esophagus was drawn downward, bringing into view the left (anterior) vagus nerve. It was seen to course along the front of the esophagus in the direction of the lesser curvature of the stomach. The right (posterior) vagus nerve was felt on the posterior aspect of the esophagus. By blunt finger dissection, the right vagus was separated from the esophageal wall. It was brought out on the left where it was ligated and divided between silk sutures, after it had been clamped superiorly. A 5 cm. segment of the nerve was resected. The left vagus was similarly treated, also being divided 7 cm. above its entrance into the stomach on the lesser curvature aspect.

The esophagus was drawn down further to facilitate investigation for additional vagus branches. None were found and the esophagus was therefore permitted to retract into the mediastinum. A few interrupted catgut sutures were used to close the opening in the diaphragm. The left lobe of the liver was returned to its former position without resuturing the coronary ligament.

A posterior gastroenterostomy was then performed with the anastomosis situated about 5 cm. from the pylorus. A satisfactory stoma was obtained.

THE SMALL BOWEL

The small bowel is made up of the second, third and fourth portions of the duodenum, the jejunum and the ileum. The average length of this segment of the gastrointestinal tract is 22 feet. The duodenum accounts for about 1 foot, the jejunum about 9 feet, and the ileum about 12 feet. These intestines are freely movable within the abdominal cavity, being anchored at the jejunum and ileum to the posterior abdominal wall by a mesentery through which they receive their blood, lymphatic and nerve supply.

The function of the small intestine is dilution, digestion, absorption and conduction of foodstuffs. The jejunum receives approximately 8-10 quarts of ingested food, fluid and intestinal secretions each day. Jejunal secretions are added to this mixture and digestion begins. Food substances are absorbed as the mixture moves into the ileum.

Conduction of the intestinal contents through the bowels takes place by a process called *peristalsis* (a wave of contraction) which moves along the tube. Interference with this forward motion results in intestinal obstruction, and is usually produced by tumors, strangulated hernia, peritoneal adhesions, intussusception, etc.

DISEASES OF THE SMALL BOWEL

Abscess
Actinomycosis infection
Adenocarcinoma of the intestine
Ancylostomiasis infestation
Ascariasis infestation
Atresia
Cyst of mesentery
Diphyllobothriasis infestation
Displacement of gastric mucosa
   into duodenum
Duodenal fistula
Duodenal spasm
Duodenal stasis
Duodenal ulcer (with perforation)
Duodenitis
Duodenojejunal obstruction
Echinococcosis of mesentery
Endometriosis
Enteric cyst
Enteritis
Epidermoid carcinoma
Fat necrosis of mesentery
Fecal fistula

Fibroma
Filariasis of mesentery
Gallstone obstruction of small bowel
Gangrene of small bowel
Gas cysts of mesentery
Granulocytopenic ulcer
Granuloma
Helminthiasis infestation
Hemangioma of intestine
Hematoma of mesentery
Hymenolepsis infestation
Ileitis, regional
Ileus, paralytic (neurogenic)
Infarction of small bowel
   due to embolism or thrombosis
   of mesenteric artery
Intestinal adhesions
Intestinal obstruction
Jejunal ulcer (with perforation)
Leiomyoma of mesentery
Lipoma
Lymphangioma
Lymphosarcoma

DISEASES OF THE SMALL BOWEL (continued)

Marginal ulcer (stomal ulcer; jejunal ulcer)
Meckel's diverticulum
Mesenteric adhesions
Pancreatic tissue in abdominal wall
Perforation
Polyp
Reticulum cell sarcoma
Redundancy of small intestine
Rupture of intestine
Sarcoma of intestine
Sarcoma of mesentery
Schistosomiasis, intestinal
Sparganosis, intestinal
Spasm of sphincter of Oddi
Strangulation of bowel
Stricture
Strongyloidiasis infestation
Syphilis
Taenia saginata (beef tapeworm)
Taenia solium (pork tapeworm)
Torsion of mesentery
Trichostrongyliasis
Tuberculosis
Ulcer of duodenum
Ulcer of jejunum
Ulcer of Meckel's diverticulum
Valve formation
Volvulus

SURGERY OF THE SMALL BOWEL

The small bowel begins at the duodenum with its sphincter of Oddi and papilla of Vater, followed by the jejunum, ileum and ileocecal valve. The gastrointestinal tract beyond this point is regarded as the colon or large intestine. Resection of the small bowel is referred to generally as an enterectomy whereas resection of the large bowel is termed colectomy. The same is true of anastomosis of the small bowel which is referred to as enterostomy or enteroenterostomy. The terms colostomy, colocolostomy, etc., are applied only to anastomoses of the large bowel.

An anastomosis may assume any of the following combinations:

ENTEROENTEROSTOMY
(small bowel to small bowel)

Duodenoduodenostomy
Duodenojejunostomy
Duodeno-ileostomy
Jejunojejunostomy
Jejuno-ileostomy
Ileoileostomy

ENTEROCOLOSTOMY
(small bowel to large bowel)

Jejuno-ileostomy
Jejunocolostomy
Ileocecostomy

Ileocolostomy
Ileosigmoidostomy

COLOCOLOSTOMY
(large bowel to large bowel)

Cecocolostomy
Cecosigmoidostomy
Colocolostomy

Colosigmoidostomy
Coloproctostomy
Sigmoidoproctostomy

A variety of methods have been devised to provide anastomosis between sections of the bowel following resection. The end-to-end method probably affords the most satisfactory anatomic continuity when the caliber of both segments of the bowel to be joined is alike. A number of factors dictate the surgeon's choice of techniques, some of which have been listed below.

CLOSED METHODS
OF ANASTOMOSIS

Basting stitch method
Bulkhead method
Dennis two-clamp & one layer silk
Furniss clamp method
Moskowitz & Rankin
   three-bladed clamp
O'Hara two-clamp method

Parker & Kerr basting stitch method
Parlavecchio & Halsted
   bulkhead method
Perret & Babcock one-clamp method
Schoemaker & Wangensteen
   modified two-clamp

OPEN METHODS
OF ANASTOMOSIS

End-to-end
Side-to-side

End-to-side
Side-to-end

Gastrojejunostomy

Gastrojejunostomy is a short-circuiting operation in which the pylorus leading into the duodenum is occluded and a new opening created between the stomach and the jejunum. The digestive route thereafter moves from the stomach to the jejunum rather than through the normal route of stomach, duodenum and jejunum. One of the most common indications for this operation is chronic duodenal ulcer. The operation is often utilized alone in the elderly, debilitated patient with a chronic duodenal ulcer or obstruction. In most instances, gastrojejunostomy is preceded by a vagotomy.

GASTROJEJUNOSTOMY
TECHNICS

Antecolic
Anterior
Antiperistaltic
Brenner
Isoperistaltic
Kocher

Lahey anterior
Mayo
Moynihan
No-Loop
Posterior

ANATOMIC
STRUCTURES ENCOUNTERED

Antral stoma
Duodenojejunal flexure
Gastrocolic ligament
Gastrocolic omentum
Gastroenteric stoma
Greater curvature
Incisura angularis
Jejunal loop

Ligament of Treitz
Mesocolon
Middle colic artery
Omentum
Proximal jejunum
Pylorus
Stoma
Vascular epiploic arch

Anterior Gastrojejunostomy

Anterior or antecolic gastrojejunostomy is sometimes indicated in cases of inoperable cancer involving the antrum of the stomach and pylorus, particularly when there is associated obstruction. The anterior gastrojejunostomy is performed more commonly than the posterior.

Technique:

Under spinal anesthesia, a semilunar incision was made approximately 1½ inches below the xiphoid. The incision extended directly over both recti. The anterior rectus sheath was dissected and transected transversely. The posterior rectus sheath and peritoneum were entered.

Upon entering the peritoneal cavity, there was a large tumor mass involving the prepyloric area, the pylorus and the first portion of the duodenum. The mass measured 14-15 cm. in diameter. It was hard and indurated. There was edema of the remaining portion of the stomach. The liver contained several hard nodules on the right, at the midportion. The tumor mass appeared to involve the hepatoduodenal ligament as well as the head of the pancreas and the hepatic triad. The entire hepatic triad was hard and firm upon examination through the foramen of Winslow. The tumor was also kissing into the pancreas. In view of these findings, resection of the stomach seemed advisable.

The jejunum was identified with the ligament of Treitz and brought anterior to the stomach. The stomach was brought into the operative field, toward the midportion, and an anastomosis accomplished anterior to the transverse colon using 000 cotton suture for the posterior seromuscular layer. The stomach and the jejunum were then incised for the anterior gastrojejunostomy.

A through-and-through 000 chromic suture was used for the posterior layer utilizing this as a continental anterior leaf. A second row of seromuscular sutures was placed. The stoma measured approximately 5-6 cm. in diameter.

The peritoneal cavity was closed with a continuous 00 chromic suture. The fascia was closed with 000 suture and the skin with subcuticular nylon suture.

Jejunostomy

In certain cases of gastric malignancy, a jejunostomy operation is indicated for feeding purposes. An opening is made in the abdominal wall and in a loop of jejunum which is anchored to the abdominal wall. A catheter is introduced through the opening and sutured in place. The feeding tube is usually fixed in the opening in such a way that it cannot be removed. The procedure serves the purpose of maintaining nourishment in far advanced, inoperable cases of cancer of the stomach where survival is not expected to exceed four to five months.

JEJUNOSTOMY TECHNIQUES

Marwedel	Travel
Mayo-Robson	Witzel

Marwedel Jejunostomy

The patient is prepared and draped sterilely in a routine manner. Under general anesthesia, a vertical 2 inch incision is made just below the tip of the ninth costal cartilage on the left. The incision is carried through the anatomic layers of the abdomen following which, the peritoneum is picked up and incised.

A loop of jejunum about 10 inches from the duodenojejunal flexure is selected for the jejunostomy. A 2 inch incision is carried down to the mucosa on the antemesenteric border of the loop of jejunum. The seromuscular layer is dissected from the mucosa on either side of the incision forming the trough in which the catheter will be implanted. Careful identification of the distal portion of the bowel is ascertained and a purse-string of 00 chromic catgut is placed. An opening made in the center of the bowel with a bistoury for insertion of the catheter. A # 14 French catheter is introduced for a distance of 11 cm., following which, suction is applied. The purse-string is drawn closed and tied with the ends being left long.

The seromuscular layer is closed over the catheter using interrupted fine silk sutures, the ends of which are also left long. A stab wound is then made through which the catheter and long ends of the purse-string are brought up, positioning the jejunum adjacent to the peritoneum. The long ends of the catgut used in the purse-string are fixed to the fascia. The seromuscular sutures are threaded on a free needle and sutured to the adjacent peritoneum. The jejunum is anchored to the abdominal wall for a distance of 3 inches to reduce the likelihood of angulation. The catheter is fixed permanently in place and sutured to the skin.

SURGERY OF THE COLON

The large bowel or colon extends beyond the ileocecal valve for about five or six feet. It consists of the cecum, ascending colon, transverse colon, descending colon, sigmoid and rectum, which have a noticeably larger caliber than the preceding small intestine. The average diameter of the large bowel is approximately two and one-half inches, diminishing somewhat toward the end of the tract.

Resection of any portion of the colon is termed a colectomy; however, excision of the cecum, sigmoid and rectum may be more specifically designated as cecectomy, sigmoidectomy and proctectomy, respectively. Total colectomy includes removal of the entire large bowel from its beginning at the cecum to its termination with the rectum.

Some other operations performed on the colon include *cecostomy,* performed for rupture of the cecum or colonic obstruction with severe distention; *loop colostomy,* for decompression and defunctioning of the bowel; and, *primary resection and anastomosis of the colon* for resectable lesions.

Malignant growths of the colon which cannot be resected in their entirety often require a palliative type procedure. Resection of the primary lesion and a short-circuiting operation such as an ileocolostomy or lateral colocolostomy, etc., are usually performed in cases where there is hope of extending survival for three or more years. In such cases, where the parent lesion cannot be removed, palliation may be afforded by a short-circuiting operation such as a lateral ileocolostomy.

In a colostomy procedure, an artificial opening is surgically formed, bringing the colon up to an opening in the abdominal wall. A single opening may be made in the colon or a double opening known as a double-barrel colostomy. Bowel contents are ejected through this newly formed opening into a pouch worn by the patient. A colostomy may be temporary for the purpose of defunctioning the bowel in preparation for a later resection, or may be a permanent opening. Regardless of which form it assumes, it is essentially a short-circuiting operation.

ANATOMIC FEATURES IN COLON SURGERY

Anastomotic site
Appendices epiploicae
Ascending colon
Cecum
Colic flexure
Colic valve
Descending colon
Duodenocolic ligament
Frenula of the valve
Gastrocolic omentum
Gastrosplenic omentum
Hepatic flexure
Houston's valves
Ileocecal junction
Ileocecal valve
Ileocolic junction
Ileum
Iliac colon
Iliacus
Lumen
Mesentery
Mesocolon
Omentum
Phrenicocolic ligament
Psoas major
Quadratus lumborum
Rectal ampulla
Rectosigmoid
Sigmoid colon
Sigmoid flexure
Sigmoid mesocolon
Splenic flexure
Stoma
Stump
Superior aperture of lesser pelvis
Taenia
Terminal ileal segment
Transverse colon
Transverse mesocolon
Vermiform process

ARTERIAL SUPPLY IN COLON SURGERY

Anterior cecal
Appendicular
External iliac
Ileal
Ileocolic
Inferior hemorrhoidal
Inferior mesenteric
Left colic
Marginal
Middle colic
Middle hemorrhoidal
Piriformis
Posterior cecal
Right colic
Sigmoidal br. of inf. mesenteric
Spermatic
Superior hemorrhoidal
Superior mesenteric

GENERAL SURGERY 325

Anatomy of the Colon

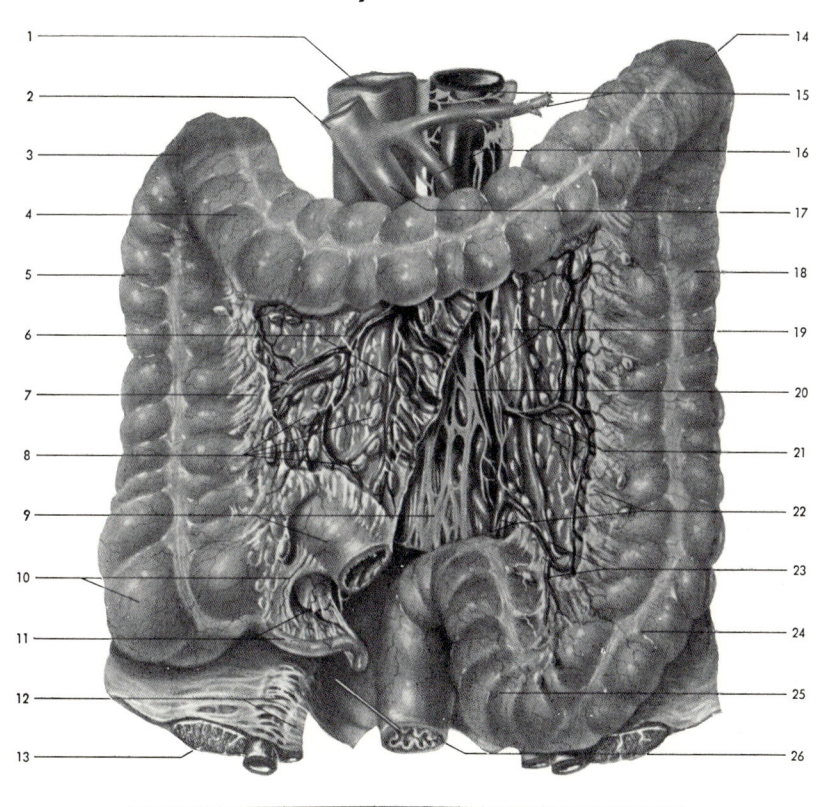

1 Inferior vena cava
2 Portal vein
3 Hepatic flexure
4 Transverse colon
5 Ascending colon
6 Branches of ileocolic artery and vein
7 Ascending mesocolon
8 Ileocecal lymph nodes
9 Ileum and hypogastric plexus
10 Cecum and ileocecal fold
11 Vermiform appendix and appendicular artery and vein
12 External iliac artery and vein
13 Psoas major muscle
14 Splenic flexure
15 Abdominal aorta and splenic vein
16 Superior mesenteric artery and inferior mesenteric vein
17 Superior mesenteric vein
18 Descending colon
19 Inferior mesenteric artery and vein
20 Inferior mesenteric plexus
21 Left colic artery and vein
22 Descending mesocolon and superior hemorrhoidal artery and vein
23 Sigmoid artery and vein
24 Iliac colon
25 Sigmoid colon
26 Rectum

Figure 45   Anatomy of the colon
Courtesy Lederle Laboratories

DISEASES OF THE LARGE INTESTINE (Colon)

Abscess of the colon wall
Actinomycosis of the colon
Adenocarcinoma of the colon
Adhesions
Appendicitis, acute
  with gangrene
  with perforation
Appendicitis, chronic recurrent
Argentaffinoma of appendix
Atony of colon
Bacillary dysentery
Carcinoid appendix
Cecum mobile
Colitis
Colostomy
Dilatation of colon
Diverticulitis, pulsion, colon
Diverticulosis, pulsion, colon
Diverticulum of appendix
Duplication of cecum, congenital
  with duplication of appendix
Endometriosis of appendix
Enterolith
Fecalith of appendix
Fistula of colon
Fistula between bladder and colon
Foreign body in appendix
Foreign body in colon
Gangrene of appendices epiploicae
Gangrene of colon
Granulocytopenic ulcer of colon
Hernia of colon
Impacted feces
Infarction of appendices epiploicae
Intussusception of appendix
Intussusception of colon
Irritability of colon
Lymphoid hyperplasia of appendix
Malfunctioning colostomy
Microcolon
Mucocele of appendix
Mucous colitis
Mucous cyst of colon
Nondescent of cecum
Obstruction of colon
Oxyuriasis of colon
Oxyuriasis vermicularis of appendix
Periappendicitis
Polyp of colon
Ptosis of colon
Redundancy of colon
Retrocecal appendix
Rotation of colon (incomplete)
Rupture of cecum
Rupture of colon
Sigmoiditis
Stercoraceous ulcer
Strangulation of colon (hernia)
Stricture of colon
Syphilis of colon
Transposition of colon
Trichuriasis of colon
Tuberculosis of colon
Typhlitis
Ulcer of colon, simple
Ulcerative colitis (left-sided
  universal)
Ulcerative colitis (right-sided,
  regional)
Valve formation of colon
Varix (pl. varices)
Volvulus

GENERAL SURGERY 327

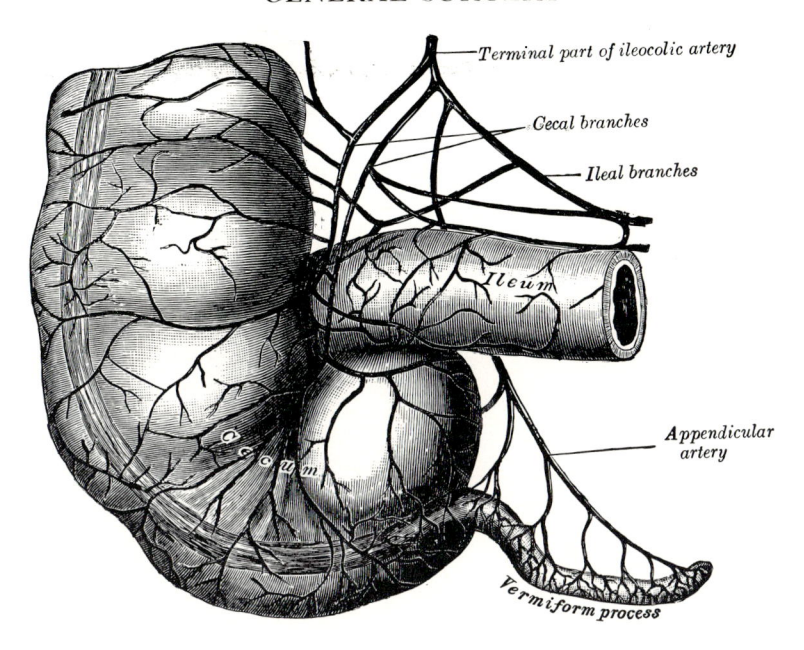

Figure 46 The cecum, vermiform appendix and ileum
From Gray's Anatomy 28th edition Courtesy Lea & Febiger.

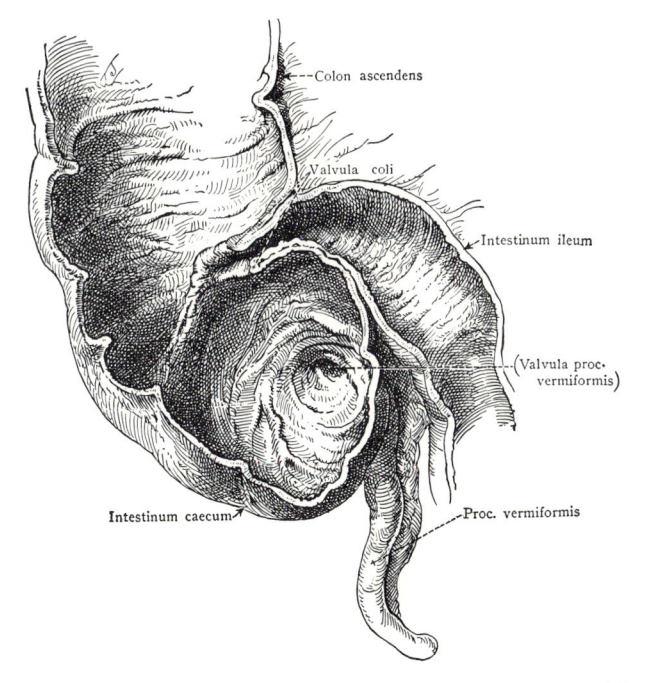

Figure 47 Interior view of the cecum, vermiform appendix and ileum
From Gray's Anatomy, 28th edition Courtesy Lea & Febiger.

Left Segmental Colectomy

Under spinal anesthesia, the patient was placed in the supine position, prepared and draped in the usual manner.

An infraumbilical midline incision, measuring approximately 3 inches in length, was made. The incision was taken down through the subcutaneous tissues and down to the anterior rectus sheath, which was incised transversely. The left and right recti muscles were retracted laterally and the peritoneum was grasped and entered.

Upon entering the abdominal cavity, palpatory examination of the abdominal contents was carried out. A small 3 x 3 cm. lesion in the rectosigmoid about 2 inches above the peritoneal reflection was discovered. The lesion was freely movable. It was not adherent. No lymph nodes were palpable although there were some areas of pericolonic induration. Examination of the liver failed to disclose any metastatic implants. The remaining abdominal organs were found to be within normal limits. There were some adhesions in the right upper quadrant from previous gallbladder surgery.

The lateral attachment of the colon to the parietal peritoneum was divided from below the brim of the pelvis, up to and just above the sigmoid colon. As the colon was mobilized medially, the spermatic vessels came into view. The left ureter, close to the spermatic vessels, was identified and carefully reflected. After complete and adequate mobilization, the rectosigmoid was divided about 1.5 cm. below the lesion. Kocher clamps were also placed across the colon in antemesenteric fashion at the elected sites of resection, just at the level of the sigmoid colon. The adjacent tissues were carefully protected with laparotomy pads. The colon was divided and the specimen removed.

An anterior anastomosis was then performed using a two layer closure. Following this, the defect in the mesentery was closed by using a continuous 000 chromic catgut suture. Again, after rechecking the anastomotic sites and obtaining hemostasis, closure of the wound was begun. Closure was carried out by approximating the peritoneum with 00 general closure, the fascia with interrupted figure-of-eight 00 dacron sutures, the subcutaneous tissues with interrupted 000 chromic catgut sutures and the skin with 00 continuous dermalon suture.

500 cc. of 5% glucose in water and 500 cc. of whole blood were used during the operation.

Surgery of the Vermiform Appendix

The appendix is a worm-like projection of the cecum. It is a blind sac subject to inflammation, abscess, gangrene, perforation and tumors. The operation for removal of the appendix is called an appendectomy.

TERMS USED
IN APPENDECTOMY REPORTS

Appendiceal
Appendicular artery
Caput caeci
Cecum
Diffuse inflammation
Exudate
Fecalith
Fecopurulent
Friable tissue
Gangrenous
Intramural artery

Invaginated stump
Meckel's diverticulum
Meso-appendix
Oxyuriasis vermicularis (pin worms)
Peritonitis
Retrocecal
Seromuscular coat
Sheath of rectus muscle
Stump of appendix
Vermiform process

APPENDECTOMY INCISIONS

Battle's pararectal
Fowler-Weir
Kocher's Modified McBurney
McBurney's gridiron
Median

Paramedian
Rectus muscle splitting
Suprapubic
Transverse

Appendectomy

Under spinal anesthesia the patient was prepared and draped in a sterile manner.

A right lower quadrant McBurney incision was made and carried through the skin and anterior sheath, transversalis, posterior sheath and peritoneum.

The appendix was located in a retrocecal position. It was noted to be acutely inflamed. The meso-appendix was clamped and ligated with a 000 cotton suture. A purse-string suture of 000 cotton was applied around the base of the appendix; the appendix was excised and the base treated with phenol and alcohol. The base was inverted and the purse-string drawn taut and tied. Further inversion was accomplished with a Z-suture.

The cecum was examined and no Meckel's diverticulum was found. The peritoneum was closed with 000 intestinal. The transversalis, internal oblique and external oblique were closed with interrupted 000 chromic. The skin was closed with subcuticular nylon.

THE RECTUM AND ANUS

The colon ends in a 5 inch segment below the sigmoid colon which is called the rectum. The distal end of the rectum, which consists of the external aperture, is called the anus. The opening to the outside of the body is guarded by an internal and external sphincter which remains closed except to permit passage of feces during defecation.

The entire length of the rectum and anus is only $6\frac{1}{2}$ inches but this short terminal segment of the gastrointestinal tract is susceptible to certain pathologic conditions. Internal and external hemorrhoids probably constitute the most common pathology of this area. Other common anorectal conditions include anal fissure, anal fistula and ischiorectal abscess. Adenocarcinoma is the most frequently encountered malignancy in this region.

ANORECTAL STRUCTURES

Anal canal
Anal orifice
Anal valves
Anococcygeal body
Anus
Columns of Morgagni
External sphincter
Houston's valves
Internal sphincter
Lateral ligaments
Levator ani
Mucocutaneous junction

Mucous membrane
Pelvic colon (sigmoid)
Rectal ampulla
Rectal columns
Rectal sinuses
Rectococcygeal muscles
Rectosigmoid
Sigmoid (pelvic colon)
Rugae
Sphincter ani
Transverse rectal folds

ANORECTAL CIRCULATION

Hemorrhoidal plexus
Hypogastric artery
Inferior hemorrhoidal artery
Inferior rectal vein
Internal iliac vein
Internal pudendal artery

Left colic vein
Middle hemorrhoidal artery
Middle hemorrhoidal vein
Superior hemorrhoidal branch
    of inferior mesenteric artery
Superior rectal veins

Incision and Drainage of Ischiorectal Abscess

Under spinal anesthesia the patient was prepared and draped. An ischiorectal abscess of the right buttocks was then drained in the following manner. A sinus was probed on the lateral middle surface of the abscess. It was approximately $1\frac{1}{2}$ inches from the rectal surface. Following the probing, a crypt was made in the posterior one half of the anus.

Sims retractors were then placed in the rectum. Using a knife, the skin and subcutaneous tissue along with the rectal sphincter were transected. The redundant portion of the sinus tract was dissected free with blunt and sharp dissection using Metzenbaum scissors. The area was packed with Iodoform gauze. Bleeders were clamped and ligated with 000 chromic suture.

Sigmoidoscopy With Rectal Polypectomy

Under spinal anesthesia, the patient was placed in the prone jackknife position, prepared and draped in the usual manner.

A sigmoidoscope was introduced into the anus and passed to a level of about 13 cm. without difficulty. At this level, a small broad sessile type polyp, somewhat necrotic in appearance and bleeding moderately, was noted. The lesion was irregular in size and shape and had an extremely broad base. It measured 2 cm. in its greatest diameter. It was initially believed to be malignant and a biopsy was therefore taken. Bleeding was minimal and required no cautery or coagulation.

The scope was passed a little further and another small polyp was seen at approximately 15 cm. This polyp was also sessile but only measured 3 mm. in diameter. This was also removed. Without any further manipulation, the scope was removed. The specimens were sent to the laboratory for histopathologic examination.

Hemorrhoidectomy

Under spinal anesthesia the patient was placed in the prone jackknife position, prepared and draped in routine fashion.

Examination of the rectum and anus revealed that there were hemorrhoids located in the usual positions, right anterior and posterior and left lateral. With the Fansler anoscope in place, internal and external hemorrhoid tags were noted in the right anterior position. A 00 chromic catgut suture was placed through the apex of the internal hemorrhoidal tag, pulled taut and tied. The hemorrhoidal tissue was excised. Excision was carried down to the external sphincter. Distally, excision extended to the level of the mucocutaneous junction.

Hemostasis was obtained by approximating the mucous membrane with a continuous 00 chromic catgut suture. Bleeding was minimal and controlled with hemostats and ligatures, as necessary.

The hemorrhoidal tags and tissue located at the other positions were treated in a similar manner. After adequate hemostasis, a rubber glove filled with Pontocainal ointment was placed in the rectum for comfort and dilatation.

CANCER OF THE COLON AND RECTUM

Approximately 73,000 cases of carcinoma of the colon and rectum are diagnosed in the U.S.A. each year where about 45,000 persons die of this disease annually. In terms of incidence, it is the most common malignancy after cancer of the skin, occurring most frequently in the age range from forty-five to seventy-five. Colonic carcinomas affect women more often than men, whereas men develop more carcinoma of the rectum.

Symptoms are vague early in the disease. In left colon lesions changes in bowel habits develop which include changes in frequency, a diminished caliber in the stool and a feeling of incomplete evacuation. About 70 per cent of these patients also complain of bleeding.

It is estimated that about three out of four of these patients might be saved each year if they had the benefit of an annual physical examination with a proctoscopy or sigmoidoscopy. In these examinations a lighted tube is inserted into the rectum enabling the physician to visualize the walls for possible newgrowths. Such examinations are available free of charge or for a nominal donation at Cancer Detection Centers located in most large cities.

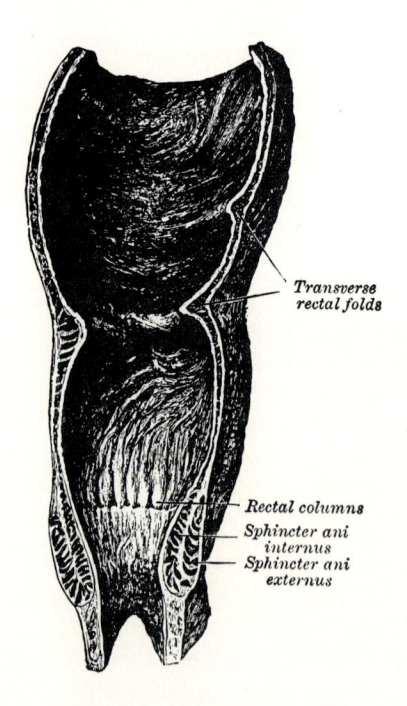

Figure 48   Rectum and anus
From Gray's Anatomy 28th Ed.
Courtesy Lea & Febiger

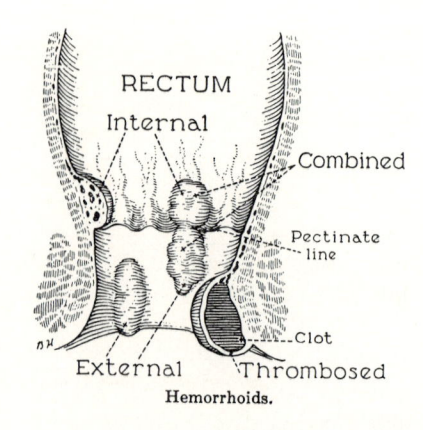

Figure 49   Anus containing hemorrhoids
Courtesy W. B. Saunders Co.

DISEASES OF THE ANUS

Aberrant sebaceous glands of anus
Abscess of perianal tissue
Absence of anus, congenital
Actinomycosis of anus
Adenocarcinoma of anus
Anal papillae, infected
Anal tags, fibrous
Atresia of anus
Chancroid of anus
Chemical burn of anus
Cicatrix of anus
Condyloma acuminatum of anus
Cryptitis
Epidermoid carcinoma of anus
Fibroma of anus
Fissure of anus
Fistula of anus
Foreign body of anus
Foreign body of anal crypt
Hemorrhoids, internal and external
Hemorrhoids, thrombosed
Hypertrophy of anal papillae
Incontinence of sphincter ani
Ischiorectal abscess
Laceration of sphincter ani
Marginal abscess of anus
Oxyuriasis of anus
Papilloma of anus
Pigmented nevus of anus
Prolapse of anal canal
Pruritis ani
Relaxation of sphincter ani
Skin tabs
Spasm of sphincter ani
Stricture of anus
Syphilis of anus
Thrombophlebitis of hemorrhoidal vein
Tuberculosis of anus
Ulcer of anus

DISEASES OF THE RECTUM

Abscess of perirectal tissue
Actinomycosis
Adenocarcinoma
Amebic proctitis
Anal crypt, enlarged
Chancroid of rectum
Chemical burn
Endometriosis
Epidermoid carcinoma
Fistula, rectal
Fistula, perirectal
Fistula, rectovesical
Foreign body
Granuloma
Lipoma
Lymphogranuloma venerum
Lymphoid polyp
Lymphosarcoma
Melanoma
Oxyuriasis
Perforation
Phlebitis of rectum
Polyp
Proctitis
Prolapse
Rectovesical fistula
Rupture of rectum
Schistosomiasis
Stercoraceous ulceration
Stricture
Syphilis
Tuberculosis
Ulcer of rectum
Varicose ulceration

OPERATIONS ON THE ANUS
For definitions see glossary at back of the book

Anoplasty
Anoscopy
  with biopsy
  with cutting into
  with excision
  with insertion of radioactive substance
  with removal of foreign body

OPERATIONS ON THE ANUS (continued)

Cauterization of anal lesion
Curettage of anal lesion
Dilation of anal sphincter
Excision of anus
Excision of lesion of anus
Fissure excision
Fistulectomy
Fistulotomy
Fulguration of anal lesion
Hemorrhoidectomy
  internal and/or external
Incision of fistula
Incision and drainage of
  perianal abscess
Sphincteroplasty
Sphincterotomy

OPERATIONS ON THE RECTUM

Anastomosis of the rectum
Closure of rectourethral fistula
Closure of rectovaginal fistula
Closure of rectovesical fistula
Dilation of rectum
Exteriorization of rectum
Fistulectomy
Incision and drainage, perirectal abscess
Proctectomy (excision of rectum)
  complete
  partial
Proctoscopy
  with biopsy
  with dilation
  with incision into
  with insertion of radioactive
    material
Proctopexy
Proctoplasty
Proctorrhaphy
Proctosigmoidectomy
Proctostomy (rectostomy)
Proctotomy (rectotomy)
  with decompression of
    imperforate anus
  with drainage of perirectal abscess
  with exploration
Resection of exteriorized rectum
Rectoplasty
Reduction of rectal prolapse
Sigmoidoscopy
  with biopsy
  with dilation
  with incision into
  with insertion of radioactive
    material

Anal Sphincterotomy and Excision of Hemorrhoidal Tags

Under spinal anesthesia, the patient was placed in the prone position and the buttocks retracted. Manual dilatation of the anal canal revealed some external hemorrhoidal tags at the 12, 3 and 6 o'clock positions. There were also a few internal hemorrhoids present.

The hemorrhoidal vessels were ligated with 000 chromic catgut suture. A partial dissection of the external and internal hemorrhoids was carried out. The sphincter was completely dissected, posteriorly. A partial sphincterotomy was done. Following resection of the mucus membrane of the internal and external hemorrhoids, the mucous membrane was anastomosed to the skin with 0000 chromic intestinal suture.

Abdominal-Perineal Resection—Proctosigmoidectomy (Miles Operation)

The patient is placed in the Trendelenburg position, prepared and draped. The abdominal cavity is entered through a right paramedian incision which begins at the crest of the pubis and is carried upward to a point 2 inches above the umbilicus. The skin margins are protected and a self-retaining retractor is introduced for the abdominal portion of the operation.

Exploration of the abdominal and pelvic cavity is carried out. There is no evidence of peritoneal implants. The liver is normal. The colon is thoroughly examined and no other area of pathology noted. The gallbladder is within normal limits with no evidence of stones. There are no palpable nodes along the inferior mesenteric vessels.

The intestines are packed away out of the operative field and the pelvic colon is drawn up through the wound. Scissors are used to lyse the adhesions which attach the sigmoid loop to the lateral wall of the pelvis. This lysis is carried out on the outer side of the pelvic mesocolon to facilitate delivery of the colon out of the abdominal cavity. The stem of the inferior mesenteric artery is ligated close to the aorta. The inferior mesenteric vein is then isolated and ligated as high up as is possible. The lateral peritoneal leaf of the mesosigmoid is then divided and the incision carried down into the pelvis, along the rectum, across the base of the bladder and then upward on to the other side of the mesentery. This provides better mobilization of the sigmoid and rectum. The pelvic mesocolon is completely divided, followed by the peritoneum, as far as the promontory of the sacrum. Care is taken to avoid injury to the ureter. Following division of the peritoneum on both sides, the fingers of the operator's left hand are introduced into the cellular space between the terminal pelvic mesocolon and anterior surface of the sacrum. The terminal pelvic colon and rectum are stripped from their attachments as far down as the sacrococcygeal articulation. Adhesive bands, extending from the sacrum to the fascia propria, are lysed with scissors. With the operator's left hand in the presacral space, the rectum is pressed upward and forward. The pelvic peritoneum, elevated in this process, is divided on either side following the brim of the true pelvis to the base of the bladder. The ureters are carefully identified and kept out of the way. The incisions in the peritoneum are extended until they come together anteriorly behind the base of the bladder. Separation of the rectum from the base of the bladder and from the vesiculae seminales is carried out. The separation of the rectum anteriorly is extended as far as the upper limits of the prostate gland. The lateral ligaments, attaching the rectum, are completely divided down to the upper surfaces of the levator ani muscles. The middle hemorrhoidal artery is divided and ligated.

Using three deMartel clamps, the pelvic colon is crushed approximately 3 inches from the end of the descending colon. The middle clamp is removed and a cautery used to burn through the colon between the two remaining clamps. The divided ends of the bowel are wrapped in waterproof sheeting which is securely tied to avoid spillage. The peritoneum is then mobilized for reconstruction of the floor of the pelvis. The edges of the defect in the peritoneum are approximated posteriorly, in front of the promontory of the sacrum and are then sutured to the stump of the pelvic mesocolon. Peritoneum is brought up from the base and lateral aspects of the bladder to cover the remaining defect. The newly constructed pelvic floor is sutured securely.

A permanent colostomy is created by bringing the proximal pelvic colon, which was severed, up through a circular opening (2 inches in diameter) in the abdominal wall. Silk sutures are used to fix the stump into position. The stump is allowed to protrude for about 3 inches beyond the skin level. A few interrupted catgut sutures are placed between the lateral wall of the pelvis and the cut edge of the pelvic mesocolon. Packs and swabs are removed and the incision is sutured in layers. The wound is dressed and the patient repositioned in the Sims' position on his left side for the perineal procedure.

The anus is closed with a purse-string suture. A transverse incision, about four inches in length, is made at the level of the sacrococcygeal articulation. From the center of this, a longitudinal incision is made in the internatal furrow and extended to a point one inch from the posterior margin of the anus. Radiating from the inferior extremity, incisions are made to the left and to the right of the anus in a horseshoe-shaped fashion, and the extremities of these are joined by a transverse cut. As a precaution against recurrence, the incision is made to embrace a wide area of perianal skin.

The coccyx is exposed by reflecting and retracting the gluteal skin flaps. An opening is made in the sacrococcygeal joint and the coccyx dissected out. The incisions around the anus are deepened to include as much of the ischiorectal fat as possible. A small transverse incision is made in the connective tissue below the sacrum. The index finger is then introduced into the space containing the isolated bowel. A transverse incision is made through the Coccygeus muscle on either side and carried to the sacrosciatic ligaments. The isolated bowel is drawn down through this opening. Traction is made on the bowel with the left hand causing the Levatores ani to come into view. The anterior wall of the anal canal is then dissected away from the central aspect of the perineum. The rectum and isolated portion of the pelvic colon are removed.

The skin incision is closed with sutures and the wounds dressed. The deMartel clamp on the proximal end of the pelvic colon is removed and the open end of the bowel wrapped in a protective covering and a pad of gauze. A Foley type bag-catheter is inserted into the dead space and brought out of the most dependent anterior portion of the wound.

The Anatomical Relationship of the Duodenum, Pancreas and Gallbladder

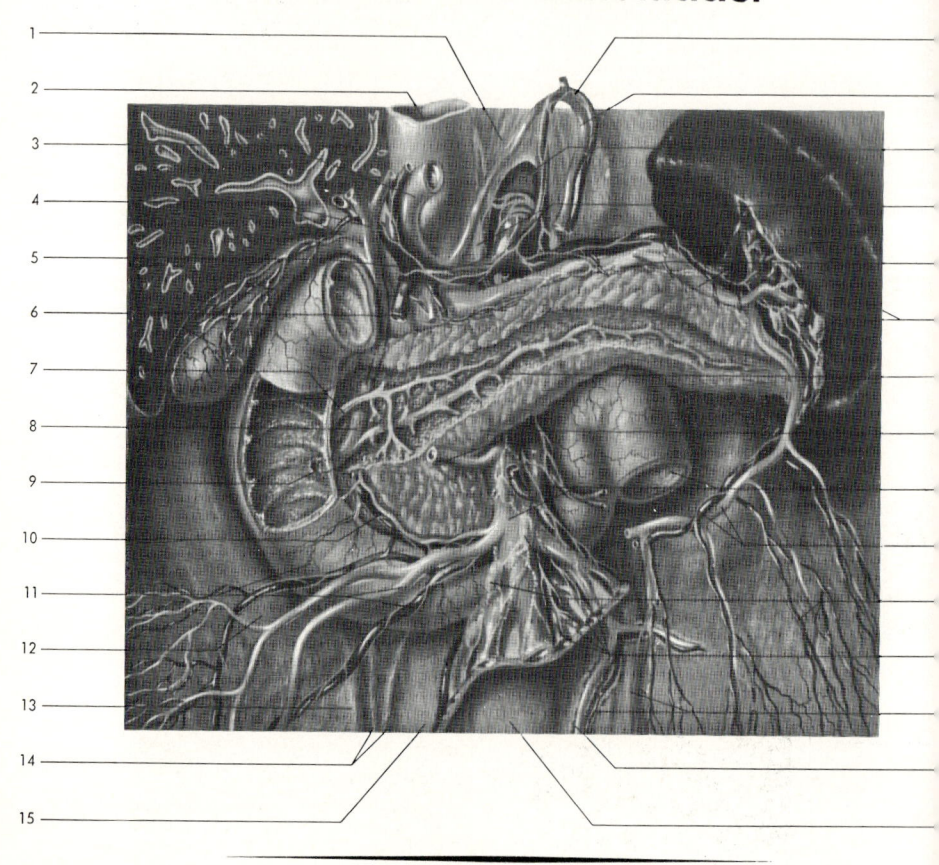

1 Crus of diaphragm
2 Inferior vena cava
3 Liver and portal vein
4 Hepatic duct and cystic artery and vein
5 Cystic duct and hepatic artery
6 Gastroduodenal artery and gallbladder
7 Lesser pancreatic duct
8 Common bile duct
9 Duodenal papilla (papilla of Vater)
10 Superior pancreaticoduodenal artery and vein
11 Duodenum and right colic artery and vein
12 Right kidney (in retroperitoneum)
13 Right ureter
14 Spermatic artery and vein
15 Vena cava (in retroperitoneum)
16 Left gastric artery
17 Coronary vein
18 Abdominal aorta
19 Celiac artery and right ganglion of celiac plexus
20 Superior pancreatic lymph node and splenic artery and vein
21 Spleen and splenic lymph nodes
22 Greater pancreatic duct
23 Pancreas and gastroduodenal vein
24 Jejunum and superior mesenteric artery and vein
25 Left gastroepiploic artery and vein
26 Superior mesenteric lymph nodes and omental vessels
27 Intestinal arteries and veins
28 Left ureter and left colic artery
29 Inferior mesenteric vein
30 Aorta (in retroperitoneum)

Figure 50   The biliary system and related structures
Courtesy Lederle Laboratories

GENERAL SURGERY

THE BILIARY TRACT

The biliary tract consists of the gallbladder, right and left hepatic ducts, common hepatic duct, cystic duct, common bile duct and sphincter of Oddi. Function of this system is the storage and conduction of hepatic (liver) secretions to the duodenum in the process of digestion.

The bile duct and hepatic ducts are essential to life; the gallbladder is not since it only serves the purpose of storage for bile. Following surgical removal of the gallbladder (cholecystectomy), this bile flows directly from the liver to the duodenum.

The most common surgical conditions of the gallbladder include cholecystitis and cholelithiasis (gallstones). The stones may be single or multiple in number and are often troublesome. They may become impacted in the cystic duct or ampulla where they cause obstruction. Smaller stones sometimes pass from the cystic duct into the common bile duct. For this reason exploration of the common bile duct for stones is performed at the time of cholecystectomy. Larger stones have been known to work themselves through the wall of the gallbladder and neighboring intestine to form a cholecystoduodenal or cholecystocolic fistula. These stones may also cause intestinal obstruction.

DISEASES OF THE GALLBLADDER AND BILIARY DUCTS

Aberrant cystic duct
Aberrant hepatic duct
Abscess, pericholecystic
Absence of bile passages, congenital
Absence of gallbladder
Accessory hepatic ducts
Adenocarcinoma
Adenoma
Adhesions, pericholecystic
Atresia of bile ducts
Bifurcation of gallbladder
Biliary dyskinesia
Calcification of gallbladder
Calculus of gallbladder
Catarrhal jaundice
Cholangiolitis
Cholangioma
Cholangitis
Cholecystitis, acute
   with gangrene
   with perforation
Cholecystitis, chronic

Cholelithiasis
Dilatation of common bile duct
Displacement of gallbladder
Distomiasis of bile passages
Duplication of common bile duct
Duplication of cystic duct
Duplication of gallbladder
Elongation of common bile duct
Elongation of cystic duct
Empyema of gallbladder
Epidermoid carcinoma
Fistula (gallbladder-cystic duct)
   cholecystogastric
   cholecystointestinal
Hernia of gallbladder
Hourglass gallbladder
Hydrops of gallbladder
Kinking of cystic duct
Mucocele of gallbladder
Papilloma
Shortening of common bile duct
Shortening of cystic duct

DISEASES OF THE BILIARY DUCTS (continued)

Syphilis
Tuberculosis
Torsion of gallbladder
Ulceration of common bile duct
Ulceration of gallbladder

OPERATIONS ON THE BILIARY TRACT
For definitions see glossary at back of the book

Biopsy of the biliary tract
Cholangiography
Cholecystectomy
Cholecystoduodenostomy
Cholecystogastrostomy
Cholecystojejunostomy
Cholecystorrhaphy
Cholecystostomy
Cholecystotomy
Choledochectomy
Choledocholithotomy (transduodenal)
Choledochoplasty
Choledochorrhaphy
Choledochostomy

Choledochotomy
Closure of biliary fistula
Duodenocholedochotomy
Excision of ampulla of Vater
Exploration of bile ducts
Hepaticostomy
Hepaticotomy
Implantation of biliary
  fistulous tract into stomach
  or intestine
Incision of bile ducts
Incision of sphincter of Oddi
Insertion of T-tube

ANATOMIC STRUCTURES ENCOUNTERED IN GALLBLADDER SURGERY

Ampulla of Vater
Bile duct
Common duct
Cystic artery
Cystic duct
Ductus choledochus
Ductus hepaticus
Foramen of Winslow
Fossa in the liver

Fundus of gallbladder
Gallbladder bed
Hartmann's pouch
Heister, spiral valve of
Hepatic artery
Hepatic duct
Hepatic fossa
Liver bed

Cholecystectomy

Under spinal anesthesia the patient was prepared and draped in the supine position.

A right subcostal Kocher incision was made. The skin was incised and the incision carried down through the anterior rectus sheath, rectus muscle, posterior sheath and peritoneum. Bleeders were clamped and ligated with 000 chromic suture.

The gallbladder was found to be markedly edematous, thickened and hyperemic. It measured approximately 15 cm. in length and 4 cm. in diameter. There were numerous adhesions around the gallbladder which were lysed by blunt dissection.

Exploration of the abdominal contents was normal. The finger could be inserted into the foramen of Winslow. The common duct was free of stones.

The gallbladder was removed by using Carmel clamps to grasp the fundus and Hartmann's pouch. The cystic duct was then clamped, divided and doubly ligated with 000 cotton. The cystic artery was likewise clamped, divided and ligated with 00 cotton and the gallbladder removed. The gallbladder bed was oversewn with a continuous locking 00 chromic. A medium sized Penrose drain was placed into the foramen of Winslow and brought out through a separate stab wound in the abdomen.

The peritoneum was closed along with the posterior sheath using chromic. The fascia was closed in layers with cotton, the subcutaneous tissue with chromic and the skin edges were approximated with dermalon.

Transduodenal Excision of Common Duct Stone; Sphincterotomy of Oddi

The patient had sustained a cholecystectomy 18 months previously. She has had repeated episodes of right upper quadrant intermittent abdominal pain associated with nausea and vomiting since. I.V. cholangiograms revealed a large calculus within the common duct with dilation of the duct.

Under spinal anesthesia, an incision was made through a previous scar and extended through the anterior rectus sheath, posterior rectus sheath and peritoneum. Multiple dense adhesions were encountered. The adhesions were lysed from the peritoneum. The renal vessels were visualized. Small bleeders were ligated. The duodenum and the common duct were identified.

The ampulla was palpated by inserting two fingers in the foramen of Winslow and getting the duodenum and pancreas in front of the fingers. A calculus measuring 1½ cm. was felt within the second portion of the duodenum near the sphincter of Oddi. It appeared to be firmly stuck at this point.

A longitudinal incision was made in an avascular area. The incision extended down through the sphincter. A calculus measuring 1½ cm. was extracted from the ampulla of Vater. The sphincter was cut in removing the stone. Bile was expressed very easily following removal of the stone. It appeared to be clear.

The duodenum was closed with a Connell 0000 continuous chromic suture and an interrupted three layer of cotton suture. All bleeding points were ligated. A through-and-through # 30 wire suture was used to approximate the various layers. A drain was inserted in the gallbladder bed and brought out through a separate stab wound.

THE LIVER

The liver is the largest organ of the body, its average weight being approximately 1,500 grams. It is located in the right upper quadrant of the abdominal cavity where it is largely protected by the ribs. It is an organ of many functions and is essential to life. The liver is the main reservoir of sugar in the body, converting it from glucose to glycogen for storage. This sugar is made available to the body, as required, between meals. The liver is also involved in the production and maintenance of the plasma and tissue proteins. Albumin, fibrinogen and prothrombin are produced in the liver which also produces and excretes bile, an important product in the digestion of fat. It is an important factor in carbohydrate, fat and protein metabolism. The full extent of its role in the many metabolic processes of the body is not yet completely known.

Surgical conditions of the liver consist of traumatic injuries, primary and metastatic neoplasms and abscesses. Most of these conditions are not readily treated by surgical procedures. The organ is an extremely vascular one. Even prior to needle biopsy through the abdominal wall, preparation of the patient with Vitamin K is necessary to promote blood clotting, and thus prevent excessive bleeding.

DISEASES OF THE LIVER

Abscess
Abscess, amebic
Accessory livers, congenital
Adenocarcinoma
Adenoma
Amebic abscess
Amyloid disease
Catarrhal jaundice
Cholangioma
Cirrhosis, alcoholic
Cirrhosis, Laennec's
Cirrhosis, nodular, coarse
Cirrhosis with lenticular
   nuclear degeneration
Coccidiosis
Cystic disease
Cysts
Fatty liver
Fibroma
Fistula
   hepatopleural
   hepatopulmonary
Hanot's hypertrophic cirrhosis

Hemangioma
Hepatitis
Hepatoblastoma
Hepatoma
Hepatomegaly
Hepatorenal syndrome
Hernia of liver
Homologous serum jaundice
Hypoplasia
Infarction of liver
   due to embolism
   due to periarteritis nodosa
   due to thrombosis
Intrahepatic calculosis
Laennec's cirrhosis
Lobulation, abnormal
Passive congestion
Portal hypertension
Ptosis
Syphilis
Tuberculosis
Yellow atrophy

OPERATIONS ON THE LIVER

Biopsy, excisional
Biopsy, needle
Excision of lesion
Hepatectomy, partial
Hepatorrhaphy (suture)
Hepatotomy (incision into)
   with drainage
   with exploration
   with foreign body removal
   Incision and packing (first stage
     drainage of liver abscess)
Marsupialization of cyst
   or liver abscess
Needle biopsy of liver

THE PANCREAS

The pancreas is a digestive as well as an endocrine gland which is anatomically described in terms of a head, a body and a tail. The organ is situated retroperitoneally at about the level of the first lumbar vertebra. Anteriorly, the pancreas is located at the level of the stomach and transverse colon. Posterior to the superior mesenteric artery lies a small portion of pancreas called the uncinate process, sometimes called the lesser pancreas, Willis pancreas or Winslow's pancreas. The gland is supplied with a duct system which carries the pancreatic secretions to the intestine. These include the **main pancreatic duct** (duct of Wirsung) which extends for the length of the pancreas and enters either the duodenum, ampulla of Vater or the papilla of Vater, and the **accessory pancreatic duct** (duct of Santorini) which usually courses from the upper head of the pancreas, connecting with the main pancreatic duct within the organ, and often emptying into the duodenum through a separate opening, proximal to the papilla of Vater.

The largest portion of the gland is concerned with the elaboration and transportation of its digestive enzymes to the intestine (duodenum). The endocrine function of the gland is concerned with the production of insulin, so important in carbohydrate metabolism. The hormone is secreted in the beta cells of the islets (or islands) of Langerhans which are present in greatest numbers in the tail and body of the organ. Glucagon, a secretion of the alpha cells, is another pancreatic endocrine product. Its purpose is the splitting up of glycogen (storage form of carbohydrate) for use by the body when the blood sugar level drops. These endocrine substances are released directly into the blood stream.

The most important surgical lesions of the pancreas include: pancreatitis, acute and chronic, cystic lesions, and tumors.

Islet cell tumors are adenomas which are usually benign. They may be functioning, i.e. producing excessive amounts of insulin, or nonfunctioning. Two syndromes associated with the nonfunctioning islet cell tumor are called the Zollinger-Ellison syndrome and the Wermer syndrome.

Cancer of the pancreas usually occurs after the age of forty, with the incidence in men three times greater than in women. The head of the pancreas is more commonly involved than the body or tail. Most surgery for such lesions is palliative rather than curative. Resectable growths of the head of the pancreas and of the ampullary region are treated by radical pancreatoduodenectomy (radical resection of the proximal pancreas, distal common bile duct, duodenum and distal stomach). Another name for the procedure is a Whipple operation. This is not a commonly performed operation because only the early and favorable cases are selected for resection. During the exploration which precedes and determines resectability, the surgeon examines the liver for neoplastic studding, the portal fissure for malignant nodes and the peritoneum, pelvic shelf, omentum and mesentery for malignant seedlings. The surgeon further determines whether or not there is any extension or invasion of the vena cava, portal vein or superior mesenteric vessels which would contraindicate surgery.

In nonresectable lesions, surgical palliation usually consists of creating a passage or by-pass for obstructed bile passages. Operations performed for this purpose include: cholecystoenterostomy (anastomosis of gallbladder to intestine), cholecystoduodenostomy (anastomosis of gallbladder to duodenum), or cholecystogastrostomy (anastomosis of the gallbladder to the stomach). Survival following such operations may be six to eight months.

A description of the Whipple operation follows to illustrate the terminology encountered in descriptions of this procedure.

PANCREATODUODENECTOMY TECHNIQUES

Brunschwig	Two-Stage
Cattell	Warren
Child's	Watson
One-Stage	Waugh
Poth	Whipple

Whipple Operation (Pancreatoduodenectomy)

Under general and spinal anesthesia, the patient was prepared and draped in the usual manner.

An epigastric transverse incision was made subcostally, approximately 14 to 16 inches in length. The anterior rectus sheath was incised, rectus muscle transected on the right and the posterior sheath and peritoneum opened.

It was noted on exploration that the area of the pancreas was somewhat enlarged and the head of the pancreas was quite hard in consistency. Upon palpation of the ampulla of Vater, a small nodule was detected. The liver was free of implants. There was no evidence, on inspection and palpation, of metastases or involvement of the great vessels. Resection was decided upon.

The peritoneal reflection of the duodenum was incised and a Kocher's maneuver used to reflect the peritoneum laterally. The common duct was dissected free. It was noted that the common duct and the gallbladder were also greatly enlarged, the duct being approximately a half inch in diameter.

The greater curvature of the stomach was dissected free and bleeders were clamped and ligated with 0 chromic suture. The lesser curvature was isolated in a similar fashion. The stomach was then transected and approximately 40% of it was removed. A clamp was left in the proximal segment distally with the common duct being transected approximately 2 inches from its terminal portion. With blunt and sharp dissection, the duodenum was dissected free. In the area of the ligament of Treitz, dissection was performed. Bleeders were clamped and ligated with 000 intestinal. The mesentery was then dissected from the jejunum to the superior mesenteric artery. With blunt and sharp dissection, the duodenum was carried, in a retrograde fashion, behind the superior mesentery and brought out anteriorly. It was noted that the head of the pancreas was then easily dissectible. Dissection was therefore carried out in a blunt and sharp manner. There was no invasion in the area of the superior mesentery or celiac axis. There were two nodes present in the area of the common duct which were removed with the dissection. On pathologic examination they were reported as possibly malignant.

On transection of the head of the pancreas, it was noted that the ducts of Wirsung and Santorini were greatly dilated. A stem of a # 14 rubber catheter was placed in the duct of Wirsung. Santorini's duct was ligated. With a through-and-through suture, the rest of the pancreas was ligated so that no evidence of any leakage was present at this point. This completed the dissection of the duodenum, the first portion of the jejunum, and the head of the pancreas along with part of the common duct. The terminal portion of the jejunum was placed over the duct of Wirsung with an interrupted row of 000 cotton sutures. Another row was used for further inversion in a circumferential fashion. The common duct was tied with two 00 cotton sutures and the fundus of the gallbladder was then anastomosed to the jejunum with a posterior row of 000 cotton sutures. A musculomucosal row of 000 chromic intestinal posteriorly, locked anteriorly, was Connelled to anastomose the gallbladder and the jejunum. Further inversion was performed with 000 cotton, anteriorly.

The jejunum was grasped and brought up the proper length to the stomach. A Polya anastomosis was then accomplished posteriorly with 000 cotton. A musculomucosal row of 000 continuous chromic posteriorly, locked anteriorly, Connell type suture was placed. Further inversion was accomplished with 000 cotton. Upon completion of this procedure, a drain was placed in the area of the duodenum and the head of the pancreas, brought out through a separate stab wound incision and tied in place with an interrupted row of 000 cotton. There was no evidence of bleeding.

The posterior sheath and peritoneum were closed with 00 chromic general type closure anteriorly. The anterior rectus sheath and external oblique were closed with # 32 wire. The skin was closed with interrupted 000 silk suture.

The patient tolerated the procedure well. During the operation, 1000 cc. of 5% glucose in water and 1000 cc. of whole blood were administered. The patient left the operating room in satisfactory condition.

DISEASES OF THE PANCREAS

Abscess of the pancreas
Accessory pancreas
Adenocarcinoma
Adenoma
Aneurysm of pancreatic artery
Annular pancreas
Arteriosclerosis of pancreatic artery
Atrophy of pancreas
Bifurcation of part of pancreas
Calculus of pancreatic duct
Cyst of pancreas due to obstruction
Distomiasis
Dorsal pancreas
Ductal carcinoma
Echinococcosis
Embolism of pancreatic artery
Fibrocystic disease
Fistula
Hemorrhage due to embolism
Hemorrhage due to blood dyscrasia
Hemorrhage due to scurvy
Interstitial pancreatitis
Ischemic necrosis
Islet cell tumor
  functioning
  nonfunctioning
Necrosis
Pancreas divisum
Pancreatic infantilism
Pancreatic necrosis
Pancreatic necrosis, aseptic
Pancreatitis
  acute hemorrhagic
  acute suppurative
  chronic
Parasitic obstruction of
  pancreatic duct
Passive congestion
Pseudocyst due to pancreatic necrosis
Pseudocyst due to aseptic necrosis
Rupture of pancreas
Senile atrophy
Steatorrhea
Stricture of pancreatic duct
Syphilis
Tuberculosis
Wound of pancreas

OPERATIONS ON THE PANCREAS

Excision of adenoma
Marsupialization of cyst of pancreas
Pancreatectomy
  complete with excision
    of duodenum
  partial
Pancreatoduodenectomy
Pancreatotomy
  with drainage
  with exploration
  with removal of calculus
Pancreaticoduodenostomy
Pancreaticogastrostomy
Pancreaticojejunostomy
Pancreolithotomy
Suture of pancreas

8 Gynecology

Gynecology is that branch of general surgery which concerns itself with diseases of the external and internal female genitalia. The gynecologist is also trained in the practice of obstetrics, gynecologic pathology and female endocrinology.

Some of the procedures performed in this specialty along with their eponymic titles are reviewed in this section to assist the secretary with her vocabulary.

EXTERNAL FEMALE GENITAL ANATOMY

Bartholin's glands
Bulbus vestibuli
Canal of Nuck
Clitoris
Crura of clitoris
Fourchette
Frenulum
Hymen

Labia majora
Labia minora
Mons pubis
Navicular fossa
Perineum
Vaginal orifice
Vestibule of vagina
Vulva

INTERNAL FEMALE GENITAL ANATOMY

Anterior ligament
Areolar tissue
Broad ligaments
Cardinal ligaments (Mackenrodt)
Cervical canal
Cervix
Cervix uteri
Corpus albicans
Corpus hemorrhagicum
Corpus luteum
Corpus of the uterus
Cul-de-sac of Douglas

Endometrium
Epoophoron
External os
Fallopian tubes
Fimbriae
Fimbriated ends
Follicular cysts
Fornix (pl. fornices)
Fundus of uterus
Graafian follicle
Hydatids of Morgagni
Infundibulopelvic ligament

INTERNAL FEMALE GENITAL ANATOMY (Continued)

Internal os
Interstitial tissues
Lateral ligament
Levator ani
Ligamentum ovarii proprium
Mackenrodt's ligament
Mesosalpinx
Mesovarium
Mucous membrane
Myometrium
Ovarian artery
Ovarian vein
Ovary (pl. ovaries)
Oviduct
Pampiniform plexus
Parametrium
Paroophoron
Pelvic floor
Portio supravaginalis
Portio vaginalis
Posterior ligament
Pouch of Douglas
Rectouterine ligaments
Round ligament of uterus
Sacrogenital ligaments
Sacrouterine ligaments
Suspensory ligament of ovary
Tunica albuginea
Uterine artery
Uterine nerves
Uterosacral ligaments
Uterus
Vagina
Vesicouterine ligaments

FEMALE GENITAL ANATOMY

The female genitalia are broadly classified into the external and internal organs. The external genitals are referred to collectively as the pudendum or vulva. They comprise the mons veneris, labia majora, labia minora, clitoris, urethral meatus, urogenital vestibule with glands and the vaginal introitus. These structures are situated below the urogenital diaphragm as well as below and in front of the pubic arch.

The internal genitals, consisting of the vagina, uterus, fallopian tubes and ovaries, are situated within the pelvis.

The External Female Genitalia

The mons veneris is that prominent triangle of subcutaneous fat just above the opening to the female genital tract which after puberty becomes covered with coarse hair. The pattern of this hair distribution is referred to as the **escutcheon** and may be described by the physician as being of male or female type. The area between the thighs generally is called the **perineum** while the narrow bridge of tissue between the outer openings of the anus and vagina is more specifically called the **perineal body.** The large outer lips of the vulva are the **labia majora.** The outer borders contain coarse hair. The inner surfaces are nonhairy. The mucocutaneous folds found at the sides of the vaginal opening are secondary folds of the upper inner portion of the labium majus and are called the **labia minora** (nymphae). They begin as a double fold below the anterior junction of the labia majora, passing above and below the clitoris. The folds which meet above the clitoris form the prepuce. The delicate fold which unites the posterior extremities of the labia minora and extends between them is called the **fourchette.** It is frequently torn in childbirth or even in sexual intercourse. Between the fourchette and the hymen there is a small depression called the **fossa navicularis.**

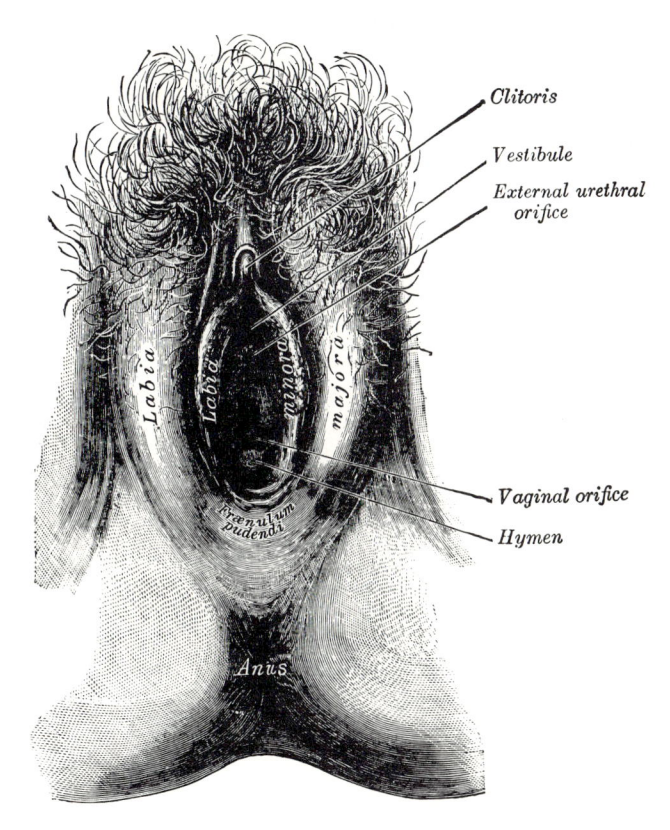

Figure 51 The external female genitalia
*From Atlas and Textbook of Human Anatomy by Sobotta and McMurrich.
Courtesy W. B. Saunders Company.*

Another feature of the external female genitals is the **clitoris,** the female analogue of the penis. Like the penis, it consists of erectile tissue which responds to sexual stimulation. At the symphysis its two lateral halves separate to form the **crura.**

When the labia are separated a shallow triangle-shaped depression is noted. This is the **urogenital vestibule** which represents a remnant of the lower portion of the urogenital sinus in the fetus. Another vestigial structure which sometimes persists is the canal of Nuck which remains along the round ligament.

Of surgical importance are the two major vestibular glands known as the **Bartholin glands** or vulvovaginal glands. Their purpose is to produce a clear mucoid secretion which acts as a lubricant in coitus. These glands are a common site of infection, abscess and cyst formation. Other genital glands include the **Skene** which are two small tube-like structures located on the posterior surface of the urethra, at the meatus.

Another important anatomic feature of the external female genitals from a surgical standpoint is the **hymen,** a circular mucosal fold which partially covers the vaginal opening (introitus). This membrane, in some persons, completely covers the opening, a condition known as imperforate hymen. Surgical incision is required, particularly with the onset of menses, to permit normal menstrual flow. When the hymen is particularly thick and rigid it may interfere with coitus. This condition is corrected by enlarging the opening with incisions of the hymen. When the membrane is of normal consistency it is simply stretched during sexual relations.

The Internal Female Genital Organs

The internal female genitalia consisting of the vagina, uterus, fallopian tubes and ovaries are illustrated in Fig. 52 in their anatomic relationship to surrounding structures. Careful study of this plate should enhance the student's understanding of these relationships.

The Vagina

The vagina is situated in proximity to the urinary bladder, rectum and intestines. The bladder and proximal urethra lie upon the vagina. The anterior vaginal wall is separated from the distal urethra by a connective tissue partition called the urethral vaginal septum. Beneath the distal urethra it becomes the more delicate vesicovaginal septum. The upper fourth of the posterior vagina is separated from the rectum by the cul-de-sac of Douglas. The thin wall of connective tissue which separates the bladder, rectum and intestines from the vaginal canal is frequently the site of herniations or protrusions, called cystocele, rectocele and enterocele.

The Uterus

The uterus is a hollow inverted pear-shaped organ situated in the pelvic cavity between the urinary bladder and the rectum. Its average length is about three inches and its weight about 30–45 grams. It is larger and heavier (about 70 grams) in women who have borne children. After

GYNECOLOGY 353

the menopause the uterus enters a phase of progressive atrophy shrinking in some aged women to the size of a dime.

The upper fullest portion of the uterus is called the **corpus uteri** or **body of the uterus.** The lower narrowed portion, which at its midpoint extends into the vagina, is called the **cervix,** or **cervix uteri.** The portion of the cervix above the level at which the vagina attaches is referred to as **supravaginal** while that portion below the attachment point, which extends into the vagina between the anterior and posterior fornices, is called the **vaginal portion** or **portio vaginalis.**

The uterine cavity opens, through the cervix, into the vaginal passage. The point at which the cervix opens into the vagina is known as the **external os.** This opening is surrounded by lips referred to as the anterior or posterior lip of the cervix.

The wall of the uterus consists of a muscular layer called the **myome-**

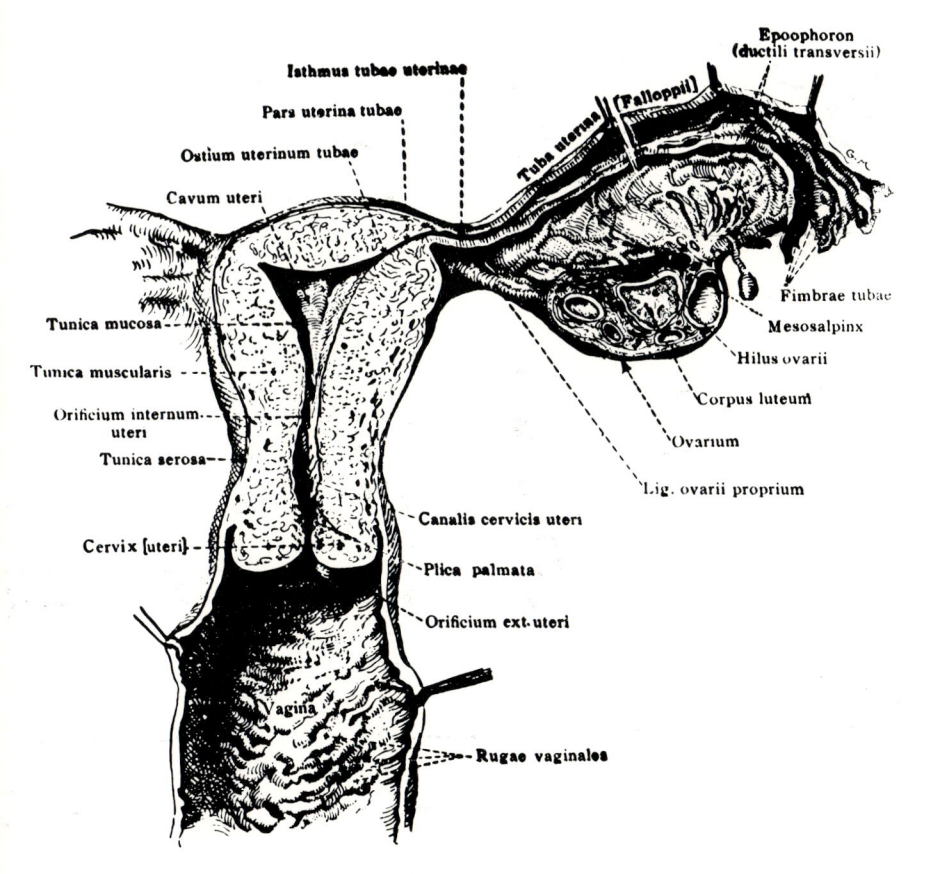

Figure 52 Internal female genitalia with section through the vagina, uterus, fallopian tube and ovary.
(Eyeleshymer and Jones) Hand Atlas of Clinical Anatomy. Courtesy Lea & Febiger.

trium. The inner lining of the body of the uterus is called the **endometrium.** It is this layer which is scraped in a D & C. This is also the lining which during childbearing years undergoes a continuous process of growth and sloughing (menstrual cycle) except during pregnancy. This layer also serves as an implantation area for the fertilized ovum when pregnancy occurs.

The tissue lining the cervix of the uterus is called the **endocervical mucosa.**

Another anatomic feature of the uterus are the horn-like projections extending from each side called the **cornua** (singular: cornu). These are the points where the fallopian tubes open into the uterus.

The Fallopian Tubes (uterine tubes)

The fallopian tubes are two muscular passages, one end of which opens into the uterine cavity while the other end opens into the peritoneal cavity. This direct opening from the outside of the body, through the vagina, cervix uteri, uterus and fallopian tubes into the peritoneal cavity explains the high incidence of peritonitis in women. Infections high in the internal female genital tract, particularly of the tubes, sometimes eventuate in peritonitis. The continuity of the genital passage also predisposes it to infection. Internal cleansing, when carried out under too great a pressure, can introduce infection into the upper genital tract. The adnexa or appendages to the uterus, consisting of the tubes and ovaries, are frequently involved in a pelvic inflammatory disease (P.I.D.)

The upper opening of each tube into the peritoneal cavity is called the **fimbriated extremity** or **infundibulum** because of the fringed-like projections they bear. These fimbria are in contact with the ovary and serve to propel the discharged ovum from the ovary to the fallopian tube and into the uterine cavity. They have also been observed to set up a fluid wave within the pelvic cavity to further propel the ovum toward the ostium or opening of the tube. The ovary is not situated anatomically to provide direct access to the fallopian tube. The discharged ovum actually finds its way to the tubal opening with the aid of tubal fimbria.

The tubes also serve the purpose of providing a passage for the sperm injected into the uterus. Union of sperm and ovum generally takes place in the tubes from which the fertilized ovum proceeds to the uterus for implantation.

The Ovaries

The ovaries are two glandular organs situated on each side of the uterus, projecting from the posterior wall of the broad ligament. The fold thus formed is called the **mesovarium.** The ovary receives its blood supply through this attachment. Each ovary weighs between 5 and 10 grams. They consist of many microscopic ova, each contained within a tiny sac called the **graafian follicle.** These sacs are separated by a meshlike arrangement of connective tissue which also serves as the framework of the ovary. This is called the **ovarian stroma.** It forms a dense capsule near the periphery of the ovary called the **tunica albuginea.** This layer is situated beneath the outer surface of the ovary called the **cortex** or cortical portion. The cortex contains the graafian follicles. The small young follicles are found near the surface and are present by the thousands. The older follicles are less abundant and are found at a deeper level. Most of the follicles never reach maturity and simply degenerate. During childbearing years usually one follicle develops to maturity each month. After the ovum has fully matured, the follicle (enclosing sac) ruptures releasing the egg into the abdominal cavity. This process is known as **ovulation.** The remaining ruptured follicle soon becomes filled with cells containing a yellow pigment (lutein cells) forming a mass called the **corpus luteum.** When pregnancy does not occur, these cells disappear leaving only a scar of white tissue called the **corpus albicans.** This is the final stage in which the ruptured follicle remains. When pregnancy occurs, the corpus luteum remains for several months before receding. It becomes problematic to the pregnancy when it persists, as it sometimes does.

The parovarium is a remnant of the wolffian body in the fetus. It consists of a group of tubules in the broad ligament, situated between the ovary and fallopian tube. The wolffian body serves as an excretory organ in the fetus. Other residual fetal structures sometimes encountered include the mullerian ducts which give rise to cysts called **hydatids of Morgagni.**

The Uterine Ligaments

The ligaments related to the uterus are also considered with the internal female genitalia since they figure prominently as supporting structures.

The uterus is held forward in its normal position by the broad and uterosacral ligaments as well as by the pelvic floor. The broad ligament holds the uterus in a central position by extending laterally from the uterus to the pelvic floor. The uterosacral ligaments are strands of fibrous tissue with some muscle fibers which project from the posterolateral surface of the cervix to the anterior surface of the sacrum. Plication (pleating procedure used for shortening) of the uterosacral ligaments is carried out for repair of enterocele and positional replacement operations. The cardinal ligament (Mackenrodt's) is the lower portion of the broad ligament which is attached to the supravaginal portion of the cervix. The round ligaments (ligamentum teres uteri) extend from the anterior surface of the lateral border of the uterus, through the inguinal canal, to the labium majus, preventing backward displacement of the uterus. They also prevent torsion or twisting of the uterus. The vesicouterine ligament is a peritoneal fold extending from the uterus to the urinary bladder. The infundibulopelvic ligament (suspensory ligament of the ovary) is the superior lateral portion of the broad ligament enclosed in a fibrous cord. It attaches the infundibulum of the tube to the lateral pelvic wall and also encloses the ovarian vessels as they enter the broad ligament.

OPERATIONS ON THE VAGINA AND VULVA

Operations performed on the vulva (external genitalia of the female) are primarily operations of excision for benign and malignant lesions.

Cancer of the vulva accounts for approximately three to four per cent of all carcinomas of the genital tract. It is a slow growing malignancy which metastasizes to the inguinofemoral lymph nodes and later to the more centrally located lymphatics. Metastases are often bilateral. Incidence of this lesion increases with age. The tumor is often radioresistant and therefore cannot be effectively treated with radiation. Radioactive gold seeds implanted into the tumors and into the inguinal lymph nodes are being used with good results. Bervan, Bickenbach and Mueller report a five year cure rate of about 40 per cent using simple vulvectomy or electrocoagulation combined with radiation of the regional lymph nodes. A 60 per cent five year cure rate is reported by Way, Green, Ulfelder, Meigs, Wimhofer and Isaac using radical extended vulvectomy with block dissection of the lymph nodes. The mortality attending the latter procedure is understandably higher.

Operations on the vagina consist primarily of repairs (colporrhaphy) of the vaginal wall for cystocele and rectocele, excision of fistulas as well as excision of benign and malignant lesions.

Primary carcinoma of the vagina accounts for less than two per cent of all genital malignancies. Radiotherapy is usually the only form of treatment used. It consists of vaginal radium application followed by deep X-radiation. Tumors which are very low lying are treated in the same manner as carcinoma of the vulva. Extensive vaginal vault carcinomas may be treated with pelvic exenteration (radical excision of the cancer, lymph nodes and surrounding tissues and involved organs).

The average five year cure rate for treated carcinoma of the vagina is about 25 per cent.

Vaginal Wall Prolapse

Prolapse (falling down) of the vaginal wall is uncommon. It may develop following an abdominal or vaginal hysterectomy. It is sometimes associated with a cystocele or enterocele. Corrective operations usually result in a shortening and narrowing of the vagina, an undesirable condition in sexually active women. For this reason, in younger women, a combined abdominovaginal suspension of the vaginal vault to the lower abdominal wall using fascial strips is used.

COLPORRHAPHY

Common surgical problems of the vaginal wall include the cystocele and rectocele; less often they also include the enterocele and urethrocele. Repair of the vaginal wall (colporrhaphy) is designated as anterior or posterior.

In a cystocele there is a protrusion of the urinary bladder through the anterior vaginal wall. In the rectocele there is a protrusion of the rectum through the posterior vaginal wall. These defects usually occur together and are repaired surgically in a procedure called an anterior and posterior colporrhaphy (A & P colporrhaphy).

Enterocele is a hernia of the pouch of Douglas into the rectovaginal space extending toward the introitus and occasionally to the vulva. It may be congenital in origin or secondary to fixation operations on the uterus. It is usually accompanied by a rectocele.

A urethrocele is an outpocketing of the urethra encroaching upon the vaginal wall. It is often associated with a cystocele and is treated by plication of the urethra.

Stress incontinence (involuntary loss of urine on laughing, sneezing, etc.) is a condition present in approximately twenty per cent of all gynecological patients. It is often treated by surgical techniques plicating the bladder neck and urethra, particularly with colporrhaphy. Although the operation is frequently performed by the gynecologist, we will consider the subject in the chapter on urology.

Anterior and Posterior Colporrhaphy

Under spinal anesthesia the patient was placed in lithotomy position and sterilely prepared and draped.

Bimanual pelvic examination was performed. The uterus was found to be normal in size. No descensus uteri was found by traction with a tenaculum. A large cystocele, urethrocele and rectocele were noted. The uterus was otherwise normal in size, shape and form. No adnexal masses were palpable.

The vaginal mucosa surrounding the external cervix was incised transversely. The mucosa was incised at the midportion creating an inverted T up to the urethral meatus. The vaginal mucosa was sharply dissected from the fascia. The bleeders were clamped and tied with 000 chromic suture. The pubocervical fascia was reapproximated in the midline using 00 interrupted chromic sutures. The urethra was plicated with 000 chromic intestinal suture. A Kelly type suture was placed at the angle of the neck of the bladder using 00 chromic intestinal suture. The bladder was well elevated with good angulation and absence of the urethrocele. The excess vaginal mucosa was excised in a triangular fashion bilaterally. The vaginal mucosa was then reapproximated in the midline with interrupted 000 chromic sutures. The mucosa was resutured to the cervix at the inverted T with interrupted 00 chromic suture.

Posterior repair was performed with an incision at the mucocutaneous portion of the posterior fourchette. The vaginal mucosa was freed from the perirectal fascia in a tunneling fashion thus creating two pillars laterally which were clamped with Kochers. The vaginal mucosa was incised. The pillars were approximated in the midline with figure-of-eight chromic sutures. The excess vaginal mucosa posteriorly was then excised in an angular manner. The vaginal mucosa was approximated with a continuous locked 00 chromic suture. The Levator ani were reapproximated in the midline with interrupted 00 chromic. The perineal bodies were approximated with the same material and the skin was closed with interrupted figure-of-eight 00 chromic suture.

A vaginal pack was introduced into the vagina. A Foley catheter was left in the bladder. The urine was clear and no bleeding was encountered following this procedure.

Hirst Operation for Dyspareunia

Under general Surital anesthesia, the patient was prepared and draped in the usual manner in a lithotomy position. The bladder was catheterized.

Preliminary examination under anesthesia revealed a uterus located in the midline, anteflexed, normal in size and consistency. The adnexal areas were negative. The marital introitus only admitted two fingers with difficulty.

The posterior lateral aspect of the introitus was grasped with Allis forceps and a skin incision made in the midline in the posterior vaginal wall and perineal body. The mucosa was reflected away from the underlying tissue until the levator muscle on each side was identified. These were cut bilaterally. Following this, the apex of the posterior vaginal wall was approximated to the midline of the posterior fourchette and the corresponding edges were approximated with interrupted 0 Gyn. sutures without difficulty.

There was a moderate blood loss. A vaginal pack was placed in the vagina for purposes of hemostasis. Furacin Cream was applied to the vaginal pack.

CERVICAL AND VAGINAL FISTULAS

Fistulas are abnormal communications or openings which develop between two internal organs or cavities or between an internal organ and the external body wall. Some of the most commonly encountered fistulas are those involving the female genital tract. These defects are usually caused by obstetrical injuries, trauma sustained in gynecological operations, or radiation to the genital regions. They usually communicate from the cervix and vagina to the bladder or rectum, structures with which they are intimately associated. Repairs in many instances are problematic, particularly in those cases where the fistula develops after radiation therapy and the tissues are scarred and fibrotic. Recurrences of these defects is not uncommon.

Rectovaginal Fistula

These are low lying fistulas which most often result from an incompletely healed third degree tear during labor. They may also result from trauma or tissue damage sustained during gynecological operations for carcinoma of the cervix or prolapse. Radiation damage to tissues is another cause.

The smaller fistulas may be troublesome only in that they permit the escape of flatus via the vagina. Larger openings may permit the excursion of liquid and even solid feces into the vagina with all of the problems inherent in such a situation. The condition is treated surgically if spontaneous healing of the fistula fails to occur. Healing may occur over a period of from several weeks to two years. When there is a concomitant carcinoma, repair is not undertaken until the carcinoma has healed locally.

Some cases are operated on using a combined abdomino-vaginal surgical approach. These are the highly situated fistulas. A pull-through procedure is also used in some instances.

Uretero-Vaginal Fistula

These are communications which develop between the ureter and vagina. They are likewise caused by radiation necrosis or injury and are described as complete or incomplete. The lower 5 cm. of the ureter is usually involved. Spontaneous healing of these fistulas sometimes results in stenosis of the ureter with resulting back-pressure atrophy of the associated kidney eventuating in a nonfunctioning kidney.

Surgical repair consists of transperitoneal ureterovesical implantation (removal of the defective segment of ureter and reimplantation of the ureter into the urinary bladder). When the fistula exists on both sides, double implantation may not be possible. In such cases a uretero-intestinal-cystoplasty after the technique of Michalowski, Foret, Heusghem, Scheele is performed with side-to-side anastomosis of an isolated ileal loop to the bladder and implantation of the ureters into the loop. A bilateral Boariplasty is used in some cases with reimplantation of the ureter into the bladder using a flap from the anterior wall of the bladder as a substitute for the lower portion of the ureter.

Vagino-Perineal Fistula

These defects consist of an abnormal communication between the vagina and the perineum (bridge of skin and tissue between the vagina and anus). The cause is usually a perineal tear sustained in an obstetrical delivery or colpoperineorrhaphy. When they become symptomatic they are treated by total excision.

Vesicocervical Fistula

This is an abnormal communication between the urinary bladder and the cervix. It is a rare occurrence which sometimes follows low segment cesarean section. Symptoms sometimes include urinary incontinence and menstruation into the bladder. The condition is corrected by surgical repair closing the opening in the bladder.

Operations for repair include the following techniques:

1. Total colpocleisis (surgical closure of vaginal canal)
2. Tissue covering operations such as:
    Doderlein rollflap operation
    Bastiaanse, Chiricuta omentum cover operation
    Ingelman-Sundberg gracilis muscle operation
3. Temporary blocking with artificial prosthesis such as the inflatable catheter (Ehrlich).

Vesicovaginal Fistula

The majority of these defects between the vagina and urinary bladder are postoperative; however, they may also be caused by untreated cervical carcinoma, delivery injuries or radiologic treatment for carcinoma.

Surgical approach may be either suprapubic or vaginal. A combined approach is sometimes used in those cases where the fistula is fixed in scar tissue.

Operations generally used for repair include:

1. Mayo-Fueth inversion operation
2. Simon modification of Marion Sims with extensive scar tissue excision.
3. Latzko's high colpocleisis (obliteration of the vagina)

OPERATIONS ON THE UTERUS

Numerous diagnostic and therapeutic procedures are performed on the uterus for a variety of conditions related to pregnancy, congenital anomalies, mechanical abnormalities, tumors, endometriosis, adenomyosis, etc.

The surgeon's decision relative to the nature and extent of uterine surgery is influenced by a consideration of malignancy in this organ. It is estimated that one per cent of all women die of cancer of the uterus. It is further estimated that one to two per cent of uterine fibroids are associated with endometrial carcinoma (Gruenberger, Kofler, et al.) Although cancer of the body of the uterus (endometrial carcinoma) is less common than cervical cancer among young women, both types occur with about equal frequency in postmenopausal women. The single earliest and most important symptom is usually intermenstrual or postmenopausal vaginal bleeding. Abnormal vaginal bleeding always requires investigation.

Cancer of the endometrium is treated by a combination of pre- and postoperative radiation with total hysterectomy after fractional curettage. When the carcinoma encroaches on the cervix, radiation is used or radical (Wertheim) hysterectomy. Bilateral salpingo-oophorectomy is performed along with the total hysterectomy because of the incidence of metastases to the adnexa. Preoperative radium or cobalt implantation is commonly used to devitalize the tumor. There follows shrinking and sclerosis of the uterus with destruction of the regional lymphatic vessels. Hysterectomy is usually performed between the fourth and sixth week following radiation. The operation is not delayed any longer than this because of the fibrosis which develops in the area making surgery hazardous. Earlier surgery is not performed in order that the results of radiation have time to develop. Patients treated by this method have higher five year cure rates (between 70% and 85%) reports Corscaden.

DILATATION AND CURETTAGE (D & C)

The D & C consists of a scraping of the inside of the uterus for the purpose of removing endometrial tissue for histologic examination. It is also performed following incomplete abortion for removal of the remaining products of conception.

INSTRUMENTS USED FOR D & C:

- Allis tissue forceps
- Auvard weighted speculum
- Backhaus towel clamp
- Bond placenta forceps
- Bozeman uterine dressing forceps
- Braun uterine tenaculum
- Curet (curette)
- Deaver retractor
- Eastman vaginal retractor
- Goodell dilator
- Graves vaginal speculum
- Hegar dilator
- Henrotin vulsellum forceps
- Hurtig dilator
- Jacobs vulsellum forceps
- Kelly placenta forceps
- Ovum forceps
- Schroeder uterine tenaculum
- Sims vaginal speculum
- Sims uterine curet
- Sims uterine probe
- Sims uterine sound
- Skene uterine spoon curet
- Sponge forceps
- Starlinger dilator
- Thomas uterine curet
- Uterine sound
- Vulsellum forceps

Operative Technic (Diagnostic D & C)

The patient was placed in the lithotomy position. The lower abdomen, inner thighs, perineum and vaginal vault were prepared and draped in a sterile manner.

Bimanual examination revealed a parous outlet. The cervix was clear. The uterus was slightly enlarged, anterior, smooth and firm. The adnexa were negative.

The anterior lip of the cervix was grasped with a single tooth tenaculum and drawn downward. The uterine cavity was sounded to a depth of 4 inches. The cervical canal was dilated with Starlinger and Goodell dilators. The uterine cavity was then well curetted with large and small curets. A moderate amount of endometrial tissue was obtained and sent to the pathologist for histologic examination.

HYSTEROPEXY

Mobile uterine retroversion is a common anomaly which generally produces no symptoms and requires no surgery. When indicated, intervention usually consists of replacement of the uterus to a position of anteversion and insertion of a Hodge pessary. Fixed retroversion may be associated with sterility, habitual abortion, dysmenorrhea and menorrhagia.

Operations employed for ventrosuspension of the uterus consist of abdominal shortening of the round ligaments and plication of the sacro-uterine ligaments.

When the anatomic structures supporting the uterus fail, prolapse occurs with the uterus descending through the vagina, everting the vagina in the process. A number of operations are performed for correcting this condition, the titles of which appear below. Vaginal hysterectomy is performed more universally than are the other corrective operations. The vaginal route of repair is the one generally agreed upon.

UTERINE PROLAPSE OPERATIONS

Donald operation
Fothergill
Gilliam suspension
Goodall-Power modification of LeFort
Heaney vaginal hysterectomy

LeFort operation
Manchester
Spalding-Richardson composite operation
Watkins transposition

OPERATIONS FOR SUSPENSION OF THE UTERUS

Abell modification of Gilliam
Alexander-Adams
Baldy-Webster (posterior implantation of round ligaments)
Coffey suspension
Davis's modification of Gilliam-Doleris
Gilliam suspension
Gilliam-Doleris
Interposition operation

Leopold modification
Manchester operation
McCall's modification of Baldy-Webster
McCall-Schumann modification
Olshausen operation
Simpson's modification of Gilliam-Doleris
Subperitoneal Baldy-Webster
Ventrofixation of uterus
Watkins interposition

Hysteropexy — Abell modification of Gilliam

The patient was prepared and draped in the Trendelenburg position. A four inch midline suprapubic incision was made.

Guy sutures of catgut were placed through each round ligament, midway between their origin and exit through the internal abdominal rings. Each suture was held by an artery forceps and not tied.

After the rectus sheath was opened on each side of the midline incision, the Rectus abdominis was separated from the under surface of the anterior rectus sheath. A curved artery forceps with blunt ends was passed under the fascia, above the rectus muscle, through the posterior end of the sheath of the rectus to the outer aspect of the internal ring. After the abdominal wall on the same side was elevated, the inner aspect of the internal ring was elevated by traction on the guy sutures in the round ligament. The artery forceps was introduced through the internal ring, under the peritoneum and on the upper surface of the round ligament, penetrating the peritoneum when well within the limits of the parietal peritoneum. After separation of the blades of the artery forceps, the guy suture in the round ligament was grasped and drawn through the internal ring, into the midline incision. By exerting further traction, the elongated round ligament was doubled on itself, through the internal ring, over the upper surface of the rectus and along the under surface of the fascia to the midline incision.

The round ligament was stretched out in the form of a triangle. It was tacked to the undersurface of the fascia with three catgut sutures with the apex at the cut edge of the fascia, in the midline incision, and the base looking outward toward the outside of the rectus. The procedure was repeated with the round ligament on the opposite side.

The midline incision was closed in tiers. The apex of each round ligament was sewn together with closure of the fascia. No. 1 chromic catgut was used to suture the round ligament. No. 2 chromic catgut was used for the peritoneum and fascia and stay sutures of silkworm gut were used to close the skin.

Modified Gilliam Suspension of the Uterus

The patient is prepared and draped in the supine position. The abdomen is entered with a midline incision. The incision is carried through the anatomic layers of the abdominal wall. The peritoneum is picked up and incised. The peritoneal cavity is entered. Allis clamps are applied to the edges of the rectus fascia and the peritoneum at approximately the level of the anterior superior spine of the ilium. The uterus is raised and its round ligaments identified. A # 1 chromic gut ligature is placed around one of the round ligaments but not tied. This is elevated with a hemostat. The same procedure is carried out on the opposite round ligament and traction applied bringing the uterus up to the abdominal wall. Following this, the rectus muscle on the left is retracted toward the midline and the subcutaneous tissue retracted away from this. A curved Kelly clamp is introduced through the internal inguinal ring to the peritoneum. The clamp is open and the peritoneum extending over the clamp is opened. The clamp is introduced further through this rent in the peritoneum and picks up the traction ligature on the left. The ligature is pulled up through the opening and through the internal inguinal canal bringing the round ligament to the outside of the anterior rectus fascia. This brings the uterus up firmly to the abdominal wall. The round ligament brought up through the opening is sutured to the anterior rectus fascia with three interrupted cotton sutures. The ligature is then removed without damage to the round ligament. The same procedure is carried out on the right side.

The peritoneum is closed with 00 chromic catgut suture, continuous; the fascia with a continuous 0 chromic catgut, and the skin with vertical mattress 000 silk sutures.

HYSTERECTOMY

Removal of the uterus is called **hysterectomy**. It may be total including the uterus and cervix (panhysterectomy) or subtotal, including only the uterus. The latter is called a supracervical hysterectomy since the uterus is amputated above the cervix. Hysterectomy may be performed by either an abdominal or a vaginal route. When the tubes and ovaries are also removed with the uterus and cervix, the operation should be designated as a panhysterectomy with salpingo-oophorectomy. Total hysterectomy is no longer defined as including the tubes and ovaries.

Subtotal hysterectomy is no longer a common procedure because of the high incidence of carcinoma which develops in cervical stumps. The procedure is reserved for those cases where the patient is in poor general condition, or where there is extreme adiposity, dense adhesions or paracervical tumors which make removal of the cervix particularly hazardous.

The principal indications for hysterectomy, other than uterine malignancy, are fibroids and dysfunctional metrorrhagia in the premenopausal patient, removal with the adnexa in cases of chronic adnexitis, adenomyosis, endometriosis, extensive genital tuberculosis and in ovarian malignancy. When pathology indicates removal of both ovaries, the uterus becomes useless and therefore is also removed. On the other hand, ovarian function continues normally after hysterectomy so long as the ovarian blood supply is adequate. For this reason the ovaries are usually spared in women under the age of 50 years when they are normal in appearance and function.

Fibroid tumors are not all treated by hysterectomy. If they are not symptomatic, the surgeon may choose only to observe them through periodic follow-ups. Whenever possible, myomectomy is performed rather than hysterectomy, particularly in women of childbearing age. Where there is rapid growth of the tumor, severe menorrhagia and pressure symptoms, hysterectomy may be indicated. These tumors are most often myomas or leiomyomatas.

The vaginal route for hysterectomy is performed in severe uterine prolapse, particularly where childbearing functions are no longer a consideration. The operation is sometimes approached through this route for small fibroids, adenomyosis or preinvasive carcinoma of the cervix. The vaginal approach permits coincident colporrhaphy or operation for correction of stress incontinence. One problem in young women is that it leaves the patient with a shortened vagina. Abdominal hysterectomy enables the surgeon to explore the peritoneal cavity for additional pathology.

All vaginal hysterectomies are total except for the Spalding-Richardson technique.

TYPES OF HYSTERECTOMY

Abdominal hysterectomy
Doyen's vaginal hysterectomy
Latzko radical abdominal
  hysterectomy
Panhysterectomy (total)
Radical hysterectomy

Ries-Wertheim operation
Spalding-Richardson
Supracervical hysterectomy
Vaginal hysterectomy
Wertheim radical

Vaginal Hysterectomy

The patient was placed in the lithotomy position with legs and hips elevated. The cervical canal was asepticized and the bladder catheterized.

The external uterine opening was closed with silkworm gut sutures which were tied and left long for tractors. Circumcision was carried out on the vaginal mucosa at its junction with the cervix uteri. The anterior vaginal cuff was separated from the bladder by sharp and blunt gauze dissection. This was carried out until the broad ligaments were exposed on both sides. The vesicouterine reflection was identified after the bladder was reflected upward and out of the way.

The peritoneal fold was identified and opened. Both indices were introduced and spread laterally. A warm lap sponge was introduced through the opening and the bowels packed away. The ureters were identified and displaced upwards and out of the way.

The cervix was pulled upwards. The anterior vaginal cuff was dissected away from the uterus up to the peritoneal pouch. The posterior cuff was treated similarly. The broad ligaments were isolated. The uterus was held suspended in the pelvis by the broad, uterosacral, infundibulopelvic and round ligaments.

A curved Mayo needle with a # 2 chromic catgut engaged the lower end of the broad ligament which was ligated, tied and left long to be used temporarily as a traction suture. This portion of the broad ligament was divided close to the uterus. Another segment of tissue above the first ligature was treated similarly. The needle was introduced under the guidance of the finger to suture a large segment of the broad ligament. The broad ligament on the other side was treated in a similar manner. A finger was hooked over the top of the broad ligament on the right. After placing safety sutures, the ligament was severed from the uterus. The same procedure was repeated on the opposite side.

A frequent check was made for thorough hemostasis. Inspection of the pedicles of the ligamentous structures held by the traction sutures disclosed no bleeding. The gauze pack was removed from the anterior cul-de-sac. The divided edge of the bladder peritoneum was isolated.

The sutures of the round ligament on each side were tied to each other. The same was done with the broad ligaments. The vaginal vault was closed with interrupted sutures. The vagina was lightly packed.

Total Abdominal Hysterectomy; Bilateral Oophorectomy; Left Salpingectomy

A right paramedian scar was present and excised. The right tube and the appendix had been removed previously. The anterior fascial sheath was incised in a vertical fashion. The recti muscles were separated. The posterior fascial sheath and peritoneum were picked up and incised vertically.

The pelvic and abdominal viscera were examined. Multiple uterine fibroids were noted. There was also a fibroid of the cervix, lying at the base of the broad ligament, measuring approximately 6 x 10 cm. in diameter. The uterus, the left tube and both ovaries were severely bound down with adhesions. The gallbladder was normal as were the kidneys and bowel. The pelvic adhesions were lysed.

The bowel was pushed back and the pelvic organs were exposed. The round ligaments were picked up with Kocher clamps, incised and ligated with chromic 00 catgut. The bladder reflection was peeled away from the lower uterine segment. The right ovary was picked up and the infundibulopelvic ligament clamped with Buies and the right ovary was removed. The infundibulopelvic ligament was sutured with a chromic 0 catgut suture. The left tube and ovary were then removed by clamping the infundibulopelvic ligament and tying same with chromic 0 catgut sutures. The uterosacral ligaments were then clamped, cut and tied with chromic 0 catgut sutures.

The uterine arteries were doubly clamped and cut using chromic # 1 catgut sutures. A double ligature was placed on each uterine artery. The pericervical vaginal fascia was then circumcised in a circular fashion and the uterus removed in toto. The vaginal mucosa was then sutured together utilizing chromic 0 catgut in a continuous suture.

The perivesical vaginal fascia was sutured together utilizing chromic 00 catgut suture in a continuous manner. The base of the left broad ligament and the left uterosacral ligament as well as the right uterosacral ligament and the base of the right broad ligament were sutured into the angles of the dome of the vagina. Reperitonealization of the pelvis was carried out with 0 intestinal suture. After a correct sponge count, the abdominal peritoneum was closed with a 00 chromic intestinal catgut everting type suture. The posterior fascial layer was then sutured with a continuous chromic 00 intestinal catgut suture. The recti muscles were then approximated with chromic 2 intestinal catgut suture. The anterior fascial layer was sutured together with figure-of-eight chromic 0 catgut sutures. The skin was approximated with 000 silk sutures.

OPERATIONS ON THE CERVIX UTERI

The cervix, situated in the upper vaginal canal at the lower portion of the uterus, is particularly vulnerable to infection (cervicitis), erosion, polyps and carcinoma. These conditions are treated by a variety of techniques which include cervical biopsy, cauterization, coagulation, conization and cervical amputation.

Superficial coagulation or linear electrosurgical cauterization is used in the treatment of severe cervical erosions. The resultant cicatrization (scarring) of the wound produces a narrowing of the external os and a diminution in the amount of cervical discharge. When chronic infection exists and carcinoma has been ruled out, conization (electrosurgical excision) of the cervix is performed. The electrode is rotated 360 degrees in a complete circle to remove a cone of tissue. The patient is observed postoperatively for possible stenosis. Both procedures result in an increased blood stained discharge for several weeks before healing takes place. Diathermy conization is used in preference to superficial cervical amputation; however, when the cervix is grossly hypertrophied it is usually amputated.

Cold conization consists of use of a scalpel for excision of the distal portion of the cervical canal. The chief indication for this operation is a biopsy or smear from the cervix positive for carcinoma in-situ in a premenopausal patient. The operation is performed for curative reasons as well as for purposes of determining the extent of invasion, the latter being determined after serial section study of the removed tissue by a pathologist. Conization is often followed by removal of the uterus.

Cancer of the Cervix

More than two per cent of all women over 20 years of age will develop cancer of the cervix (Gruenberger, Kofler, et al.). This malignancy ranks second in incidence only to cancer of the breast. It is more common in women who have borne children, women who married when young and among women of a low socioeconomic status. The disease is far more common among prostitutes than among celibate women. It also is more common among wives of uncircumcised men than among spouses of circumcised men. It is comparatively rare in virginal women and in Jewish women. Cancer specialists have long theorized that cancer of the cervix might be caused by some agent transmitted venereally. Researchers consisting of a team of virologists and epidemiologists from the Baylor University College of Medicine in Houston have turned up evidence linking cervical cancer with a virus.

Studies have long suggested that something associated with cervical cancer might be in the smegma of the male. Smegma is a thick, cheesy, foul smelling secretion consisting primarily of desquamated epithelial cells found under the prepuce. Proper male hygiene reduces the accumulation of smegma which accumulates in the uncircumcised male. The Baylor researchers have succeeded in isolating a virus from smegma which has been labeled Type 2 herpesvirus. The same team have reported finding a far greater infection with Type 2 herpesvirus in women who have cervical cancer than in persons without this malignancy. The virus is described as being related to the common Type 1 herpesvirus known to cause "cold sores." While Type 1 herpesvirus is found around the mouth, Type 2 is found around the genitals.

There is no conclusive proof that viruses cause cancer in man, although it has been established that several kinds of cancer in various animals are caused by viruses. Researchers strongly suspect that leukemia might be caused by a virus.

Reporting in Science Magazine, the research team represented by W. E. Rawls, W. A. F. Tompkins, M. E. Figueroa and J. L. Melnick published results of a survey screening cervical cancer patients for antibodies against Type 2 herpesvirus. Antibodies are bits of protein the body produces in an attempt to defend itself against a virus. Presence of these antibodies in the blood would indicate that the person had at some time been infected by the herpesvirus. Their testing revealed that 15 of the 18 women or 83 per cent had antibodies against Type 2 herpesvirus. In a control group consisting of 44 women without cervical cancer, only nine, or 20 per cent had Type 2 herpesvirus antibodies. They also observed that only one out of 10 persons suffering with other types of cancer had Type 2 herpesvirus antibodies, and that none of 37 adults and children selected at random had such antibodies. The findings, they said, are compatible with the theory that the Type 2 herpesvirus either causes cervical cancer or plays an important role in its cause.

Investigators currently believe that an area of cancer nonapparent to the naked eye may exist in the cervix for as long as five to 10 years before invasive carcinoma develops. This is called carcinoma in-situ or Stage 0 carcinoma. The condition may be detected by Papanicolaou smear of cells wiped from the cervix. The condition is completely curable. Pelvic examinations with Pap smears should be performed at least yearly on all women over the age of 20 years.

The Cancer Committee of the League of Nations in 1929 developed a classification system dividing carcinomas of the cervix into Stages I to IV based on manifestations of the disease. The pathologist in reporting cervical malignancy usually specifies the stage, an important factor in prognosis. The stages are as follows:

STAGE I—carcinoma of the cervix shows the growth confined strictly to the cervix.

STAGE II—the growth has spread to the upper portion of the vagina or parametrium, but not to the pelvic wall.

STAGE III—the growth has spread to the pelvic wall or the lower third of the vagina.

STAGE IV—the lesion has invaded the bladder or rectum, or has metastasized beyond the pelvis.

Carcinoma of the cervix usually progresses beyond stage I before symptoms of intermenstrual, postmenopausal or postcoital bleeding develop. Hope of cure lies in early detection by Pap smear.

Treatment of carcinoma in-situ varies with surgeons. Some treat the condition by simple conization while others prefer simple amputations of the cervix or radical hysterectomy with pelvic lymphadenectomy. Invasive carcinoma is most frequently treated by external irradiation with supervoltage X-ray and by implantation of radium, iridium or cobalt within the cervical cavity. Surgery is generally confined to Stage O and some Stage I cases although a select few with advanced disease and some patients with recurrence after irradiation therapy are also treated surgically. The operation includes total hysterectomy with bilateral salpingo-oophorectomy and excision of the pelvic lymph nodes. When the urinary bladder and rectum are involved, removal of the bladder and/or rectum with implantation of the ureters into an isolated segment of small intestine or colon is performed. Urine thereafter passes from an opening (stoma) in the abdominal wall into a bag glued about the opening. When the ureters are implanted into the ileum the operation is called a ureteroileostomy. When the operation assumes the radical proportions of en masse excision of the urinary bladder, lower ureters, vagina, uterus, tubes, pelvic and lower sigmoid colon, pelvic lymph nodes and all pelvic peritoneum it is called a total pelvic exenteration.

The cure rate for cancer of the cervix in Stage I lesions is about 70 per cent. Among all women with cancer of the cervix, the cure rate is about 50 per cent.

OPERATIONS FOR CERVICAL INCOMPETENCE

Operations to correct incompetence of the cervix have received popular acceptance in recent years. The most commonly performed of these operations include the "cerclage" (Shirodkar's operation) and the isthmorrhaphy (Lash's operation).

Insufficiency of the internal cervical os is a common cause of late spontaneous abortion. This condition is sometimes congenital, being associated with a malformed uterus. More frequently, it is caused by previous obstetrical trauma or forcible overdilation of the cervix preliminary to curettage. Women in whom this condition prevails become habitual aborters. The cervix, rather than closing in pregnancy, continues to gap permitting protrusion of the amniotic sac which finally ruptures. Such circumstances eventuate in abortion.

The Lash operation is another procedure designed to correct the incompetent cervix. The operation consists of plication (pleating) of the internal os in the nonpregnant uterus. Cerclage is the operation generally employed for cervical incompetency during pregnancy. It is usually performed between the 14th and 16th week of gestation. The operation is also used on the nonpregnant uterus. Another technique used is the McDonald operation.

Shirodkar Operation for Incompetent Cervix

An injection of adrenalin and saline was performed under the bladder, at the sides of the cervix and posteriorly, where the incision was made. The incision was made in front of the cervix. The area above the external os was exposed by dissecting the anterior vaginal wall and bladder away from the cervix. A fold of posterior vaginal wall was raised with an Allis forceps and a vertical incision made in the fold. Curved artery forceps were used to stretch the incision.

A right Shirodkar isthmorrhaphy needle was directed in and under the right pillar of the bladder adhering to the cervix. It was introduced under the mucosa and backward toward the posterior incision. Linen thread holding one end of a Mersilene tape was placed on a Mayo needle and was threaded through the eye of the Shirodkar needle on a handle. The right limb of the Mersilene tape was then drawn forward.

A left Shirodkar needle was used to take up the other end of the Mersilene tape. The two ends of the tape were then tied into a reef knot and the knot transfixed with a fine linen suture. The redundant ends on either side were sutured to the circular part of the tape to prevent slipping. The vaginal mucosa was then closed with interrupted 00 chromic. Blood loss was minimal.

Lash Operation for Incompetent Cervix

The patient was prepared and draped in the lithotomy position. A semicircular incision of 3 cm. was made above the external os. A vaginal mucosal flap was elevated and the urinary bladder retracted from the cervix. A stay suture was introduced above the upper border of the defect, the defect excised and the cervical canal opened.

A Hegar dilator was introduced through the cervical canal to the uterine cavity. Four interrupted # 1 surgical gut sutures were taken through the inner half of the cervical wall, avoiding the endocervix. Interrupted sutures were then placed in the outer half of the cervical wall. The anterior portions of the cardinal ligaments were then approximated and sutured in the midline to the cervical wall. The vaginal flap was closed. No blood replacement was necessary.

Insertion of Radium into the Cervix Uteri

The anterior lip of the cervix is grasped with a tenaculum and drawn downward. The cervical canal is dilated with Hegar dilators up to # 10. Using an Ernst applicator, a tandem containing radium is inserted into the uterine cavity and cervical canal. The cervical canal is firmly packed with ½ inch gauze and the vagina packed with a 1 inch gauze. The cord extending from the tandem is attached to the inner thigh with adhesive. Paracervical irradiation is obtained by means of a colpostat comprised of three corks containing radium tubes. One cork is placed in the right vaginal vault and another in the left vaginal vault. The third cork is placed midway between the other two. The two lateral corks are connected by a rubber covered spring.

A 2 inch gauze packing is placed between the rectum and the colpostat, into the vaginal fornices and between the bladder and the anterior lip of the cervix.

A total of 4,000 roentgen gammas is delivered by intracervical tandem and 4,000 more by colpostat.

Electrocoagulation of the Cervix

With the patient in lithotomy position, the perineum was prepared and draped. I.V. Sodium Pentothal was used for anesthesia.

With the tip of the coning instrument placed against the cervical external os, the combined cutting and coagulating current was used. As the wire cut into the cervix the instrument was twisted to enucleate a cone of tissue. Crucial incisions were made with coagulation at the 12, 9, 6 and 3 o'clock points.

Operations for Control of Pain

Operations for control of pain in gynecological disorders such as endometriosis, intractable dysmenorrhea and inoperable carcinoma consist of presacral neurectomy (Cottle), extended presacral neurectomy, ovarian denervation, alcohol injection of the pelvic plexus, intraspinal alcohol injection or resection of the uterosacral ligaments.

THE TUBES AND OVARIES

The fallopian tubes and ovaries are referred to collectively as the **adnexa**. Removal of the tubes is called **salpingectomy,** removal of the ovaries is called **oophorectomy** and removal of both tubes and ovaries is known as **salpingo-oophorectomy** (bilateral or unilateral).

Tumors of the ovary represent the most important pathology of this organ. These lesions represent a threat of torsion of the ovary and in older women, of malignant change. Benign tumors and cysts are sometimes only enucleated (shelled out) in younger women. In malignant ovarian tumors, total hysterectomy with bilateral salpingo-oophorectomy is performed. When unilateral excision of an ovary discloses the lesion to be malignant, the patient is irradiated and this is followed by removal of the other ovary, tube and the uterus. Cancer of the ovary is not usually discovered until late in the disease when ascites or intra-abdominal symptoms develop. Symptoms include weight loss, abdominal enlargement, difficulty in breathing due to the pressure of the ascites, occasional vaginal bleeding, constipation, urinary frequency due to pressure on the urinary bladder, and abdominal pain. Metastases are usually to the liver. Over-all five year survival rate of patients with ovarian carcinoma is about 25 per cent.

Salpingo-oophorectomy is also carried out for chronic inflammation of the adnexa. Wedge resection of the ovaries is performed for polycystic ovaries (Stein-Leventhal syndrome). Many benign lesions such as follicle cysts, corpus luteum cysts, cystomas and dermoids can simply be enucleated.

Prolapse of one or both ovaries in the pouch of Douglas often is associated with uterine retroversion. This condition is treated by repositioning and suspension of the uterus followed by replacement of the ovaries in their normal anatomical position and suturing them to the adjacent peritoneum of the lateral pelvic wall or to the uterine fundus.

The main indications for salpingectomy (excision of fallopian tubes) are tubal pregnancy, chronic inflammation in conditions such as pyosalpinx or hydrosalpinx and tuberculous salpingitis.

Ligation or transection of the tubes is performed bilaterally in sterilization operations on the female.

Tubal insufflation and hysterosalpingography are procedures performed on the tubes for evaluation of their patency. They represent an important segment of the sterility work-up. Insufflation with carbon dioxide (Rubin test) provides information relative to pressure differences within the tubes. These results are registered on a manometer or on a written record. Hysterosalpingography is a complimentary examination which provides a pictorial report of tubal patency, condition of the cervical canal, competence of the internal os, tone of the uterus and location of any tubal obstruction.

Ectopic pregnancies are most often seen in the tubes. They are generally treated by salpingectomy in order to avoid the hazard of tubal rupture and hemorrhage. Ruptured tubal pregnancy is a condition easily mistaken for other gynecologic conditions, particularly P.I.D. (pelvic inflammatory disease). In making a differential diagnosis, the surgeon looks for Cullen's sign, a blue discoloration of the periumbilical skin which results from intraperitoneal hemorrhage. Unfortunately, the sign is not always present and deaths due to this condition are high. National statistics for 1959 showed that of 1588 maternal deaths, 128 were due to ectopic pregnancy, a ratio of 1:12.

At the time of salpingectomy for tubal ectopic pregnancy the ovary is preserved whenever possible. Both tubes are examined for although it is a rare occurrence, double tubal gestations have been found. Twin pregnancies have been found in a single tube. Ectopic pregnancies may also be peritoneal, ovarian, ampullary (near fimbriated end of tube), or interstitial (at the point where the tube joins the uterus). Ovarian pregnancy is rarer than tubal pregnancy. Treatment consists of partial or total oophorectomy or salpingo-oophorectomy.

Prophylactic bilateral oophorectomy is performed in some breast cancer cases to suppress estrogen production and provide palliative relief of symptoms.

DISEASES OF THE FEMALE GENITALIA
(Excluding obstetrical conditions)

Amenorrhea
BARTHOLIN'S GLAND
  abscess
  adenitis
  cyst
  retention cyst
Canal of Nuck, patent
CERVIX
  abscess
  absence
    complete
    partial
  adhesions
    cervicovaginal
    annular detachment
  atresia
  atrophy
  calcification
  cicatrix
  cyst
  diverticulum
  division of external os
  embryonal cyst
  epidermoid carcinoma
    in situ
  erosion
  eversion
  hemorrhage
  hypertrophy
  hypoplasia
  laceration
  leukoplakia
  mucous polyp
  nabothian cyst
  oxyuriasis
  persistence of fetal form
  polyp
  prolapse of hypertrophied
  pseudoerosion, congenital
  sarcoma
  stenosis
  stricture
  syphilis of

CERVIX (continued)
  Trichomonas infection
  tuberculosis of
CLITORIS
  absence
  adhesions
  bifid
  concretion in
  epidermoid carcinoma
  hypertrophy
Colpitis, adhesive
Cystocele
Dysfunctional uterine bleeding
Dysmenorrhea
Dyspareunia
Endometrial carcinoma
Endometrial dysfunction
Endometrial hyperplasia
Endometriosis of
  broad ligament
  fallopian tube
  ovary
  rectovaginal septum
  uterus
Epoophoron cyst

FALLOPIAN TUBES
  absence of one tube
  absence of both tubes
  adenocarcinoma
  atresia
  cyst
  duplication of tubes
  ectopic tubal pregnancy
    with rupture
  endometriosis
  fistula
  hydatid of Morgagni
  mesothelioma
  occlusion of
  polyp
  pregnancy, ectopic
  stricture
  supernumerary

DISEASES OF THE FEMALE GENITALIA (continued)

triplication of ostiums
tuberculosis of
volvulus
Fetal oophoritis
Fibromyoma of broad ligament
Hematocolpos
Hematometra
Hematosalpinx
Hernia of cul-de-sac of Douglas
Hydatid of Morgagni
Hydrocele of Canal of Nuck
Hydrocele of round ligament
Hydrosalpinx

HYMEN
absence
atresia
circular
cribriform
cyst of
displacement upward
division of
embryonal cyst
falciform
fenestrate
hypertrophy
labiate
punctiform fimbriate
septate
supernumerary
thickened
Hyperplasia of endometrium
Hypertrophy of clitoris
Hypertrophy of hymen

LABIA MAJORA
absence of
adhesion
hypertrophy

LABIA MINORA
absence of
adhesion
division into three folds
division into four folds
elongation
Leiomyoma of broad ligament

Leiomyoma of parametrium
Leiomyoma of round ligament
Leiomyoma of sacrouterine ligament
Leiomyomata uteri
Menometrorrhagia
Menorrhagia
Metrorrhagia
Mittelschmerz
Myometrial hyperplasia
Nabothian cyst
Obliteration of endometrium
Oophoritis

OVARY
absence of
abscess
accessory
adhesions
arrhenoblastoma
Brenner tumor
cyst
corpus albicans
corpus luteum
of graafian follicle
cystadenocarcinoma
cystadenoma
disgerminoma
displacement of
fibroma
granulosa cell tumor
hematoma
hemorrhage
hernia
into Canal of Nuck
into inguinal canal
into labium majus
hypertrophy
hypofunction
hypoplasia
Krukenberg tumor
mesonephroma
necrosis
pregnancy of (ectopic)
pseudomucinous cystadenoma
pseudomucinous cystadeno-
carcinoma
senile involution

DISEASES OF THE FEMALE GENITALIA (continued)

serous papillary cystadeno-
  carcinoma
serous papillary cystadenoma
strangulation
supernumerary
syphilis of
teratoma
thecoma
torsion of pedicle
tuberculosis of
Ovotestis
Parametritis
Paraoophoron
Parauterine adhesions
Paravaginal abscess
Paravaginitis
Perioophoritis
Perisalpingitis
Premenstrual tension
Primary amenorrhea
Primary dysmenorrhea
Primary menorrhagia
Primary metrorrhagia
Proliferative endometrium
Pruritis vulvae, neurogenic
Pyocolpos
Pyometria
Pyosalpinx
  with rupture
Rectocele
Rectolabial fistula
Rectovaginal fistula
Relaxation of pelvic floor
Relaxation of perineum
Salpingitis
  acute
  chronic
  gonococcic
  nodular
Tear of rectovaginal septum
Torsion of ovarian pedicle

TUBES (See: Fallopian tubes)
Tubo-ovarian abscess
Two uteri
Ulcus vulvae acutum
Uterorectal fistula

UTERUS
  absence of with absence
    of adnexa
  adenocarcinoma
  adenomyosis
  anteflexion
  arcuatus
  atresia
  bicornis
  biforis
  carcinosarcoma
  didelphys
  displacement
  double uterus
  embryonal cyst
  endometriosis
  fetalis
  fistula
  hypoplasia
  instrumentation wound of
  lateral flexion
  lateral version
  laterocession
  leiomyoma (pl. leiomyomata)
    (leiomyomata uteri)
  leiomyosarcoma
  membranacea
  mucous polyp
  myoma
  perforation
  prolapse
  puncture
  retrocession
  retrodisplacement
  retroflexion
  retroversion
  rudimentary
  senile atrophy
  septus
  stricture of
  subseptus
  supra simplex
  syphilis of
  tuberculosis of
  unicollis
  unicornis

DISEASES OF THE FEMALE GENITALIA (continued)

    unicorporeus
    uniforis

VAGINA
  abscess
  absence
  atresia
  chemical burn
  double vagina
  embryonal cyst
  epidermoid carcinoma
  fibroma
  foreign body in
  inclusion cyst
  kraurosis
  lymphogranuloma venerum
  melanoma, malignant
  mesenchymal mixed tumor
  necrosis
  oxyuriasis
  prolapse
  rudimentary
  senile atresia
  senile atrophy
  septum of
  stenosis
  stricture
  Trichomonas infection
  tuberculosis of

Vaginismus

Vaginitis
  circumscribed
  emphysematous
  exfoliative
  gonococcic
  senile

Vaginocutaneous fistula
Varicosities of broad ligament
Varicosities of pampiniform plexus
Vesicovaginal fistula

VULVA
  abscess
  absence
  adenocarcinoma
  adenoma
  atresia
  basal cell carcinoma
  cellulitis
  chancroid
  condyloma acuminatum
  cyst of
  diphtheria
  elephantiasis
  embryonal cyst
  epidermoid carcinoma
  fibroma
  gangrene
  hemangioma
  hematoma, nonpuerperal
  hemorrhage
  herpes
  infantile
  kraurosis
  leiomyoma
  leukoplakia
  lipoma
  melanoma, malignant
  pediculosis
  pigmented nevus
  polyp
  sarcoma
  scabies
  sebaceous cyst
  senile atrophy
  sweat gland tumor
  syphilis of
  thrush
  tuberculosis of
  ulcer
  varix
  vitiligo

Vulvitis
  acute
  adhesive
  chronic
  diabetic
  gonococcic
  intertriginous

Vulvorectal fistula
Vulvovaginitis

OPERATIONS ON THE FEMALE GENITALIA
(Excluding pregnancy)

Amputation of the cervix
Amputation of the clitoris
A & P colporrhaphy (anterior and
  posterior repair of cystocele and
  rectocele)
Biopsy of cervix
Biopsy of vagina
Cauterization of cervix
Cervicectomy
Clitoridectomy
Clitoridotomy
Closure of rectovaginal fistula
Closure of ureterovaginal fistula
Closure of vesicovaginal fistula
Colpectomy
  complete
  partial
Colpocleisis
Colpoperineoplasty
Colpoperineorrhaphy
Colpopexy
Colpoplasty
Colporrhaphy
Colpotomy
Conization of cervix
Cystocele repair (ant. vag. wall)
Dilation of cervix
D & C (dilation and curettage)
  diagnostic
  therapeutic
Drainage of ovarian abscess
Drainage of ovarian cyst
Episioperineoplasty
Episioperineorrhaphy
Episioplasty
Episiorrhaphy
Episiotomy
Excision of labia majora
Excision of labia minora
Excision of lesion of cervix
Fundectomy of uterus
Hymenotomy
Hysterectomy
  supracervical
  total (pan hysterectomy)
Hysterolysis
Hysteromyomectomy
Hysterorrhaphy
Hysterosalpingostomy
Hysterotomy
Hysterotrachelotomy
Insertion of vaginal pack
Incision and drainage of
  Bartholin's glands
Incision and drainage of
  Skene's glands
Incision and drainage of vulva
Insufflation of uterus
Interposition operation
Ligation of fallopian tubes
Myomectomy
Oophorectomy
  partial
  bilateral complete
Oophoropexy
Oophoroplasty
Panhysterectomy
Perineoplasty
Perineorrhaphy
Perineotomy
Radical hysterectomy
Rectocele repair (post. vag. wall)
Salpingectomy
  complete
  partial
Salpingo-oophorectomy
  bilateral
  unilateral
Salpingoplasty
Salpingostomy
Shortening of endopelvic fascia
Shortening of round ligaments
Shortening of sacrouterine
  ligaments

OPERATIONS ON THE FEMALE GENITALIA (continued)

Supracervical hysterectomy
Suspension of the uterus
Trachelectomy
Tracheloplasty
Trachelorrhaphy
Trachelotomy
Tubal ligation
Uterocentesis
Vaginal hysterectomy

Vaginotomy
Ventrofixation of uterus
Ventrosuspension of uterus
Vulvectomy
  complete
  partial
  radical
Wertheim's operation

EPONYMIC TITLES OF GYNECOLOGIC OPERATIONS

Abell modification of the Gilliam uterine suspension
Aldridge temporary sterilization
Alexander-Adams uterine suspension
Baldy-Webster uterine suspension
Ball technic for omentectomy
Basset radical vulvectomy
Coffey uterine suspension
Donald operation for uterine prolapse
Donald-Fothergill operation for uterine prolapse
Doyen vaginal hysterectomy
Falk technic for vesicovaginal fistula
Fleming instrument conization of cervix
Fothergill operation for uterine prolapse
Frangenheim-Goebell-Stoeckel operation for urinary incontinence
Freund operation for uterine prolapse; cystocele
Fritsch modification of Freund operation
Gilliam uterine suspension
Giordano operation for urinary incontinence
Goodall-Power modification of LeFort operation
Grant-Ward operation for vaginal prolapse
Green-Armytage pursestring cervical closure
Heaney technic for vaginal hysterectomy
Hirst operation for dyspareunia
Irving sterilization
Kelly operation for urinary stress incontinence
Kennedy operation for urinary stress incontinence
Lash operation for incompetent cervix
Latzko repair of the bladder
LeFort colpocleisis
Leopold uterine suspension

EPONYMIC TITLES OF GYNECOLOGIC OPERATIONS (Continued)

Madlener technic for sterilization
Manchester operation for uterine prolapse
Marshall-Marchetti-Krantz operation for urinary stress incontinence
McIndoe reconstruction of the vagina
Moschowitz enterocele repair
Munnell bilateral oophorectomy
Olshausen uterine suspension
Peterson insufflation of tubes
Pomeroy sterilization operation
Poro cesarean section
Radium application technics, intrauterine and intravaginal
    Ernst applicator method
    Manchester ovoid method
    Stockholm box method
Ries-Wertheim hysterectomy
Rizzoli operation for congenital rectovaginal fistula
Rubin tubal insufflation
Schauffler removal of bartholin cyst
Schauta radical vaginal hysterectomy
Schuchardt incision in carcinoma of the cervix
Shirodkar operation for incompetent cervix
Spalding-Richardson composite operation
Spinelli operation for inversion of the uterus

Stockholm radium application
Strassman-Jones operation for double uterus
Sturmdorf amputation of the cervix
Sturmdorf trachelorrhaphy
Taussig-Morton node dissection
TeLinde operation for vaginal prolapse
Twombly operation for vulvar carcinoma
Twombly-Ulfelder operation for carcinoma of the cervix
Waters cesarean section
Watkins interposition uterine suspension
Watkins-Wertheim operation for uterine prolapse
Wertheim radical hysterectomy and node dissection
Wharton technic for construction of an artificial vagina
Whitacre sterilization operation
Williams vaginal occlusion
Williams-Richardson operation for vaginal prolapse

9 } *Neurosurgery*

Neurosurgery, the specialty dealing with surgical lesions of the nervous system, might well be considered one of the most modern surgical specialties. Although archaeologic evidence has been uncovered to indicate the earliest efforts of man to operate on the brain, it was not until the beginning of this century that modern neurosurgery had its inception. In the half century which has followed, the scope of this specialty has been magnified many times and its store of knowledge enlarged to an extent which could not have been anticipated by its most enthusiastic forefathers.

Neurosurgery is no longer limited to the removal of brain tumors, treatment of brain and spinal cord injuries and alleviation of pain. Procedures are being performed today which thirty years ago would have been regarded as daringly experimental. Modern anesthesia, new drugs and modern supportive treatment based on advances in our knowledge of morphology, physiology, ultrabiophysics and biochemistry have made possible these more radical operations. Radioactive isotopes, electroencephalography, electrocorticography, depth recordings, bioelectric potentials and new radiographic methods have facilitated earlier detection and localization of neurosurgical lesions.

The fund of scientific knowledge relating to this specialty is being swelled by contributions from bioscientists and neurosurgeons all over the world, each lending his genius to unraveling the mysteries of this all important organ, the brain.

The complexity of the brain and its associated structures can be better appreciated if we consider the brain proper and the spinal cord separately. No attempt will be made to elaborate further on the nerves which have been discussed in Chapter 6.

ANATOMY OF THE BRAIN

The brain can be divided grossly into three parts: the forebrain, the midbrain and the hindbrain. Each of these sections is subdivided into major subdivisions as must be the case with an organ as complex morphologically and physiologically as the brain. No attempt can be made to review the anatomy of this system other than superficially in the confines of this chapter; however, salient features of the brain and its major divisions are listed to provide the secretary with an anatomic reference.

The forebrain comprises the largest portion of the brain. It consists of the diencephalon and the cerebrum. A longitudinal fissure divides the cerebrum into halves called *cerebral hemispheres.* Each of these hemispheres are further divided into lobes: *the insula* (island of Reil), *limbic, occipital, temporal, parietal,* and *frontal.* The outer surface (cortex) of the cerebrum consists of numerous convolutions or folds (gyri) separated by fissures or sulci.

The midbrain is a short section which connects the forebrain with the pons and cerebellum. It is situated just below the inferior aspect of the cerebrum.

The hindbrain consists of the pons, cerebellum and the medulla oblongata. The cerebellum is the second largest section of the brain. It is located just beneath the posterior aspect of the occipital lobe of the cerebrum, in the back of the skull. The medulla oblongata is a 3 cm. segment of brain connecting with the spinal cord below and with the pons above. The pons situated just above the medulla serves as a connection for the neural pathways between the cerebellum and the cerebral cortex.

The anatomy of the brain is more complex than that of any organ in the body. No attempt will be made to list all of its features; however, the structures which might be identified in a surgeon's report have been included in the following list.

SALIENT FEATURES OF THE BRAIN AND ITS INVESTING TISSUE

Accessory cuneate nucleus
Accessory nerves
Ala cinerea
Anterior central gyrus
Anterior cerebrospinal fasciculus
Anterior external arcuate fibers
Anterior median fissure
Anterior medullary velum
Anterolateral sulcus
Aqueduct of Sylvius
Arachnoid mater
Arachnoid space
Arbor vitae
Area acoustica
Area postrema
Calcarine fissure
Cerebellum
Cerebral aqueduct
Cerebral hemisphere
Cerebral peduncle
Cerebrum
Choroid plexus
Cingulate sulcus
Clava
Colliculus facialis
Corpora quadrigemina
Corpus callosum
Corpus cerebelli
Cortex
Corticopontile fibers
Corticospinal tract
Crura
Crusta
Cuneate tubercle
Deep transverse fibers
Dentate fascia
Diencephalon
Dorsal fasciculus of Schütz
Dorsospinocerebellar fasciculus
Dura mater
Epithalamus
Falx cerebri
Fasciculus cuneatus
Fasciculus gracilis
Fibrae propriae
Fissure prima

Fissure of Sylvius
Flocculonodular lobe
Foramen cecum
Formatio reticularis
Fornix
Fourth ventricle
Frenulum veli
Frontal lobe
Frontopontile fibers
Funiculus separans
Furrow
Fusiform gyrus
Geniculate body
Genu
Glia
Gyrus (gyri)
Gyrus of Broca
Hippocampal gyrus
Hook bundle of Risien Russell
Hypoglossal nucleus
Hypothalamic area
Hypothalamus
Incisura temporalis
Inferior cerebellar peduncle
Inferior fovea
Inferior frontal gyrus
Insula lobe (island of Reil)
Interpeduncular fossa
Interpeduncular ganglion
Interventricular foramen
Intraparietal sulcus of Turner
Lateral aperture
Lateral cerebral fissure
Lateral ventricle
Lateral cerebrospinal fasciculus
Lateral hemispheres
Lateral sulcus
Limbic lobe
Lingula
Lobus simplex
Locus caeruleus
Longitudinal cerebral fissure
Mammillary bodies
Marginal gyrus
Medial aperture
Medial eminence

SALIENT FEATURES OF THE BRAIN AND ITS INVESTING TISSUES (Continued)

Medial frontal sulcus of Eberstaller
Medial lemniscus
Medial lobule
Medial longitudinal fasciculus
Median sulcus
Medulla oblongata
Medulla spinalis
Metathalamus
Middle cerebral peduncle
Middle frontal gyrus
Nucleus ambiguus
Nucleus arcuatus
Nucleus cuneatus
Nucleus gracilis
Nucleus lacrimalis
Nucleus of Schwalbe
Nucleus salivatorius
Occipital lobe
Oculomotor sulcus
Olive
Opercula of the insula
Orbital operculum
Paramedial sulcus
Parietal lobe
Parieto-occipital fissure
Pars optica
Pia mater
Pineal body
Pons
Posterior commissure
Posterior median fissure
Posteromedian lobule
Primary fissure
Pyramid
Pyramidal decussation
Raphe
Recess
Recessus infundibuli
Recessus suprapinealis
Restiform bodies
Rhomboid fossa
Rubrospinal tract
Septum pellucidum
Splenium
Striae medullaris
Subdural space
Substantia ferruginea
Substantia nigra
Subthalamus
Sulcus basilaris
Sulcus circularis
Sulcus limitans
Sulcus lunatus
Superficial transverse fibers
Superior fovea
Superior frontal gyrus
Taenia pontis
Tectospinal tract
Tegmental part of pons
Tegmentum
Tela choroidea
Telencephalon
Temporal lobe
Thalamus
Transverse occipital sulcus
Trigonum hypoglossi
Tuber cinereum
Tubercle of Rolando
Tuberculum acusticum
Uncinate fasciculus
Ventral spinocerebellar tract
Ventral spinothalamic fasciculus
Ventricle
Ventriculus quartus
Vermis
Zona compacta
Zona reticulata

ARTERIES OF THE BRAIN

Anterior cerebral
Anterior choroidal
Anterior communicating
Arterial circle of Willis
Basilar
Lateral striate arteries
Middle cerebral
Posterior cerebral
Posterior communicating

Anatomy of the Brain

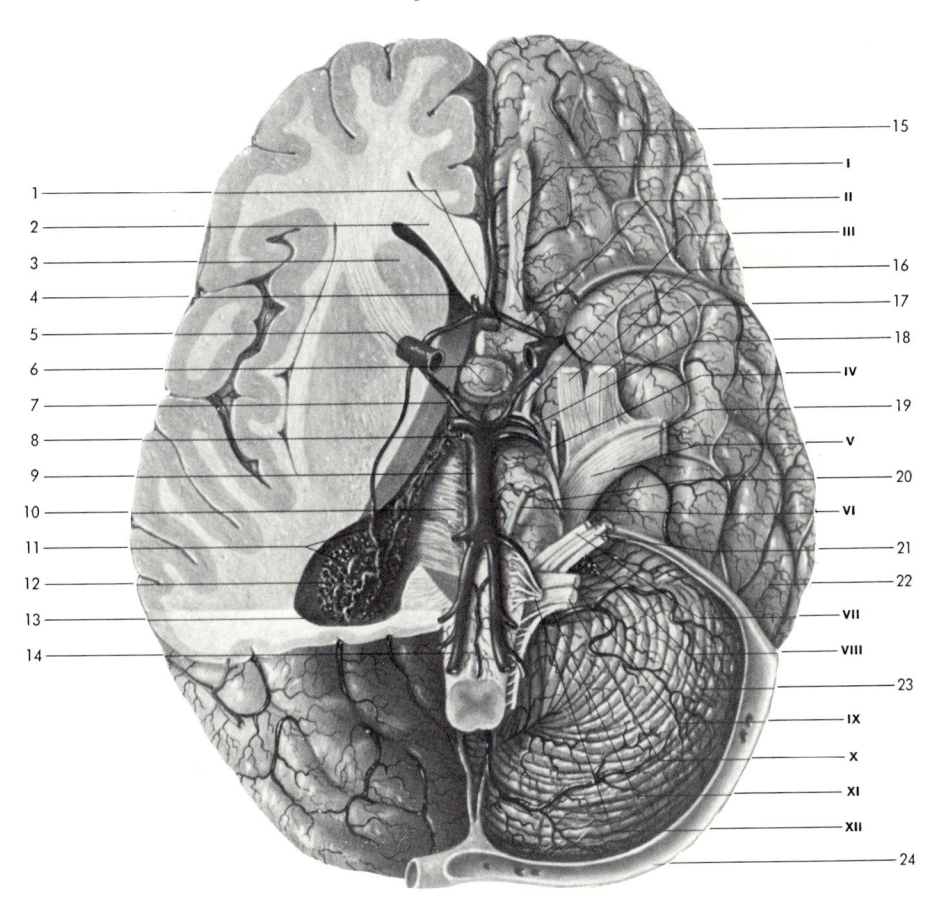

1 Anterior cerebral artery
2 Trunk of corpus callosum
3 Head of caudate nucleus
4 Anterior communicating artery
5 Middle cerebral artery
6 Hypophysis
7 Posterior communicating artery
8 Superior cerebellar artery
9 Basilar artery
10 Internal cerebral vein
11 Choroid artery and vein
12 Choroid plexus of lateral ventricle
13 Inferior cornu of lateral ventricle
14 Vertebral artery
15 Frontal lobe
16 Ophthalmic nerve
17 Maxillary nerve
18 Posterior cerebral artery
19 Mandibular nerve
20 Pons
21 Intermediate nerve
22 Temporal lobe
23 Cerebellum
24 Left transverse sinus

CRANIAL NERVES

I. Olfactory nerve
II. Optic nerve
III. Oculomotor nerve
IV. Trochlear nerve
V. Trigeminal nerve
VI. Abducens nerve
VII. Facial nerve
VIII. Acoustic nerve
IX. Glossopharyngeal nerve
X. Vagus nerve
XI. Accessory nerve
XII. Hypoglossal nerve

Figure 53 Anatomy of the brain
Courtesy Lederle Laboratories

The Ventricles of the Brain

SUPERIOR VIEW

- Superior sagittal sinus
- Frontal lobe
- Anterior cornu of lateral ventricle
- Corpus callosum
- Body of lateral ventricle
- Inferior cornu of lateral ventricle
- Thalamus
- Choroid plexus of lateral ventricle
- Terminal stria
- Choroid glomus
- Fornix (reflected)
- Posterior cornu of lateral ventricle
- Occipital lobe
- Transverse sinus

- Bodies of lateral ventricles
- Suprapineal recess
- Choroid plexus of third ventricle
- Perforation for massa intermedia
- Interventricular foramen
- Anterior cornua of lateral ventricles
- Third ventricle
- Aqueduct of Sylvius
- Optic recess
- Inferior cornu of lateral ventricle
- Posterior cornua of lateral ventricles
- Fourth ventricle

LATERAL VIEW

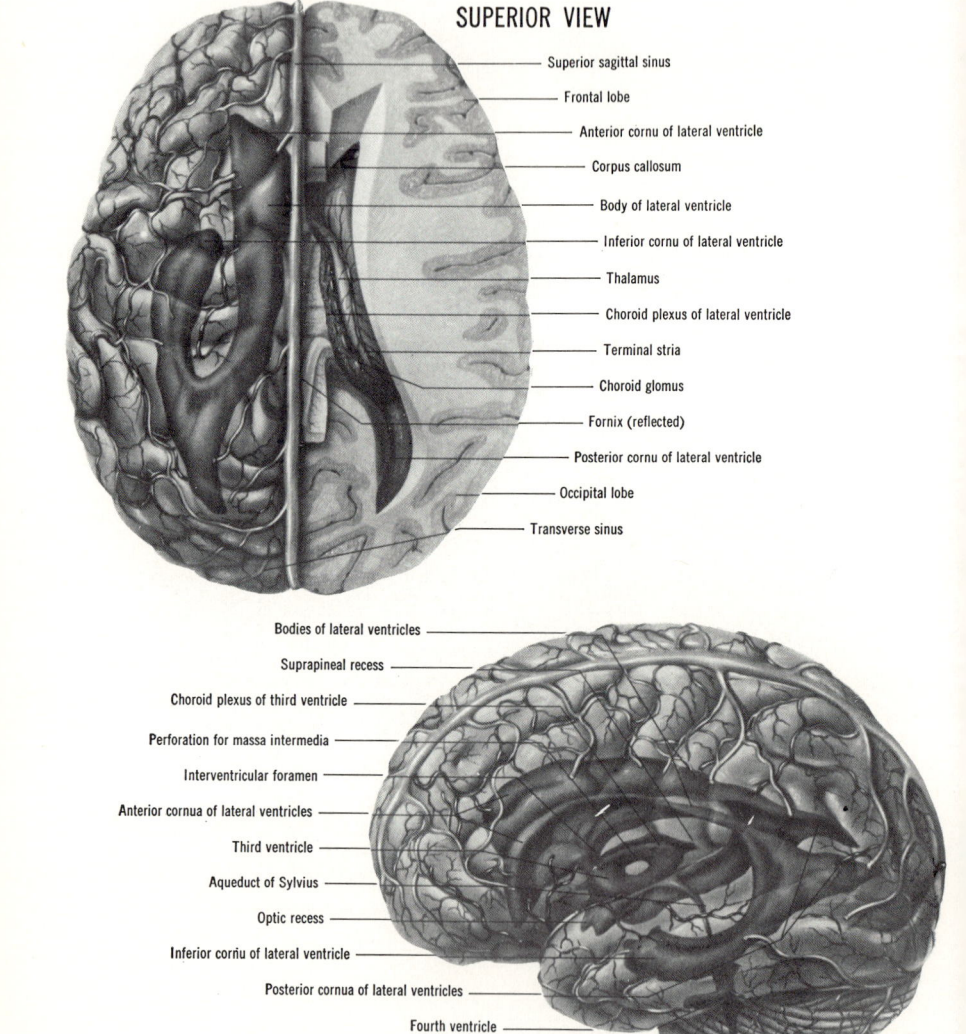

Figure 54   The ventricles of the brain
Courtesy Lederle Laboratories

CRANIOTOMY

Unlike most surgeons, the neurosurgeon operating on the brain cannot reach his operative site by simply deepening his skin incision. He has the bony protective incasement of the brain confronting him before he can gain access to the cranial cavity and the brain. Limited access to his objective makes it necessary that he accurately localize the lesion through preliminary diagnostic examinations. Sometimes it is possible for him to operate through one or more bur holes; however, when a more extensive lesion is involved, it may be necessary to turn down a skull flap.

The operation in which a hole is cut in the skull is called a *trephination* or *craniotomy*. It is performed with an instrument resembling a corkscrew (trephine) which has a short nail-like tip above which is situated a threaded cutting disk. In this procedure an opening is made through which the surgeon may operate. These openings range in size from about 5/8ths of an inch to 1½ inches in diameter and are enlarged, as necessary, with a rongeur. Such openings are adequate for the introduction of needles, exploring cannulas and the removal of subdural hematomas.

When a portion of the skull must be removed and cannot be replaced, the operation is called a *craniectomy*. When such a procedure is extensive as in certain skull fractures, the defect in the cranium is corrected by insertion of a vitallium skull plate such as the Hoen skull plate. Plastic materials, usually acrylics, are also used to cover cranial defects.

CRANIOTOMY INSTRUMENTS (for additional listings see Chapter 5)

Adson brain forceps
Adson brain suction tip
Adson dura hook
Adson hemostatic forceps
Adson saw guides
Allis forceps
Bayonet thumb forceps
Blair saw guides
Cone wire twister
Crile hemostatic forceps
Cushing brain retractor
Cushing brain spatula
Cushing flat drill
Cushing vein retractor
Dandy scalp hemostats
D'Errico bur
DeVilbiss cranial rongeur
DeVilbiss cranial trephine
Ferguson bone grasping forceps
Frazier dura elevator
Frazier dura hook
Galt trephine
Gigli saw
Hajek-Ballenger elevator
Horsley dura separator
Horsley bone wax
Hudson cranial drill
Kanavel exploring cannula
Kirmisson periosteal raspatory
Klemme retractor
Kolodny scalp hemostats
Langenbeck periosteal elevator
Love-Gruenwald rongeur
Lucae bone mallet
McKenzie clip applying forceps
Oldberg retractor
Raney cranial drill
Sachs exploring cannula
Seletz ventricular cannula
Senn small rake retractor

CRANIOTOMY INSTRUMENTS (Continued)

Smithwick clip applying forceps
Smithwick nerve hook
Spurling rongeur
Stille-Gigli wire saw
Stille-Liston bone cutting forceps
Stille-Luer cutting forceps
Stille-Luer rongeur

Stille osteotome
Strully scissors
Sweet clip applying forceps
Taylor scissors
Verbrugghen retractor
Volkman curet
Weitlaner retractor

HEMOSTATIC AGENTS AND METHODS IN NEUROSURGERY

Bone wax
Bovie electrocautery
   coagulating current
   cutting current
Cellulose gauze
Clips
   Adson
   Cushing
   Köln
   Mayfield
   McKenzie
   Michel
   Olivecrona
   Raney
   Silver

Tantalum
Tonnis
Crushed muscle
Fibrin film
Fibrin foam
Gelfoam
Gelita B
Horsley's bone wax
Ligatures
Muscle graft
Muscle stamp
Oxycel
Spongostan
Suction

Trigeminal Rhizotomy, Right

With the patient in a sitting position under general anesthesia, a vertical incision was made over the right temporal region about 2 cm. anterior to the external auditory canal on the right side. Retraction was obtained.

The squamous portion of the temporal bone was identified. A trephine opening was made. This opening in the temporal bone was enlarged with rongeurs until it was about 1½ inches in diameter. The dura was separated from the base of the middle fossa until the middle meningeal artery was identified. The middle meningeal artery was cauterized at its point of emergence from the foramen spinosum and the foramen spinosum was packed with cotton. The middle meningeal artery was then cut across.

The dura was reflected from the base of the middle fossa medial to the foramen spinosum until the foramen ovale was identified. The external dura was then stripped away from its trigeminal ganglion until the whole of the trigeminal ganglion was identified. The maxillary and mandibular roots of the trigeminal ganglion were then cut leaving the ophthalmic root intact.

Bleeding was controlled by packing.

Temporal Craniotomy with Exploratory Trephine

Under general anesthesia, the patient was placed in the supine position, prepared and draped in the usual manner.

A left frontal temporal craniotomy incision was marked out. After instillation of ½% Xylocaine with ephedrine, local, a skin incision was made over the coronal suture approximately 3 cm. in length and held open with self-retaining retractors. No. 1, 2 and 3 burs were used and a trephine was done. The dura was not noted to be under tension. It was incised in a cruciate manner. Bleeding was controlled by the use of bone wax and electrocautery.

The surface of the brain was noted to be bulging somewhat. An exploratory needle was passed inferiorly, superiorly, anteriorly and posteriorly. The anterior horn of the lateral ventricle was entered and 10 cc. of air instilled. As the needle was passed inferiorly toward the middle fossa, increased resistance was encountered which possibly represented a tumor. It was felt that any such lesion in this area would be inoperable.

The wound was closed in two layers with 000 black silk interrupted sutures.

The biopsy specimen was sent to the pathologist for histologic examination. It was reported back as an Astrocytoma, Grade 1.

Left Temporal Craniotomy with Removal of Subdural Hematoma

Under general anesthesia, a horseshoe-shaped flap was turned down on the left temporal region. The flap was approximately 2½ inches in diameter.

The dura was found to be under increased tension. The dura was opened and underneath it, a subdural hematoma was found. The membrane was ruptured. There was a gush of liquid, consisting of old changed dark blood, from the opening. The hematoma extended from the tip of the frontal lobe to the tip of the occipital lobe, over the whole surface of the hemisphere. The maximum depth of the subdural hematoma was approximately 1¼ inches.

The hematoma cavity was completely washed out. All bleeding points were controlled. There was no large single bleeding point.

A silver clip was placed on the surface of the left hemisphere for x-ray control in the future. The dura was closed with interrupted silk. The bone flap was replaced and the scalp closed in two layers with silk.

Exploration for Extracerebral Hematoma

The scalp was shaved and then surgically prepared and draped. Under local anesthesia using Avertin as a basal anesthetic, a vertical incision was made above and 2 cm. in front of the ear. The first bur hole was made just below the superior insertion of the temporal muscle. No hematoma was found. A similar bur hole was then made in the same position, on the opposite side. A clot was found. The bur hole was enlarged with rongeurs. The clot was removed in its entirety using suction.

Bleeding was traced and the incision extended down to the floor of the temporal fossa. Bleeding was noted to be originating from the foramen spinosum. The incision was extended, the bone rongeured away and the bleeding point exposed. Bleeding was controlled with electrocoagulation. All of the clot was evacuated by suction and irrigation. Bleeding was controlled from the emissary veins between the dura and the bone. Hemostasis was obtained.

The temporal muscle and scalp were closed in layers with interrupted silk. No drainage was necessary.

Craniectomy

The scalp was shaved, prepared and draped and the patient was positioned in the face down position. The head was supported on an Adson outrigger type headrest.

After local infiltration of the operative site with Novocain, a curved incision was made in the scalp, starting just opposite the middle of one mastoid process, curving upward and around to the middle of the other mastoid process. The incision paralleled the superior nuchal line. An incision was then made in the occipital muscle and fascia parallel to the scalp incision, 5 mm. below its insertion on the occipital bone. The musculocutaneous flap thus formed was reflected downward until the rim of the foramen magnum was exposed. The occipital muscles were divided in the midline down to the arch of the atlas.

A bur hole was made in the occipital bone, rongeuring away bone up to the insertion of the occipital fascia above, downwards to the foramen magnum and laterally to the mastoid processes. An accidental incision into the mastoid cells was immediately sealed with bone wax.

The dorsal rim of the foramen magnum was removed along with the arch of the atlas. Next, the bone in the middle was removed. This was followed by profuse bleeding which was controlled by generous application of bone wax.

The dura was noted to be under increased tension. The lateral ventricle was tapped.

NEUROSURGERY

Traumata of the Brain

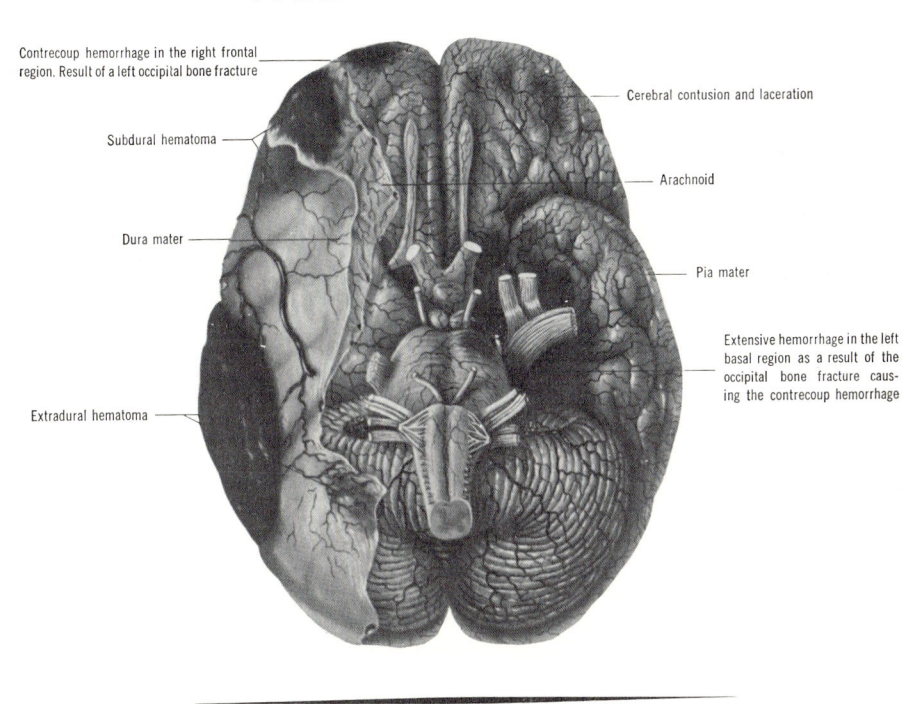

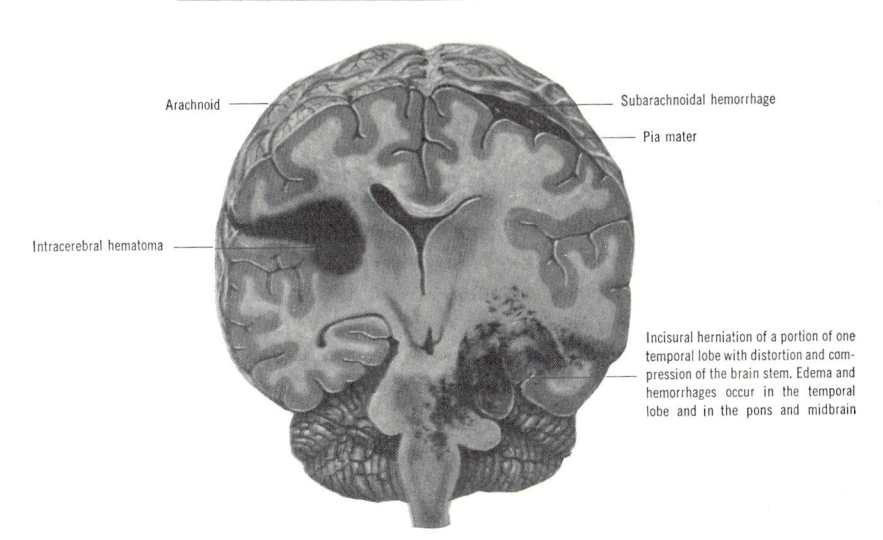

Figure 55 Traumata of the brain
Courtesy Lederle Laboratories

A 4 cm. vertical incision was made in the scalp about 7 cm. above the external occipital protuberance and 4 cm. toward the midline followed by a bur hole with incision of the dura. A cannula was inserted into the posterior horn of the lateral ventricle. A flanged cannula was left in situ during the operation for continuous drainage.

The dura was opened down to the foramen magnum with ligation of the occipital sinus. Hemostasis was obtained. After exploration of the posterior fossa had been carried out, the dural flaps were replaced without sutures. The deep occipital muscles were sutured in the midline with interrupted sutures of silk being sutured back to the fascial margin along the superior nuchal line. The fascia was then sutured in a similar manner. The galea and skin were closed using interrupted sutures of silk. drainage was used.

Elevation of Depressed Skull Fracture

The scalp was shaved and the head surgically prepared and draped. A bur hole was made to one side of the depressed bone. All depressed fragments of the inner table were removed with rongeur forceps. It was noted that the fracture was situated above the superior longitudinal dural sinus. Hemorrhage followed removal of the bone fragments. This was controlled by application of a muscle stamp, held in place with a suction tip against wet cottonoid which adhered to the dura.

The bone fragments were fitted into place, the larger fragments being anchored by silk sutures passed through gimlet holes in the bone edges.

The scalp wound was closed with a layer of interrupted silk sutures in the galea and another row in the skin

Subtemporal Decompression

After the scalp had been surgically prepared and the area draped, a hockeystick incision was made in front of the ear. The resulting scalp flap was reflected anteriorly. Using a vertical incision, the temporal fascia was incised by beginning at the zygoma. A 3 mm. horizontal incision at the zygoma from the vertical incision permitted better retraction of the temporal fascia. The upper end of the vertical incision was then converted into a Y-shape and the resulting flap retracted superiorly. The temporal muscle was incised in the direction of its fibers and the edges were retracted. A bur hole was then made in the exposed temporal bone, rongeuring away the bone in all directions. The underlying dura was opened by a cruciate incision.

Hemostasis was obtained. The exposed cortex was covered with fibrin film to prevent adhesions between the cortex and overlying structures.

The galea and then the skin were closed with interrupted silk sutures.

Clipping of Middle Cerebral Artery

Under general anesthesia, with the patient on his right side, a horseshoe-shaped flap was turned down over the left temporal region. The incision was carried down to the zygoma. The bone flap, involving the squamous portion of the temporal bone, was reflected and the bone was further rongeured away down to the base of the middle fossa.

When adequate exposure of the dura over the temporal lobe had been obtained, a curved incision was made through the dura centering over the Sylvian fissure. The dura was reflected downward and the Sylvian fissure was identified. The arachnoid over the Sylvian fissure (sulcus lateralis cerebri) was then split so that the frontal lobe could be separated from the temporal lobe by splitting the tissues through the Sylvian fissure.

Small bleeding points were coagulated as the fissure was opened. The branches of the middle cerebral artery were identified. These were followed medially until the aneurysm was encountered. The aneurysm was carefully dissected away from its bed. It was found to be about 5 or 6 mm. in diameter. When the actual aneurysm had been identified along with its feeding branches, a clip was placed across the base of the artery. There was a hematoma in the tip of the temporal lobe. This was punctured and evacuated with suction. Bleeding points were coagulated and clipped.

The dura was closed with interrupted black silk. The bone flap was replaced and the scalp closed with silk throughout.

Cistern Puncture

With the patient on his side at the edge of the bed and the suboccipital area properly prepared, the spine of the second cervical vertebra was identified by palpation. A 2% Novocain solution was injected intradermally 1 cm. above this. An 18 gauge spinal puncture needle was inserted in the midline as well as in the plane of the outer canthus of the eye and external auditory meatus. The needle was advanced very carefully to a depth of 5 cm. until it was felt to penetrate the fused atlanto-occipital membrane and dura. The stylet was removed and fluid permitted to escape. The manometric pressure was measured and fluid was withdrawn for further studies.

THE SPINAL CORD (Myelon)

The spinal cord is the elongated portion of the central nervous system extending from the foramen magnum, at the level of the upper part of the atlas, down to the upper border of the second lumbar vertebra. At this level it gives off a terminal strand of nonnervous tissue called the filum terminale which projects extradurally down to the first coccygeal vertebra. At its upper (intradural) portion, the filum terminale is surrounded by the lumbar, sacral and coccygeal spinal nerve roots which are referred to collectively as the cauda equina (horse's tail).

The average length of the spinal cord is about 18 inches, extending from the base of the brain down to the upper border of the second lumbar vertebra. The cord is situated within the spinal canal of the vertebral column where it is invested by three layers of membranes (meninges) continuous with those covering the brain. The outermost layer is called the *dura mater* or dura; the middle layer is the *arachnoid mater,* and the innermost layer is the *pia mater*. The pia mater extends beyond the spinal cord and is joined with dura mater at the level of the third sacral segment.

Spinal fluid circulates between the meninges particularly in the subarachnoid space situated between the pia and the arachnoid membranes.

An epidural cavity separates the dura mater from the vertebral canal wall and an intervening space called the *subdural cavity* separates the dura from the underlying arachnoid. The arachnoid, in turn, is separated from the underlying pia mater by a wide space known as the *subarachnoid cavity* which is filled with spinal fluid.

The *ligamentum denticulatum* (dentate ligament) extends as a narrow band on either side of the spinal cord for its entire length. Its medial border is continuous with the pia mater and its lateral border with the dura mater, at intervals. It separates the anterior and posterior nerve roots.

The spinal nerves, consisting of thirty-one pairs, project from the spinal cord. Each of these nerves has a ventral (anterior) root and a dorsal (posterior) root. The dorsal roots contain a spinal ganglion. The spinal nerves are paired into 8 cervical, 12 thoracic, 5 lumbar, 5 sacral and 1 coccygeal.

A longitudinal median groove incompletely divides the spinal cord into halves. This groove is called the anterior median fissure and the posterior median sulcus.

The anatomic terms for structures associated with the spinal cord and for the cord proper have been listed below to provide a ready reference.

Cervical and Thoracic Regions of the Spinal Cord

Inferior cerebellar veins

Cerebral dura (cut); posterior inferior cerebellar artery

Sternocleidomastoid muscle; deep cervical vein

Transverse process of atlas; nodose ganglion

Superior cervical ganglion

Vagus nerve; posterior spinal artery and vein (cut)

Middle cervical ganglion

Brachial plexus

Inferior cervical ganglion

Third thoracic vertebra

Sympathetic trunk

Left lung

Sixth thoracic ganglion

Posterior median sulcus

Post. root, ninth thoracic nerve

Ninth thoracic ganglion; tenth thoracic vertebra

Arachnoid (cut)

Twelfth thoracic vertebra

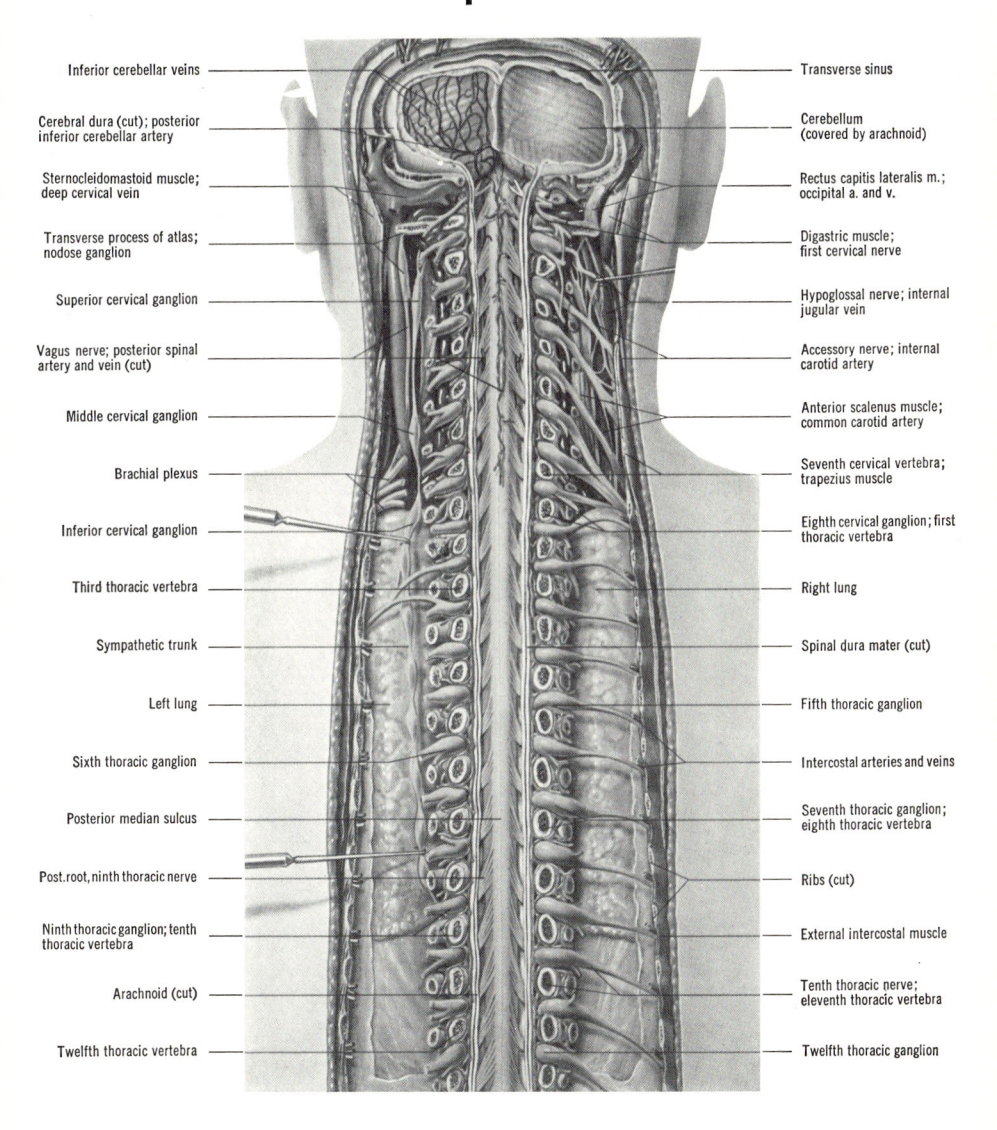

Transverse sinus

Cerebellum (covered by arachnoid)

Rectus capitis lateralis m.; occipital a. and v.

Digastric muscle; first cervical nerve

Hypoglossal nerve; internal jugular vein

Accessory nerve; internal carotid artery

Anterior scalenus muscle; common carotid artery

Seventh cervical vertebra; trapezius muscle

Eighth cervical ganglion; first thoracic vertebra

Right lung

Spinal dura mater (cut)

Fifth thoracic ganglion

Intercostal arteries and veins

Seventh thoracic ganglion; eighth thoracic vertebra

Ribs (cut)

External intercostal muscle

Tenth thoracic nerve; eleventh thoracic vertebra

Twelfth thoracic ganglion

Figure 56 Cervical and thoracic regions of the spinal cord
Courtesy Lederle Laboratories

The Vertebral Column

The vertebral column is made up of a series of bones called vertebrae, usually thirty three in number, which are designated as cervical, thoracic, lumbar, sacral and coccygeal depending upon the area they occupy. Each bony segment in each area is numbered. The fourth lumbar vertebra is referred to as L-4, the first sacral as S-1, etc. The smoother segmented outline of the vertebral column faces toward the interior and front of the body. The surface containing the projections faces toward the back. In addition to supporting the skeleton the vertebral column serves as a bony enclosure protecting the spinal cord.

The cartilaginous cushion between each vertebra is called the intervertebral disc. The pulpy center of the disc is called the nucleus pulposus. Protrusion or herniation of these discs represents one of the most common causes of severe and chronic or recurrent low back and leg pain. The most common site of such ruptures is between L-5 and S-1. It occurs with lessening frequency with each segment up the lumbar vertebrae, and is virtually nonexistent in the thoracic area. The most common site of cervical discs is between C-6 and C-7 and between C-5 and C-6.

Fig. 57 and 58 are used here to demonstrate that access to a ruptured disc, the spinal cord or spinal meninges (membranes enveloping the spinal cord) can only be gained through the creation of a defect in the vertebral column. When the vertebral laminae are removed on one side only as in disc removal, the operation is called a **hemilaminectomy.** When the posterior arch of the vertebra must be removed to provide access to the spinal cord or spinal meninges, the operation is called a **laminectomy.**

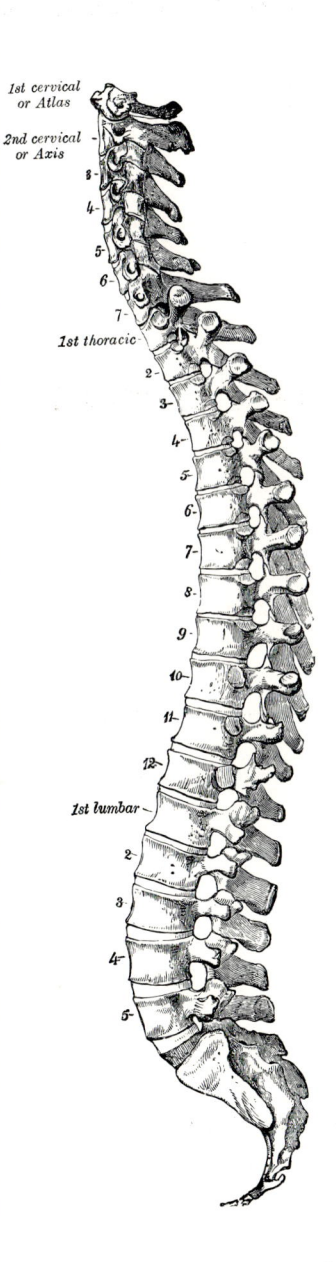

Figure 57 Lateral view of the vertebral column
*From Gray's Anatomy 28th Ed.
Courtesy Lea & Febiger Publ.*

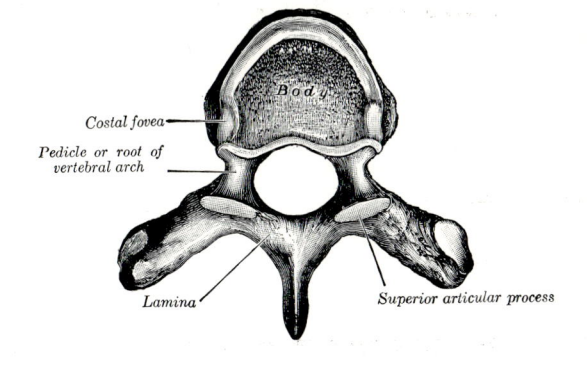

Figure 58 View of thoracic vertebra from above.
*From Gray's Anatomy 28th edition
Courtesy Lea & Febiger Publishers*

FEATURES OF THE SPINAL CORD AND ASSOCIATED STRUCTURES:

Anterior column
Anterior cornu
Anterior funiculus
Anterior gray commissure
Anterior median fissure
Anterior nerve roots
Anterior white commissure
Anterolateral region
Arachnoid
Cauda equina
Central canal
Cisterna magna
Conus medullaris
Dentate ligament
Dorsal nerve root
Dura mater (dura)
Epidural cavity
Fasciculus cuneatus
Fasciculus gracilis
Filum terminale
Filum terminale externum
Filum terminale internum
Formatio reticularis
Glial sheath
Lateral column
Lateral funiculus
Ligamentum denticulatum
Ligamenta flava (plural)
Ligamentum flavum
Medulla oblongata
Medulla spinalis
Meninges
Nerve rootlet
Pia-glial membrane
Pia mater
Posterior column
Posterior funiculus
Posterior gray commissure
Posterior median sulcus
Posterior nerve roots
Postero-intermediate sulcus
Posterolateral sulcus
Spinal ganglion
Subarachnoid cavity
Subarachnoid cisterna
Subarachnoid septum
Subarachnoid space
Subdural space
Substantia gelatinosa centralis
Substantia gelatinosa of Rolando
Terminal ventricle
Tract of Burdach
Tract of Goll
Tract of Lissauer
Transverse commissure
Vertebral canal

Lumbar Hemilaminectomy for Ruptured Disc (Herniated Nucleus Pulposus)

The patient was surgically prepared and draped in a prone, semiflexed position on the operating table.

A midline incision was made in the lower back over the spinous processes of the 3rd, 4th, and 5th lumbar and 1st sacral vertebrae. The spinous processes of L-4, L-5 and S-1 were exposed. An incision was made in the thoracolumbar fascia just lateral to the spinous processes on the side where the hemilaminectomy was planned. Bleeding was controlled by coagulation.

A periosteal elevator was used to separate the Erector spinae and Multifidus muscles from the spinous processes and laminae. The laminae and the articular processes of the vertebrae were exposed. A coagulating cur-

The Intervertebral Disks

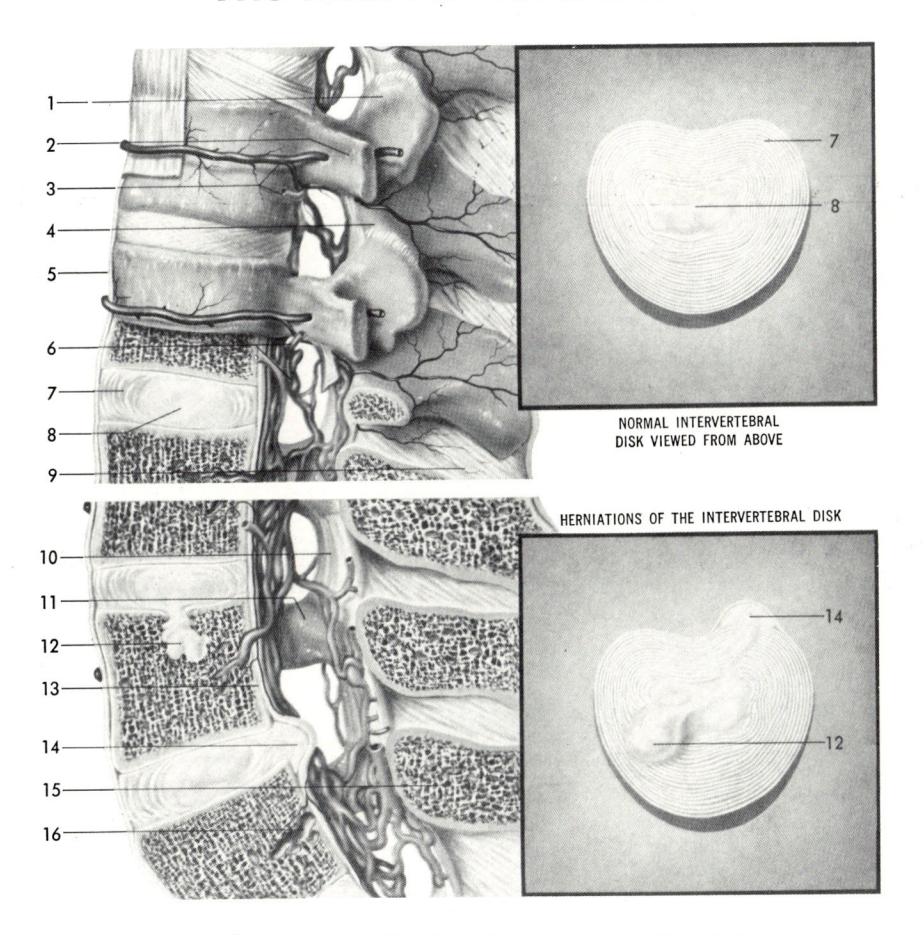

NORMAL INTERVERTEBRAL DISK VIEWED FROM ABOVE

HERNIATIONS OF THE INTERVERTEBRAL DISK

1 Superior articular process
2 Transverse process
3 Lumbar artery and vein
4 Inferior articular process
5 Anterior longitudinal ligament
6 Internal vertebral venous plexus
7 Fibrous ring of intervertebral disk
8 Nucleus pulposus
9 Interspinous ligament
10 Ligamentum flavum
11 Lamina
12 Herniation of nucleus pulposus into the spongiosa (Schmorl lesion)
13 Posterior longitudinal ligament
14 Herniation of nucleus pulposus beneath the posterior longitudinal ligament
15 Spinous process
16 Basivertebral vein

Figure 59

rent was used to control bleeding. All bleeding from the cut ends of the bone was controlled with Horsley's bone wax. The interspaces were visualized after the muscle had been removed. The ligamenta flava were seen between the vertebrae.

The proposed hemilaminectomy was outlined on the 4th and 5th lumbar laminae on the left. A gooseneck rongeur was used to remove this portion of the lamina. After the hemilaminectomy had been performed at the 5th and 4th lumbar areas, the ligamentum flavum was grasped with a hook at the 4th interspace. Cottonoid was introduced under this area to protect the dura. The ligamentum flavum was excised by incision of its attachments. It was completely removed in its lateral attachment.

The nerve root was identified and retracted following which the ruptured disc was identified at the level of L-5. It was noted to be compressing the outgoing nerve. Using a Love retractor the 1st sacral nerve was retracted. The disc was removed piecemeal from the epidural space using pituitary forceps. Bleeding was controlled by electrocautery on vessels and Gelfoam at the sites of oozing.

The 4th interspace was then explored and no pathology was found. The dura was tightly closed with a running suture of fine silk with stitches 4 mm. apart. The Erector spinae muscles were closed with interrupted chromic catgut sutures. The fascia was treated in a similar manner. The subcutaneous tissues and skin were closed with interrupted silk sutures.

Hemilaminectomy for Cervical Disc

The patient was prepared and draped in a sitting position. An incision was made over the spinous processes of the 4th, 5th, 6th, and 7th cervical vertebrae to the 1st dorsal vertebra. Following the incision of the midline of the posterior neck and thorax, the ligamentum nuchae and the spinous processes of the lower cervical and 1st dorsal vertebrae were exposed. The incision was made on the side of the lesion. The spinous processes of the 7th cervical and the 1st dorsal were exposed. Bleeders were coagulated with electrocautery. Further dissection with scissors was carried out to expose the spinous processes of C-5 and C-6. The bifid portions of the spinous processes of C-5 and C-6 were separated from their muscle attachments on the side of the ruptured disc. A periosteal elevator was used to further dissect the muscles away from the spinous processes and the laminae. A Scoville self-retaining retractor was used to retract the muscles. The laminae were removed. A dental drill was used to bite off the shelf of bone on the lateral aspect of the opening.

By gentle palpation, the ruptured disc was located under the outgoing nerve; however, to avoid trauma to the outgoing nerve, a transdural approach was elected. The dura was transfixed with a pair of silk sutures at the ends of the proposed incision, following which, the dura was elevated and incised. Following retraction of the dura, the denticulate ligament was identified. This was cut with scissors exposing the ruptured disc. The outgoing nerve was gently retracted downward and the disc removed with pituitary forceps.

The anterior dural opening was closed with a single interrupted silk suture. The muscles and fascia were closed with a chromic catgut. The subcutaneous tissues and skin were closed with interrupted silk sutures.

Chordotomy (Sectioning of the lateral spinothalamic tract)

After satisfactory preparation, draping and anesthesia, a median incision was made in the back and a laminectomy performed involving the 3rd and 4th thoracic vertebrae. Using a Kerrison rongeur the lateral portion of the canal was removed. Full exposure was accomplished on both sides. The dura was then opened and retracted with sutures. The outgoing anterior and posterior nerve roots as well as the ligamentum denticulatum were visualized. The attachment of the denticulate ligament was severed bilaterally and grasped with a hemostat on the side of the section. The spinal cord was carefully rotated by means of the denticulate ligament. In an avascular area, at a depth of 4 mm., the anterolateral portion of the cord was sectioned with a # 11 Bard-Parker blade. The arachnoid in the area for section was removed. The section was carried anteriorly at a point just medial to the outgoing anterior nerve roots.

The dura was closed with interrupted 0000 silk ties. The muscles were reapproximated with interrupted 00 chromic. The subcutaneous tissue was closed with interrupted chromic and the skin edges were brought together with interrupted silk. A dressing was applied.

Cervical Sympathectomy

An incision was made in the skin parallel to the posterior border of the sternocleidomastoid muscle, extending from the tip of the mastoid process toward the lower border of the clavicle. The spinal accessory nerve was identified and retracted. The external jugular vein was divided and hemostasis secured. The muscle incision was made longitudinally. The carotid-vagus-jugular bundle was freed without entering its sheath and retracted medially along with the sternocleidomastoid muscle.

The cervical sympathetic chain was identified and followed up to the fusiform superior cervical ganglion. The superior cervical ganglion was freed and dissection carried downward. The superior ganglion was avulsed from its cranial attachments. The cervical chain was seen to course around the inferior thyroid artery and was found in proximity to the vertebral artery. The vertebral artery was freed and retracted. The thyroid axis, vertebral and subclavian vessels, scalenus anticus muscle along with the sternocleidomastoid muscle, pleura, carotid sheath and contents were likewise retracted. The lateral branches of the ganglion were divided and the sympathetic trunk followed upward to the first thoracic ganglion.

Following hemostasis, the wound was closed using fine silk.

Lumbar Sympathectomy

A midline incision was made through the skin and fat extending from the symphysis pubis to one inch below the umbilicus. The incision was extended into the shape of a Y with its upper limbs on either side of the umbilicus. The superficial fascia was then separated from the inner halves of the rectus sheaths on each side, in the lower incision, to a level in the same plane as the upper extensions of the incision. A longitudinal incision in each rectus sheath was then made in such a fashion that a third of the muscle was medial and two-thirds of the muscle was lateral to each incision.

The rectus muscle was incised in the same plane extending to the posterior sheath of the rectus in the upper three-fourths, and the peritoneum in the lower one-fourth of the incision. Using a finger, the posterior sheath was gently separated from the peritoneum. This was continued inward, toward the midline. The posterior sheath was incised just lateral to the deep epigastric artery, leaving the artery medial to the incision.

The patient was repositioned in a low Trendelenburg position. The peritoneum was then separated laterally from the abdominal fascia. The abdominal contents were retracted to facilitate exposure of the aorta and iliac vessels on the left and the vena cava and iliac vessels on the right.

The incision was closed in layers using a single continuous chromic catgut suture in the posterior sheath and muscle. Single chromic interrupted catgut sutures were used in the anterior sheath reinforced with figure-of-eight silkworm gut sutures. The Y extensions of the incision were closed with figure-of-eight sutures, the lower loops of these sutures alternating on opposite sides with one suture passing through the skin and fat and looping through the right rectus to exit through the skin and fat on the opposite side. The same procedure was carried out, in an alternating fashion, on the opposite side. After emerging from the skin, one end of each loop was passed through the margins of the skin incision and tied to one side of the skin incision. Dead space within the incision was obliterated by rubber tubing passed under the silkworm loops above the skin. The sutures were tied over the rubber tubes. The skin was closed with clips.

DISEASES OF THE NERVOUS SYSTEM
(brain, meninges, spinal cord and related structures)

Abscess of the brain
Abscess of the spinal cord
Adenocarcinoma
Adhesions of cauda equina
Air embolism
Amyelia
Amyotonia congenita
Amyotrophic lateral sclerosis
Anencephaly
Aneurysm
Aneurysmal varix
Angioneurotic edema of vessels
Angiospasm
Aplasia
Arachnoiditis
Arteriovenous aneurysm
Aseptic meningitis
Astrocytoma
Atelomyelia
Athetosis, bilateral
Atrophy
Basal cell carcinoma
Bell's palsy
Birth injury of brain
Bulbar palsy
Calcification of choroid plexus
Caudal displacement of brain
    stem, cerebellum and spinal cord
Cerebellar sclerosis
Cerebral cortical atrophy
Cerebral dysplasia
Cerebral hemihypoplasia
Cerebral hemorrhage
Cerebral sclerosis, familial
Cerebral thrombosis
Cerebrospinal arteriosclerosis
Cerebrospinal endarteritis
Cerebrospinal thromboangiitis
    obliterans
Cerebrospinal syphilis
Cholesteatoma
Chondroma
Chordoma
Chorea
    chronic progressive

Choriomeningitis, lymphocytic
Compression of spinal cord
Concussion of brain
Corticostriatal encephalopathy
Corticostriato-spinal degeneration
Craniopharyngioma
Cyst of cavum septi pellucidi
Cyst of meninges
Cyst of tentorium
Degenerative tic
    generalized
    localized
Dermal sinus, congenital
Dilation of cavum septi pellucidi
Dorsal sclerosis
Dysplasia of nervous system
Dystonia musculorum deformans
Embolism
Encephalitis
Encephalomalacia
Encephalomeningopathy
Encephalomyelitis
Encephalomyeloneuropathy
Encephalomyelopathy
    with kernicterus
Encephalomyeloradiculitis
Encephalomyeloradiculopathy
Encephalopathy
Encephalorrhagia, pericapillary
Ependymoma
Epidermoid carcinoma
Epidural abscess
Epidural aerocele
Epidural hematoma
Erythredema polyneuropathy
Essential polyangiitis
Fat embolism
Fibroma
Fibrosarcoma
Ganglioneuroma
Glial membrane of 4th ventricle
Glioblastoma multiforme
Glioma
Gliosis of cerebral aqueduct
Grand mal

DISEASES OF THE NERVOUS SYSTEM (continued)

Hemangioendothelioma
Hemangioma, meningeal vessels
Hemangiomatosis, meningeal vessels
Hemangiosarcoma
Hematomyelia
Hemianencephaly
Hemisection of spinal cord
Hepatolenticular degeneration
Hereditary sclerosis
Herniation of the brain
Herpes zoster
Heterotopia cerebralis
Hydrencephalomeningocele
Hydrocephalus
Hydromicrocephaly
Hyperplasia
Hypertensive meningeal hydrops
Hypoplasia
Jacksonian seizures
Labioglossopharyngeal paralysis progressive
Laceration of middle meningeal artery
Lenticular degeneration progressive
Leptomeningitis
  circumscribed
  nonserous
  serous
  syphilitic
  tuberculous
Leptomeningopathy
Leukodystrophia cerebri
  Progressiva hereditaria
Lipoma
Lymphangioma
Lymphocytic choriomeningitis
Lymphosarcoma
Macrogyria
Marantic thrombosis
Medulloblastoma
Melanoma of meninges
Meningeal adhesions
Meningeal hemorrhage
Meningioma

Meningismus
Meningitis
  acute
  cerebrospinal
  chronic serous
  sympathica
Meningocele
Meningoencephalomyelitis
Meningoencephalomyelopathy
Meningoencephalopathy
Meningomyelitis
Meralgia paresthetica
Microcephaly
Microgyria
Micromyelia
Migraine
Multiple sclerosis
Muscular atrophy
  hereditary familial spinal
  myelopathic
  progressive neuropathic
Mycotic aneurysm
Myelitis
  acute ascending
  chronic
  disseminated
Myelodysplasia
Myelomalacia
Myelomeningocele
Myelopathy
Myeloradicular dysplasia
Myeloradiculitis
Myeloradiculodysplasia
Myeloradiculopathy
Necrosis of spinal cord
Neuralgia
  facial
  geniculate
  glossopharyngeal
  sphenopalatine
  trigeminal
Neuritis
Neuroepithelioma
Neurofibroma (neurofibromatosis)
Neuroma

DISEASES OF THE NERVOUS SYSTEM (continued)

Neuropathy
  diabetic
  multiple
  peripheral
  progressive hypertrophic
    interstitial
  toxic
Oligodendroma
Olivopantocerebellar atrophy
Optic atrophy, hereditary
Optic neuroencephalomyelopathy
Ossification of meninges
Osteoma
Pachymeningitis
Papilloma
Paraganglioma
Paralysis agitans
Petit mal
Pheochromocytoma
Phlebitis
  of cavernous sinus
  of cranial sinus
  of lateral sinus
Plexiform neuroma
Pneumocephalus
Polioencephalitis
  bulbar acute
  inferior
  superior hemorrhagic
Polioencephalopathy
Poliomyelitis, acute
  bulbospinal
Porencephaly
Presenile sclerosis
Primary lateral sclerosis
Pseudosclerosis

Radiculitis
Radiculoneuritis
Radiculoneuropathy
Radiculopathy
Rupture of congenital aneurysm
Sarcoma
Schwannoma
Septic phlebitis of cranial sinus
Sinus pericranii
Spastic torticollis
Status convulsivus
Subarachnoid hemorrhage
Subcortical encephalopathy
Subdural abscess
Subdural hematoma
Subdural hygroma
Sympathicoblastoma
Sympathicogonioma
Syphilis, cerebrospinal
Syphilis, meningovascular
Syringobulbia
Syringomyelia
Tabes dorsalis
Tabo-paresis, tabetic form
Teratoma
Thromboangitis obliterans, cerebral
Thrombosis
  of cavernous sinus
  of jugular bulb
  of lateral sinus
  of sigmoid sinus
Trypanosomiasis of nervous system
Tuberous sclerosis
Varix of
Virus encephalomyelitis
  (Guillain-Barré syndrome)

OPERATIONS ON THE NERVOUS SYSTEM
(brain, meninges, spinal cord and related structures)

Acoustic neurotomy
Biopsy of meninges
Biopsy of nerve
Biopsy of spinal cord
Chordotomy
Cranial puncture
Craniectomy

Cranioplasty
Craniotomy
Crushing of nerve
Decompression of spinal cord
Debridement of compound skull
  fracture

OPERATIONS ON THE NERVOUS SYSTEM (continued)

Decompression
  suboccipital
  subtemporal
Division of cortical adhesions
Drainage of cerebral epidural space
Drainage of cranial sinus
Drainage of lateral sinus
Drainage of meninges
Drainage of sigmoid sinus
Drainage of spinal cord
Drainage of spinal epidural space
Drainage of subarachnoid space
Drainage of subdural space
Duraplasty
Encephalography
Excision of choroid plexus
Excision of lesion of meninges
Excision of neuroma
Excision of lesion of spinal cord
Excision of lobe of brain
  frontal
  occipital
  parietal
  temporal
Excision of tumor of brain
Exploration of brain
Exploration of meninges
Exploration of nerve
Exploration of spinal cord
Ganglionectomy
  cerebral nerve
  gasserian
  sphenopalatine (Meckel's)
Glossopharyngeal neurotomy
Graft of nerve
Hemilaminectomy
Laminectomy
Ligation of meningeal vessels
  middle meningeal artery
  superior longitudinal sinus
Lobotomy
Marsupialization of lesion
Myelography
Neurectasia
Neurectomy
  cranial nerves
  spinal nerves

Neurexeresis
Neuroanastomosis
  hypoglossal-facial
  spinal accessory-facial
  spinal accessory-hypoglossal
Neurolysis
Neuroplasty
Neurorrhaphy
Neurotomy
  acoustic
  cranial nerves
  glossopharyngeal
  retrogasserian
  spinal nerves
Neurotripsy
Open reduction of skull fracture
Phrenemphraxis
Phrenicectomy
Phrenicoexeresis
Phrenicotomy
Phrenicotripsy
Presacral neurectomy
Puncture of brain
Puncture of subarachnoid space
Puncture of ventricles
Removal of foreign body
Repair of spina bifida
  with meningocele
  with meningomyelocele
Retrogasserian neurotomy
Rhizotomy
  dorsal nerve roots
  ventral nerve roots
Spinal puncture
Splanchnicectomy
Splanchnicotomy
Suture of meninges
Sympathectomy
Sympathicotripsy
Topectomy
Tractotomy
Vagotomy
Ventriculocisternostomy by tube
  (Torkildsen's operation)
Ventriculography
Ventriculostomy

10 | Obstetrics

The language of obstetrics is unique and peculiar to that specialty, borrowing little from general surgical terminology. It provides for technical and precise communication without recourse to nonprofessional expressions.

The course of pregnancy from conception until delivery is divided into **trimesters** (three periods of three months each) and is called the **prenatal** or **antepartum period**. Delivery is called **parturition** and the mother in labor, the **parturient**. The duration of a pregnancy is spoken of as the **length of gestation**. The six to eight weeks following delivery constitutes the **postpartum period,** otherwise known as the **puerperium.**

The medical record of the obstetrical patient is quite different from that of the medical or surgical patient in that it contains a much more extensive obstetrical history, a prenatal record, delivery record and postpartum record with notations of examinations and observations incident to the postpartum course.

An important part of every obstetrical history is the obstetrical index, abbreviated as GPMAL. The letters represent the terms GRAVIDA, PARA, MULTIPLE BIRTHS, ABORTIONS and LIVE BIRTHS. The letters are replaced by appropriate numbers separated by dashes to represent the specific information.

Gravida refers to the number of times the patient has been pregnant regardless of whether the pregnancy ended in abortion or a viable birth. By a viable birth is meant a pregnancy beyond 22 weeks gestation. There is no chance for survival of fetuses delivered earlier than this and for this reason deliveries short of 22 weeks are classified as abortions. A woman who is pregnant for the first time is classified as a **primigravida** while a woman who has been pregnant more than once is considered a **multigravida.**

The term **para,** referring to parity, is a record of the pregnancies which have reached a viable stage (over 22 weeks). The number of pregnancies which ended in abortion would not be reflected in this number.

To further exemplify use of the terms gravida and para, we classify a woman who is pregnant for the first time, prior to delivery as a gravida I para O. After delivery, whether the child was born dead or alive so long as it exceeded 22 weeks of gestation, the mother is classified as a gravida I para I. If her pregnancy ended in abortion, she remains a gravida I para O. During her second pregnancy, if she delivered a viable infant rather than aborted in her first pregnancy, she is classified as a gravida II para I prior to delivery. After delivery of a viable infant, she would be regarded as a gravida II para II. If her first two pregnancies ended in abortions and she becomes pregnant a third time, she is considered a gravida III para O. If she delivers a viable infant in this third pregnancy, she becomes a gravida III para I. The terms gravida and para refer to the number of pregnancies and viable conclusions of pregnancy, respectively. Neither index refers to the number of fetuses. A woman who delivers twins in her first pregnancy is still considered a gravida I para I after delivery.

A woman who has never borne a viable infant (para O) is known as a **nullipara** while a woman who has had two or more viable deliveries is classified as a **multipara.**

Classifications of Prematurity

For purposes of uniform reporting certain criteria have been established by the medical profession to distinguish three stages of infant prematurity. On this basis deliveries are classified as abortion, immature delivery, premature delivery or full term birth.

An abortion is said to have occurred when the length of gestation is less than 22 weeks, the weight of the fetus is less than 17 ounces (500 grams) and/or the length of the fetus from crown to heel is less than 28 centimeters. There is no liklihood of survival in these cases.

A later stage of prematurity is the immature delivery. In these instances survival of the fetus is possible but the mortality rate is understandably high. These are pregnancies delivered between 22 and 28 weeks. The weight of the fetus may range from 17 ounces to two pounds.

Premature delivery is the classification reserved for deliveries occurring between the 28th and 37th week of gestation. The weight of the infant may range from two to five and a half pounds (5 lbs. 8 ounces) or 1000 to 2499 grams.

Full term pregnancy is classified on the basis of infant weight, i.e. over five pounds and eight ounces or 2500 grams.

ABORTIONS

Premature interruption of a pregnancy before the fetus has arrived at a viable stage of development constitutes an abortion. Although a variety of adjectives are used to describe abortions, the main types are:

Threatened abortion—A pregnancy threatened prior to the viable stage. This is not actually an abortion unless it progresses to that stage. Such cases often go on to deliver a viable infant.

Missed abortion—Death of the fetus occurs in utero prior to a viable stage with retention of the fetus and placenta within the uterus. In such cases the uterus must be emptied of its contents using an oxytocin (a hormone which causes uterine contraction) or by dilation and evacuation. In later pregnancy, hysterotomy (incision into the uterus) with removal of products of conception is sometimes necessary.

Incomplete abortion—An abortion in which only part of the products of conception are expelled. The retained tissue usually consists of a part of the placenta which has remained attached to its bed in the uterus. A D & C is performed to empty the uterus of any residual tissues of conception.

Complete abortion—There is expulsion of the fetus and all chorionic tissue. A D & C is frequently performed to insure against retention of any placental tissue.

Therapeutic abortion—This is deliberate interruption of a pregnancy for legally acceptable reasons.

The Diagnosis of Pregnancy

A number of circumstances may simulate pregnancy, either by causing amenorrhea or suggestive secondary signs. These situations include uterine tumors, ovarian cysts, hematometra, pseudocyesis (imagined pregnancy), hydatidiform mole, etc. Although pregnancy can be ruled out eventually in these conditions, an early diagnosis may not be possible.

Various laboratory examinations are used for confirming a diagnosis of pregnancy. None of these tests are absolutely conclusive since "false positives" and "false negatives" will occur. For this reason, the results of at least two of these tests are used as a basis for diagnosis.

Tests for pregnancy include biological methods injecting urine from the patient into a laboratory animal. These are summarized below.

TEST	RESULTS IN ANIMAL	LAB ANIMAL	RESULT IN (hours)
Ascheim Zondek	Hemorrhagic follicles	Immature mouse	96 - 120
Friedman	Hemorrhagic follicles	Female rabbit	24 - 48
Galli-Mainini	Ejection of spermatozoa	Frog or toad	2
Hogben	Ovulation and oviposition	Female toad	24
Kupperman	Ovarian hyperemia	Female rat	2

Other pregnancy tests utilize the following techniques:

Ultrasound—This test utilizes equipment for detection of ultrasound echoes. It may be used without toxic effect to outline normal and abnormal pregnancies, multiple pregnancies, intrauterine hydatidiform mole and the biparietal diameter (widest part of fetal head) of the fetus.

Progesterone test—This is a nonharmful physiologic pregnancy test effective in about 95 per cent of cases. A strong progestin (substance which causes changes in the endometrium) is given for two days. In two or three days after the last dose menstruation occurs in nonpregnant women. In most women who are pregnant bleeding will not develop.

Immunologic test—This test is based on the premise that the human chorionic gonadotropin hormone (HCG) is a protein and therefore antigenic. The patient's urine and anti-HCG serum obtained from rabbits immunized by HCG are mixed in a tube to which sensitized sheep cells are added. If hemagglutination of the sheep cells occurs the test is considered negative for pregnancy. In the absence of hemagglutination, the test is considered positive. It is about 95 per cent accurate for pregnancy and about 98 per cent accurate for nonpregnancy.

Fetal electrocardiogram—Tracings may be obtained as early as the twelfth week before heart tones can be heard by auscultation or movement can be felt by the mother. This technique can also establish an early diagnosis of multiple pregnancy.

Multiple Pregnancies

Multiple births constitute an exceptional circumstance in the human female. Twins occur about once in every 90 births, triplets about once in every 1,800 births, and quadruplets about once in every 729,000 births. There appears to be a hereditary tendency to twins with a history on either side of the family. A mother may give birth to several sets of twins or triplets throughout her obstetrical career. The highest incidence of multiple births has been observed to occur in Negroes, the lowest incidence among Mongoloids (yellow races), with a frequency between these two races prevailing among Caucasians.

Twin pregnancy may arise either from the fertilization of two separate and distinct ova or from a single ovum. The first results in double-ovum dizygotic or fraternal twins which may be of different sex and not necessarily resemble each other. The latter produces single-ovum monozygotic or identical twins.

Premature labor is common in multiple pregnancies, occurring even earlier in triplets, etc. Twins are usually smaller at term than the single fetus. Presentations may differ for each infant or be the same. One infant usually follows the other by about a half hour in delivery.

Determination of the E.D.C. (estimated date of confinement)

Ovulation, the period when fertilization of the discharged ovum by the sperm can occur, is a time about midway in the menstrual cycle, usually about 14 days prior to the end of the menstrual cycle. Impregnation or fertilization is supposed to prevent further ovulation. Since the actual date of fertilization cannot be determined prior to delivery except where pregnancy develops after a single act of coitus, the first day of the last menstrual period is used as an index to determine the estimated date of confinement. In actuality, delivery occurs about 266 days after fertilization. The calculation used, however, is based on 10 lunar months, 280 days or 40 weeks.

The E.D.C. may be calculated by counting forward 280 days from the first day of the last menstrual period. Another method involves adding seven days to the date of the onset of the last menstrual period and counting back three months. For example, if the first date of the L.M.P. (last menstrual period) was August 14, seven days added to this would yield 21 days. Counting back three months would result in an E.D.C. of May 21. It should be pointed out that only about 10 per cent of patients deliver on their E.D.C., with about 50 per cent delivering within about a week of this date. It has been observed that women who have longer intervals between menstrual periods may have longer durations of pregnancy while those with shorter intervals may have shorter pregnancies.

Antepartum Complications

Pregnancy is a normal development which, with modern prenatal care, usually proceeds to fruition uneventfully. The complications which may develop, however, are many and varied. They may be attributed to mechanical factors involving the placenta, uterus and/or fetus, or to physiologic causes, the latter often being the most serious. Some of these circumstances are mentioned here to acquaint the secretary with their significance in the course of pregnancy and the reason for their use in some cases as an indication for cesarean section.

Acute toxemia—This is a condition peculiar to pregnancy characterized by hypertension, edema and proteinuria. In the nonconvulsive stage it is called **pre-eclampsia.** It is classified as **eclampsia** when convulsions and coma ensue, often resulting in death of the patient. The occurrence of this complication increases with the length of gestation, the incidence being highest in the third trimester. Patients who survive to become pregnant again risk recurrent toxemia, the incidence running as high as 94.5 per cent in some surveys (Brown and Dodds, Peters). The overall recurrence rate of toxemia in recently published surveys is about 45 per cent. It has been observed that many of the toxemias are simply chronic hypertension. Repeated studies have borne out the observation that nearly all women who develop recurrent toxemia ultimately become hypertensive.

Dystocia (difficult childbirth)—This condition may complicate labor as a result of abnormalities in position, presentation or development of the fetus. Fetal size is generally not a problem. The average weight of full term infants is about seven pounds. Infants weighing more than 10 pounds are regarded as excessively large. Diabetic mothers have a tendency to produce large infants. The largest baby written up in the literature was one reported by Belcher, a stillborn female weighing 25 pounds.

Pelvic contracture is a cause of dystocia as are abnormalities of the genital tract including pelvic tumors, ovarian cysts, etc.

Abruptio placenta—This is a condition where separation of a normally situated placenta from its attachment occurs after about the twenty second week of pregnancy. If the detachment occurs earlier it eventuates in abortion. There is an attending hemorrhage which may be external (80 per cent of cases) or internal or concealed (20 per cent of cases), the latter being the most hazardous. The condition is classified as toxic when there is associated acute or chronic hypertension.

Marginal sinus rupture—This condition results from the placenta separating at its margin, disrupting the marginal sinus, a vein which courses along the edge of the placenta, causing hemorrhage. Delivery is usually initiated several hours after the onset of bleeding, often by elective cesarean section.

Placenta previa—In this condition the placenta rather than being inserted on the anterior or posterior wall or fundus of the uterus is situated in the lower uterine segment where it overlaps the internal os. It is associated with hemorrhage in the first stage of labor. Cesarean section has become the accepted method of delivery. The incidence is about once in every 200 deliveries.

Total placenta previa is diagnosed when the internal os is covered, partial placenta previa when it is only partially covered and marginal placenta previa (low implantation of the placenta) when it only encroaches upon the internal os.

Labor

Uncomplicated labor is contingent upon certain considerations in which the following factors figure prominently:

1. Size and shape of maternal pelvis, the principal types being gynecoid, anthropoid, android (masculine) and platypelloid. An inadequate outlet coupled with a large fetal head often results in a cephalopelvic disproportion (CPD), one of the indications for cesarean section. Pelvimetry is performed when such circumstances are suspected. See Fig. 19 in Chapter 3.
2. Size of the fetal head
3. Moldability of the fetal head

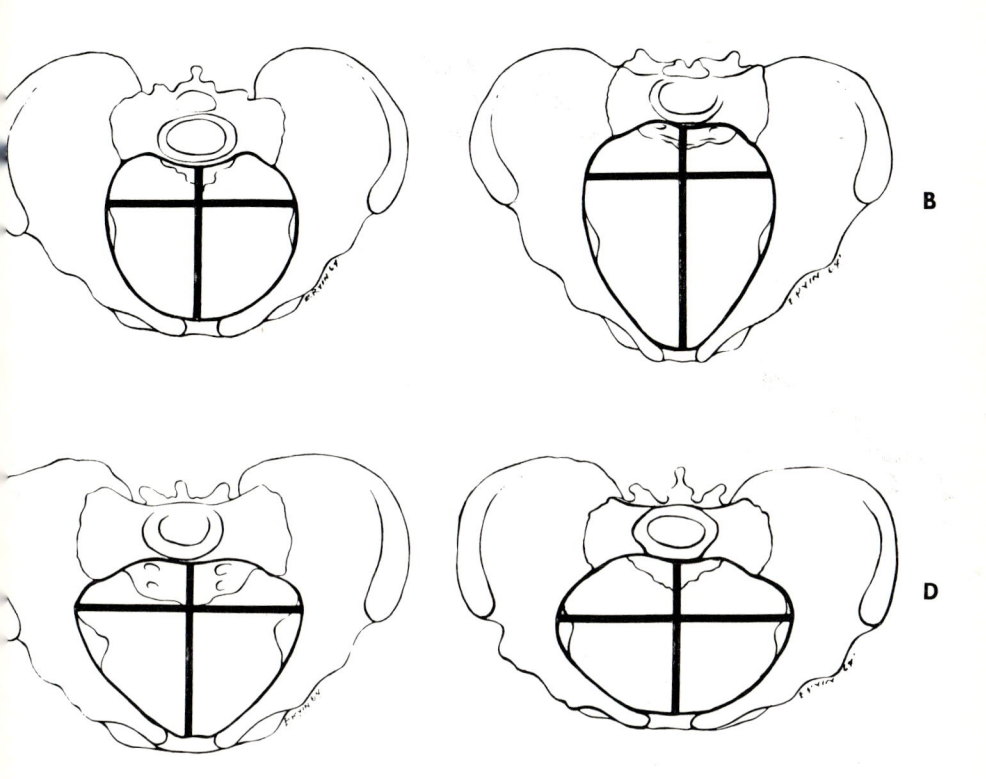

Figure 60 The four basic types of pelves. A line drawn through the widest transverse diameter divides the inlet into anterior and posterior segments. A line drawn through the longest anteroposterior diameter helps to show the inlet of the basic types: *A*, gynecoid; *B*, anthropoid; *C*, android; and *D*, platypelloid.

From Textbook of Obstetrics (C. V. Mosby Publishers)
Courtesy Drs. John C. Ullery and Zeph Hollenbeck.

4. Presentation and position
5. Force of uterine contractions

The Stages of Labor

Labor which may extend over a period of 14 or more hours in the primipara, to a much lesser duration in the multipara, is divided into three stages:

FIRST STAGE—labor begins with regular rhythmic uterine contractions until dilatation of the cervix is complete. The average duration is 12 hours for primiparas and seven hours for multiparas.

SECOND STAGE—extends from the time of complete cervical dilatation to rupture of the membranes and birth of the fetus. The duration is about one hour in primiparas and about 20 minutes in multiparas.

THIRD STAGE—covers the period from birth of the fetus to expulsion of the placenta and membranes. The duration is about 15 minutes for primiparas as well as multiparas.

Some patients deliver en route to the hospital or immediately following admission; however, the majority of patients are admitted to a pending room in the delivery suite where their labor is managed by an attending or house physician. Periodic examinations and notations are made in the medical record relative to the degree of effacement, station, fetal heart tones, presentation, position and progress of labor. Effacement refers to the gradual stretching of the cervical canal until only an aperture remains in place of the canal. See Fig. 61.

EFFACEMENT OF THE CERVIX

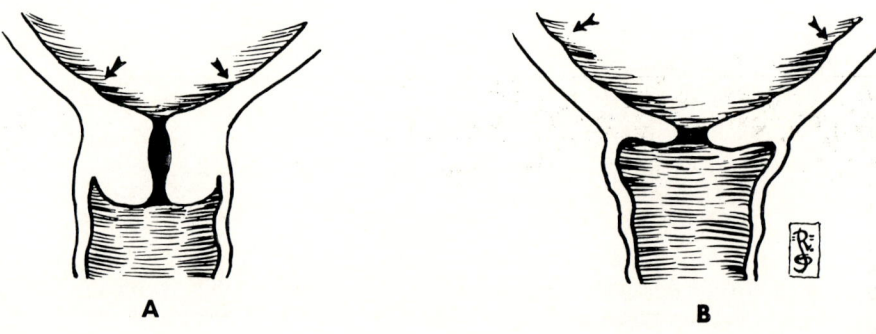

Figure 61 Effacement of the cervix. *A*, Near term the cervix is thick; only the internal os is dilated. *B*, Later the cervix is thinner; dilatation of the external os of the cervix has just begun. (Arrows indicate upper limit of the "lower segment.") (Original drawing by Anthony J. Ruppersberg, Jr.)

From Textbook of Obstetrics (C. V. Mosby Publishers)
Courtesy of Drs. John C. Ullery and Zeph Hollenbeck.

Effacement is expressed in terms of percentages. As a result of pressure from the fetal presenting part (that part of the fetus which is lowest in the maternal pelvis), the lower segment stretches and the external os opens.

Station refers to the degree of descent of the fetus in the birth canal. The degree of descent is recorded in numbers from one to five in combination with the following symbols:

○ location of the greatest diameter of the fetal presenting part at the level of the maternal ischial spine.

OBSTETRICS

— level above the maternal ischial spine.

+ level below the ischial spine.

The range of observations extends from — 1 to 5 to + 1 to 5, the plus symbol and higher number indicating the later stages of labor.

DETERMINATION OF STATION

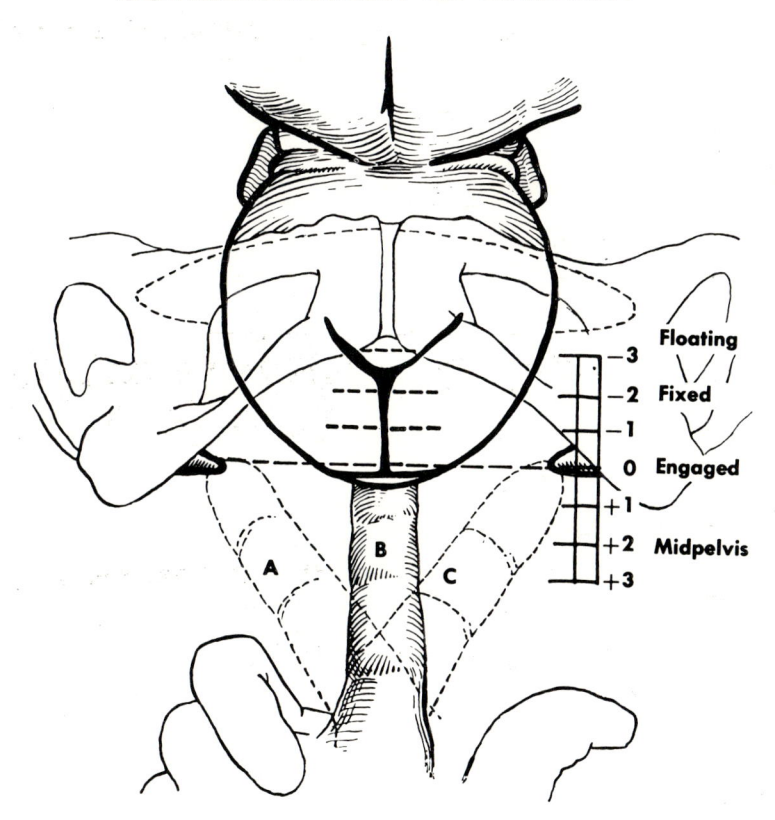

Figure 62 Diagrammatic representation of digital determination of the station of the presenting fetal part. (Original drawing by Anthony J. Ruppersberg, Jr.)

From Textbook of Obstetrics (C. V. Mosby Publishers)
Courtesy Drs. John C. Ullery and Zeph Hollenbeck.

Presentation

With the progress of labor, the physician takes note of the presentation, also called the fetal lie. This term refers to the relationship of the long axis (length) of the fetus to the long axis of the birth canal. Presentation may be longitudinal or transverse. In a longitudinal presentation, the infant is lined up parallel with the birth canal with either the head or buttocks presenting. This is the usual lie relationship. A transverse lie is much less common, occurring in only about 0.5 per cent of all deliveries. In the transverse lie the fetus rests crosswise to the birth canal with neither the head nor the buttocks presenting. These presentations are best exemplified by Fig. 63 and 64.

Presentation is determined by the first part of the fetus to descend into the birth canal. The variations may be summarized as follows:

CEPHALIC (vertex)—The incidence is about 96 per cent of all deliveries. The head presents at the pelvic inlet in any of the following manners:

Vertex—Usual presentation in 99 per cent of cephalic presentations. The top of the head enters the pelvic inlet. See Fig. 65

Brow—The incidence is about one in every 1,500 cephalic cases. The forehead presents at the pelvic inlet. See Fig. 66

Face—The incidence is about 0.5 per cent of cephalic cases. The fetal face is the presenting part. See Fig. 67

Parietal—The back portion of the top of the fetal head is the presenting part. See Fig. 68

BREECH (caudal)—The incidence is about four per cent of all deliveries. In this presentation the buttocks present at the pelvic inlet in any of the following variations:

Full breech (double or complete breech)—This occurs in about 7 per cent of all breech presentations. The thighs of the fetus are flexed upon the abdomen and the legs of the fetus are flexed on the thighs. See Fig. 69

Frank breech (single breech)—This occurs in about 63 per cent of breech deliveries. The legs of the fetus are straight up in front of the face with the fetus in a V-shape, the bottom of the V being the buttocks. See Fig. 70

Footling breech (incomplete breech)—This occurs in about 29 per cent of breech presentations. This may involve a double or single footling presenting. See Fig. 71

Knee breech—This is a rare occurrence with the fetus in a kneeling position at the pelvic inlet. See Fig. 72

LATERAL—This presentation involves the fetus in a transverse lie with shoulder, arm or side of the body presenting. The incidence is about 0.5 per cent of all deliveries.

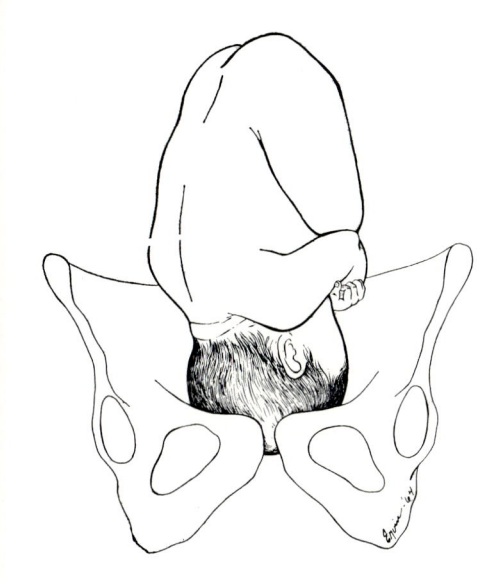

Figure 63 Longitudinal lie.

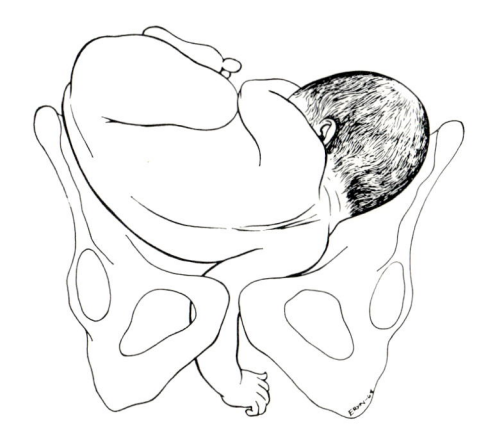

Figure 64 Transverse lie with the arm prolapsed.
*From Textbook of Obstetrics (C. V. Mosby Publishers)
Courtesy Drs. John C. Ullery and Zeph Hollenbeck.*

CEPHALIC PRESENTATIONS

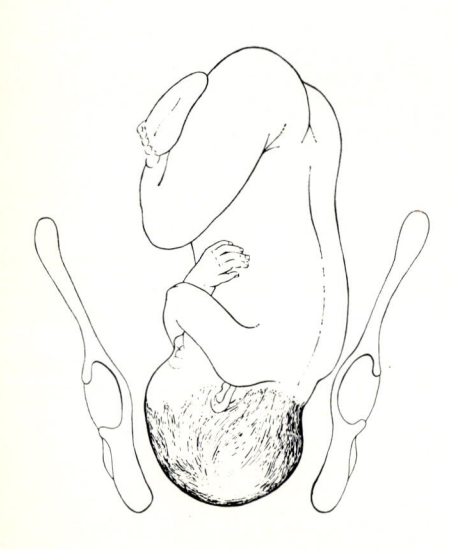

Figure 65   Vertex presentation.

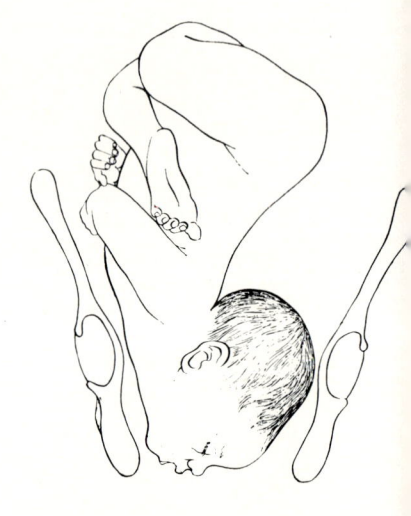

Figure 67   Face presentation.

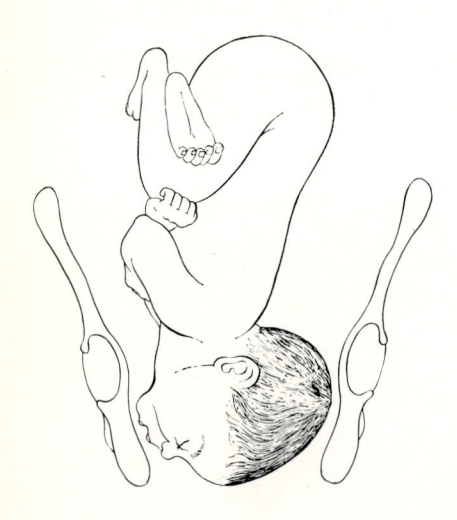

Figure 66   Brow presentation.

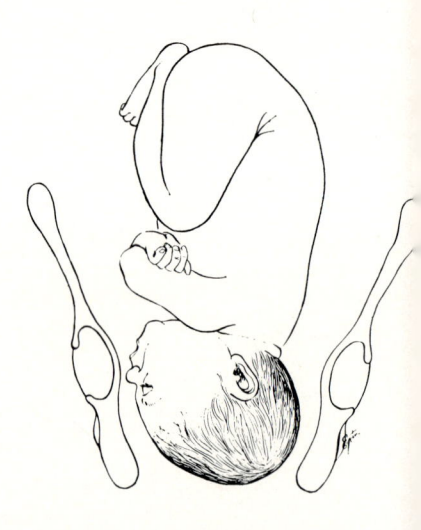

Figure 68   Parietal presentation.

From Textbook of Obstetrics (C. V. Mosby Publishers)
Courtesy Drs. John C. Ullery and Zeph Hollenbeck

OBSTETRICS

BREECH PRESENTATIONS

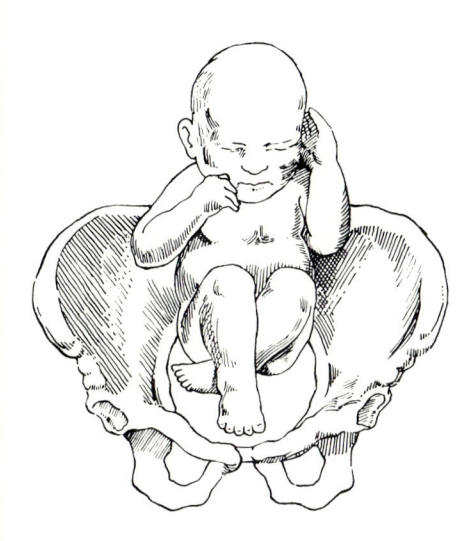

Figure 69 Full breech presentation.

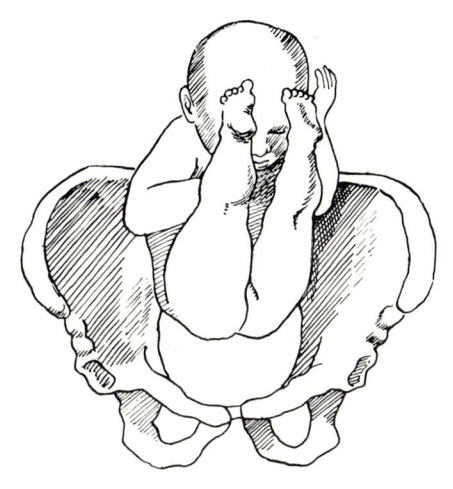

Figure 70 Frank breech presentation.

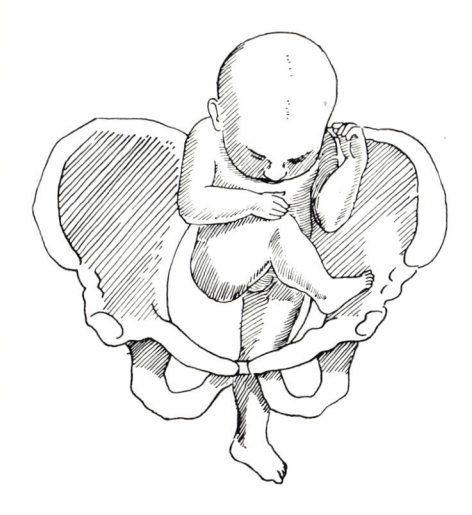

Figure 71 Single footling breech presentation.

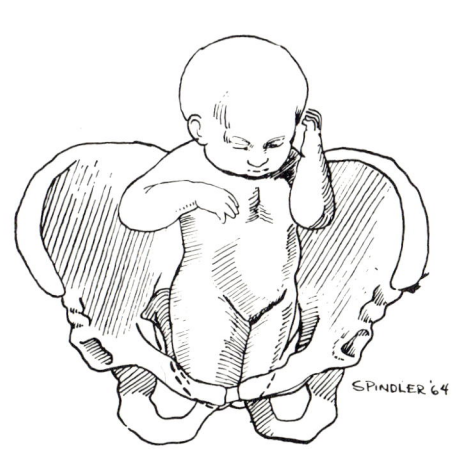

Figure 72 Knee-breech presentation.

From Textbook of Obstetrics (C. V. Mosby Publishers)
Courtesy Drs. John C. Ullery and Zeph Hollenbeck

Position

The maternal pelvis is divided into four quadrants and a right and left oblique landmark. The relationship of the presenting part of the fetus to the divisions and landmarks of the maternal pelvic inlet is called the **position**. The presenting part is usually in the obliquely anterior, transverse or obliquely posterior aspect of the left or right side of the pelvis. The six positions usually considered are: left anterior, left transverse, left posterior, right anterior, right transverse and right posterior. Transverse is used to indicate the halfway point between the anterior and posterior.

Position is indicated by a three letter abbreviation, e.g. L.O.A., R.O.P., L.O.T., etc. The first and last letter refer to the maternal pelvis and are abbreviations for right, left, anterior, posterior and transverse The middle initial indicates the presenting part of the fetus to include: O for occiput, M (mentum) for face, S for sacral (breech) and Sc. for scapula (transverse lie).

All of the abbreviations used are listed below:

I. Longitudinal presentations
   Cephalic (head)
      Vertex (occipital)

L.O.A.	left occipito-anterior
L.O.T.	left occipito-transverse
L.O.P.	left occipito-posterior
R.O.A.	right occipito-anterior
R.O.T.	right occipito-transverse
R.O.P.	right occipito-posterior

   Face (mental or mentum)

L.M.A.	left mento-anterior
L.M.T.	left mento-transverse
L.M.P.	left mento-posterior
R.M.A.	right mento-anterior
R.M.T.	right mento-transverse
R.M.P.	right mento-posterior

   Pelvic (Sacral; Breech)

L.S.A.	left sacro-anterior
S.A.	sacro-anterior
L.S.P.	left sacro-posterior
R.S.A.	right sacro-anterior
S.P.	sacro-posterior
R.S.P.	right sacro-posterior

II. Transverse Lie

Scapular (shoulder)

L. Sc. A.	left scapulo-anterior
L. Sc. P.	left scapulo-posterior
R. Sc. A.	right scapulo-anterior
R. Sc. P.	right scapulo-posterior

In breech presentations one of the hips rather than the sacrum is the presenting part; however, the sacrum continues to be used as a reference factor.

Version

When the fetal position is not favorable to delivery, the physician may elect to rotate the fetus to another position. When this maneuver is carried out manually it is known as **version.** External version is performed by manipulation of the fetus through the abdominal wall. Internal version is performed by the obstetrician's hand within the uterus.

In a cephalic version, the head of the fetus is rotated into the pelvic inlet. In a podalic version, the feet and buttocks are made to present at the pelvic inlet.

Attempts are sometimes made to convert the breech position to a vertex position by external version. Some of these positions correct themselves spontaneously before the thirty-fourth week. After that they are permanent unless they can be rotated and this is not often successful.

Rotation is sometimes accomplished by forceps applied to the fetal head. The Scanzoni double application of forceps for occiput posterior positions is one such example. Luikart-McLean forceps, sometimes supplemented by the Bill axis-traction handle are used in forceps rotations. In breech presentations, Piper forceps are used on the aftercoming head.

Induction of Labor

When circumstances dictate the delivery of an infant before normal spontaneous delivery has occurred, parturition is sometimes initiated by artificial means. This is usually accomplished after the thirty fifth week of gestation when a live infant is desired. Normal delivery occurs at about 40 weeks.

Indications for induction of labor include maternal complications such as toxemia, placenta previa, abruptio placenta, borderline pelvic disproportion, polyhydramnios, tuberculosis, kidney damage, heart disease, diabetes and malignancy. Fetal causes include diabetes in the mother, erythroblastosis and postmaturity.

The methods of inducing labor include: (1) stripping of membranes from cervix, (2) rupture of membranes (amniotomy) usually performed after the vertex is engaged to prevent prolapse of the cord, or (3) I.V. oxytocin drip when the cervix is ripe but the presenting part is not yet in the pelvis. Dührssens incision (incisions of an incompletely dilated cervix at 10, 2 and 6 o'clock) followed by forceps delivery and cervical repair are rarely used today.

Episiotomy

An episiotomy is an incision made in the perineum between the vulvar orifice and the anus. Two types of incision are used:

Median episiotomy—a midline incision is made from the posterior vaginal opening to the anus.

Mediolateral—begins at the posterior vaginal opening but is carried sideways away from the anus at about a 30 degree angle.

This operation is performed to prevent lacerations of the perineal tissues, as well as excessive stretching of the muscles and fascia of the perineum. It shortens the second stage of labor by 15 to 30 minutes. Another advantage is that the incision is easier to repair than is a ragged laceration.

Delivery

Obstetrical delivery may assume the form of a spontaneous normal delivery or that of an assisted procedure requiring instruments or surgical intervention.

Spontaneous—This is a delivery which takes place without instrumentation by the obstetrician. Such deliveries are most frequent with premature infants or in multiparas with large pelves and rapid labors.

Forceps—These are scoop-like instruments placed about the head of the fetus in order to extract it from the birth canal or to rotate its head within the vagina. Forceps are never applied to any part of the fetal body other than the head.

Low forceps—These are used when the skull of the fetus has reached the pelvic floor, the position is direct L.O.A. or R.O.A. and the scalp of the infant can be seen with each contraction. Elective low forceps are usually combined with episiotomy to eliminate the last 15 to 30 minutes of labor during which time injury may occur to the fetal head and/or the distended perineum.

Midforceps—These are rarely used unless there is a definite indication for termination of labor. Cesarean section is usually employed when delivery must be carried out before the fetal head is engaged in the pelvis.

High forceps—The presenting part lies between the plane of the inlet and the ischial spines.

Breech delivery occurs in about three per cent of all deliveries when the infant weighs five pounds eight ounces or more.

Spontaneous breech delivery—This is more likely to occur with premature infants.

Complete breech extraction—The entire infant is manually extracted from the birth canal. This method of delivery is more common in complete (full breech) than with frank breech because in complete breech the feet and buttocks lie in the vagina while in the frank breech they must be brought out from within the uterus. The Mauriceau maneuver is sometimes used to deliver the aftercoming head.

Partial breech extraction (assisted breech delivery)—This describes spontaneous delivery of the infant from feet to umbilicus after which the shoulders and head are extracted by the obstetrician. Piper forceps are sometimes used.

Perinatal mortality (infant deaths occurring between the 28th week of gestation and one week postpartum) for all breech deliveries averages about 20 per cent, the principal causes being anoxia, injury and complications or prematurity. The figure is still considerably higher than that for vertex deliveries if it is corrected to exclude premature and malformed infants as well as those already dead at the onset of labor.

The Placenta

Anatomically, the placenta connects the fetus to the uterine wall and is the organ by means of which the fetal nutritive, respiratory and excretory functions are carried out. It consists of a fetal and a maternal portion. The chorion (fetal portion) or superficial portion is covered by a smooth glistening membrane continuous with the amnion (sheath or covering of the umbilical cord). The maternal or deep portion of the placenta is composed of lobes of irregular outline covered by a transparent membrane of fetal origin. At the edge of the placenta there is a large vein, the marginal sinus, which serves as a return route for some of the maternal blood from the organ.

A short time after the birth of the infant, the placenta and membranes are expelled. Rupture of uterine vessels occurs in the process; however, postpartum hemorrhage is avoided as a result of firm contractions by the uterine muscular fibers. In addition, oxytocins such as pitocin are used to insure contraction of the uterus.

The placenta sometimes exhibits anomalous formation, attachment and surface markings. The following terms are used to describe such abnormalities.

Types of Placenta

Accessory—placental tissue apart from the main placenta.

Accreta (placenta accreta)—anomalous adherence of the placenta to the uterine wall.

Adherent—a placenta which adheres closely to the uterine wall.

Annular—a placenta extending within the uterus in a ring-like fashion.

Battledore—a placenta with the cord inserted at its edge.

Bidiscoidal—a placenta consisting of two flat circular masses.

Bilobed (bilobate)—a placenta made up of two lobes.

Bipartite (placenta bipartita)—a placenta consisting of two lobes.

Circumvallate (placenta circumvallata)—a placenta in which the attached membranes are doubled back over the edge of the placenta containing a ringed infarct raised from its surface.

Cirsoid (placenta cirsoides)—a placenta with varicose-like vessels.

Dimidiate (placenta dimidiata)—two lobed placenta.

Discoid (placenta discoidea)—disc shaped placenta.

Duplex—a two lobed placenta.

Fundal—a normally attached placenta.

Furcate—a lobed placenta.

Horseshoe—a half moon-shaped placenta sometimes seen in twin pregnancies.

Incarcerated—a retained placenta as a result of irregular uterine contractions.

Increta (placenta increta)—a placenta with abnormal adherence to, and penetration of the uterine wall.

Lobed—a placenta consisting of a lobe-like formation.

Marginalis (placenta marginalis or marginata)—a placenta around which is found a more than usual amount of raised infarcted tissue.

Multilobed (placenta multipartita)—a placenta made up of more than three lobes.

Nappiformis—same as circumvallata.

Panduriform (placenta panduriformis)—two placental halves arranged in a shape resembling a violin.

Percreta—an abnormally adherent placenta with invasion of the uterine wall to the serosa often eventuating in uterine rupture.

Reflexa (placenta reflexa)—a placenta with a thickened edge which appears to turn back upon itself.

Reniformis—a kidney-shaped placenta.

Schultze's—a placenta with its central portion coming before the outer border.

Spuria—an accessory placenta with no vascular attachment to the main placenta.

Stone—a calcified placenta.

Succenturiate (placenta succenturiata)—an accessory placenta with an artery and vein connecting it to the main placenta.

Trilobate (placenta triloba)—a three lobed placenta.

Triplex—a three lobed placenta.

Truffee—a placenta dotted with small dark red infarcts.

Velamentous—the umbilical cord is attached on the adjoining membranes.

Zonular—same as annular.

Cesarean Section

Cesarean section consists of the delivery of the newborn infant through an incision in the abdominal wall and uterus. There are numerous indications for this operation which include: CPD (cephalopelvic disproportion), previous cesarean section, previous operation for prolapse, anomalies of fetal posture and position, primary uterine inertia, antepartum hemorrhage from placenta previa or abruptio placentae with undilated cervix, failed trial of labor, some cases of toxemia or diabetes, elderly primigravida with previous abortions, failed forceps, cord prolapse, previous incisions in the uterus which might have left a weakening scar, previous cervical repairs, and some cases of iso-immunization.

The lower segment operation (low cervical cesarean section) is most commonly preferred for a number of reasons. The incision runs parallel to the muscle fibers in the cervix instead of across them in the body, peritonealization is carried out more effectively, the scar is less likely to rupture in future pregnancies, but if it does, there is less danger to mother and child. When rupture of the uterus occurs hysterectomy is not always necessary. If the rent is not extensive and is favorably situated, it is simply sutured. There remains the risk of rupture through the scar with future pregnancies.

The classical cesarean section is used in cases where hysterectomy or tubal sterilization will follow delivery. Other operations sometimes performed with cesarean section include appendectomy, herniorrhaphy, ovarian cystectomy, and uterine myomectomy.

Postoperative complications most often seen in cesarean section include pulmonary embolism, hemorrhage, infection and anesthetic hazards. The mortality rate shown in a survey of 16,000 sections performed in New York City from 1954-1955 (Ehrhardt et al.) was 0.2 per cent. Infant mortality varies between 4 and 8 per cent.

Cervical Cesarean Section Technic

The patient is placed in the Trendelenburg position and catheterized. A midline incision is made extending from a point immediately below the umbilicus to the symphysis pubis. The wound edges are retracted to expose the lower uterine segment along with the bladder and its uterine reflection. The vesicouterine peritoneum is incised transversely just below the firm attachment of the peritoneum to the upper uterine segment. Using finger dissection, the inferior flap is gently dissected toward the pelvis along with the bladder. A rounded retractor is used to hold the bladder out of the operative field.

The lower uterine segment is incised at the upper pole of the intended incision. Care is taken to avoid opening the amniotic sac. Bandage scissors are used to extend the incision to the lower pole. Bleeding is controlled with ring forceps.

A finger is introduced into the baby's mouth and the infant's face is brought into the incision. The chin is delivered first, over the upper angle of the incision, and then the rest of the head by flexion.

Bleeding is controlled with hemostatic clamps. Pituitrin is injected into the uterus. The placenta is removed manually after delivery of the infant. The uterus is packed with gauze with an end allowed to project out through the vagina.

Interrupted sutures of # 1 20-day catgut are placed down to the mucosa. A second row of sutures is placed external to the first which also include the fascia. The fascia is closed with interrupted sutures with one side slightly overlapping the other. Insert mattress sutures are used as required to control bleeding. The reflected vesicouterine peritoneum is closed by fastening the superior flap over the upper pole of the uterine incision with a few stitches and then bringing the inferior flap over the entire incision, closing it with continuous suture of # 1 chromic catgut. The knot is buried under the peritoneum.

DIAGNOSES IN PREGNANCY

Abdominal pregnancy
Abortion
  complete
  habitual
  incomplete
  inevitable
  missed
  therapeutic
  threatened
Abruptio placentae
Adherent placenta
Amniotic adhesions of fetus
Amniotic cyst
Caput succedaneum
Cephalopelvic disproportion
Cervical pregnancy (ectopic)
Chorioadenoma
Choriocarcinoma
Chorioepithelioma
Cornual pregnancy (ectopic)
Cyst of placenta
False labor

Fetal asphyxia
Fetus papyraceus
Fibrosis of placenta
Hematoma of placenta
Hydatidiform mole
Hydrorrhea gravidarum
Infarction of placenta
Intraligamentous pregnancy (ectopic)
Lithopedion
Low insertion of placenta
Missed abortion
Oligohydramnios
Omphalomesenteric duct
Ovarian pregnancy (ectopic)
Patent vitelline duct
Pelvic deformities (maternal)
  android
  assimilation
  coxalgic
  cretin
  dwarf type
  flat

DIAGNOSES IN PREGNANCY (continued)

    kyphotic
    masculine
    Nagele's
    obliquely contracted
    osteomalacia
    rachitic
    Robert's
    scoliotic
    separation of symphysis pubis
    spondylolisthetic
    tuberculous funnel
Placenta accreta
Placenta duplex
Placenta circumvallata
Placenta fenestrata
Placenta membranacea
Placenta multipartita
Placenta previa
    partial
    total
Placenta spuria
Placenta succenturiata
Placenta tripartita
Placentitis
Polyhydramnios
Pregnancy uterine delivered
    double ovum twins
    single ovum twins

Pregnancy uterine, delivered
    premature
    term
Pregnancy, uterine, undelivered
Premature birth, living child
Premature birth, neonatal death
Premature delivery, antepartum
    death
Premature delivery, intrapartum
    death
Premature rupture of membranes
Premature separation of normally
    implanted placenta
Premature separation of placenta
Retention of decidual fragment
Retention of membranes
Retention of placenta
Retention of placenta & membranes
Retention of placental fragment
Retention of portion of membranes
Syphilis of placenta
Term delivery, antepartum death
Term delivery, intrapartum death
Term delivery, neonatal death
Threatened abortion
Threatened premature delivery
Vasa previa

OPERATIONS IN PREGNANCY

Artificial rupture of membranes
Basiotripsy, fetal
Biopsy of placenta
Breech delivery
Breech extraction
    partial
    total
Cesarean section
    classic
    extraperitoneal
    low cervical
    Porro's
    vaginal
Cleidotomy, fetal
Conversion of position

Cranioclasis, fetal
Craniotomy, fetal
Dührssen's incision
Embryotomy
Episiotomy, LML
High forceps
Low forceps
Mid forceps
Podalic version
Removal of hydatidiform mole
Version
    external
    internal
    combined int. & ext.

11 { *Ophthalmology (Eye)*

Ophthalmology is the surgical specialty concerned with diseases of the eye and its associated structures to include the eyelids, ocular muscles and lacrimal apparatus. Surgery of the eyelids is not confined exclusively to ophthalmology since lid surgery is also performed by the plastic surgeon. Eye surgery is otherwise the exclusive domain of the ophthalmologist.

ANATOMY OF THE EYE AND ACCESSORY STRUCTURES

The eyes are spherical shaped organs with an anterior rounded projection which bulges from the globe proper. This is the portion of the eye which can be seen when the eyelids are open. The major part of the eye is housed in the cavity of the orbit which is lined by fat to afford further protection to the eyeball. The actual socket in which the eyeball moves consists of a thin membranous sac, the *fascia bulbi* (Tenon's capsule) which extends from the optic nerve at the back of the eyeball to the ciliary region toward the front of the eyeball.

The eyeball, per se, consists of three tunics or coverings which include:
(1) a fibrous tunic (sclera behind and cornea in front)
(2) a vascular, pigmented tunic (choroid, ciliary body and iris)
(3) a nervous tunic (retina)

The sclera (white of the eye) is the outermost tough layer which gives the eyeball its shape. It covers the entire eyeball as the sclera on the back and sides and continues as the transparent cornea over the front of the eye. The point at which the sclera continues as the cornea is called the sclerocorneal junction.

The middle (vascular) tunic contains an abundance of pigment and blood vessels. The posterior five-sixths of the middle layer consists of the choroid, while the anterior portion is comprised of the ciliary body, suspensory ligament and iris. The iris is that portion of the eye around the pupil which we refer to when we speak of the color of the eyes.

The innermost tunic of the eye, consisting of the retina, does not cover the entire eyeball. It extends from the optic nerve at the back of the eyeball as far forward, toward the front of the eyeball, as the ciliary body where it terminates in the ora serrata. Beyond this point it extends only as a non-nervous, pigmented membrane over the back of the ciliary processes and iris.

The eyegrounds (fundus of the eye) may be examined by the physician with an instrument called an ophthalmoscope. This is a fundoscopic examination of the eyes which permits the physician to see through the cornea, pupil, lens and eye fluids into the retina. The optic disc is also visible in this examination, representing the point at which the optic nerve enters the retina.

The eyeball is not a solid organ. It actually contains a large hollow interior consisting of the anterior and posterior cavities. The posterior cavity is the greater of the two, consisting of all of the area behind the lens. It contains a gelatinous substance, the vitreous humor, which provides intraocular pressure and helps to support the layers of the eyeball.

The anterior cavity, situated in front of the lens, consists of an anterior and posterior chamber. A clear fluid called the aqueous humor fills the entire anterior cavity.

The muscles of the eye are extrinsic and intrinsic in type. The intrinsic muscles consist of the ciliary muscles and iris and are involuntary. The extrinsic muscles are voluntary muscles which control the movements of the eye. They are the inferior, superior, lateral and medial rectus and the inferior and superior oblique muscles.

ACCESSORY STRUCTURES OF THE EYE

The accessory structures of the eye consist of the eyelids, eyebrows, cilia (eyelashes) and lacrimal apparatus.

The opening between the eyelids through which the eye can be seen is known as the *palpebral fissure*. The point at which the upper and lower lids come together, closest to the upper nose, is the *inner canthus*. The outer corner of the lids is the *outer canthus*. The thickened margin of the eyelids is called the *tarsal plate*.

An important accessory structure of the eye is the lacrimal apparatus consisting of the lacrimal gland which secretes tears, lacrimal ducts (lacrimal canals), lacrimal sac and the nasolacrimal duct through which the secretions are carried into the nasal cavity.

These passages sometimes become occluded to the point where surgery is indicated. The operation for drainage of the lacrimal sac is called a dacryocystostomy. When a channel must be established between the lacrimal sac and the nasal cavity an operation called a dacryocystorhinostomy is performed.

OPHTHALMOLOGY

SECTION THROUGH RIGHT EYE.

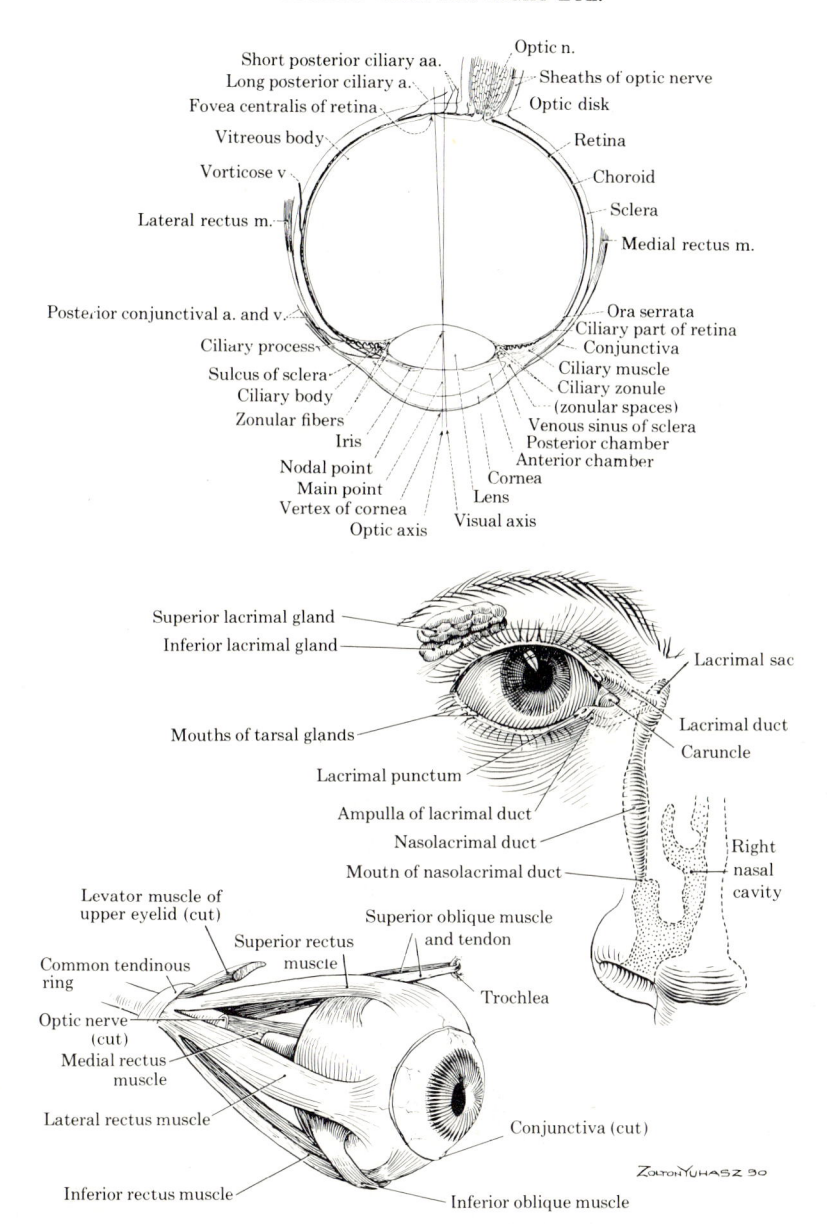

THE EYE AND RELATED STRUCTURES

Figure 73   The Eye and related structures

*From Dorland's Illustrated Medical Dictionary 24th Edition
Courtesy W. B. Saunders Company*

ANATOMIC FEATURES OF THE EYE AND ACCESSORY STRUCTURES

Ampulla (pl. ampullae)
Annular plexus
Anterior chamber
Aqueous humor
Bowman's membrane
Canal of Schlemm
Canthus
Capsula lentis
Capsule of the lens
Capsule of Tenon
Caruncle
Choroid
Cilia (eyelashes)
Ciliaris muscle
Ciliary body
Ciliary processes
Ciliary veins
Conjunctiva
Cornea
Crystalline humor
Crystalline lens
Cul-de-sac
Descemet's membrane
Eyeball
Fascia bulbi (capsule of Tenon)
Fovea centralis
Hyaloid canal
Hyaloid membrane
Inferior fornix
Infratrochlear nerve
Intraepithelial plexus
Iris
Jacob's membrane (rods & cones)
Lacrimal duct
Lacrimal gland
Lacrimal papilla
Lacrimal sac
Lacus lacrimalis
Lamina basalis
Lamina choriocapillaris
Lamina cribrosa sclerae
Lamina suprachoroidea
Lamina vasculosa
Lens
Ligament of Zinn

Limbus
Macula lutea
Meibomian glands (tarsal)
Membrane of Demours
Membrane of Descemet
Muscles of the eye
    Levator palpebrae superi
    Obliquus inferior
    Obliquus superior
    Rectus inferior
    Rectus lateralis
    Rectus medialis
    Rectus superior
Nasolacrimal duct
Optic disk
Optic nerve
Ora serrata of retina
Orbicularis ciliaris
Orbicularis oculi
Palpebral commissure
Palpebral fissure
Pars ciliaris retinae
Pars iridica retinae
Pars optica retinae
Pectinate ligament of the iris
Pectinate villi
Periscleral space
Plica semilunaris
Posterior chamber
Punctum lacrimale
Pupil
Retina (tunica interna)
Sclera
Scleral spur
Sclerocorneal junction
Sinus venosus sclerae
Space of Tenon
Spaces of Fontana
Spatia zonularia (canal of Petit)
Sphincter pupillae
Stratum intermedium
Subepithelial plexus
Substantia propria
Superior tendon of Lockwood
Suspensory ligament of lens

ANATOMIC FEATURES OF THE EYE AND ACCESSORY STRUCTURES (Continued)

Tapetum
Tarsal plates (tarsi)
Tarsus
Tendon of Lockwood
Tendon of Zinn
Tenon's capsule
Trochlea
Tunica vasculosa
Uvea
Vaginae bulbi (Tenon's capsule)
Vascular tunic
Venae vorticosae
Vitreous body
Vitreous humor
Zonula ciliaris
Zonule of Zinn

EYE ABBREVIATIONS

O.D. — right eye (oculus dexter) O.U. — both eyes (oculi unitas)
O.S. — left eye (oculus sinister)

SOME MEDICATIONS USED IN EYE SURGERY

Acetylcholine 1:10,000
Alpha Chymar Trypsin
Atropine
Cocaine
Cortisone
Dexametazone
Epinephrine
Hyaluronidase
Methylcellulose
Neosporin
Novocain-Suprarenin
Pilocarpine
Ringer's solution
Saline solution
Sodium Sulamyd 10% Ointment
Suprarenin
White's Ointment
Yellow Oxide of Mercury
Xylocaine

Simple Iridectomy

After satisfactory anesthesia, the eyeball was fixed with fixation forceps. The tip of the keratome was placed about 1 mm. above the limbus at the 12 o'clock position and gently directed forward until the point could be detected in the anterior chamber. The handle of the keratome was positioned downward somewhat until the blade was parallel to the plane of the iris and projected forward to a point approximating the center of the pupil. The handle of the keratome was lowered somewhat and the instrument gently withdrawn.

A closed iris forceps was inserted through the original incision to a point almost at the pupillary border where the forceps was opened to bite a small fold of iris. This tissue was brought out through the wound and removed with the aid of de Wecker scissors creating a small coloboma as the scissors were applied in the vertical meridian of the cornea.

The iris pillars were repositioned with the aid of a spatula. The anterior chamber was irrigated with saline.

Iridencleisis

Under local anesthesia and after a subconjunctival injection of 2% cocaine above the upper limbus, a conjunctival flap including the conjunctiva and episclera was made.

A limbal incision was made with a keratome through which an iris forceps was inserted. The iris was grasped near the edge of the pupil and drawn out until the pigment epithelium on the back of the iridial tent could be seen. The sphincter pupillae was cut on either side of the forceps. A piece of sclera adjacent to the limbal incision was snipped off with the use of a scleral punch. A continuous silk suture was placed through the conjunctival flap.

Peripheral Iridectomy

After routine preparation and draping of the lids, a 00000 black silk bridle suture was placed through the superior rectus muscle. A conjunctival flap was made approximately 5 mm. in depth and dissected down to the limbus. A keratome incision was made and enlarged slightly with scissors. The anterior capsule was grasped and pulled free. Lens material was expressed. A small basal iridectomy was performed. In attempting to remove more of the posterior capsule, a small amount of vitreous was lost.

The conjunctiva was closed with a running 00000 black silk suture. Sodium Sulamyd Ointment and atropine drops of 1% were instilled. An eye pad and shield were applied.

Extracapsular Cataract Extraction

After satisfactory anesthesia, preparation and draping of the operative area, a capsule forceps was introduced through the coloboma and the teeth of this forceps used to grasp the anterior capsule just below the pupillary center. A piece of capsule was removed from the lens in a gentle maneuver after the capsule was incised in two directions with a cystotome. A strabismus hook was used to express the lens, applying pressure from below. During this procedure the assistant pulled the corneal lip downward with gentle traction on the corneal suture and the surgeon held a spoon on the upper lip of the wound. The lens was delivered by elevating the lens from behind as it was withdrawn. The sutures were tied and the remnants of the lens washed out. The pillars of the iris were replaced with a spatula.

Atropine and White's Ointment were applied to the operated eye and both eyes were bandaged.

Cryogenic Eye Surgery

The clinical application of extremely cold temperatures produced in specialized surgical instruments through the use of special refrigerants such as Freon 12 or liquid nitrogen is called cryosurgery. Although this technique has found acceptance in various surgical specialties, its greatest value has been recognized in the delicate surgery of the eye. The surgical use of cold for cataract extraction, particularly intumescent cataract was introduced in 1961 by Dr. T. Krwawicz of the Medical Academy in Lublin, Poland. The technique is widely accepted in Europe and South America, but is just being recognized in the United States. It is gaining further acceptance in the treatment of retinal detachment, dendritic ulcers of the cornea, glaucoma, tumor biopsy, tumor therapy and iris prolapse.

Pictured below is the Thomas Cryoptor, specially designed for cataract surgery.

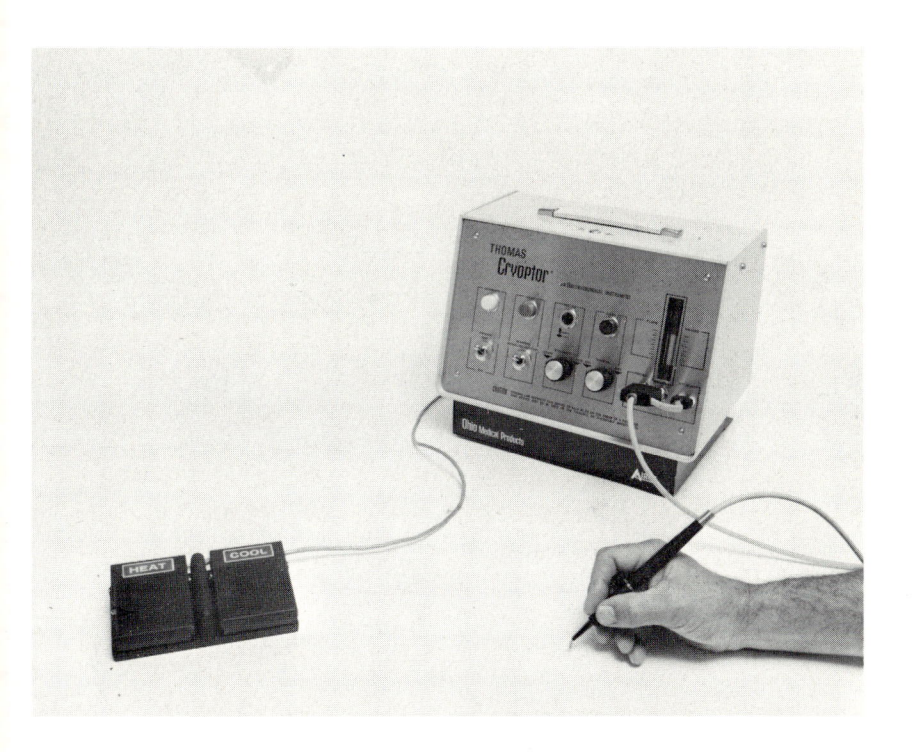

Figure 74 Thomas Cryopter designed for cryogenic cataract extraction.

Courtesy Ohio Medical Products, 1400 East Washington Avenue, Madison, Wisc. 53701

Intracapsular Cataract Extraction

After satisfactory akinesia of the lids and injection of Novocain-Suprarenin, the superior rectus was anesthetized by a cocaine soaked applicator.

A bridle suture was inserted beneath the superior rectus muscle. A Desmarres lid elevator was used to keep the eye open during the procedure.

A conjunctival flap was developed by dissecting the conjunctiva in the region of the upper limbus and undermining it. A needle of a double armed suture was introduced through the episclera and superficial sclera horizontally at the 12 o'clock position about 3 mm. above the cornea. Another needle was then inserted through the superficial layers of the cornea in a vertical manner. Both needles were brought out through the conjunctival flap 8 mm. from its free border.

A Graefe knife was used for the corneal section being introduced into the cornea at the limbus. As the tip of the knife entered the anterior chamber, the handle was lowered somewhat and the blade advanced parallel to the plane of the iris to the opposite limbus. The knife was then advanced upward and section carried out in a back and forth fashion bringing the cutting edge of the knife toward the surgeon. The lens was extracted with the use of Arruga's forceps in a tumbling fashion. The sutures were tied and the iris reposited.

Intracapsular Cataract Extraction With Iridectomy

The patient was admitted with a senile cataract of the right eye. She had a postsurgical aphakia of the left eye as well as a postoperative coloboma of the left iris.

After routine preparation and draping of the area, a 00000 black silk superior rectus bridle suture was placed. A Beaver blade was used to make a limbal groove superiorly from 3 to 9 o'clock. Three interrupted 0000000 black silk sutures were placed at 10, 12 and 2 o'clock.

A keratome incision was made and enlarged with scissors. A basal iridectomy was performed at 12 o'clock. The lens was delivered by a tumbling procedure with an erisophake. Sutures were tightened. Two additional sutures were placed to completely close the wound. An air bubble was instilled in the anterior chamber and the iris pillars replaced. An eye pad and shield were applied.

Recession of Ocular Muscles—correction for strabismus

Local anesthesia is obtained using cocaine instillation and 2% Novocain-Suprarenin injection into the muscle and its insertion.

A vertical incision is made through the conjunctiva 6 mm. from the limbus which is freed from the underlying Tenon's capsule. A strabismus hook is inserted under the muscle through a buttonhole made in Tenon's capsule, below the lower edge of the muscle. A similar opening is made where the point of the hook causes the capsule to bulge. The point of the hook is then introduced through this second opening following which another hook is also placed into this buttonhole. It is carried in the opposite direction, under the muscle, until its point comes up through the first hole. The muscle belly and tendon now rest on the hooks.

An incision is made on both edges of the tendon and the muscle tendon freed of its capsular sheath. The recession suture is placed at the proximal end of the tendon. The tendon is cut from its scleral insertion and the capsular adhesions under the muscle belly are lysed. The two ends of the sutures are passed through the superficial layers of the sclera and then through the tendon stump and tied.

The conjunctival wound is sutured and binocular dressing applied.

Kuhnt-Szymanowski Operation for Spastic Ectropion of the Lower Eyelid

After routine preparation and draping of the area and 2% Xylocaine local infiltration anesthesia, the lower lid was split between the skin surface and the conjunctivotarsal area in the lateral two-thirds of the lid. A skin triangle was then excised from the conjunctivotarsal surface of the lower lid and this surface was brought together with the other using 00000 black silk suture.

The skin was undermined so as to present a sliding flap which could be moved up into the triangular defect laterally and pulled up and closed with seven interrupted 00000 black silk sutures.

The previously split lid was then reapproximated by a through-and-through 00000 black silk suture onto a button.

Sodium Sulamyd 10% Ointment was instilled and pressure dressing was applied.

Flapping of Conjunctiva, Rt. Eye

After routine preparation and draping of the lids, the conjunctiva was excised at the limbus from 3 o'clock to 9 o'clock. It was then dissected free up into the superior cul-de-sac. Two 00000 black silk sutures were placed at 10 o'clock and 2 o'clock and hooked into the conjunctiva in the lower cul-de-sac so as to pull a flap of the conjunctiva over the corneal ulcer. The central suture was also incised so as to give complete corneal coverage. Sodium Sulamyd Ointment was instilled and an eye pad applied.

Excision of Chalazion

The area of the right eye was prepared and draped in the usual manner. Several drops of 4% cocaine were instilled. The portion of the eyelid containing the tumefaction was grasped in a chalazion forceps. The lid was everted and several drops of Novocain-Suprarenin were placed around the chalazion.

After a few minutes, a vertical incision was made on the conjunctival side, with care, to avoid injury to the lid margins. The contents of the chalazion were evacuated with a small curet. The cystic wall was gently removed with scissors. No excessive bleeding was encountered.

Transplant of Pterygium

Under general anesthesia, the head of the pterygium was grasped with a forceps and it was removed from the cornea on which it was encroaching with a fine knife. The portion of the cornea from which the pterygium had been removed was carefully curetted.

The pterygium was undermined along with the conjunctiva proximal to it. This extended toward the lower cul-de-sac. The head of the pterygium was then slightly elevated. A double-armed mattress suture was inserted through the head of the pterygium. Two needles were passed through the conjunctival pocket which had been formed beneath. The suture was tied and the pterygium buried.

Partial Penetrating Keratoplasty

With the trephine centered on the pupil and the host eye in myosis (or: miosis) the Paufique trephine was applied perpendicularly to the surface of the cornea and a graft removed with care to insure regular corneal margins. The graft measured 7 mm.

A vertical incision was made with the trephine and scissors in the host eye, without bevel. The graft was sutured in place using direct radial sutures, edge-to-edge, placed 1 mm. from the corneal margins and passing through the middle portion of the stroma.

A Grieshaber 83/4 needle with virgin silk and a Barraquer mosquito needle holder were used to seal the anterior chamber.

Three milligrams of Dexametazone were injected under the conjunctiva to reduce postoperative reactions.

Reattachment of Retina by Electric Cautery

A conjunctival incision was made inferiorly about 3 to 9 o'clock. The inferior rectus muscle was dissected free. The conjunctiva and Tenon's capsule were dissected back to the posterior globe area. Multiple $\frac{1}{2}$ mm.

retinal cautery punctures were made with good fluid drainage in both inferior quadrants. The conjunctiva was closed with a running 00000 black silk suture. Sodium Sulamyd 10% Ointment was instilled in the conjunctival sac.

Discission of the Lens

A sickle-shaped Ziegler knife was introduced at the limbus subconjunctivally. Keeping its flat surface parallel to the plane of the iris, it was further introduced through the cornea until the tip of the instrument extended to the upper border of the pupil. The cutting edge was directed towards the lens making a deep vertical cut into the capsule and anterior lens. A horizontal incision was made and the instrument removed via the route of introduction.

Removal of Meshed Ball Implant; Insertion of Polyethylene Implant with mucous membrane graft to conjunctiva covering the implant

After routine preparation and draping of the lids, enucleation scissors were used to dissect free the meshed implant ball that showed about an 8 mm. exposure anteriorly. A 15 mm. polyethylene ball was inserted.

Tenon's capsule and the scleral area were dissected free from the conjunctiva. Interrupted 0000 chromic sutures were used to close this defect. A mucous membrane graft approximately 1 cm. wide by 3 cm. long was then removed from the inner side of the lower lip. It was attached to the existing conjunctiva so as to give a complete closure using interrupted 00000 black silk sutures. Gentle pressure bandages were applied.

Evisceration of the Right Eye; Insertion of Plastic Ball

The patient was given a local anesthetic and a topical anesthetic was introduced into the conjunctival sac. A Good retractor was introduced. It was noted that the eye was considerably engorged and the conjunctiva was quite reddened. The iris was cloudy and the eyeball was under considerable tension.

The conjunctiva was incised in an elliptical fashion near the limbus. Dissection was then continued to the region of the limbus where the anterior chamber was entered with a keratome. Fluid from the anterior chamber was released and the eyeball relaxed.

By means of forceps the retina was removed. The iris was scraped free. The incision was enlarged in a T-shaped fashion.

A Lucite plastic ball was introduced. The sclera was approximated with interrupted 00000 plain suture. The conjunctiva was sutured similarly and closed with 00000 silk suture.

Dacryocystorhinostomy (Toti Operation)

Anesthesia was obtained by blocking the infratrochlear nerve with 2 cc. of a 2% solution of Novocain Hydrochloride with epinephrine hydrochloride. In addition to this, a cocaine-Suprarenin pledget was inserted on the inside of the nasal mucosa against the middle turbinate. This was followed by packing of this side of the nose.

An incision was made in the skin beginning from 3 to 5 mm. above the internal canthal ligament, curving outward as it was carried downward along the anterior lacrimal crest to a point immediately below the nasal duct.

A Mueller speculum was then introduced into the wound. The canthal ligament was then identified, beneath which, we were able to identify the lacrimal sac. The ligament was then incised vertically. The sac was gently teased away from the ligament. A longitudinal incision was then made the entire length of the sac on its nasal side. The periosteum beyond the lacrimal crests was then elevated and the anterior crest chiseled away. The mucous membrane of the nose was exposed and care was taken to avoid injury to this tissue. A 2 cm. piece of bone was removed from the ascending process of the maxilla and lacrimal bone with the use of a chisel and mallet.

A longitudinal incision was then made in the nasal mucosa opposite the one made in the lacrimal sac. The anterior and posterior lips of the nasal mucosa were then sutured with the matching sides of the sac in apposition.

The outer wound was closed by a few deep catgut sutures. Interrupted silk was used for the outer wound edges.

McLaughlin Canthoplasty, Lateral, Left

Following suitable premedication, the patient was taken to surgery and the face prepared with pHisoHex and draped. 1% Xylocaine containing ½ cc. of adrenalin to the ounce was used for local anesthesia.

A wedge-shaped area of tissue on the lateral canthus of the left eye, to include some of the lash margin, was excised in both the upper and lower lid areas. These areas were based with the narrow portion of the triangle medially. They were trimmed so that they would overlap accurately and give a new canthus. This would permit tears to flow out over the cheek from the lateral angle of the eye.

A 00000 dermalon suture was used to close the canthoplasty. It was sutured through-and-through the lid and tied over a small piece of polyethylene tubing used as a bolster. The remainder of the incision was closed into a crow's foot using 00000 dermalon cuticular suture and twists to follow, as necessary.

An ellipse of tissue in the left nasolabial fold measuring 2 cm. in width and 4 cm. in length was excised with skin, subcutaneous fat and scar. This was suitably defatted and undermined. Closure was accomplished with interrupted subcutaneous nylon sutures followed by 00000 dermalon cuticular sutures and twists, as necessary.

Fine moistened mesh gauze was placed over the wound. Some Terramycin Ointment was placed in the eye and an eye pad applied. A light pressure dressing was placed over the wound and the mouth was immobilized on the left side.

DISEASES OF THE EYE AND ORBIT

Abrasion of the cornea
Abscess of conjunctiva
Abscess of cornea
Abscess of orbit
Abscess of vitreous
Absence of eyeball
Achromatopsia (total color blindness)
Acne rosacea conjunctivitis
Acne rosacea keratitis
Actinomycosis of cornea
Adhesions of the conjunctiva
Albinism
Allergic pannus
Amaurosis
Amblyopia ex anopsia
Amyloidosis of conjunctiva
Anastomosis of retinal and
    choroidal vessels
Aneurysm in orbit
Angiopathy of retina
Aniridia
Aniseikonia
    anisometropsia predominating
    due to unilateral aphakia
Anisocoria
Anisometropia
Annular scleritis
Anomalous trichromatopsia
Anomalous vessels of papilla

Anomaly of optico-ciliary vessels
Anophthalmos
Anterior synechia
Aphakia (absence of lens)
Aplasia of fovea centralis
Arcus juvenilis
Arcus senilis
Argyrosis of cornea
Arteriosclerotic disease of retina
Arteriovenous aneurysm of retina
Astigmatism
    corneal irregular
    hypermetropic
    hypermetropic compound
    lenticular, irregular
    mixed
    myopic
    myopic compound
    due to asymmetric refraction
        of lens
    due to tilting of lens
Atropia gyrata of choroid
Atrophy of choroid
Atrophy of eyeball
Atrophy of iris
Atrophy of optic nerve
Atrophy of retina
Avulsion of eyeball
Avulsion of optic nerve

DISEASES OF THE EYE AND ORBIT (continued)

Band keratitis
Basal cell carcinoma of conjunctiva
Blastomycosis of cornea
Blennorrhea, inclusion
Blood staining of cornea
Blue sclera
Burn of cornea
Canal of Cloquet remnants
Cataract
  anterior polar
  anterior and posterior axial
    embryonal
  black
  central
  coralliformis
  diabetic
  floriformis
  heterochromic
  hypermature
  incipient
  lamellar zonular perinuclear
  mature
  morgagnian
  myotonic dystrophy
  nuclear
  polar, diabetic
  pyramidal
  secondary
  senile
  spindle-shaped
  syphilitic
  tetany
  total
  traumatic
Cataracta cerulea
Cataracta complicata
Cataracta congenita membranacea
Cataracta coronaria
Cataracta membranacea accreta
Cataracta neurodermatica
Cataracta ossea
Cavity of optic papilla
Chalcosis of cornea
Chemical burn
Cholesterol in retina
Cholesterol in vitreous

Chorioretinitis
  central
  senile
Cicatrix of limbus
Cilioretinal artery, persistent
Cilioretinal vein, persistent
Coloboma of choroid
Coloboma of ciliary body
Coloboma of iris, typical
Coloboma of iris, atypical
Coloboma of lens
Coloboma of optic nerve
Coloboma of vitreous
Color blindness
Commotio retinae
Concretions in conjunctiva
Conjunctival cyst
Conjunctivitis
  follicular
  infectious
  due to lagophthalmos
Contusion of cornea
Conus, congenital
  lateral
  oblique
  underlying
Corectopia
Cornea guttata
Cornea plana
Corneal degeneration
Corneal infiltrate
Corneal ulcer
Crescent
Crushing of optic nerve
Cyanosis of retina
Cyclophoria
Cyclopia
Cyclotropia
Cyst of iris
Cyst of retina
Cysticercosis of optic papilla
Cystoid cicatrix of limbus
Descemet's membrane defect
Descemetocele
Detachment of choroid
Detachment of retina

DISEASES OF THE EYE AND ORBIT (continued)

Detachment of vitreous
Diabetic iritis
Diabetic melanosis of cornea
Dichromatopsia
Disorganized globe
Distortion of lens
Drusen of choroid
Drusen of optic papilla
Dystrophy of cornea
  endothelial
  epithelial
  marginal
Eclipse blindness
Ectasia of cornea
Ectasia of sclera
Ectopia of lens
Ectropion uveae
Eczematous pannus
Edema of iris
Edema of macula
Embolism of retinal artery
Embryotoxon
Emmetropia
Emphysema of conjunctiva
Emphysema of orbit
Endophlebitis of retinal veins
Endophthalmitis
Enophthalmos
Epidermoid carcinoma of conjunctiva
Epidermoid carcinoma of cornea
Erosion of cornea
Esophoria
Esotropia
  alternating
  left
  right
  periodic
Excyclophoria
Excyclotropia
Exophoria
Exophthalmos
  due to pressure
  due to tower skull
Exotropia
  alternating
  left
  right
  periodic
Facet of cornea
Fibroma of conjunctiva
Fibroma of orbit
Fibroma of sclera
Fibrosarcoma of orbit
Fibrosis choroideae corrugans
Filariasis of orbit
Fistula of cornea
Fistula of orbit
Fistula of sclera
Foreign body in anterior chamber
Foreign body in ciliary body
Foreign body in cornea
Foreign body in iris
Foreign body in lens
Foreign body in optic nerve
Glaucoma
  absolute
  congestive
  noncongestive
  primary
Glioma
Gouty episcleritis
Gouty iritis
Granuloma of orbit
Hemangioma of choroid
Hemangioma of conjunctiva
Hemangioma of iris
Hemangioma of orbit
Hemangioma of retina
Hemangiomatosis of retina
Hematoma of orbit
Hemorrhage in orbit
Hemorrhage in retina
Hemorrhage in vitreous
Hemorrhage of iris
Hemosiderin deposit in old
  corneal scars
Hereditary atrophy of optic nerve
Hernia of vitreous into
  anterior chamber
Herpes iris of conjunctiva
Herpes ophthalmicus
Herpes simplex

DISEASES OF THE EYE AND ORBIT (continued)

Herpes zoster of cornea
Herpes zoster of iris
Heterochromia iridis
Heterochromic uveitis
Heterophoria
Heterotropia
  alternating
  left
  right
  periodic
Hole in retina
Hyaline degeneration
Hyaline formation in cornea
Hydrophthalmos
Hyperemia, conjunctival
Hyperemia of iris
Hyperemia of retina
  active
  passive
Hypermetropia
Hyperphoria
  left
  right
  alternating sursumduction
Hypertropia
  right
  left
  periodic
Hypoplasia of zonule
Hypopyon
Hypotony
  following loss of aqueous
  following loss of vitreous
Implantation cyst of iris
Incarceration of iris
Incyclophoria
Incyclotropia
Infantile glaucoma
Infarction of retina
  due to embolism
  due to thrombosis
Injury to cornea
Inversion of optic papilla
Iridencleisis
Iridocyclitis
Iridodialysis

Iridodonesis
Iridotasis
Iris bombe
Iritis
  sympathetic
  tuberculous
Irregular astigmatism
Ischemia of retina
Keloid of cornea
Keratectasia
Keratitis
  band
  bullosa
  deep
  dendritic
  disciformis
  due to lagophthalmos
  neuroparalytica
  parenchymatosa anaphylactica
  parenchymatous
  phlyctenular
  postvaccinulosa
  punctata leprosa
  punctata profunda
  purulent
  pustuliformis profunda
  superficial
  syphilitic
  tuberculous
  varicella
Keratocele
Keratoconjunctivitis sicca
Keratoconus
Keratomalacia
Keratomyosis
Lamellar separation of lens
Large angle gamma
Large angle kappa
Large physiologic cup
Late prolapse of iris
Lateral displacement
Lead incrustation of cornea
Leiomyoma of iris
Leiomyoma of orbit
Leiomyosarcoma of orbit
Lens with double focus

DISEASES OF THE EYE AND ORBIT (continued)

Lenticonus anterior
Lenticonus posterior
Lenticular astigmatism
Lentiglobus, posterior
Leprosy of cornea
Leptotrichosis of cornea
Leukemic infiltration of retina
Leukoma
Linea corneae senilis
Lipid degeneration of cornea
Lipoma of conjunctiva
Liposarcoma of orbit
Loss of vitreous
Luxation of eyeball
Luxation of lens
Lymphangiectasis of conjunctiva
Lymphangioma of conjunctiva
Lymphoma of conjunctiva
Lymphoma of orbit
Lymphosarcoma of conjunctiva
Lymphosarcoma of orbit
Macula
Macular degeneration
Macular displacement
Macular heredodegeneration
Megalocornea
Megalophthalmos
Melanoma, malignant of choroid
Melanoma, malignant of conjunctiva
Melanoma, malignant of orbit
Melanoma, malignant of uveal tract
Melanosis of cornea
Melanosis of iris
Melanosis of sclera
Membrana capsularis lentis posterior
Membrana epipapillaris
Microcornea
Microphakia
Microphthalmos
Miosis
Muscae volitantes
Mydriasis
Myiodesopsia
Myopia (near sightedness)
   axial
   curvature
   due to lens displacement
   due to increased refraction
     of nucleus of lens
   progressive
Nebula
Neuroepithelioma of retina
Neurofibroma of conjunctiva
Neurofibroma of cornea
Neurofibroma of optic nerve
Neurofibroma of orbit
Nevoid pigmentation
Night blindness
Notch of iris
Nystagmus
   of amblyopia, horizontal
   due to fatigue of nucleus
   rotary
   of labyrinthine origin
Occlusion of pupil
Opacity of cornea
Opacity in vitreous
Ophthalmia electrica
Optic neuritis
Orbital cellulitis
Orbital periostitis
Ossification of vitreous
Osteoma of orbital bone
Osteoma of sclera
Overaction of inferior oblique
Pannus degenerativus
Pannus trachomatosus
Panophthalmitis
Papilledema
Papilloma of caruncle
Papilloma of conjunctivitis
Paralysis of conjugate lateral
   movement (cortical)
Paralysis of conjugate lateral
   movement (supranuclear)
Paralysis of convergence (nuclear)
Paralysis of divergence (nuclear)
Paralysis of extrinsic muscles
Paralysis of intrinsic muscles
Paralysis of iris
Pemphigus
Penetrating wound of eyeball

DISEASES OF THE EYE AND ORBIT (continued)

Perforation of cornea
Peripheral wedge shaped opacities
Periphlebitis
Persistence of tunica vasculosa lentis
Persistent hyaline artery
Persistent pupillary membrane
Phakocele (hernia of lens)
Photophthalmia
Phthisis of eyeball
Pigment deposit in limbus
Pigmentation of choroid
Pigmentation of ciliary body
Pigmentation of conjunctiva
Pigmentation of iris
Pigmentation of optic papilla
Pigmented nevus of orbit
Pinguecula
Polycoria
Polyp of conjunctiva
Presbyopia
Presenile melanosis of cornea
Primary pigmented degeneration
   at retina
Prolapse of iris
Prolapse of vitreous
Protrusion of orbital fat
Pseudoneuritis of optic papilla
Pseudopterygium
Pterygium
Pupillary membrane
Radium necrosis of conjunctiva
Retinal hemorrhage
Retinal lipemia
Retinitis
  circinata
  diabetic
  disciformis
  exudativa
  gravidarum
  nephritica
  proliferans
  septic
Retinoblastoma
Retrobulbar neuritis
Retrolental fibroplasia
Rhabdomyoma of orbit

Rheumatoid scleritis
Ring ulcer of cornea
Rudimentary eye
Rupture of choroid
Rupture of cornea
  due to trauma
  due to increased intraocular
    pressure
Rupture of sclera
Sarcoma of ciliary body
Sarcoma of conjunctivitis
Sarcoma of iris
Scar of cornea
Scleritis, anterior
Sclerosed lens
Seclusion of pupil
Senile atrophy
Shrinking of vitreous
Siderosis of eyeball
Siderosis of iris
Siderosis of vitreous
Spasm of retinal artery
Staphyloma of cornea
Staphyloma of sclera
Strabismus
Subconjunctival hemorrhage
Subendothelial striped corneal
  opacity
Subepithelial striped corneal
  opacity
Superficial marginal ulcer
Symblepharon
Sympathetic irritation of
  optic nerve
Synchysis of vitreous
Synechia
  anterior
  posterior
Syphilis of conjunctiva
Syphilis of iris
Syphilis of optic papilla
Syphilis of uveal tract
Syphilitic angiopathy of retina
Syphilitic keratitis
Thrombosis of retinal vessel
Toxic amblyopia

DISEASES OF THE EYE AND ORBIT (continued)

Trichomatopsia
Tuberculoma of iris
Tuberculosis of optic papilla
Ulcus serpens
Uremic amaurosis
Uremic amblyopia
Uveitis, sympathetic
Vascular loop on papilla
Vitreous opacities
Vossius' ring
Water fissures in lens
Wound of eyeball
Xerophthalmia
Zinc incrustation of cornea

DISEASES OF THE LACRIMAL TRACT

Absence of canaliculus and punctum
Achroacytosis of lacrimal gland
Adenocarcinoma of lacrimal gland
Atresia (stenosis) of lacrimal passage
Atresia (stenosis) of lacrimonasal duct
Calculus of lacrimal gland
Cyst due to supernumerary
   lacrimonasal ducts
Dacryoadenitis
Dacryocystitis
   acute
   chronic
   phlegmonous
   syphilitic
   trachomatous
   tuberculous
Dacryops
Dislocation of lacrimal gland
Displacement of canaliculus and
   punctum
Epidermoid carcinoma of lacrimal
   gland
Epiphora due to hypersecretion of
   lacrimal glands
Eversion of punctum
Fistula of lacrimal gland
Fistula of lacrimal sac
Fistula of lacrimonasal duct
Foreign body in canaliculus
Foreign body in lacrimal sac
Granuloma in canaliculus
Granuloma in lacrimal sac
Luxation of lacrimal gland
Lymphosarcoma of lacrimal gland
Mixed tumor of lacrimal gland
Multiple benign cystic epithelioma
Polyp in canaliculus
Polyp in lacrimal sac
Retention cyst of lacrimal gland
Rhinoscleroma of lacrimal sac
Senile eversion of punctum
Sporotrichosis of canaliculus
Sporotrichosis of lacrimal sac
Stenosis of canaliculus, cicatricial
Stenosis of lacrimonasal duct
   cicatricial
Streptotrichosis of canaliculus
Streptotrichosis of lacrimal sac
Supernumerary lacrimal gland
Supernumerary lacrimonasal duct
Syphilis of lacrimal gland
Tuberculosis of lacrimal gland

OPERATIONS ON THE EYE AND ORBIT

Advancement of ocular muscle
   superior rectus muscle
   inferior oblique muscle
   medial (internal) rectus muscle
   inferior rectus muscle
   superior oblique muscle
   lateral (external) rectus muscle
Aspiration of vitreous
Biopsy of choroid
Biopsy of orbit
Capsulectomy
Capsulotomy
Coreoplasty
Cryoextraction of cataract
Cyclodialysis
Cyclodiathermy

OPERATIONS ON THE EYE AND ORBIT (continued)

Decompression of orbit
Discission of lens
Enucleation of eyeball
Evisceration of eyeball
Exenteration of orbital contents
Extracapsular extraction of cataract
Goniotomy
Graft of cornea
Intracapsular extraction of cataract
Iridectomy
Iridencleisis
Iridodialysis
Iridotasis
Iridotomy
Keratectomy
  complete
  partial
Keratocentesis
Keratoplasty
Keratotomy
  delimiting (Gifford's operation)
Myectomy of ocular muscle
Myotomy of ocular muscle
Needling of lens
Optical iridectomy
Orbital implant
Peripheral iridectomy

Plastic operation on eyeball
Plastic repair of orbit
Preliminary iridectomy
Reattachment of choroid
Reattachment of retina
Recession of ocular muscle
Removal of foreign body from cornea
Scleral fistula operation
Scleral shortening
Sclerectomy
  with punch (Holth operation)
  with scissors (LaGrange operation)
  with trephine (Elliot operation)
Scleroplasty
Sclerotomy
  with drainage
  with exploration
  with removal of foreign body
Suture of cornea
Suture of eyeball
Suture of iris
Suture of sclera
Tattoo of cornea
Tenotomy of ocular tendon
Transfixion of iris (iris bombe)
Transplantation of ocular muscle

OPERATIONS ON THE LACRIMAL TRACT

Catheterization of the lacrimonasal duct
Dacryoadenectomy
Dacryocystectomy
Dacryocystorhinostomy
Dacryocystostomy
Dacryocystotomy
Dilation of punctum

Drainage of lacrimal gland
Drainage of lacrimal sac
Excision of lacrimal gland
Excision of lacrimal sac
Plastic operation on canaliculi
Probing of lacrimonasal duct
Splitting of lacrimal papilla

EPONYMIC TITLES OF EYE OPERATIONS

Agnew canthoplasty
Ammon canthoplasty
Arlt epicanthus repair
Arruga cataract extraction
Arruga dacryostomy
Arruga keratoplasty

Arruga tenotomy
Bardelli lid ptosis operation
Barkan double cyclodialysis
Barkan goniotomy
Barrio iridencleisis
Basterra dacryostomy

EPONYMIC TITLES OF EYE OPERATIONS (continued)

Berens sclerectomy
Bielschowsky strabismus operation
Blasius lid operation
Blaskovics canthoplasty
Blaskovics dacryostomy
Blaskovics inversion of tarsus
Blaskovics lid operation
Blaskovics tarsectomy
Blatt pterygium operation
Bossalino blepharorrhaphy
Briggs strabismus operation
Büdinger blepharoplasty
Casanellas operation on lacrimal canaliculi
Castroviejo keratoplasty
Celsus lid operation
Celsus spasmodic entropion operation
Csapody orbital cavity repair
Czermak pterygium operation
Daviel cataract extraction
Dupuy-Dutemps dacryostomy
Dupuy-Dutemps lid operation
Dürr non-penetrating keratoplasty
Duverger and Velter dacryostomy
Elliott corneoscleral trephination
Elschnig blepharorrhaphy
Elschnig canthorrhaphy
Elschnig central iridectomy
Elschnig cicatricial entropian operation
Elschnig ptosis operation
Elschnig total keratoplasty
Filatov keratoplasty
Filatov-Marzinkowsky keratoplasty
Franceschetti keratoplasty
Franceschetti upward deviation of pupil
Fricke lid operation
Friede keratoplasty
Friedenwald ptosis operation
Fuchs canthorrhaphy
Fuchs transfixion of iris

Fukala lens extraction
Gayet operation for trichiasis
Georgariou cyclodialysis and sclerectomy
Gifford's delimiting keratotomy
Gomez-Marquez operation for obstructed lacrimal canaliculi
Gonin cautery of retinal detachment
Gradle keratoplasty
Gutzeit dacryostomy
Guyton ptosis operation
Hasner lid operation
Hess ptosis operation
Hippel (Von) keratoplasty
Hogan dacryostomy
Holth iridencleisis
Holth punch sclerectomy
Horay muscle and tendon advancement
Horvath muscle and tendon advancement
Hotz cicatricial entropion operation
Hughes lid operation
Imre blepharochalasis
Imre canthoplasty
Imre epicanthus operation
Imre keratoplasty
Imre lid plasty
Imre spasmodic entropion operation
Jaesche-Arlt trichiasis operation
Jameson tenotomy
Key iridodialysis
Kirby cataract extraction
Knapp lid operation
Knapp pterygium operation
Knapp-Imre lid operation
Kofler endonasal dacryostomy
Kraupa keratoplasty
Kreiker blepharochalasis
Kreiker blepharorrhaphy
Kriebig lid operation
Krönlein orbit operation
Kuhnt dacryostomy

EPONYMIC TITLES OF EYE OPERATIONS (continued)

Kuhnt lid operation
Kuhnt ectropion operation
Kuhnt epicanthus operation
Kuhnt tarsectomy
Lacarrere strabismus operation
Lagleyze cicatricial entropion operation
Lagrange sclerectomy
Lagrange modification of Arruga
Lagrange modification of Berens
Lagrange strabismus operation
Langenbeck plastic lid operation
Lindner corneoscleroconjunctival suture
Lindner posterior sclerotomy
Lindner shortening of eyeball
Löhlein keratoplasty
Londermann trephination of cornea
Lopez Enriquez trephine of the sclera
Löwenstein dacryostomy
Machek trichiasis operation
Magitot keratoplasty
Majewsky keratoplasty
Mauksch cyclodialysis
McGuire advancement in strabismus
McReynolds pterygium operation
Meller operation for coloboma of the lids
Morax keratoplasty
Mosher-Toti dacryostomy
Motais ptosis lid operation
Nida ptosis operation
Nizetic inversion of tarsus
Nizetic keratoplasty
O'Connor strabismus operation
O'Connor-Peter muscle operation
Paufique detachment of retina
Paufique lamellar keratoplasty
Paufique shortening of the eyeball
Peter tenotomy
Polyak endonasal dacryostomy
Poulard operation for spasmodic entropion
Raverdino dacryostomy
Richet cicatricial ectropion operation

Rowinski dacryostomy
Rubbrecht extirpation of cornea segmentally
Silva-Costa lacrimal operation
Smith extraction of cataract
Snellen entropion operation
Soria dacryostomy
Sourdille ptosis operation
Sourdille total lamellar keratoplasty
Spaeth pterygium operation
Speas strabismus operation
Spencer-Watson trichiasis operation
Stock dacryostomy
Suarez Villafranca plastic lid operation
Szymanowski spastic ectropion lid operation
Szymanowski-Kuhnt lid operation
Terson pterygium operation
Thomas keratoplasty
Thomas strabismus operation
Toti operation dacryostomy
Toti-Mosher dacryostomy
Trantas tarsectomy
Verhoeff advancement operation
Verhoeff corneoscleral trephination

Verwey epicanthus operation
Waldhauer trichiasis operation
Wecker, de anterior sclerotomy
Wecker, de posterior sclerotomy
Weekers iridencleisis
West dacryostomy
Weve dacryostomy
Weve shortening of the eyeball
Wheeler advancement of the inferior oblique
Wheeler advancement of the superior oblique
Wheeler operation for coloboma
Wheeler iridectomy
Wiener keratoplasty
Wilmer central iridectomy
Wolfe sclerectomy and cyclodialysis
Worth strabismus operation

12 | Orthopedic Surgery

Orthopedics is that branch of surgery which is concerned with preservation and restoration of the function of the skeletal system, its articulations and associated structures.

Tables of the bones, joints, ligaments and muscles are presented in Chapter 6.

In this chapter we will include a consideration of fractures, dislocations, bony deformities, amputations, arthroplastic procedures and surgery of the muscles, ligaments and tendons. This material is designed primarily to assist the secretary with technical terms encountered in dictations of these various procedures, including eponymic titles of the operations.

APPROACHES TO ORTHOPEDIC OPERATIONS

Abbott
Abbott and Lucas
Avila
Badgley
Banks and Laufman
Bosworth
Boyd
Callahan
Cave
Coonse and Adams
Cubbins
Darrach and McLaughlin
Fahey
Fisher "U"
Gatellier
Gibson
Guleke–Stookey
Harmon
Henderson
Henry
Heuter
Jones and Brackett
Kocher
Koenig
Luck
Ludloff
MacAusland
McFarland and Osborne
McWhorter
Milch
Ollier
Osborne
Osgood
Phemister
Putti
Radley, Liebig and Brown
Ralston
Roberts
Rowe
Saber-cut
Smith-Petersen
Thompson
Van Gorder
Wagoner
Watson-Jones
Yee

AMPUTATIONS

In the broadest consideration of amputations of the extremities, they may be divided into two main types: *open* and *closed*. The open amputation is a temporary procedure where the surface of the wound is not covered over with skin. The wound is left open to promote drainage. The closed type of amputation is a final operation where the resulting stump may be fitted with a prosthesis.

A further refinement of the closed amputation is a *cineplastic amputation* in which the stump is formed to permit the patient to activate the prosthesis directly by a muscle "motor" placed within the muscle belly. The "motor" consists of an inverted tube skin flap, lined on the inside by skin, which is pulled up transversely through a muscle canal, at right angles to the line of muscular pull, and attached to the opposite end. A peg is fixed in the tube, with cables attached to either end, for the purpose of transmitting muscle action to the prosthesis. The amputee thus obtains active control of the artificial limb or hook. This is specialized orthoplastic surgery usually confined to orthopedic centers equipped for proper limb fitting and rehabilitation.

An amputation may be performed through the body of a bone or through a joint. When the latter method is used, the operation is termed a *disarticulation*.

The "phantom" limb phenomenon, where pain and sensation is experienced in the limb which has been removed, is one of the undesirable effects following some amputations. The development of a painful terminal neuroma is another such occurrence. Revision of the amputation stump is often necessary when these conditions exist.

AMPUTATION TECHNIQUES

Aperiosteal supracondylar tendoplastic
Batch, Spittler, McFadden
Boyd
Callander
Carnes
Chopart's
Gritti-Stokes
Hey's
King and Steelquist
Kirk
Kutler
LeMesurier
Lisfranc's
Littlewood
Pedersen and Day
Pirogoff
Rogers
Silbert and Haimovici
Slocum
Sorondo and Ferre
Spittler
Stokes-Gritti
Syme
Vasconcelos
Woughter

Anatomy of the Hand

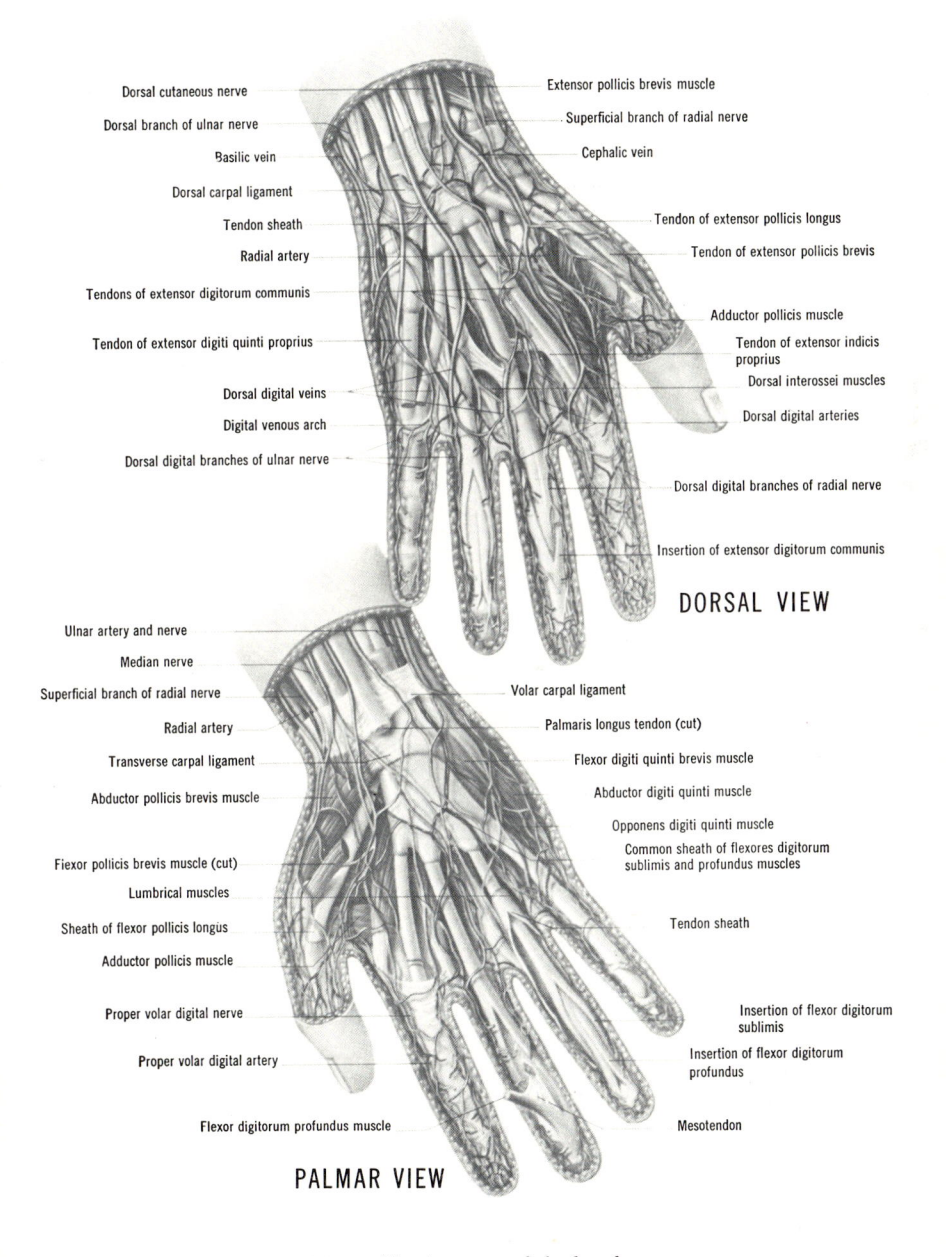

DORSAL VIEW

PALMAR VIEW

Figure 75 Anatomy of the hand
Courtesy Lederle Laboratories

Anatomy of the Foot

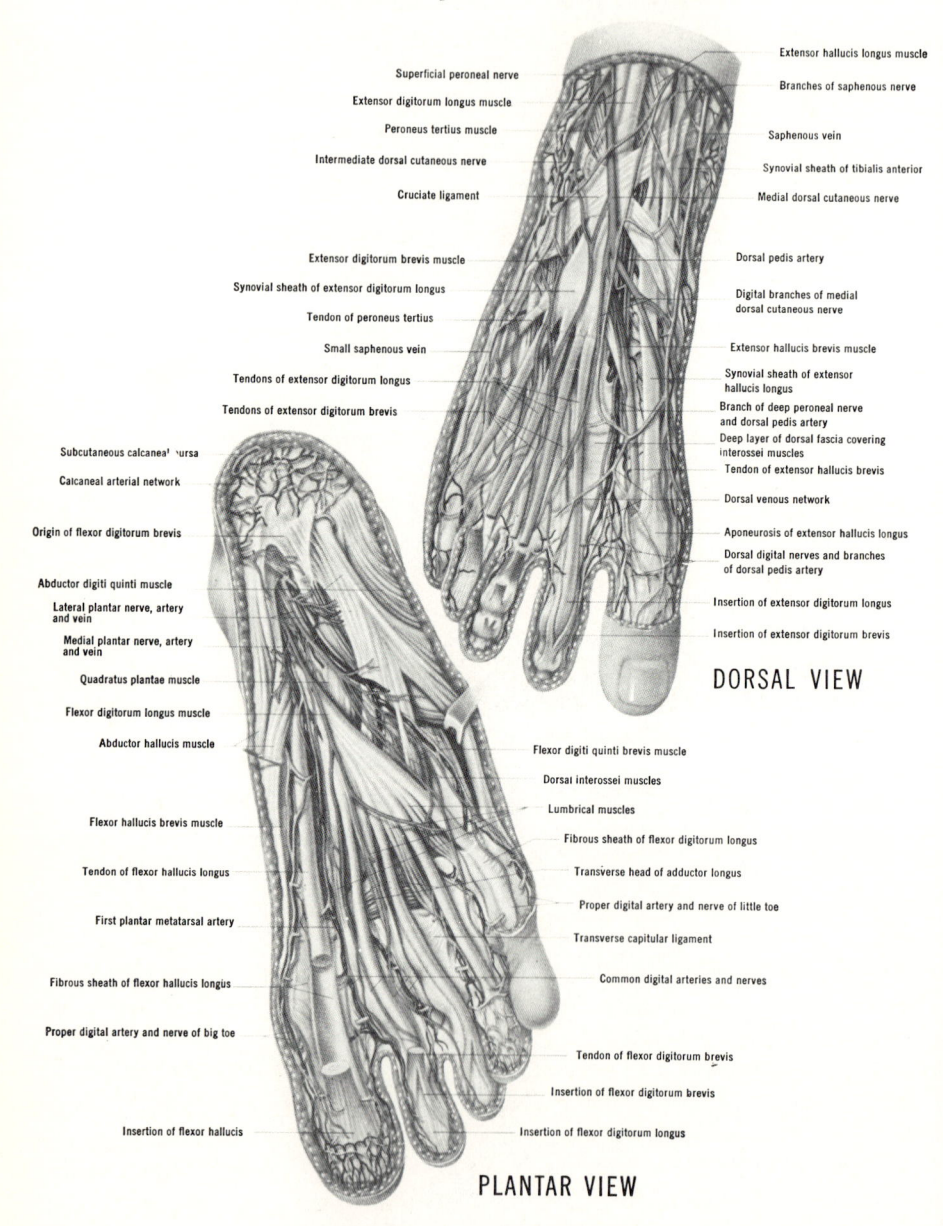

DORSAL VIEW

- Extensor hallucis longus muscle
- Branches of saphenous nerve
- Saphenous vein
- Synovial sheath of tibialis anterior
- Medial dorsal cutaneous nerve
- Dorsal pedis artery
- Digital branches of medial dorsal cutaneous nerve
- Extensor hallucis brevis muscle
- Synovial sheath of extensor hallucis longus
- Branch of deep peroneal nerve and dorsal pedis artery
- Deep layer of dorsal fascia covering interossei muscles
- Tendon of extensor hallucis brevis
- Dorsal venous network
- Aponeurosis of extensor hallucis longus
- Dorsal digital nerves and branches of dorsal pedis artery
- Insertion of extensor digitorum longus
- Insertion of extensor digitorum brevis

- Superficial peroneal nerve
- Extensor digitorum longus muscle
- Peroneus tertius muscle
- Intermediate dorsal cutaneous nerve
- Cruciate ligament
- Extensor digitorum brevis muscle
- Synovial sheath of extensor digitorum longus
- Tendon of peroneus tertius
- Small saphenous vein
- Tendons of extensor digitorum longus
- Tendons of extensor digitorum brevis

PLANTAR VIEW

- Subcutaneous calcaneal bursa
- Calcaneal arterial network
- Origin of flexor digitorum brevis
- Abductor digiti quinti muscle
- Lateral plantar nerve, artery and vein
- Medial plantar nerve, artery and vein
- Quadratus plantae muscle
- Flexor digitorum longus muscle
- Abductor hallucis muscle
- Flexor hallucis brevis muscle
- Tendon of flexor hallucis longus
- First plantar metatarsal artery
- Fibrous sheath of flexor hallucis longus
- Proper digital artery and nerve of big toe
- Insertion of flexor hallucis

- Flexor digiti quinti brevis muscle
- Dorsal interossei muscles
- Lumbrical muscles
- Fibrous sheath of flexor digitorum longus
- Transverse head of adductor longus
- Proper digital artery and nerve of little toe
- Transverse capitular ligament
- Common digital arteries and nerves
- Tendon of flexor digitorum brevis
- Insertion of flexor digitorum brevis
- Insertion of flexor digitorum longus

Figure 76 Anatomy of the foot
Courtesy Lederle Laboratories

Amputation Through the Surgical Neck of the Humerus

The patient was placed in the dorsal decubitus position with the back supported by a sandbag. The arm and adjacent areas were sterilely prepared and draped.

The skin incision was started at the level of the coracoid process and extended along the anterior border of the deltoid muscle down to its point of insertion. An incision was then carried along the posterior aspect of the deltoid muscle to the axillary fold. A separate incision was carried through the axilla to join the previous incisions.

The Pectoralis major muscle was identified and traced to its insertion where it was sectioned and reflected medially. The neurovascular bundle between the Pectoralis minor and the Coracobrachialis muscles was exposed. The axillary artery and vein were sectioned just below the Pectoralis minor muscle. Next, the radial, ulnar, median and musculocutaneous nerves were isolated, gently drawn down and sectioned in such a way that they were able to fall above the Pectoralis minor muscle. The deltoid muscle was then sectioned at its insertion and reflected upward together with its attached lateral skin flap. Further sectioning was carried out of the Latissimus dorsi and Teres major at the bicipital groove near their insertions. At a point about 2 cm. distal to the saw line, the Coracobrachialis, biceps tendon and triceps were severed. A Gigli saw was used to cut through the humeral neck. After the bone was severed, the Coracobrachialis and long head of the biceps were sutured over the end of the remaining humerus. The Pectoralis major was carried laterally and sutured to the inferior pole of the bone. This was covered by the deltoid muscle and a skin flap carefully outlined to provide a well aligned closure. Interrupted skin sutures were used to approximate the wound edges.

Above Knee (A-K) Amputation

The patient was placed on the operating table in the supine position after infiltration of spinal anesthesia. The entire leg, groin and abdomen were prepared with alcohol and Zephiran and draped. A site for A-K amputation was chosen. Anterior and posterior skin flaps were fashioned.

The incision was carried down through the fascia and muscle layers to the femur. It was noted that the blood supply was quite adequate. The superficial femoral artery was divided and had an excellent pulsatile flow. This artery was doubly ligated, both with a free ligature and suture ligature. The sciatic nerve was identified and placed under traction. A 00 chromic ligature was placed high around the nerve and the nerve was then transected and allowed to retract high up into the thigh.

The femur was transected with a hand saw and the edges filed. The marrow cavity was packed with bee's wax. All bleeding was controlled by clamping and fine chromic ligatures. After good hemostasis was achieved, the deep fascia of the thigh was approximated with interrupted 00 chromic sutures and the skin reapproximated with interrupted 00000 Tevdek sutures.

A through-and-through thyroid drain was passed through the thigh to the fascial layer. A pressure and occlusive dressing was applied.

Revision and Closure of Partial Amputation, Right Index Finger

After the usual sterile preparation and draping and with a pneumatic tourniquet on the arm elevated to 300 mm. of mercury, the wound was thoroughly lavaged with copious amounts of saline. Meticulous debridement was carried out.

The amputation had occurred at the distal joint causing a disarticulation of the joint and a comminuted fracture of the distal end of the middle phalanx.

The skin of the dorsal aspect of the finger was amputated at the level of the joint while the volar aspect of the remaining flap extended about 1 cm. beyond the amputation level. It was shredded and severely lacerated. A midline incision was made on the radial and ulnar aspect of the finger, approximately 1 cm. from the distal end of the middle phalanx. Dorsal and volar skin flaps were retracted. The middle phalanx was amputated at the level of the flare of the condyles, at its distal end. The amputation site was smoothed off and the edges rounded.

The extensor tendon and the Flexor digitorum profundus were both pulled down and severed allowing them to retract proximally. The neurovascular bundle on each side was identified. The artery and vein were ligated. The nerve was dissected free and amputated proximal to the level of the amputated phalanx.

The skin flaps were revised in such a manner that the volar flap was brought back over the dorsal end of the stump and sutured to the end of the dorsal flap. This produced a tactile pad without a scar over the volar surface of the distal end of the stump.

A pressure dressing and dorsal plaster of Paris splint were applied.

ARTHRODESIS

Arthrodesis (fusion) is an operation performed to induce immobilization (bony ankylosis) in a joint where motion is not desired. These fusions may be intra-articular, intra- and extra-articular, or extra-articular in type. An extra-articular arthrodesis is performed when union is desired between normal bony surfaces outside of the joint capsule. A spinal fusion is the best example of this type of arthrodesis.

Intra-articular arthrodesis is performed when fusion of cancellous bony surfaces is the surgeon's goal. The articulating surfaces are devested of diseased tissue to facilitate union of cancellous bony surfaces. Autogenous cancellous bone grafts are sometimes used to promote fusion.

In the intra- and extra-articular arthodeses bone grafts are used across the joint after the articular surfaces are stripped of their investments.

SEE: Listing of orthopedic operations at the end of this chapter for assistance with the titles of specific operations.

Charnley Arthrodesis of the Ankle

An incision extending from 1 cm. proximal to the tip of one malleolus to the same point on the other is made across the anterior aspect of the ankle joint. The incision curves out distally in a semicircular fashion at its midpoint. A thick flap is formed by dissection of the skin and subcutaneous tissues proximally. The extensor tendons are thus exposed. The Extensor digitorum communis, the Extensor hallucis longus and the Tibialis anterior tendons are divided. Care is exercised to avoid the distal portion of the Peroneus tertius tendon.

The anterior tibial vessels are cut and tied, the nerve is sectioned and the joint capsule is incised transversely. Subperiosteal exposure of the posterior surfaces of the malleoli and lower portion of the tibia is carried out. Traction is obtained by introducing a periosteal elevator behind each malleolus.

The fibular and tibial collateral ligaments are divided and the foot is plantarflexed. Using a saw, the lower ends of the tibia and fibula are cut horizontally. An osteotome is used to complete the bone division. The foot is then placed in the position of choice. A one-fourth of an inch thick piece of bone is removed from the talus. A Steinman pin is then introduced through the talus and open wound, well anterior to the axis of the bone. It is positioned in such a way that it will counterbalance the pull of the tendo calcaneus posteriorly. Care is taken to avoid puncturing the subtalar joint. An upper pin is inserted through the shaft of the tibia using the compression clamps on the lower pin as a guide. The clamps are tightened to assure proper position. The sutures in the tendons are tied and the skin incision closed. A thickly padded plaster cast is applied from below the knee to the toes.

Ischiofemoral Arthrodesis of the Left Hip (Brittain Technique)

The patient was anesthetized with Pentothal Sodium and placed on the fracture table. The left leg was prepared from the hip to the ankle with G-11 and the operative area draped free in the usual fashion.

First, an incision was made parallel to an old incision of the hip. It was carried directly to the tensor fascia lata. This structure was then sectioned with a clean scalpel. The Vastus lateralis was then incised and separated from the shaft of the femur by a sharp periosteal elevator. A single guide wire was drilled through the area of the femur, just above the lesser trochanter, and an x-ray was made. The wire was found to lie in a satisfactory plane in relation to the ischium.

Next, an incision was made over the tibial crest, beginning one inch above the ankle joint, and carried proximally to the tibial tubercle. The margins were reflected. The periosteum was incised and separated from the entire tibial shaft by a sharp periosteal elevator. With a Stryker bone saw, a large arrow-shaped graft was cut from the entire width of the surface of the tibia, measuring $6\frac{1}{2}$ inches in length. The wound was closed by approximating the periosteum with interrupted 00 chromic catgut. The subcutaneous tissue was closed with interrupted 000 plain catgut and the skin with interlocking black silk suture. Dry sterile dressings were applied to this wound.

The femur was osteotomized along the wire osteotomy plane that had been established. The femur was then driven into the ischium and this bone was also osteotomized. The previously cut graft was then inserted into the osteotomy area and driven well into the ischium. The femoral shaft was displaced medially.

The wound was closed by approximating the Vastus lateralis with interrupted 0 chromic catgut, the tensor fascia lata with interrupted 00 chromicized catgut, the subcutaneous tissue with 000 plain catgut and the skin with interlocking black silk suture.

Dry sterile dressings were applied. A left hip spica was applied from the costal margin to the toes on the left leg with the leg in abduction and the knee in slight flexion. The ankle was kept in a neutral position.

Shoulder Arthrodesis

With the patient in Fowler's position with the knees flexed and the feet braced against a padded foot rest, the area of the shoulder was prepared and draped.

An incision was made over the glenohumeral joint and carried through the anatomic layers to the joint. The joint was entered anteriorly and superiorly. It was stripped of cartilage. The acromion was prepared and

ORTHOPEDIC SURGERY 463

Anatomy of the Shoulder

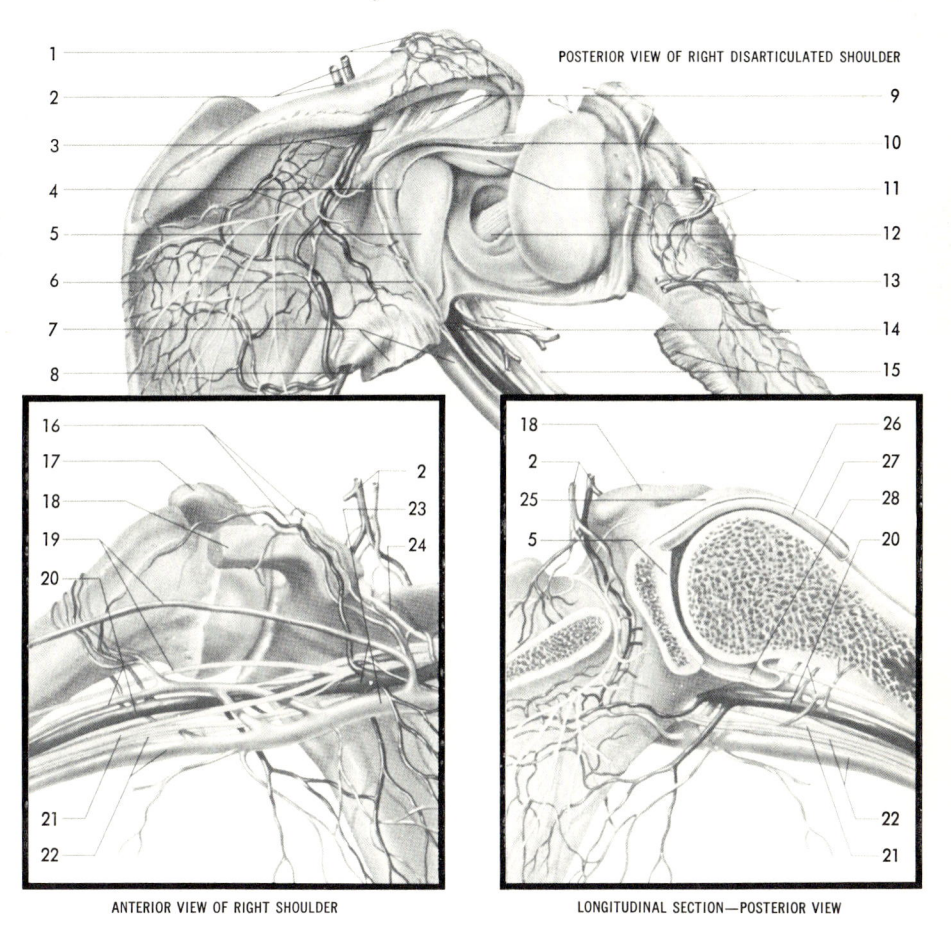

POSTERIOR VIEW OF RIGHT DISARTICULATED SHOULDER

ANTERIOR VIEW OF RIGHT SHOULDER

LONGITUDINAL SECTION—POSTERIOR VIEW

1 Acromial branches of thoracoacromial artery and vein
2 Transverse scapular artery and vein
3 Coracoclavicular ligament (conoid portion)
4 Glenoidal lip; branch of suprascapular nerve
5 Glenoid cavity
6 Cut edge of articular capsule
7 Long head of triceps brachii; basilic vein
8 Scapular circumflex artery and vein
9 Coracoclavicular ligament (trapezoid portion)
10 Cut edge of coracohumeral ligament
11 Tendon of long head of biceps brachii; anterior humeral circumflex artery and vein
12 Tendon of subscapularis
13 Posterior humeral circumflex artery and vein; teres minor muscle
14 Axillary nerve; brachial artery and vein
15 Radial nerve; teres major muscle
16 Thoracoacromial artery and vein
17 Acromion
18 Coracoid process
19 Cephalic vein; musculocutaneous nerve
20 Brachial artery and vein
21 Median nerve
22 Ulnar nerve; basilic vein
23 Axillary artery and vein
24 Suprascapular nerve
25 Coracohumeral ligament
26 Tendon of long head of biceps brachii
27 Intertubercular mucous sheath
28 Articular capsule

Figure 77   Anatomy of the shoulder
Courtesy Lederle Laboratories

Anatomy of the Elbow

ANTERIOR VIEW

Sagittal section through the right elbow joint

Frontal section of the bones and joints of the elbow

POSTERIOR VIEW

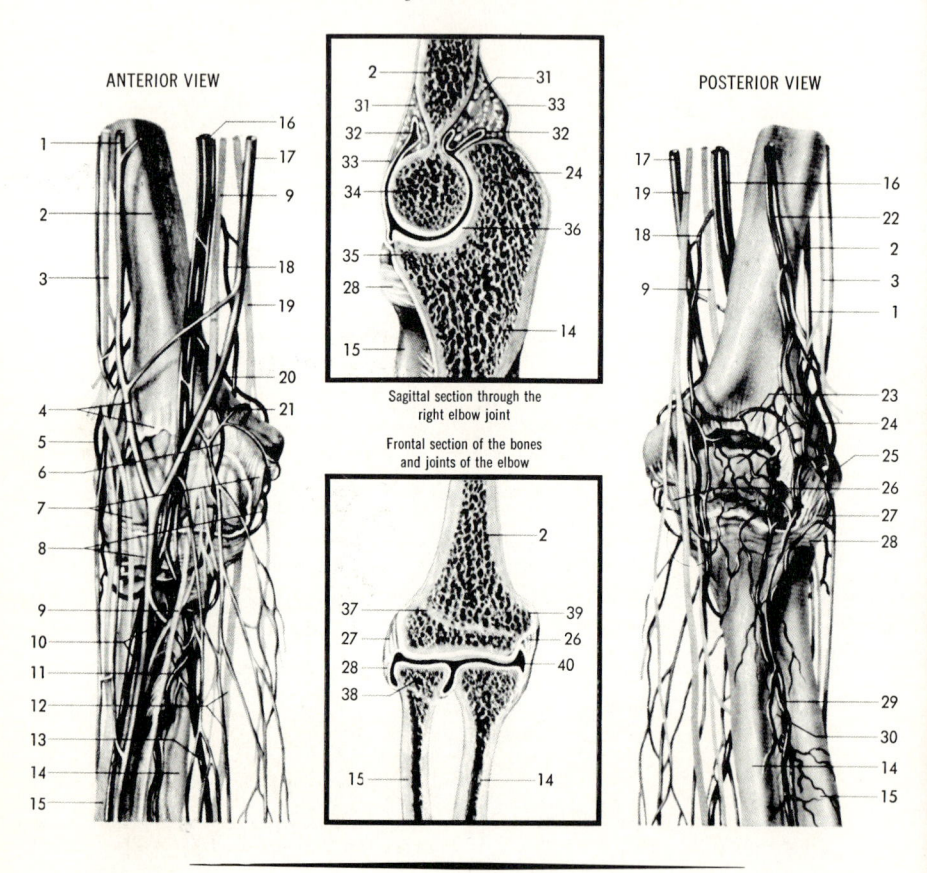

1 Brachial cephalic vein
2 Humerus
3 Radial nerve
4 Median cephalic vein; articular capsule
5 Radial collateral branch of profunda brachii artery
6 Anterior ulnar recurrent artery
7 Superficial branch of radial nerve; ulnar lateral ligament
8 Annular ligament; posterior ulnar recurrent artery
9 Median nerve
10 Antebrachial cephalic vein; radial artery
11 Volar interosseous artery
12 Antebrachial basilic vein; ulnar nerve
13 Ulnar artery
14 Ulna
15 Radius
16 Brachial artery
17 Brachial basilic vein
18 Superior ulnar collateral artery
19 Ulnar nerve
20 Inferior ulnar collateral artery
21 Median basilic vein
22 Profunda brachii artery
23 Articular capsule
24 Olecranon
25 Lateral epicondyle
26 Ulnar lateral ligament
27 Radial lateral ligament
28 Annular ligament
29 Dorsal interosseous artery
30 Interosseous membrane
31 Fat pad
32 Synovial membrane
33 Fibrous capsule
34 Trochlea
35 Coronoid process of ulna
36 Ulnar semilunar notch
37 Epiphyseal line
38 Capitulum of radius
39 Medial epicondyle
40 Articular cavity

Figure 78   Anatomy of the elbow
Courtesy Lederle Laboratories

ORTHOPEDIC SURGERY

Anatomy of the Wrist

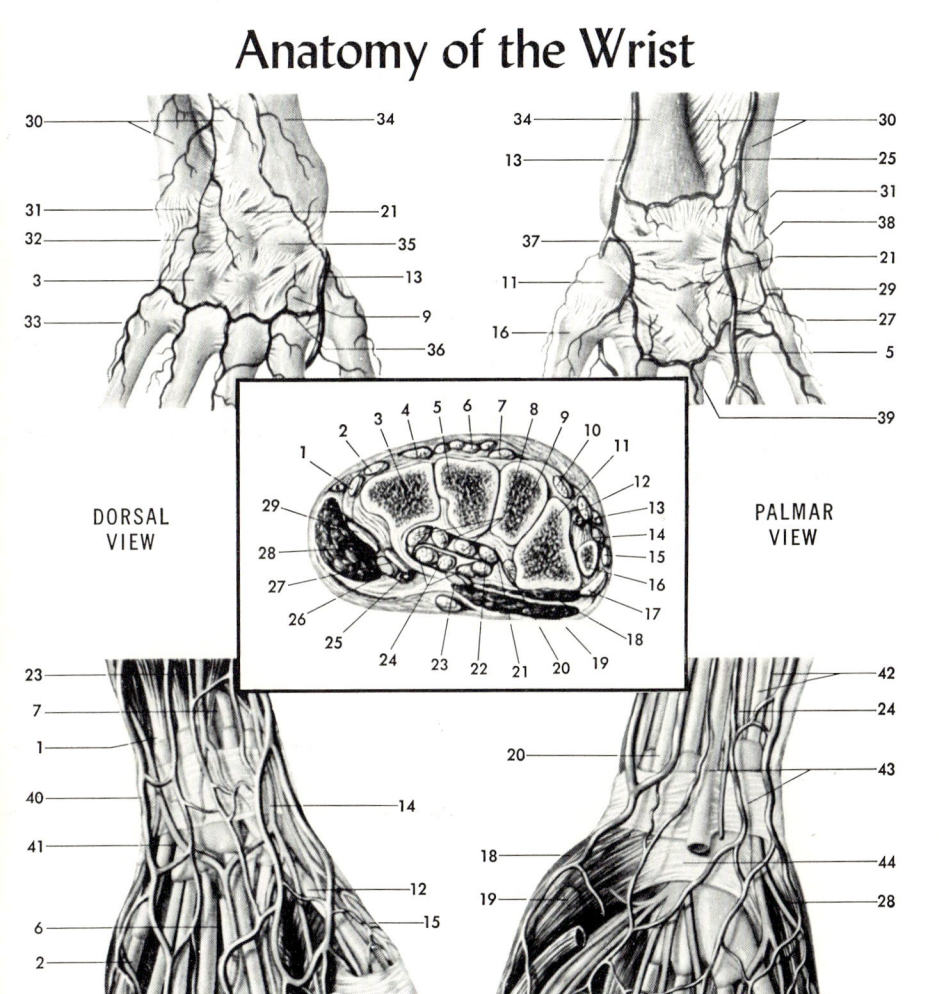

DORSAL VIEW

PALMAR VIEW

1 Tendon of extensor carpi ulnaris
2 Tendon of extensor digiti quinti proprius
3 Hamate bone
4 Tendon of extensor digitorum communis
5 Capitate bone
6 Tendon of extensor indicis proprius
7 Tendon of extensor carpi radialis brevis
8 Tendons of flexor digitorum profundus
9 Lesser multangular bone
10 Tendon of extensor carpi radialis longus
11 Greater multangular bone
12 Tendon of extensor pollicis longus
13 Radial artery
14 Superficial branch of radial nerve
15 Tendon of extensor pollicis brevis
16 First metacarpal bone
17 Tendon of abductor pollicis longus
18 Opponens pollicis muscle
19 Abductor pollicis brevis muscle
20 Tendon of flexor carpi radialis
21 Radiate carpal ligament
22 Tendon of flexor pollicis longus
23 Median nerve
24 Tendons of flexor digitorum sublimis
25 Ulnar artery
26 Volar branch of ulnar nerve
27 Pisohamate ligament
28 Abductor digiti quinti muscle
29 Pisometacarpal ligament
30 Ulna; interosseous membrane
31 Ulnar lateral carpal ligament
32 Triangular bone
33 Dorsal metacarpal artery
34 Radius
35 Navicular bone
36 Dorsal carpal branch of radial artery
37 Lunate bone
38 Pisiform bone
39 Deep volar arterial arch
40 Basilic vein
41 Dorsal branch of ulnar nerve
42 Ulnar nerve; tendon of flexor carpi ulnaris
43 Tendon of palmaris longus; volar carpal ligament
44 Transverse carpal ligament

Figure 79 Anatomy of the wrist
Courtesy Lederle Laboratories

Anatomy of the Hip

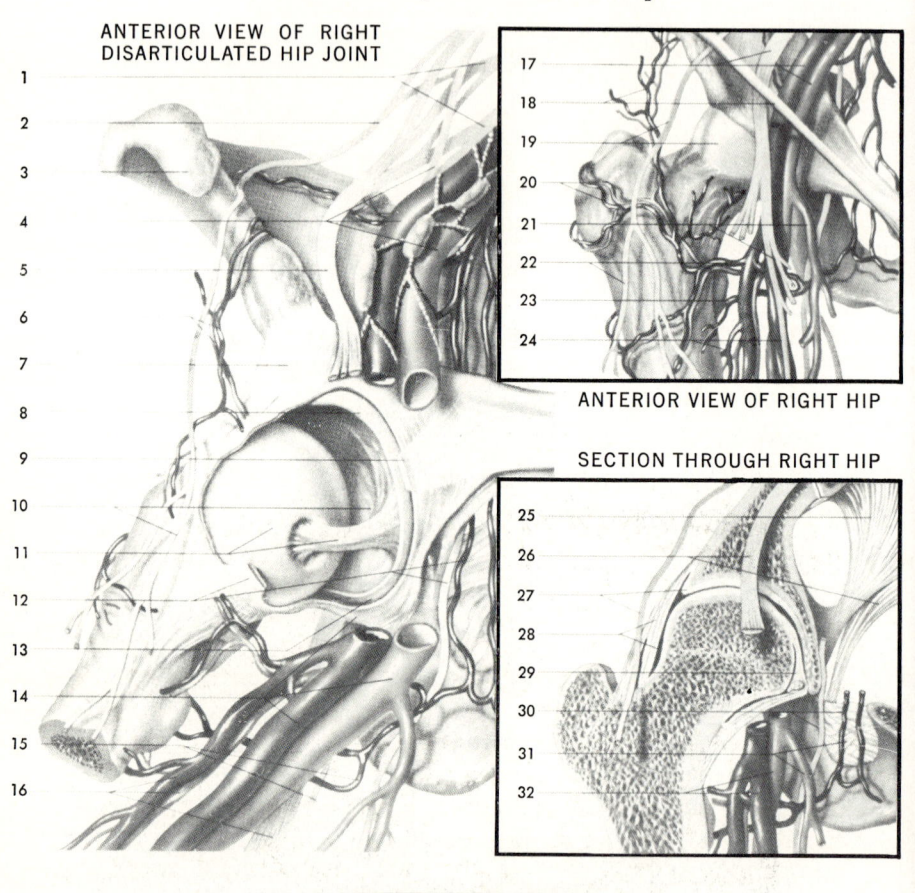

ANTERIOR VIEW OF RIGHT DISARTICULATED HIP JOINT

ANTERIOR VIEW OF RIGHT HIP

SECTION THROUGH RIGHT HIP

1 Lumbar nerves
2 Lateral femoral cutaneous nerve
3 Anterior superior spine of ilium
4 External iliac artery and vein; obturator nerve
5 Femoral nerve
6 Ascending branches of lateral femoral circumflex artery and vein
7 Iliofemoral ligament
8 Glenoid lip
9 Pubocapsular ligament (cut)
10 Anterior branch of lateral femoral cutaneous nerve; acetabular fossa
11 Head of femur; round ligament
12 Pubocapsular ligament (cut); obturator nerve and artery
13 Transverse ligament of acetabulum
14 Ischiocapsular ligament; femoral artery and vein
15 Posterior femoral cutaneous nerve; medial femoral circumflex artery
16 Deep femoral artery and vein; sciatic nerve
17 Femoral nerve; external iliac artery and vein
18 Ascending branch of lateral femoral circumflex artery; inguinal ligament
19 Lateral femoral cutaneous nerve; head of femur
20 Transverse branches of lateral femoral circumflex artery and vein
21 Muscular branch of femoral nerve; saphenous vein
22 Posterior branch of lateral femoral cutaneous nerve; lateral femoral circumflex artery
23 Medial femoral circumflex artery
24 First perforating artery; saphenous nerve
25 Sacrospinous ligament
26 Femoral nerve; sacrotuberous ligament
27 Lateral femoral cutaneous nerve; glenoid lip
28 Iliofemoral ligament; synovial cavity
29 Round ligament
30 Obturator nerve and artery
31 Saphenous vein; obturator membrane
32 Femoral artery and vein

Figure 80   Anatomy of the hip
Courtesy Lederle Laboratories

fitted into a depression formed in the greater tuberosity of the humerus. Satisfactory positioning was obtained. A shoulder spica was applied. The upper arm was placed in a position of 70 degrees abduction from the scapula with 30 degrees forward flexion and 30 degrees internal rotation.

Arthrodesis L-4 — Sacrum With Autogenous Right Iliac Graft (Modified Hibbs Technique with H-grafts)

After administration of satisfactory general anesthesia, the patient was placed in the prone position on the operating table and positioned for spinal fusion. The back area, including the posterior aspect of the right ilium, was prepared and draped in the usual fashion.

The lumbosacral spine was approached through a midline vertical skin incision which was carried down to the investing lumbar fascia. This was divided vertically in the midline. The spinous processes and lamina of the 3rd, 4th and 5th lumbar vertebrae and the upper sacral segments were exposed by subperiosteal dissection of the paravertebral muscles.

A Downing muscle retractor was positioned so as to afford proper exposure of the area. Investigation of the stability of this portion of the spine revealed that the L-4-5 segment was the most significant area of instability, although the L-5 and S-1 area did show mild instability. An arthrodesis from the 4th lumbar segment to the upper sacrum was elected and performed by the modified Hibbs technique with superimposition of two H-grafts. The spinous process of L-5 was carefully cut and prepared to act as an intermediary between the two H-grafts. The 4th lumbar spinous process was also prepared as was the upper sacral process. The laminae were carefully dissected with sharp osteotome to expose raw cancellous bone. Small shingles of cortical bone were turned over to permit this. All extraneous soft tissue was carefully removed by rongeur dissection. The facet joints were exposed and destroyed by dissection with an osteotome and prepared for packing with cancellous bone graft. The entire area of fusion was prepared for reception of the bone graft. When this preparation was completed and the area lavaged, the site was packed with sponges.

Attention was directed to the posterior crest of the right ilium. A curved skin incision was made directly over the crest. Subperiosteal dissection of the muscles on the outer aspect of the crest was utilized to expose a sufficient area from which a bone graft could be taken. Only outer table grafts were taken. Two relatively large pieces were cut in the usual fashion to be used as H-grafts. Multiple strips of cortical cancellous and cancellous bone were removed with a gouge and curet for additional bone graft material. When sufficient bone grafts had been obtained, the area was lavaged with sterile saline.

Bleeding from the bone was controlled by Gelfoam packing and a closure accomplished with 00 chromic to reapproximate the musculature 0000 chromic for the subcutaneous tissue and interrupted 000 silk for the skin.

Attention was then directed to the arthrodesis site where cancellous bone graft was packed into the facet joint spaces. Previously prepared strips of cancellous and cortical cancellous bone were laid down in the usual barrel stave manner to afford a satisfactory fusion bed. The H-grafts were carefully cut to the proper size. The patient's spine was then hyper flexed. The two H-grafts were fitted into place, one between L-4 and 5 and one between L-5 and S-1. The patient's spine was extended. The H-grafts were locked into place satisfactorily. Remaining bone graft was packed in and about the area. Another sterile lavage with saline was performed.

Anatomical closure was accomplished using 00 chromic for the muscle and lumbar fascia, 000 chromic interrupted for the subcutaneous tissue and 000 silk interrupted for the skin. A sterile compression dressing was applied over the entire area. The patient was then turned on his back on the Stryker circOlectric bed and extubated.

The patient was transfused during and after the surgical procedure with 1000 cc. of whole blood.

Harrington Spinal Instrumentation With Multilevel Spinal Fusion

The patient, a 15 year old white female with known idiopathic scoliosis was placed on the operating table in the prone position. General anesthesia was administered and both of the patient's legs were wrapped with 6 inch Ace bandages. The chest was protected with chest pads to allow free breathing of the abdominal wall. The entire width of the back and its entire length from the neck to below the buttocks were prepared with Septisol and draped free.

A long skin incision, extending from the level of T-6 to L-4, was carried through the skin, subcutaneous tissues and overlying fascia. Just before the skin incision was made, 120 cc. of ¼% Xylocaine and epinephrine were injected into the area to decrease the amount of bleeding. The incision was carried down through the underlying fascia to the spinous processes of the vertebrae. The fascia and periosteum over the vertebra were incised with each tip. Using two periosteal elevators, one team working each side of the table, the spine was simultaneously stripped of it muscle attachments by subperiosteal dissection extending from the vertebral spines back to the transverse processes and facet areas. This wa accomplished from the level of T-7 down to the level of L-4. All soft tissues were removed from this area.

A partial laminectomy, removing approximately 2 or 3 mm. of the superior surface of the left lamina L-3, was carried out which allowed the lower distraction hook to seat easily, gripping sufficient bone for strength. Attention was then directed to the upper portion of the wound at the level of T-7 where another distraction hook was placed between the facet area of T-7 and T-8. Attention was then turned to the right side of the body where compression hooks were placed at T-8, 9 and 10, and at the bottom of the wound in T-12 and L-1 and 2.

The operation was then directed to the right iliac crest. A long incision, approximately 5 inches in length, was carried through the skin, subcutaneous tissues and overlying fascia. All bleeders were clamped and cauterized. Dissection was carried down to the fascia which was incised and to the periosteum of the iliac crest which was also incised. This was stripped with a periosteal elevator revealing the external surface of the iliac bone. Using a curved and straight osteotome, a large graft measuring approximately 4-5 inches square was removed, taking only the outer table of the iliac crest and all cancellous bone to be used later in the graft area. Bleeding was minimal. The periosteal and fascial layers were closed with 00 chromic interrupted sutures. The subcutaneous tissue was closed with 000 plain interrupted sutures.

The operation was again focused on the original wound. The facets between the two distracting hooks were removed, from the facet at T-8-T-9, all the way down the left side of the spine to L-2. The facets between these areas were removed and cancellous bone packed into the area. The facets were also removed on the right side of the body between T-11 and 12 and this was also packed with cancellous bone. Now a 7 inch distraction rod was placed between the distraction hooks and directed partially into position. A completed compression rod assembly, utilizing 6 hooks and a small threaded rod, was taken to the right side of the body and the individual hooks which had been placed previously were removed. This new compression assembly was placed in the same areas. Tightening was then accomplished. First, the distraction hook was jacked out one or two notches until tightness was felt. Compression hooks were then directed in until tightness was felt. This was carried out until stability was achieved. The curve appeared straight, perhaps a little overcorrected. A point was reached where it was unwise to apply any more pressure to these hooks. The ends of the threaded rod were removed and the wire crimped so that the nuts would not back off.

The graft, originally taken from the right iliac crest, was cut up into many small segments. Using sharp gouges and osteotomes, the lamina and posterior elements of all the processes involved in the fusion were scarified and elevated into a modified Hibbs type fusion. At the same time, the spines of the vertebrae were split vertically and bent laterally and portions of the graft were inserted between the split and turned over spines and along the gutters of the vertebral bodies.

The wound was inspected for bleeding. The sponge count was correct. The deep fascia was closed with 00 chromic interrupted sutures, the subcutaneous tissue with 000 plain interrupted sutures and the skin closed with 0000 dermalon interrupted sutures as was the skin over the graft site.

The patient tolerated the procedure well. She received 5 bottles of blood for a total of 2500 cc. of whole blood. A large compression dressing was placed on her back. She was placed in a circOlectric bed and taken to the recovery room in good condition.

ARTHROPLASTY

Arthroplasty is a plastic or reconstructive operation on the joints for the purpose of restoring motion to the joint and function to the component parts of the articulation. Such operations are performed on joints where abnormal immobility (ankylosis) has occurred as a result of trauma or pyogenic infection. Ankylosis is seen most often in the joints of the hip, knee, elbow and jaw and it is in these joints that the operation can be performed most effectively. Arthroplastic procedures include plastic revisions of the soft parts and the introduction of autogenous tissues between the articular surfaces of the joint in addition to reconstruction of the osseous parts.

Reconstructive Arthroplasty of the Left Knee (including primary reconstruction of the anterior cruciate ligament, the deep medial collateral and superficial medial collateral ligaments and excision of the dislocated medial meniscus)

After administration of a satisfactory general anesthetic, the left lower extremity was prepared and draped in the usual fashion. A pneumatic tourniquet was inflated about the left thigh. A modified median parapatellar skin incision was utilized of sufficient length to permit ready inspection of the entire medial compartment and a good share of the lateral compartment. After dissection of the subcutaneous tissue and investing deep fascia, the ruptured medial collateral ligament (superficial portion) was seen. Continuing the dissection and carefully identifying both ends of the ligamentous rupture, the deep injured portions were visualized. The medial meniscus was dislocated into the adjacent soft tissue. The capsule of the joint was then very carefully opened in a median parapatellar fashion and the remaining portion of the joint inspected. The anterior cruciate ligament was obviously also involved.

The knee was flexed to 90 degrees and the patient was properly positioned for continuation of the procedure and repair. The inner surface of the patella was not significantly injured. The patella was dislocated laterally to permit better exposure. There were areas of the articular cartilage of the femur which had been acutely injured with the ligament. The medial meniscus was sharply dissected and removed, care being taken at the margins to insure removal of the total dislocated meniscus. The anterior cruciate ligament had ruptured just at its origin from the lateral femoral condyle, but there were sufficient portions of the fibers present to permit reconstruction of the ligament and end-to-end anastomosis with the proximal and distal fragments. This was accomplished with interrupted 00 cotton suture material. A satisfactory reconstruction of the ligament was obtained. The deep medial collateral ligament was repaired with interrupted 00 cotton suture and reinforcement of the superficial ligament was also performed. The wound was then lavaged with sterile saline and the knee brought into a neutral position and redraped.

A standard closure of the knee incision was performed with interrupted 00 chromic for the capsule and investing fascia and a continuous 00 nylon subcuticular suture for the skin. A Sommers compression dressing with anterior and posterior plaster molds was applied. The tourniquet was deflated.

Austin-Moore Endoprosthetic Arthoplasty

The patient was placed in the right lateral position and the left hip prepared and draped from the iliac crest to below the knee.

Under general anesthesia, a long Gibson approach was carried out with a skin incision approximately 12 inches long. The incision started posteriorly and traveled anteriorly into the previous incisional area in the old hip nailing site of two years ago. The incision was carried down through the skin, subcutaneous tissues and overlying fascia. All bleeders were cauterized.

The fascia lata was opened and the nail palpated underneath. The fascia lata was further opened in the line of the incision and the nail was visible. All five screws were removed from the Jewett nail. There was no sign of corrosion. As soon as the five screws were removed the nail could be easily extracted. This hip nailing was performed two years ago for an intertrochanteric fracture.

The reason for this operation was the pathologic fracture of the femoral neck which would not allow the Jewett nail to protrude into the superior part of the acetabulum, causing the patient a great deal of pain.

With the nail removed, attention was directed to the area of the femoral head. One half of the abductors of the Gluteus maximus and medius were released from the trochanteric region. The leg was rotated and flexed. Blunt and sharp dissection was carried over the anterior portion of the hip capsule.

It was believed that the pathologic fracture of the left femoral neck was 2½ weeks old. With some difficulty, the capsule was located and incised onto the femoral neck and head area. The femoral head was very soft. In some areas it was of egg shell thickness and had to be removed in pieces. The femoral neck was now high riding. There was no question about tumor in the femoral neck. Posteriorly, there was very little bone left.

Using what remained of the femoral neck, it was cut down and notched to admit the Austin-Moore prosthesis. A $1\frac{7}{8}$ prosthesis was inserted and fixation accomplished with a #18 wire through the bone and prosthesis

There was considerable bleeding from the tumor area with a drop in blood pressure which was rectified by the administration of additional blood.

Closure was carried out with 00 chromic for the capsule and 00 chromic for the overlying muscle and fascial layers. The incision of the fascia lata and Vastus lateralis where the Jewett nail had been removed was closed in a similar manner. The subcutaneous tissue was closed with 00 chromic interrupted sutures and the skin closed with sutures of 0000 dermalon. A large compression dressing was placed on the wound. The heels were wrapped with ABD and Ace bandages and the lower extremities immobilized with three pillows between the legs. The legs were held in a position of function.

Magnuson Modified Arthroplasty, Rt. Knee

The right lower extremity was prepared and draped following which a pneumatic tourniquet was applied and inflated to 500 mm. of mercury It was sustained at that pressure.

The right knee was approached through a median peripatellar skin incision carried through the subcutaneous tissue down to the investing deep fascia of the thigh. This was also incised in the course of the skin incision.

The insertion of the Vastus medialis muscle into the rectus and the medial patella was sharply incised and allowed to retract medially. The incision was continued along the medial border margin of the patella down to the joint line and this curved distally following the patellar tendon insertion. The capsular joint was thereby opened as was the synovium

ORTHOPEDIC SURGERY

Anatomy of the Knee

ANTERIOR VIEW

POSTERIOR VIEW

HEAD OF RIGHT TIBIA SEEN FROM ABOVE

SAGITTAL SECTION THROUGH RIGHT KNEE

1 Femoral artery and vein; saphenous nerve
2 Great saphenous vein; cutaneous branch of obturator nerve
3 Descending branch of lateral femoral circumflex artery
4 Anterior cutaneous branch of femoral nerve
5 Deep branch of highest genicular artery
6 Femur; lateral superior genicular artery
7 Tendon of quadriceps femoris muscle
8 Patella; medial inferior genicular artery
9 Fibular collateral ligament
10 Patellar ligament
11 Tibial collateral ligament
12 Anterior tibial artery and venae comitantes
13 Superficial peroneal nerve
14 Deep peroneal nerve
15 Fibula; interosseous membrane
16 Tibia
17 Sciatic nerve
18 Common peroneal nerve
19 Tibial nerve
20 Popliteal artery and vein
21 Muscular branch of tibial nerve; medial superior genicular artery
22 Lateral meniscus
23 Posterior cruciate ligament
24 Tendon of semimembranosus muscle
25 Muscular branch of tibial nerve
26 Posterior tibial artery and venae comitantes
27 Peroneal artery and venae comitantes
28 Popliteus muscle
29 Tendon of biceps femoris muscle
30 Ligament of lateral meniscus
31 Anterior cruciate ligament
32 Transverse ligament
33 Deep infrapatellar bursa
34 Articular capsule
35 Tendon of gracilis muscle
36 Tendon of sartorius muscle
37 Medial meniscus
38 Suprapatellar bursa
39 Patella
40 Anterior insertion of lateral meniscus
41 Subcutaneous prepatellar bursa
42 Infrapatellar fat pad
43 Bursa of tibial collateral ligament
44 Fibula

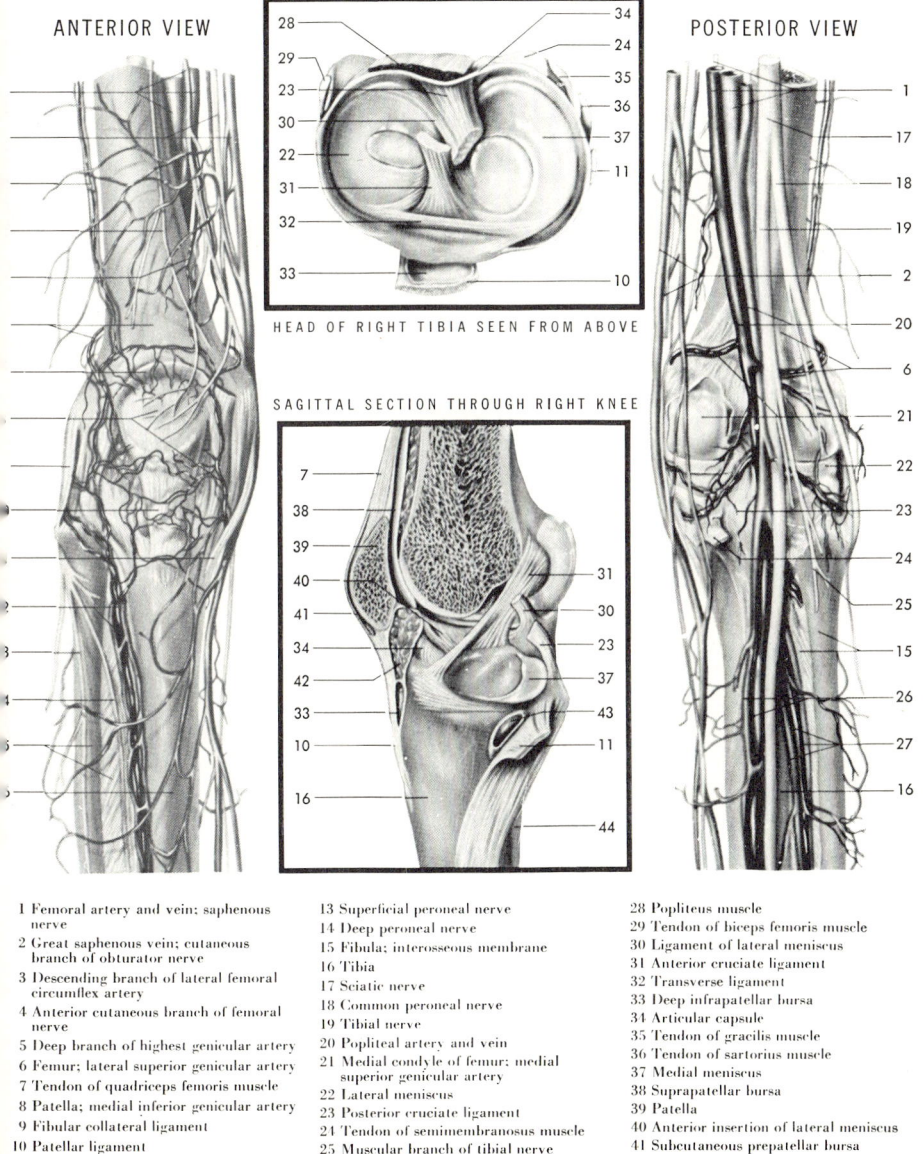

Figure 81   Anatomy of the knee
Courtesy Lederle Laboratories

474

Anatomy of the Ankle

LATERAL VIEW

MEDIAL VIEW

1 Great saphenous vein	16 Tibial nerve	29 Deltoid ligament
2 Talus	17 Posterior tibial artery	30 Sustentaculum tali
3 Tendon of tibialis anterior	18 Tendon of flexor digitorum longus	31 Long plantar ligament and lateral plantar artery
4 Tendon of extensor hallucis longus	19 Tendon of tibialis posterior	32 Sural nerve and cruciate ligament
5 Deep peroneal nerve	20 Medial malleolus	33 Superior peroneal retinaculum and sm saphenous vein
6 Anterior tibial artery	21 Fibula	34 Inferior peroneal retinaculum
7 Tendon of extensor digitorum longus	22 Perforating peroneal artery and anterior ligament of external malleolus	35 Extensor digitorum brevis muscle
8 Peroneus tertius muscle and superficial peroneal nerve	23 Peroneal artery and anterior talofibular ligament	36 Tendon of peroneus tertius
9 Lateral malleolus	24 Calcaneofibular ligament	37 Medial dorsal cutaneous nerve and cruciate ligament
10 Posterior talofibular ligament	25 External talocalcaneal ligament	38 Saphenous nerve
11 Tendon of peroneus longus	26 Tibia	39 Laciniate ligament
12 Tendon of peroneus brevis	27 Lateral tarsal artery and dorsal cuboideo-navicular ligament	40 Medial plantar nerve
13 Calcaneal tendon	28 Dorsal pedis artery	
14 Calcaneus		
15 Tendon of flexor hallucis longus		

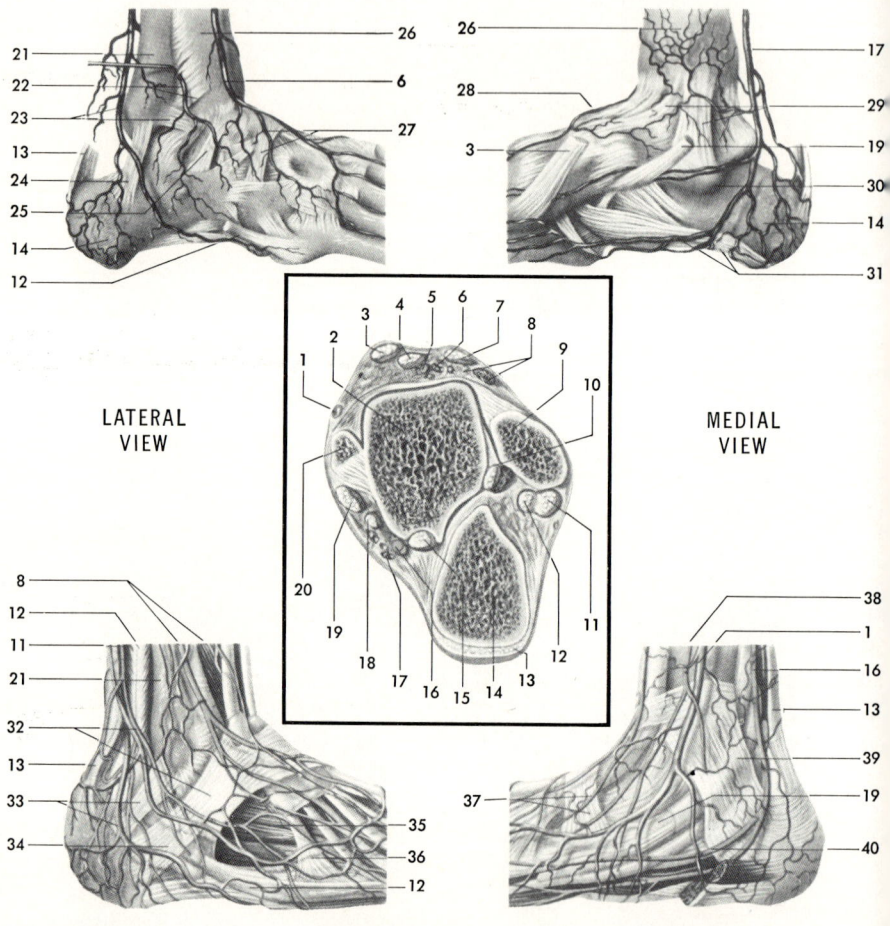

Figure 82 Anatomy of the ankle
Courtesy Lederle Laboratories

up to and including the suprapatellar pouch. Very thick redundant synovium filled the suprapatellar pouch and was therefore resected as completely as possible.

Inspection of the medial and lateral compartments was accomplished with the patella dislocated laterally, revealing detachment of the anterior third of the medial meniscus, with evidence of a chronic process. The undersurface of the patella was inspected and found to have undergone both subacute and chronic chondromalacial change. Very careful recontouring of the undersurface of the patella was accomplished, including osteotome dissection of the margins and sharp knife condyleplasty of the articular surface of the patella. The femoral condyles were treated in like fashion producing smooth, gliding articular surfaces. The medial meniscus was then removed almost totally under direct vision with the knee flexed at 90 degrees. Inspection of the anterior and posterior cruciate ligaments revealed no pathology. The two-thirds of the lateral meniscus, which could be visualized, appeared normal.

A very copious lavage of the joint was performed and all small bits of cartilage and synovium were removed. The knee was extended and the patella replaced in its normal position.

An anatomical closure was performed. The Vastus medialis muscle was reattached to the Rectus femoris tendon and the medial aspect of the newly contoured patella under a normal amount of tension. The capsule of the joint was closed with interrupted 00 chromic suture material. The subcutaneous tissue and deep fascia were approximated with interrupted 00 chromic and the skin was closed with 0000 nylon interrupted and vertical mattress sutures. A bulky Sommers compression dressing was applied with a posterior plaster splint. The tourniquet was deflated.

BONE GRAFTS

The use of autogenous and homogenous bone grafts as a means of providing fixation with osteogenesis is becoming more widely accepted. The availability of material from bone banks has further promoted the use of this technique in preference to other methods of fixation where union is apt to progress more slowly.

Bone grafts are used in a variety of situations: to promote union, to fill defects in delayed union, in cases of nonunion, to provide fixation, to bridge joints and provide arthrodesis, to fill defects following excision of lesions, to provide bone blocks which limit joint motion, and in numerous other circumstances.

Grafts are divided into three categories based on their source of origin as follows:

Autogenous — Bone removed from one site and implanted in another site in the same individual.

Homogenous — Bone obtained from a human other than the patient. Bone bank specimens belong in this group.

Heterogenous — Use of material such as boiled ox bone upon which the host deposits his own tissues.

TYPES OF BONE GRAFTS

Diamond inlay graft
Dual onlay
Hemicylindrical
Inlay
Intramedullary and spongiosa
Massive sliding
Medullary

Onlay
Osteoperiosteal
Peg
Single onlay cortical
Sliding inlay
Whole bone transplant

BONE GRAFT TECHNIQUES

Albee sliding inlay
Banks
Boyd dual inlay
Flanagan & Burem massive apposing
Gallie diamond inlay
Haldeman

Henderson
Hey-Groves and Kirk self-sustaining
Hoglund medullary bone
Phemister onlay
Ryerson medullary bone
Soto-Hall

Bone Graft to the Femur

The area of the right femur was prepared and draped. The tissues covering the site of the fracture were dissected bluntly and the tissue between the fragments carefully removed. Eburnized bone ends were trimmed until cancellous bone was reached. The fragments were pared with a motor saw, reaming out the medulla.

The site of the donor area was selected on the tibia and the periosteum stripped to each side of the proposed graft site for about an inch. A large graft was removed. The cortex and spongiosa were separated. A strip of the spongiosa along with its endosteum was inserted in the medulla bridging the fragments. The graft was fitted into place on the cortex.

Drill holes were made in the graft and receiving sites. Autogenous bone nails which had been developed from the cortical graft were then driven through the holes into the cortex.

The wound was closed in layers and dressed. A hip spica was applied

Autogenous Bone Graft to Right Tibia Donor site: Left Anterior Ilium

After administration of a satisfactory general anesthetic, a pneumatic tourniquet was inflated to 500 mm. of mercury and sustained about the right leg. The right lower extremity and the anterior crest of the ilium were prepared and draped in the usual manner.

The area of delayed union in the proximal third of the right tibia was exposed by a curvilinear incision following one of the previous skin incisions. The incision was carried directly to the bone. The periosteum was divided in the course of the skin incision. Very careful soft tissue dissection was utilized to bring the delayed union site into view. The subperiosteal dissection was carried around to the lateral aspect of the tibia. The delayed union site was then prepared in fenestra fashion by roughening and shingling the cortex by sharp osteotome dissection. Multiple drill holes were made in different directions to stimulate and provide access for new blood vessel growth. This area was then lavaged and packed and the tourniquet deflated.

Attention was then directed to the left anterior iliac crest which was exposed through a skin incision directly over the crest. Strips of autogenous cancellous and cancellous-cortical bone graft were obtained in the usual fashion and placed in a sterile saline basin. The donor site wound was then packed with Gelfoam over the bone and closed with interrupted 00 chromic to approximate the musculature over the crest. Interrupted 00000 nylon was used for the skin closure.

The bone grafts were carefully cut to proper proportion and packed in and about the area of nonunion, especially in the lateral and posterior aspects, with some anteromedially also. The periosteum was then loosely closed over the bone grafts and the skin was brought into its normal position and closed with interrupted 00000 nylon suture material.

After satisfactory lavage of the area, a sterile dressing was applied and a long leg anterior-posterior plaster mold with a Sommers compression dressing. The tourniquet was deflated. A dressing was also placed over the previously closed donor site.

Removal of Tibial Bone Grafts

With the patient in the supine position, the area of the lower right leg is prepared and draped in a sterile manner.

An incision is made along the flat portion of the tibia and carried through the skin and tissues. An osteoperiosteal graft is removed and an incision is then made through the periosteum following the shape of the proposed graft. The desired graft is further outlined with a Luck bone saw. A motor drill is then used to drill the ends. A sharp, thin osteotome is used to connect the drill holes and the tibial graft is removed. Some cancellous bone is curetted out of the medullary cavity.

The periosteum is closed with plain catgut and the wound closed in layers. Dressing and stockinette are applied.

DISLOCATIONS

The displacement of a bone from its normal anatomic position is termed a *dislocation*. Most acute or fresh dislocations are amenable to manual reduction through proper manipulation; however, dislocations which resist closed reduction or which have become habitual are treated by open reduction. Dislocations are often attended by fractures of varying degree which complicate conservative management and require surgery. The most frequently encountered injury of this type is dislocation of the shoulder with fracture of the surgical neck of the humerus. The shoulder is also the joint in which recurrent dislocations are most likely to occur. These dislocations usually occur anteriorly constituting a subcoracoid type displacement.

Numerous operative techniques have been adopted to correct dislocation, with or without fractures, by methods of open reduction. Some of the more popular methods are listed here.

OPERATIONS FOR DISLOCATION

Bankart (shoulder)
Blount osteotomy
Campbell (patella)
Campbell shelf operation
Cave (capitate bone)
Cave and Rowe (shoulder)
Conn operation
Cubbins (shoulder)
Dickson (shoulder)
Eden-Hybbinette (shoulder)
Evans (ankle)
Haas
Hauser (patella)
Kapel (elbow)
King and Richards (hip)
Levine (hip)
Lorenz bifurcation
MacAusland (lunate)

Magnuson-Stack (shoulder)
Mahorner and Mead (lunate)
McLaughlin (shoulder)
Milch (elbow)
Mumford and Gurd (clavicle)
Nicola (shoulder)
Palmer and Widen (shoulder)
Pheasant (elbow)
Putti-Platt (shoulder)
Reichenheim and King (elbow)
Reversed Eden-Hybbinette (shoulder)
Roux-Goldthwait (patella)
Schanz
Slocum (metacarpal joint-thumb)
Speed (elbow)
Watson-Jones (ankle)
Wilson-McKeever (shoulder)

ORTHOPEDIC SURGERY

DISLOCATIONS

Anterior temporal mandibular dislocation

Vertebral dislocation

Subcoracoid dislocation

Subglenoid dislocation

Dislocated carpal lunate (lateral view)

Posterior dislocation of hip

Dislocation of ankle

Posterior dislocation of elbow

Posterior dislocation of knee

Dislocation of thumb

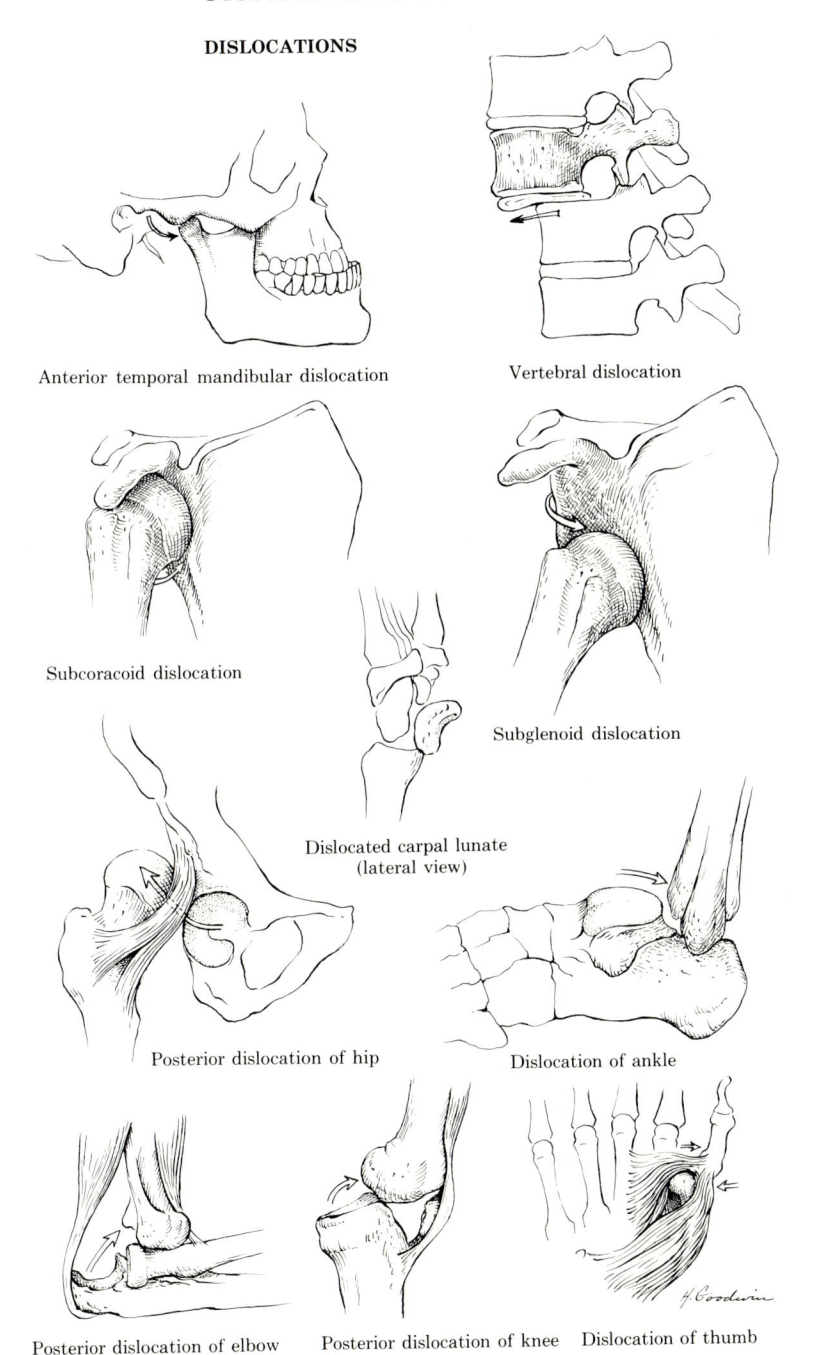

Figure 83   Dislocations
From Dorland's Illustrated Medical Dictionary 24th edition
Courtesy W. B. Saunders Co.—Philadelphia

Watson-Jones Operation for Dislocation of the Ankle

The operative area is sterilely prepared and draped. Under general anesthesia, a lateral incision is made over the posterior border of the lower third of the shaft of the fibula. It is carried around the tip of the lateral malleolus and brought out on the lateral aspect of the foot. Proximally the Peroneus brevis tendon is freed from its muscular attachment. The muscle fibers are sutured to the Peroneus longus tendon. The Peroneus brevis tendon is released as far as the lateral malleolus distally, care being taken not to disturb the annular fibers.

Beginning about one inch above the tip of the malleolus, an anteroposterior tunnel is developed for the tendon through the fibula. A vertical drill hole is made through the outer margin of the neck of the talus, just in front of the articular surface. The drill emerges in the roof of the sinus tarsi. The drill is then introduced in the outermost tip of the lateral malleolus and directed from the anterior aspect, upward and backward. The tendon is then brought from a posterior position forward, is threaded through the first hole in the lateral malleolus, through the second hole in the talus, in a direction from above downward, and then back through the hole in the malleolus. The end of the tendon is sutured to the periosteum on the posterior aspect of the external malleolus.

A cast is applied from the toes to the tibial tubercle.

Bankart Operation for Chronic Dislocation of Shoulder

The patient was placed in Fowler's position with the knees flexed and the feet supported by a padded foot rest. Sterile preparation and draping was carried out.

A deltopectoral incision was made extending from the tip of the acromion to the middle and distal third of the clavicle. The incision was curved downward following the course of the cephalic vein. A groove was created between the pectoral and deltoid muscles. The cephalic vein was ligated and retracted mesially.

Using a No. 3/32 drill, the tip of the coracoid process was drilled and an osteotomy performed.

Medial retraction of the muscles of the coracoid process was carried out. Lateral retraction of the Deltoideus and Pectoralis major muscles was obtained. The Subscapularis muscle was reflected from its insertion. The capsule was opened along the glenoid labrum. The torn glenoid labrum was attached to the bone with wire sutures which were pulled through a drill hole in the neck of the scapula and tied over a button and felt pads posteriorly.

The Subscapularis muscle was reattached to its original insertion using a heavy chromic catgut. A suture placed through a previously made drill hole served to reattach the tip of the osteotomized coracoid process. The muscles were repaired and the wound closed in layers with plain catgut.

A Velpeau dressing was applied.

FRACTURES

A partial or complete interruption in the continuity of a bone is referred to as a *fracture*. Such a break may assume many and varied forms. Definitions of the more frequently used designations for fractures are listed below to familiarize the secretary with the precise connotation of these terms.

BENNETT	A fracture through the first metacarpal of the wrist involving the carpometacarpal joint and associated with subluxation.
CLOSED	A fracture which does not involve a break in the skin.
COLLES'	Fracture of the radius at the wrist with displacement of the lower fragment.
COMMINUTED	A crushing fracture in which the fragments are splintered to pieces.
COMPOUND	Fracture of a bone with an open wound of the skin.
COMPRESSION	Fracture caused by compression and usually seen involving the spine.
COTTON'S	Trimalleolar fracture of the ankle.
DEPRESSED	A type of skull fracture where fragments are pushed inward.
GREENSTICK	An incomplete fracture of a bone.
LEFORT	Fracture of the maxilla, bilaterally, in a horizontal plane.
LINEAR	A fracture running the length of a bone.
MONTEGGIA'S	Dislocation of the head of the radius associated with fracture of the ulnar shaft.
OPEN	Same as compound fracture where there is a wound through the skin.
PATHOLOGIC	Fractures caused by disease such as malignancy.
POTT'S	Bimalleolar fracture of the ankle.
TRIMALLEOLAR	Fracture of the ankle. Cotton's fracture.

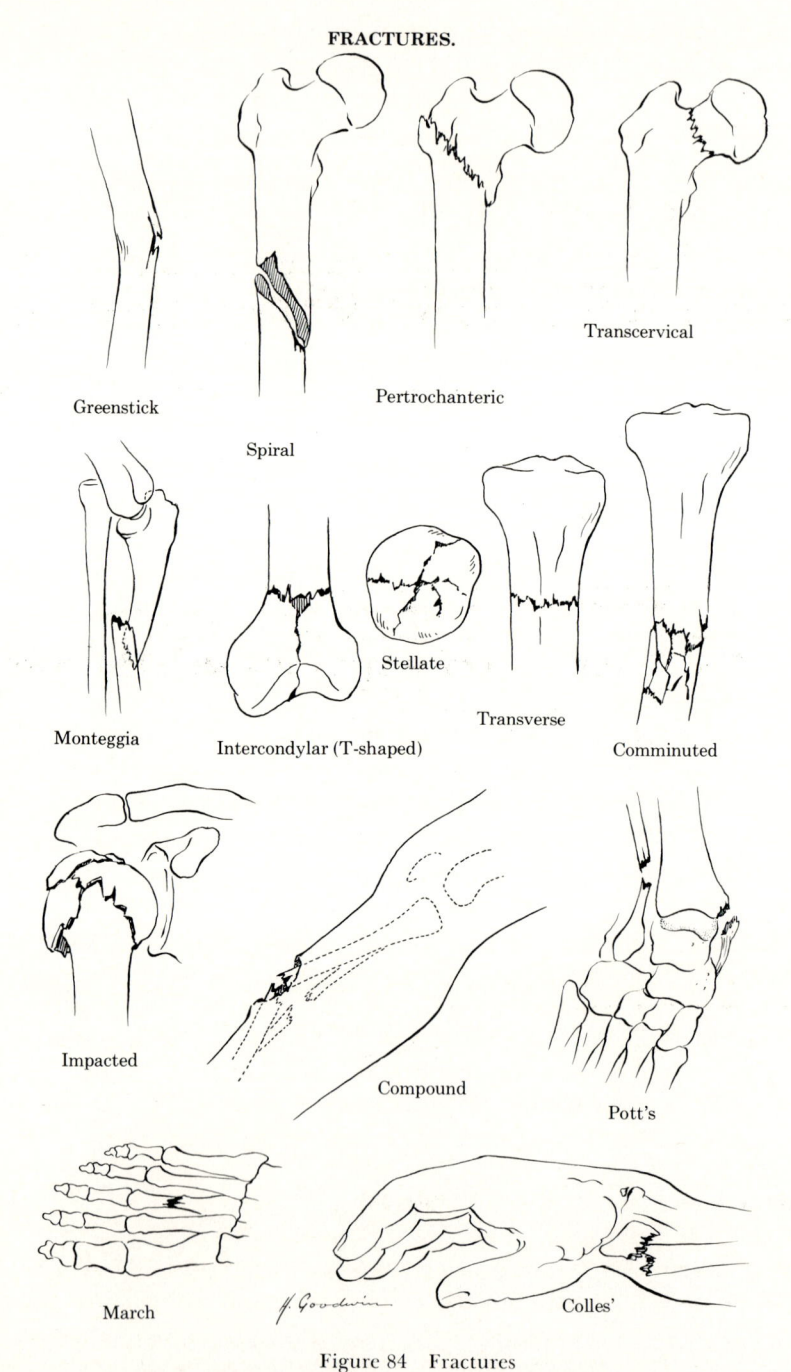

FRACTURES.

Greenstick

Pertrochanteric

Transcervical

Spiral

Monteggia

Intercondylar (T-shaped)

Stellate

Transverse

Comminuted

Impacted

Compound

Pott's

March

Colles'

Figure 84   Fractures
*From Dorland's Illustrated Medical Dictionary 24th edition
Courtesy W. B. Saunders Co.—Philadelphia*

Occasionally, fractures occur near a joint resulting in a dislocation of the joint. Such an entity is referred to as a *fracture-dislocation*.

Surgical Techniques in the Treatment of Fractures

Fractures are treated by closed or open reductions. A variety of screws, nails, plates and prostheses are used to perform internal fixations of fractures. Such equipment and instruments are listed in Chapter 5.

This section will be devoted primarily to a presentation of sample operative reports and listings of techniques employed in fracture management.

SOME REDUCTION TECHNIQUES

Crutchfield (cervical spine)
Essex-Lopresti (axial fixation of calcaneous)
Lottes (tibia)
Magnuson (patella)
Martin (patella)
Speed and Boyd (Monteggia fracture)
Thomson (patella)
Wagner (Bennett fracture)

Lottes Technique for Medullary Nailing of the Tibia

After sterile preparation and draping and after the administration of a general anesthetic, the leg is supported on a fracture table. The hip is flexed 130 degrees and the knee to 90 degrees. A traction apparatus is used.

The tibial crest is palpated. Proper alignment and apposition of the fracture is obtained by manual manipulation.

A small skin incision is made and extended proximally one fingerbreadth medial to the tibial tubercle. The incision is carried through the subcutaneous tissues; however, the bone is exposed only in the distal 3 cms. of the incision. With a three-eighths inch drill, a perforation is made in the cortex opposite the mid-portion of the tibial tubercle. The drill is introduced at right angles to the bone. The handle of the drill is gently depressed after entry into the medullary canal. The drill is kept parallel with the shaft of the tibia. A small metal shield is placed in the incision proximally to prevent soft tissue damage. A carefully positioned slotted hole is then made. The driver is attached and the tip of the nail inserted into the slotted hole with its dorsal fin pointed forward. The tip of the anterior flange is aligned with the middle and lower thirds junction of the tibial shaft. The nail is tapped down into place until resistance is encountered. The tip of the nail is then brought forward by depressing the mid-portion of the nail with the palm of the hand. The nail is driven down the medullary canal and its progress checked by a nail of the same length. Rotation and reduction of the fracture are checked again and the nail driven through the fracture site.

Roentgenograms are made to determine the course of the nail. Satisfactory position having been obtained, the nail is driven in further until the driver strikes the cortex. A small threaded portion of the nail is allowed to protrude to facilitate future extraction.

A temporary plaster cast is applied extending from the toes to the midthigh.

Open Reduction of Left Humerus with Rush Rod Insertion

With the patient under general anesthesia, the left shoulder, chest, and arm were prepared and draped in a sterile manner. A pillow was inserted under the shoulder to elevate the operative area.

An incision was made anteriorly and longitudinally between the pectoral groove. The cephalic vein was not identified. The incision was carried down to the fracture site. A moderate amount of hematoma was evacuated.

The head of the humerus was dislocated posteriorly and the base of the fracture site pointed in a lateral direction. By means of manual manipulation the head of the humerus was placed back into the glenoid fossa and rotated. Traction was applied to the extremity and by means of bone hooks the fracture was reduced. The post-reduction position was satisfactory.

A stab wound was made just lateral to the acromion tip on the shoulder and carried down to the intercondylar groove. Two 8 inch Rush rods were driven down into the humeral shaft. This stabilized the fracture.

The operative area was thoroughly irrigated with saline and the wound closed in layers with interrupted 000 chromic.

Check films of the shoulder showed it to be in satisfactory position. The extremity was bandaged in a Velpeau sling.

Open Reduction—Smith-Petersen Nailing with a Lawson-Thornton Plate, Left Hip

With the patient under suitable anesthesia, the left hip was manipulated and satisfactory reduction obtained. This was verified by x-ray examination.

A lateral incision, approximately 10 inches in length, was made starting at the level of the greater trochanter and extending distally. This was deepened through the fascia. The Vastus lateralis was reflected subperiosteally. There was marked subtrochanteric comminution.

With some difficulty, the spikes were manipulated into position and held in place with a Wilman clamp. The inferior trochanteric fossa was osteotomized and a guide wire passed. Due to the x-ray appearance of bending of the guide wire, it was removed and a 4 inch Smith-Petersen nail inserted into the neck and head of the femur. X-ray examination revealed adequate alignment of this nail. A Lawson-Thornton side plate was suitably fastened to the nail and attached to the femoral cortices with stainless steel screws. Stability was solid following this procedure.

The muscular and fascial layers were closed with interrupted 00 chromic catgut. The subcutaneous tissue was closed with 000 plain catgut and the skin with a running suture of black silk. A dressing was applied.

Austin-Moore Prosthesis, Right Hip

With the patient under spinal anesthesia in a left lateral position, the right extremity was prepared and draped in a sterile manner.

A hockey-stick incision was used to expose the capsule and head of the femur. The Gluteus maximus attachment was then separated. The capsule was entered. Using a periosteal elevator, the broken femoral head was removed. After chipping the bone over the greater trochanter, the reamer was driven into the shaft of the femur. The acetabulum was then tested for the size of the prosthesis to be used. This was inserted into the femur after packing it with cancellous bone. It was then fitted into the socket and a snug fit obtained.

The capsule was reapproximated with interrupted 00 chromic. The muscles were reattached with interrupted chromic. The skin was also closed with chromic.

OTHER ORTHOPEDIC PROCEDURES

In addition to the types of orthopedic procedures already presented, there exist a wide variety of other procedures which include osteotomy, ostectomy, osteoclasis and operations on the bursae, muscles, tendons, ligaments, and fasciae. Examples of some of these operations have also been included in this section to provide the secretary with additional exercise in orthopedic terminology.

Bunionectomy and Hammer Toe Correction

With the patient under general anesthesia, a bloodless field was created by using a blood pressure cuff on the right leg, inflated to 500 mm. of mercury, as a pneumatic tourniquet. The operative field was prepared and draped.

A semilunar incision was made just dorsal to the presenting bunion and skin flaps were raised. The subcutaneous presenting synovial cyst was removed and a triangular flap of synovium was raised exposing the joint cavity. By means of an osteotome and mallet, the exostosis was removed. An incision curving laterally and beginning at the webs of the first and second toes was made. By means of blunt dissection the sesamoid bone on the medial aspect of the first metatarsal head was removed.

A hemostat was passed beneath the first and second metatarsal heads and a 00 chromic suture was threaded completely around the first two metatarsals. It was tied snugly on the medial aspect of the first metatarsal. This helped in the correction of the metatarsus varus.

A wedge-shaped piece of skin over the interphalangeal area of the second and third toes was raised and removed. The extensor tendon was divided proximal to the joint and raised distally until the joint was exposed. By means of an electric saw the articular surface, both proximally and distally, was removed.

Hammer Toe Correction

The hammer toe defect was then corrected. A Kirschner wire of appropriate size was introduced into the joint from the tip of the distal phalanx. This held the joint in position. A Kirschner wire was also introduced into the metatarsophalangeal joint of the first toe from a distal and a medial direction. The wires were then cut leaving them exposed for a brief distance on the second and third toes and burying them subcutaneously on the first toe. The tendons of the toes were then repaired with interrupted 000000 cotton and the synovial flap was resutured in place with interrupted 000000 cotton.

A Jones procedure was performed on the second and third hammer toes. This consisted of tying the long and short extensors of the second and third toes together with a 000000 cotton, freeing the long extensor of the second and third toes approximately to this point, and abrading the surface of the tendon with a knife. The second and third metatarsals were exposed and the periosteum was raised on the lateral aspect of the metatarsal. The extensor tendons of the second and third toes were divided and threaded through a Keith needle with a 00 cotton. This was tunneled between the bone and periosteum ventrally. The sutures were then brought out through the skin in the plantar aspect of the foot.

The foot was padded with a sponge over the cotton sutures which were tied on a button. All skin incisions were closed with interrupted 00000 dermalon. A plaster boot was applied with the foot in a neutral position, maintaining compression on the metatarsal head. The blood pressure cuff was deflated.

Hauser Procedure — Bilateral transfer of tibial tubercle medially

After adequate anesthesia had been obtained, both lower extremities were prepared and draped in the usual fashion.

The right knee was corrected first. The tourniquet was inflated about the right thigh to 500 mm. of mercury and sustained.

A curvilinear skin incision crossing the knee joint in the flexion crease from the medial to the lateral aspect was utilized to expose the patella, patellar tendon and tibial tubercle. Sharp and blunt dissection were used to outline the area. A flap was cut in the periosteum about the tibial tubercle. Multiple drill holes were used to outline a small rectangular area including the tibial tubercle and the insertion of the patellar tendon. These drill holes were joined by sharp osteotome dissection and the patellar tendon insertion, including the tibial tubercle and the fragment of bone there, were lifted away from the tibia. The new insertion site for the tibial tubercle was prepared 1 cm. distally and 1 cm. medially from the previous insertion.

A sharp H incision was made and periosteal flaps raised. Multiple drill holes were used to outline the rectangular bone block. The drill holes were joined by sharp osteotome dissection and the bone block was gently elevated.

The bone block removed from the new insertion was then placed in the defect left by removing the tibial tubercle. The patellar tendon with its bone block was then inserted in this new site. It was internally fixed by means of one large bone screw. The periosteum was sewn carefully to the tibial tubercle periosteum and to the patellar tendon at its new insertion to provide additional security.

The area was lavaged with copious amounts of sterile saline. The lateral portion of the patellar retinaculum was carefully divided with a scissors up to the Vastus lateralis crossover. The medial portion of the retinaculum was then imbricated with interrupted 00 chromic. Subcutaneous tissues were closed with interrupted 000 plain suture and the skin with interrupted 00000 cotton. A compression dressing was applied. The tourniquet was deflated. Another tourniquet was inflated about the left thigh.

The same procedure was repeated on the left lower extremity with the exception that a stainless steel bone screw was not necessary to secure the tibial tubercle transplant. This was done by geometrically cutting the block and placing it in its new bed. It was fixed securely enough and therefore did not require a bone screw.

When both knees had been finished, dressings were applied. Long leg plaster splints were utilized to secure immobilization of the knees.

Medial Meniscectomy

Under general anesthesia, with tourniquet control, an arthrotomy of the left knee was performed through a medial peripatellar skin incision. The medial meniscus was found to be completely detached posteriorly with a large bucket-handle caught in the joint. A total meniscectomy was performed. The remainder of the knee appeared normal.

Following lavage with saline, an anatomical closure with 000 nylon subcuticular sutures for the skin was accomplished. The tourniquet was deflated and a Sommers compression dressing applied.

Primary Tenorrhaphy

Under general anesthesia the patient was placed in the supine position. Routine sterile preparation and draping was carried out.

Initially, the wound was irrigated with normal saline. Mild debridement of the necrotic and bruised tissue was done. The various tendons were then located and held in place with a Keith needle. Inspection of the wound made it apparent that the Flexor digitorum sublimis, the Flexor carpi radialis and ulnaris as well as the Palmaris longus tendon had been completely severed. After these tendons were found, a primary tenorrhaphy was carried out by approximating the respective tendons to their counterparts with interrupted 000000 cotton sutures.

After adequate hemostasis had been maintained, the wound was closed using interrupted 000000 cotton sutures for the subcutaneous tissue and continuous running 00000 dermalon suture for the skin. The hand was then dressed with a compression dressing and splinted in flexion and partial ulnar deviation.

500 cc. of 5% glucose in water was used during the operation.

Tendon Graft

The Flexor digitorum sublimis (superficialis) tendon was used for a graft to the Flexor digitorum profundus tendon.

Under general anesthesia, the entire right hand and forearm were thoroughly prepared with soap and water for 10 minutes. A pneumatic cuff was used as a pneumatic tourniquet to control bleeding.

A midline incision was made on the ulnar aspect of the right middle finger. It was found that the Flexor digitorum profundus and sublimis tendons had been cut into two parts. The ends were divided and separated. The proximal end of the profundus and sublimis tendons had retracted into the palm.

A longitudinal semicurved incision was made in the palm and the proximal ends of the tendon were identified here. A transverse incision was

ORTHOPEDIC SURGERY

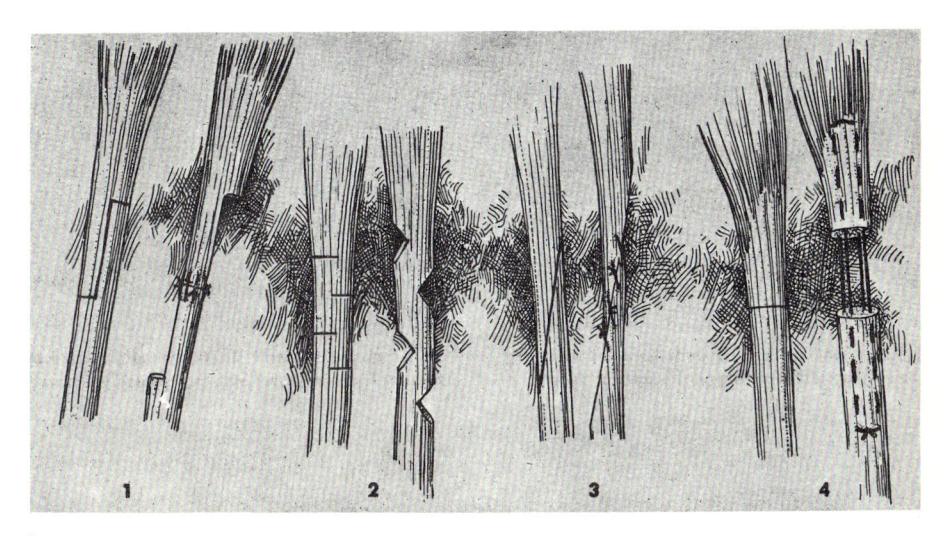

Transverse methods of tendon lengthening and repair. **1.** Half section slitting and gliding ("Z" tenotomy) method. **2.** Accordion method. **3.** Oblique section and gliding method. **4.** Lange method.

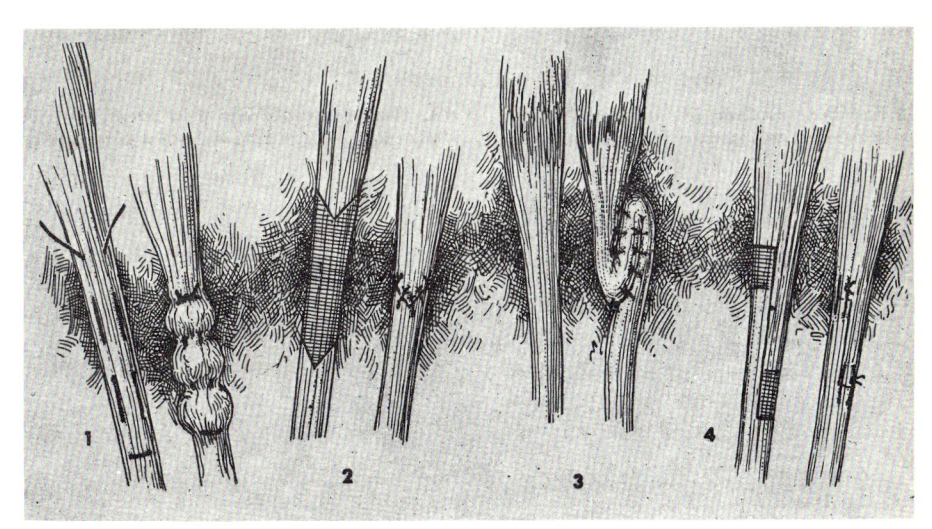

Methods of tendon shortening. **1.** Hoffa's method. **2.** Removal of section of tendon and mortise. Method of uniting ends. **3.** Doubling over method and technique of suturing folds. **4.** "Z" incision with excision of ends.

Figure 85 Tendon lengthening and shortening techniques
Courtesy Ethicon, Inc.

made in the wrist and the sublimis tendon removed at the wrist. Considerable scarring was present throughout the tendon, in the finger as well as in the palm.

The Flexor digitorum sublimis tendon was used as a graft. It was united to the insertion of the Flexor digitorum profundus in the distal phalanx of the right middle finger. The graft extended from the distal phalanx to the volar area of the palm. A pulley was reconstructed out of the remaining portion of the sublimis tendon over the middle finger.

The blood pressure cuff was removed at half hour intervals. The skin edges were carefully closed with interrupted fine 00000 nylon sutures. Several small rubber drains were inserted in each operative site. A large compression type dressing with a posterior metal splint was applied.

Split Thickness Skin Graft to Index Finger With Repair

With the patient under general anesthesia, in the supine position, the right hand and forearm were prepared and draped in the usual manner. A bloodless field was secured by means of a pneumatic tourniquet about the right arm. The tourniquet was elevated to 300 mm. of mercury.

There was an avulsion of skin and subcutaneous tissue on the tactile pad of the finger. A split thickness skin graft was taken with a razor blade from the volar aspect of the forearm, transferred to the index finger amputation stump and sutured in position with interrupted 000000 nylon.

In the case of the middle finger there was an amputation through the distal phalanx. There was adequate skin and subcutaneous tissue for direct primary closure which was performed after the digital sensory nerves had been resected back into healthy soft tissue.

In the ring finger, there was a laceration on the tactile pad. This laceration was repaired with interrupted 000000 nylon.

Section of Transverse Carpal Ligament, Right Wrist

The patient presented a carpal tunnel syndrome of the right wrist.

Under general anesthesia a tourniquet was applied to the right upper arm and the hand was surgically prepared and draped.

A curved incision was made across the flexor palmar crease extending into the palm of the hand. The dissection was carried down to the palmar fascia. The Palmaris longus was identified and retracted. An incision was made through the fascia and the transverse carpal ligament identified. With a hemostat under the transverse carpal ligament to protect the median nerve, it was sectioned. It was found to be hard and gritty. There was evidence to indicate compression of the median nerve.

A small portion of the transverse carpal ligament was removed to insure adequate passage of the Flexor sublimis and Flexor profundus tendons as well as the median nerve. The median nerve was not disturbed in any way. Except for the swelling and thickening noted proximal to the transverse carpal ligament, no abnormalities were encountered.

The wound was closed with three sutures of plain catgut for the subcutaneous fascia. The skin was closed with a subcuticular suture of 000 nylon. This was followed by the application of Telfa, dry sterile gauze and a heavy compression bandage, after the tourniquet had been removed.

DISEASES OF THE MUSCULOSKELETAL SYSTEM

Abduction contracture of the hip
Abscess of
Accessory bone
Acetabulum, pelvic protrusion of
Achondroplasia
Actinomycosis of bone
Adduction contracture of hip
Adventitious bursa
Albright's syndrome
Amyloid infiltration
Amyotonia congenita
Ankylosis, bony or fibrous
Anteversion of neck of femur
Arthritis
  allergic
  hypertrophic
  infectious
  rheumatoid
  syphilitic
Arthrodesis
Arthrogryposis
Aseptic necrosis
Atrophy
Avulsion of epiphysis
Bertolotti's syndrome
Blastomycosis
Bunion (bursitis of joint of toe)
Bursitis
Caffey's syndrome
Caisson disease of bone
Calcification of intervertebral cartilage
Calcification of medial collateral ligament of knee
Callus formation, excessive
Caries of petrous bone

Cephalohematoma
Charcot joint
Chondritis of costal cartilage
Chondritis of intervertebral cartilage
Chondroblastoma
Chondroma
Chondromalacia of patella
Chondrosarcoma
Clawfoot
Clawhand, syringomyelic
Clubfoot
Clubhand
Coccidioidomycosis
Contracture of ligament
Contracture due to flaccid paralysis
Coxa valga
Coxa vara
  due to osteitis fibrosa cystica
Craniorachischisis
Craniotabes
Curvature of radius, progressive
Cyst of
Cyst of meniscus of knee
Cysticercosis
Dermatomyositis
Detachment of medial meniscus
Diaphragmatic hernia
Diastasis of cranial bones
Diastasis of muscle
Diastasis recti
Dislocation
  compound
  incomplete
Dislocation of cartilage

DISEASES OF THE MUSCULOSKELETAL SYSTEM (continued)

Dislocation of joint
Dislocation of patella (knee)
Dupuytrens contracture
Dyschondroplasia
Dysplasia, fibrous monostotic
Dysplasia, fibrous, polyostotic
Eccentro-osteochondrodysplasia
Echinococcosis
Elevation of scapula
Elongation of styloid of temporal bone
Enchondromatosis, skeletal
Eosinophilic granuloma
Epiphysiolysis
Epiphysis, slipping
Epiphysitis
Erb disease (pseudohypertrophic muscular dystrophy)
Erb-Goldflam disease (myasthenia gravis)
Ewing's sarcoma
Exaggerated lumbosacral angle
Exostosis (pl. exostoses)
External rotation contracture of hip
Fasciitis
Fibroma
Fibrosarcoma
Flail joint
Flatfoot
Flexion contracture of hip
Foreign body of
Fracture
  chip
  closed
  Colles'
  comminuted
  compression
  depressed
  dislocation
  due to osteitis fibrosa cystica
  impacted
  Monteggia's
  open
  pathologic
  Pott's
  trimalleolar

Fracture with:
  cross union
  delayed union
  malunion
  nonunion
Fragilitas ossium
Funnel chest
Fusion defect
Genu recurvatum
Genu valgum
Genu varum
Giant cell tumor
Gluteal bursitis
Goundou
Granular cell myoblastoma
Growth arrest
Hallux rigidus
Hallux valgus
Hallux varus
Hammer toe
Hemangioma
Hemangiosarcoma
Hemarthrosis
Hemiatrophy of face
Herniation of nucleus pulposus
Hydrarthrosis, intermittent
Hyperostosis cortical
Hyperostosis frontalis interna
Hypertelorism
Hypertrophic arthritis
Hypertrophic osteoarthropathy
Hypertrophy of ligamenta flava
Hypertrophy of meniscus of knee
Hypoplasia
Internal rotation contracture of hip
Kyphosis
Lead osteosclerosis
Lipoma
Liposarcoma
Lordosis
Lumbosacral joint, incomplete sacralization
Lumbosacral joint, instability
Lumbosacral joint, transitional
Melorheostosis
Metaphysical aclasis

DISEASES OF THE MUSCULOSKELETAL SYSTEM (continued)

Metatarsal varus
Microgenia
Micrognathia
Milkman's syndrome
Moniliasis
Muscular dystrophy
Myasthenia gravis
Myoblastoma, granular cell
Myositis
   ossificans
   progressive ossifying
Myotonia acquisita
Myotonia congenita
Myotonia intermittens
Myxoma
Necrosis of bone
Neurofibroma
Neurogenic arthropathy
Neurogenic atrophy
Obstetric paralysis
Olecranon bursitis
Osteitis deformans
Osteitis fibrosa cystica
Osteoarthritis
Osteochondritis
Osteochondritis dissecans
Osteochondrosis
Osteoid osteoma
Osteomalacia
   juvenile
   senile
Osteomyelitis
Osteopetrosis
Osteopoikilosis
Osteoporosis
Overdevelopment of nasal bones
Palindromic rheumatism
Paramyoclonus multiplex
Paramyotonia congenita
Patella biparta
Pelvic obliquity fixed
Pelvic obliquity not fixed
Periarticular fibrositis
Periosteal fibroma
Periostitis
Pidgeon breast, congenital

Pigmented villonodular synovitis
Plasma cell myeloma
Platybasia
Polyarthritis due to Sickle
   cell anemia
Polyostotic fibrous dysplasia
Postpoliomyelitic atrophy
Prognathia
Pseudoarthrosis of lumbosacral
   spine
Rachitis tarda
Rarefaction of
Refracture following fracture
Relaxation of ligaments of joint
Renal osteodystrophy
Reticulum cell sarcoma
Retropatellar fat pad hypertrophy
Rhabdomyoma of muscle
Rhabdomyosarcoma of muscle
Rheumatoid arthritis
Round back due to senile atrophy
Rudimentary bone
Rupture of muscle
Sacralization of L-5
Sarcoma
Sclerotic osteitis
Scoliosis
Segmentation, incomplete
Sequestrum formation
Sesamoid bone fusion defect
Sesamoiditis
Slipped epiphysis
Slipping rib
Snapping hip
Spasmus nutans
Sporotrichosis of bone
Sprain of joint
Sprain of ligament
Stenosis of tendon sheath
Stewart-Morel syndrome
Subluxation
Subperiosteal calcification
Supernumerary cervical ribs
Supernumerary vertebra
Synostosis
Synovioma

DISEASES OF THE MUSCULOSKELETAL SYSTEM (continued)

Synovitis
Syphilis of bone
Syphilitic osteochonditis
Syringomyelia
Tabetic arthropathy of knee
Talipes calcaneovalgus
Talipes calcaneovarus
Talipes calcaneus
Talipes cavus
Talipes equinovalgus
Talipes equinovarus (clubfoot)
Talipes equinus
Talipes, flaccid
Talipes planovalgus
Talipes varus (clubfoot)
Tear of capsule
Tear of lateral meniscus of knee
Tenosynovitis
  adhesive
  crepitans
  villous
Tibia vara
Tilt of pelvis
Torticollis
Transitional lumbosacral vertebra
Trigger finger
Tuberculosis of bone
Unstable lumbosacral joint
Varus of fifth toe
Vertebral arch fusion defect
Xanthoma of joint
Xanthomatosis of bone

OPERATIONS ON THE MUSCULOSKELETAL SYSTEM

Advancement of tendon
Amputation of upper extremity
  Amputation, interthoracoscapular
  Amputation of arm through humerus
  Amputation of forearm through radius and ulna
  Amputation of hand through metacarpal bones
  Amputation of finger by disarticulation of metacarpophalangeal joint of the:
    thumb
    index finger
    middle finger
    ring finger
    little finger
  Amputation of finger by dismemberment through metacarpals (1 thru 5) or:
    through phalanges of thumb
    index finger
    middle finger
    ring finger
    little finger
Amputation of lower extremity
  Amputation of leg at thigh (through femur)
  Amputation A-K (above knee)
  Amputation of knee through condyles of femur (Gritti-Stokes amputation)
  Amputation of leg through tibia and fibula
  Amputation at ankle through malleoli of tibia and fibula (Pirogoff's amputation; Syme's amputation)
  Amputation of foot between tarsus and metatarsus (Hey's amputation)
  Amputation of foot by midtarsal disarticulation (Chopart's amputation)
  Amputation of toe by disarticulation of metatarsophalangeal joint of the:
    great toe
    second toe
    third toe
    fourth toe
    fifth toe

OPERATIONS ON THE MUSCULOSKELETAL SYSTEM (continued)

Amputation of toe by dismemberment through metatarsal (1 thru 5)
or:
  through phalanges of great toe
  second toe
  third toe
  fourth toe
  fifth toe
Aponeurorrhaphy
Arthrectomy (excision of joint)
Arthrocentesis
Arthrodesis
Arthroplasty
Arthrotomy
  with drainage (arthrostomy)
  with exploration
  with removal
Astragalectomy
Biopsy of
Bone graft
Bursectomy
Capsulorrhaphy
Capsulotomy
Carpectomy
Chondrectomy
Chondrotomy
Clavicotomy
Closed reduction of fracture
Coccygectomy
Condylectomy
Costectomy
Costotransversectomy
Debridement
Desmotomy
Disarticulation of elbow
Disarticulation of hip
Disarticulation at knee
Disarticulation of shoulder
Disarticulation of wrist
  carpometacarpal
  midcarpal
  radiocarpal
Drainage of bone
Drainage of muscle
Drainage of tendon sheath
Excision of lesion
Exploration of bone
Exploration of fascia
Exploration of muscle
Exploration of tendon
Exploration of tendon sheath
Fasciectomy
Fascioplasty
Fasciorrhaphy
Fasciotomy
Fusion of (bone)
Graft of fascia
Graft of tendon
Hemilaminectomy
Incision and drainage of:
  bursa
  distal anterior closed space
  dorsal subaponeurotic space
  hypothenar space
  middle palmar space
  thenar space
  web space
Insertion of wire, metal plate, nail, screw, pin, etc.
Interpelviabdominal amputation
Ischiopubiotomy
Laminectomy
Laminotomy
Lengthening of bone
Lengthening of tendon
Lumbosacral fusion
Manipulation of fracture
Meniscectomy
Metatarsectomy
Myectomy
Myoplasty
Myorrhaphy
Myotasis
Myotenotomy
Myotomy
Open reduction of fracture
Ostectomy (exc. of bone)
Osteoclasis
Osteoperiosteal graft
Osteoplasty
Osteotomy

OPERATIONS ON THE MUSCULOSKELETAL SYSTEM (continued)

Periosteal graft	Sternotomy
Periosteotomy	Suture of ligament
Pubiotomy	Suture of muscle (myorrhaphy)
Removal of band	Suture of tendon (tenorrhaphy)
Removal of foreign body	Synchondrotomy
Removal of metal plate, pin, nail, screw, bolt, etc.	Synovectomy
	Tenoplasty
Removal of sequestrum	Tenorrhaphy
Scapulopexy	Tenotomy
Shortening of bone	Transplantation of muscle
Shortening of tendon	Transposition of tendon
Spinal fusion	

Eponymic titles often pose a problem for the medical secretary and for this reason we have included the following list of orthopedic procedures The surgeons whose names appear in these titles often have numerous operative techniques to their credit, many of which have not been indicated here. This list is intended primarily as an index to some of the more important contributions to operative orthopedics. It will also serve to familiarize the secretary with the names of the men after whom operations in this field have been named.

Abbott arthrodesis
Albee fusion of the spine
Albee reconstruction operation
Albee shelf operation
Badgley arthrodesis of the hip
Bateman denervation of the knee
Bateman tendon transference of the shoulder
Bickel and Moe translocation of Peroneus longus
Blocker operation for elephantiasis
Blount rotation osteotomy
Blount technique for ununited fractures
Blundell Jones varus osteotomy
Boyd dual onlay bone graft
Boyd patellectomy
Brackett osteosynthesis of the femur
Brett technique for genu recurvatum
Brisement Force manipulation
Brittain extra-articular arthrodesis
Brittain fusion of the knee
Brockman operation for equinovarus
Bunnell repair of ligaments
Bunnell repair of tendons
Bunnell technique for malunited Bennett's fracture
Burman tendon transfer
Campbell bone block for paralytic equinus

ORTHOPEDIC OPERATIONS (Continued)

Campbell shelf operation
Carrell replacement of distal end of fibula
Cartilaginous cup arthroplasty
Chandler fusion of hip
Charnley compression arthrodesis
Clothespin "H" or Prop graft in spinal fusion
Cole operation for cavus deformity of the foot
Colonna arthrodesis of the wrist
Colonna arthroplasty for congenital dislocation of the hip
Colonna reconstruction operation
Colop ostectomy
Compere operation for lengthening the femur
Credo operation for congenital dislocation of the hip
Darrach resection of the distal end of the ulna
Denuse operation for congenital dislocation of the hip
Dickson shelf operation
Dickson-Diveley operation for clawtoe deformity
Dunn-Brittain arthrodesis of the ankle
Durman osteotomy and bone graft
Eden-Hybbinette bone graft
Eggers neurectomy
Eggers transplantation of hamstring tendons
Ellis Jones operation for displacement of peroneal tendons
Elmslie-Cholmeley double tarsal wedge osteotomy
Eyler flexorplasty
Fowler capsulotomy of metacarpophalangeal joints
Fritz Lange operation for congenital dislocation of the hip
Gaenslen split heel incision
Garceau anterior tibial tendon transfer in clubfoot
Ghormley arthrodesis of the hip
Ghormley osteotomy and bone graft
Ghormley shelf operation
Gibson arthroplasty
Gill arthrodesis of the shoulder
Gill operation for paralytic foot drop
Girdlestone laminectomy
Girdlestone-Taylor tendon transfer for clawtoe
Grice-Green extra-articular arthrodesis of subtalar joint
Hammond operation for hallux equinus
Hark operation for flatfoot
Harmon osteotomy
Harris-Beath operation for flatfoot
Hauser lengthening of tendo-calcaneus
Heifitz operation for ingrown toenail
Henderson arthrodesis of the hip

ORTHOPEDIC OPERATIONS (Continued)

Hendry posterior bone block of elbow
Henry and Geist spinal fusion
Heyman operation for genu recurvatum
Hibbs arthrodesis of the hip
Hibbs spinal fusion
His-Hass operation for brachial plexus injury
Hohmann operation for tennis elbow
Hoke pes planus operation
Horwitz and Adams transfibular arthrodesis
Howorth open reduction for congenital dislocation of the hip
Hueter-Mayo toe operation
Inclan bone block
Inclan osteotomy and bone graft
Joplin bunion operation
Judet prosthetic replacement arthroplasty
Judet technique for stem prosthesis
Kelikian arthroplasty of temporomandibular joint
Keller bunion operation
Kellogg-Speed operation for spondylolisthesis (anterior fusion)
Kidner pes planus operation
Kirkaldy-Willis ischiofemoral arthrodesis
Koenig-Wittek operation for congenital elevation of the scapula
Kutler plastic closure in transverse fingertip amputations
Lambrinudi drop-foot operation
Lapidus bunion operation
Lapidus operation for hallux equinus (dorsal bunion)
Legge spherical prosthesis technique
L'Episcopo osteotomy
Liebolt operation for radioulnar joint stability
Linton and Talbott operation for removal of gouty tophus
Littlewood's forequarter amputation
Lorenz bifurcation osteotomy
Lorenz operation for congenital dislocation of the hip
Lucas and Cottrell notched rotation osteotomy of the tibia
Ludloff incision for psoas abscess
MacAusland arthroplasty of the elbow
Macey technique for elephantiasis
Magnuson arthroplasty of the knee
Mayo bunion operation
Mazur patellectomy
McBride bunion operation
McCarroll rotation osteotomy
McElvenny neuroma operation
McElvenny operation for hallux varus
McLaughlin repair of musculotendinous cuff

ORTHOPEDIC OPERATIONS (Continued)

Milch cuff resection of ulna
Moyer transplantation of Trapezius
Mozicki spinal fusion
Mustard transference of Iliopsoas tendon
Naughton-Dunn arthrodesis of the ankle
Ober forward transference of Tibialis posterior tendon
Ober operation for congenital elevation of the scapula
Osgood osteotomy of the femur
Parkes tendon transplantation of Volkmann's contracture
Pauwels adduction osteotomy
Pauwels Y-osteotomy
Platou rotation osteotomy
Putti arthrodesis of knee with tibial bone graft
Putti arthrodesis of shoulder
Ridlon operation for congenital dislocation of the hip
Riordan tendon transfer of the thumb
Ruiz-Mora operation for overlapping 5th toe
Schanz osteotomy in congenital hip dislocation
Schede rotation osteotomy
Seddon arthrodesis of the wrist
Shrock operation for congenital elevation of the scapula (Sprengel's deformity)
Smith-Petersen acromioplasty
Sofield operation for congenital pseudarthrosis of the tibia
Soutter transference of crest of ilium
J.S. Speed osteotomy and bone graft
Stamm arthrodesis of the hip
Staples arthrodesis of the elbow
Steele-Stewart operation for equinovarus
Steindler flexorplasty
Steindler operation for pes cavus
Steindler operation of the shoulder joint
Trethowan operation for tennis elbow
Trumble arthrodesis
Vulpius-Compere lengthening of tendo-calcaneus
Whitman reconstruction operation
Whitman talectomy
Wickstrom arthrodesis of the wrist
Wilson trochanteric arthroplasty
Wilson-Jones arthrodesis of the shoulder
Wilson-Straub spinal fusion
Woughter sliding flap graft in transverse fingertip amputations
Yount posterior capsulotomy
Zodik operation for ingrown toenails
Zahradnicek biplane cuneiform osteotomy

13 } Otolaryngology (E.N.T.)

EAR—NOSE—THROAT

Otolaryngology, also referred to as E.N.T. (Ear, Nose and Throat) or otorhinolaryngology, is a surgical specialty which concerns itself with inflammatory and surgical lesions of the ears, nose and throat. These conditions are treated medically as well as surgically with antibiotics providing important therapeutic support.

The introduction of antibiotics has probably not influenced any surgical specialty to the extent that it has otolaryngology. Many of the conditions which were formerly common occurences in the practice of the otolaryngologist are seldom seen today as a result of early antibiotic intervention. Antibiotics have also produced many ear, nose and throat conditions which were uncommon before their use.

Advances in modes of treatment have been attended by dramatic new developments in surgical techniques which enable the modern otolaryngologist to successfully manage conditions for which, only a few years ago, no help was available.

In the field of otology (ear), some of the most spectacular progress has been made. There is possibly no more exacting and sensitive operation in any branch of surgery than the *stapedectomy,* performed for clinical otosclerosis.

In the field of rhinology (nose), pyogenic infections are better controlled; however, surgical conditions such as deviated nasal septum, nasal polyps, sinus defects and nasal fractures are no less common.

The otolaryngologist, skilled in modern surgical techniques, is equipped to care for almost all conditions of the neck with the possible exception of thyroidectomy operations. He does not routinely perform thyroidectomies unless the thyroid must be sacrificed in the course of a radical neck operation.

One of the more recent developments in laryngology (throat) is an

THE EAR AND RELATED STRUCTURES.

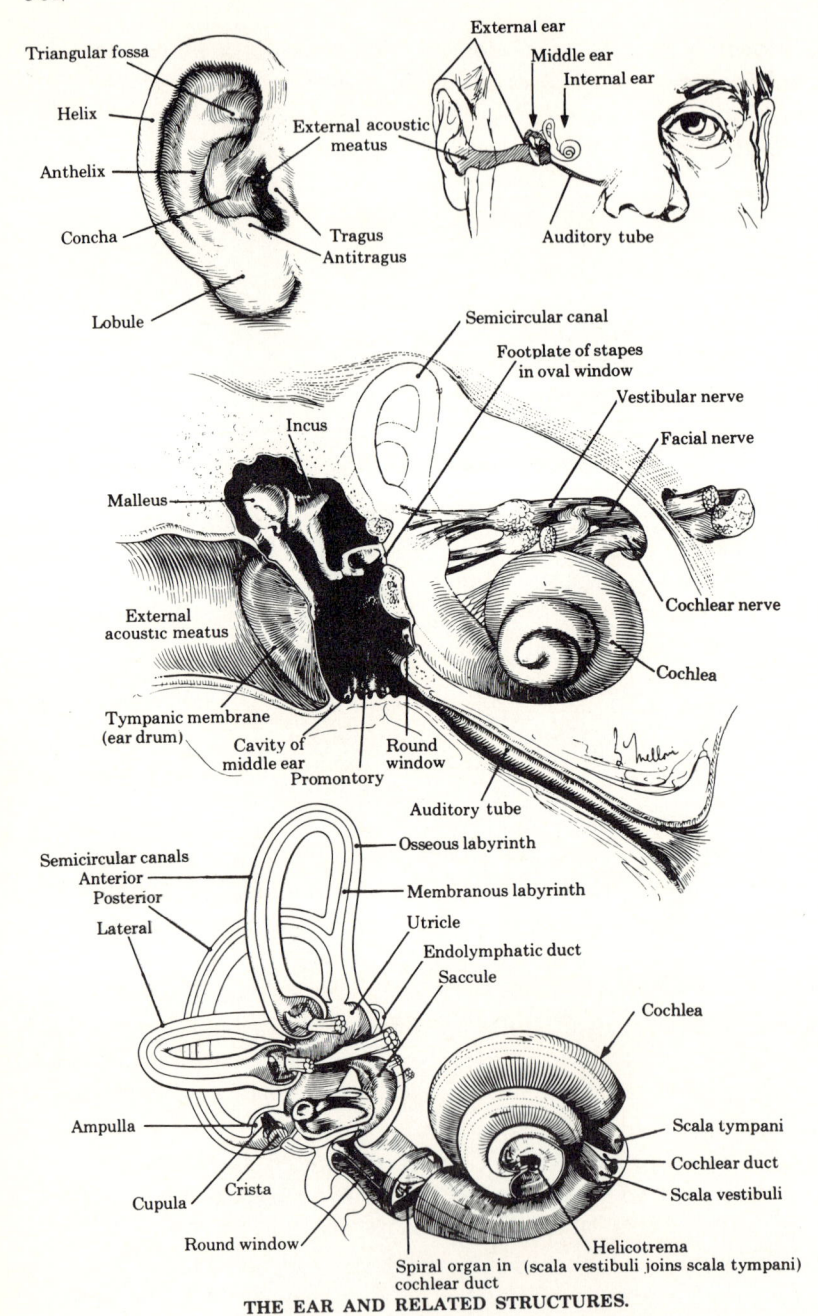

Figure 86 The Ear and related structures.
From Dorland's Illustrated Medical Dictionary 24th Edition
Courtesy W. B. Saunders Company

operation known as an *arytenoidectomy* which provides a more adequate airway to relieve respiratory obstruction in the throat. A description of this procedure has been included in this chapter under the section dealing with operations on the throat.

THE MIDDLE EAR

The ear is anatomically divided into the external ear, the middle ear and the internal ear. The internal ear is surgically inaccessible for all practical purposes. The middle ear is more important in the specialty of otolaryngology than is the external ear, the latter often being managed by the plastic surgeon. We will confine our considerations of the ear in this chapter to the middle ear.

The tympanic cavity, otherwise known as the middle ear, is a minute air cavity in the petrous portion of the temporal bone. It contains an ossicular chain of three small bones designated as the *malleus, incus,* and *stapes* which transmit vibrations of sound across the middle ear cavity to the internal ear.

The middle ear contains five openings which include: one into the external auditory canal (separated by the tympanic membrane), one into the auditory (eustachian) tube, one into the mastoid sinuses, and two into the internal ear. The latter two openings or windows are called the *fenestra rotunda* (also: fenestra cochleae or round window) and the *fenestra ovalis* (also: fenestra vestibuli or oval window).

The anatomic structures of the external ear are listed in Chapter 13. Important surgical features of the middle ear and associated structures are listed below.

ANATOMIC FEATURES OF THE MIDDLE EAR AND RELATED STRUCTURES

Aditus
Annular ligament
Annulus tympanicus
Anterior ligament of the malleus
Anterior process
Anterior wall
Articular capsule
Attic
Auditory canal
Auditory tube (eustachian)
Axis ligament
Base of the stapes
Capitulum of the stapes

Carotid canal
Cartilaginous portion
Chorda tympani nerve
Cochlea (pl. cochleae)
Cog-tooth of malleus
Columella
Crura
Crus
Deep petrosal nerve
Drumhead (tympanic membrane)
Endaural
Epitympanic recess
Epitympanum

ANATOMIC FEATURES OF THE MIDDLE EAR AND RELATED STRUCTURES (Continued)

Eustachian canal
Eustachian tube
External acoustic meatus
External ligament of the malleus
Fenestra cochleae (round window)
Fenestra ovalis (oval window)
Fenestra rotunda (round window)
Fenestra vestibuli (oval window)
Foot-plate
Fossa incudis
Fundus tympani
Glaserian fissure
Head of the malleus
Horizontal canal
Hyaline cartilage
Incudomalleolar joint
Incudostapedial joint
Incus
Isthmus
Iter chordae, anterior, posterior
Jugular wall or floor
Labyrinthic wall
Lateral ligament of the malleus
Lateral process of the malleus
Lenticular process of the incus
Long crus
Long process of the incus
Malleo-incudal joint
Malleolar folds
Malleus
Manubrium of the malleus
Mastoid
Mastoid antrum
Mastoid air cells
Mastoid wall
Medial wall
Membranous (lateral) wall
Meniscus
Notch of Rivinus
Osseous portion
Ossicles
Oval window

Oval window niche
Oval window reflex
Paries jugularis
Paries tegmentalis
Pars flassida
Petrotympanic fissure
Postauricular area
Posterior ligament of the incus
Posterior wall
Prominence of the facial canal
Promontory
Pyramidal eminence
Round window
Round window reflex
Secondary tympanic membrane
Semicanal for Tensor tympani
Semicircular canal
Septum canalis musculotubarii
Short crus of the incus
Sigmoid sinus
Sino-dural
Sinus tympanicus
Spine of Henle
Spur of the malleus
Stapedius muscle
Stapedius tendon
Stapes
Superior ligament of the incus
Tegmen tympani
Tegmental wall roof
Temporalis muscle
Tensor tympani muscle
Torus tubarius
Trautmann's triangle
Tympanic antrum
Tympanic cavity
Tympanic membrane (drumhead)
Tympanic orifice
Tympanic sulcus
Tympanomeatal
Umbo
Vestibule

Endolymphatic-Subarachnoid Shunt

After injection with 1% Xylocaine with epinephrine, a routine postauricular incision was made. The subcutaneous tissue and periosteum were divided by sharp dissection. Bleeders were clamped and electrocoagulated. The periosteum was incised and retracted. This exposed the mastoid cavity. The cortex was entered with a cutting bur at the spine of Henle. The entire operation was performed using the operating microscope.

After drilling away a few superficial cells, the antrum was reached. The anterior prominence of the lateral sinus was identified as was the semicircular canal. Trautmann's triangle was now completely exenterated with cutting burs. The posterior semicircular canal was roughly skeletonized. From this point on, the Diamond bur and continuous irrigation with Ringer's solution were used. The posterior semicircular canal was thinned down but not to a point where blue line was visible.

The dural plate overlying the posterior cranial fossa was removed partly with a Diamond bur and partly with small curettes. The endolymphatic sac was identified. Its outer layer was then incised through the dura with a House tympanoplastic knife. Care was taken to avoid opening any of the large veins in the dura.

The medial wall of the endolymphatic sac was incised and the incision continued into the subarachnoid space. A small amount of cerebrospinal fluid escaped. A Teflon endolymphatic shunt tube was inserted into the incision.

From the postauricular incision, the muscle and fascia graft was obtained by sharp dissection. The entire exposed posterior fossa region was covered with this as a free graft. The mastoid cavity was packed with Gelfoam soaked in Chloromycetin. The postauricular incision was closed with interrupted 0000 dermalon mattress sutures. A gauze wick smeared with Achromycin-Hydrocortisone Ointment was inserted into the external auditory canal. A routine mastoid dressing was applied.

Labyrinthotomy, Left Transmeatal

Under general anesthesia, the left ear was prepared and draped. After injection with 1% Xylocaine with epinephrine and using the operating microscope throughout the procedure, an incision was made in the bony external auditory canal from 6 to 12 o'clock. The tympanomeatal flap was elevated. The tympanic membrane was lifted out of its sulcus and the middle ear was exposed. Some bone was curetted away from the posterior superior annulus to expose the stapes well. The chorda tympani was displaced in a downward direction. The incudostapedial joint was cut along with the Stapedius and the stapes was removed in toto.

Suction was applied through the oval window into the vestibule of the inner ear. Immediately, as soon as suction was withdrawn, a large amount of what appeared to be spinal fluid flowed out of the oval window to fill the middle and external auditory canal. This could not be controlled well with suction but it was finally brought under control. Working with two hands, the inferior margin of the oval window was widened by curettage. The curet was used to destroy the accessible parts of the inner ear. The inner ear was packed as well as possible with Gelfoam. The tympanomeatal flap was replaced. The external auditory canal was packed with a strip of gauze smeared with Achromycin-Hydrocortisone Ophthalmic Ointment and a mastoid dressing was applied.

TYMPANOPLASTY

The middle ear is separated from the external auditory canal by the tympanic membrane (drumhead). This membrane is connected to the internal ear by a series of three small bones or ossicles known as the *malleus, incus* and *stapes*.

As a result of trauma or infection, the tympanic membrane is often ruptured. When such a perforation exists in the presence of a normal ossicular chain (malleus, incus and stapes) it may be repaired with an operation called a *myringoplasty* (same as tympanoplasty I). When the damage exceeds perforation, a *tympanoplasty* is performed in those cases amenable to surgery. Descriptions of the various types of tympanoplasty have been included here to provide the secretary with an understanding of the differences between these procedures and the criteria which dictate selection of the procedure.

Types of Tympanoplasty

TYPE I   This operation is essentially a myringoplasty with repair of the perforated tympanic membrane by means of a graft. It is done in those cases which present a perforated tympanic membrane with a normal ossicular chain.

TYPE II In this operation the malleus and complete tympanic membrane are replaced by a graft in contact with the incus or remainder of the malleus. This procedure is elected in those cases which present erosion of the malleus in addition to perforation of the tympanic membrane.

TYPE III A graft is used to replace the tympanic membrane. It is placed in contact with the stapes and also affords protection for the round window. This type of reconstruction is performed when the tympanic membrane is destroyed along with the incus and malleus, leaving only the stapes mobile and intact.

TYPE IV   A graft is attached to the promontory, extending over the tympanic orifice of the eustachian tube with attachment to the outer inferior margin of the middle ear space. A small air-containing cavity is thus developed between the round window and graft affording protection for the round window. The mobile foot-plate remains exposed. This operation is done when there is a functioning oval window membrane and mobile foot-plate even though the head, neck and crura of the stapes have been destroyed.

TYPE V   A window (fenestra) is created in the horizontal canal and is covered by a rather extensive skin graft which also forms a small tympanic cavity. The middle ear is sealed off by the skin graft thus providing sound protection for the round window. This operation is performed in cases of non-functioning oval window and fixed foot-plate.

Tympanoplasty   *Type I* — **Right Myringoplasty With Skin Graft Donor Site: External Auditory Canal**

Preliminary exposure of the middle ear was accomplished through an ear speculum with a magnifying loupe. After exposure, the Zeiss operating microscope was used for greater magnification.

Under high power magnification, using small picks and tympanoplastic knives, the remnants of the tympanic membrane were denuded of their epithelial layers.

After complete elevation of the epithelium, a longitudinal incision was made with a House knife in the bony auditory canal at 5 and 8 o'clock, respectively. Both incisions were connected about 5 mm. external to the annulus. This portion of the canal skin was elevated completely and freed. It was then shifted over the denuded portions of the tympanic membrane and external auditory canal, taking the utmost care to evert the edges of the graft.

Prior to this manipulation, the middle ear was filled with Hydrocortisone-Achromycin Ointment. The outer portions of the canal were loosely packed with a gauze strip smeared with the same ointment.

Tympanoplasty Type II — With Exploratory Meatoantrotomy

The left ear was prepared and sterilely draped. Local anesthesia was accomplished by injecting 2% Xylocaine with epinephrine in the usual manner at the entrance of the external canal. The entire operation was carried out using the Zeiss operating microscope under 6, 10 and 16 power magnification.

A Heerman endaural incision was made splitting the membranous canal at 12 o'clock and carrying the incision out parallel to the crus of the helix. Two self-retaining Wullstein retractors were inserted crosswise thus exposing the entire bony wall canal including the superior canal wall.

The usual meatal incisions for an exploratory tympanotomy were made and a tympanomeatal flap was elevated. The tympanic membrane which appeared quite thickened was elevated out of the tympanic sulcus together with the annular ligament without perforation. There were adhesions in the middle ear. These were dissected free under high power magnification. They mainly involved the long process of the incus and the tympanic membrane as well as the posterior annular region.

The mucous membrane of the middle ear appeared to be slightly thickened but there was no evidence of cholesteatoma or of irreversible pathology. The attic was explored by removing the posterior superior aspect of the annular region and thus, the lateral wall of the attic. There was no evidence of cholesteatoma. A few more adhesions around the ossicular chain were found and freed. Using a Diamond bur, a meatoantrotomy was performed, turning the bone over the aditus away and exposing the mastoid antrum. There was no evidence of cholesteatoma.

The entire middle ear and exposed part of the mastoid were thoroughly irrigated with Ringer's solution. A Teflon sheet was then placed over the areas where the adhesions were sectioned. The middle ear and mastoid antrum were filled with Achromycin-Hydrocortisone Ointment.

The tympanomeatal flap was replaced in its original position covering the defect in the bone wall. The endaural incision was closed with interrupted 00000 dermalon sutures. The external auditory canal was packed with gauze smeared with Achromycin-Hydrocortisone Ointment. A mastoid dressing was applied.

Tympanoplasty Type III

The left ear was sterilely prepared and draped in the usual manner A postauricular approach was used making an incision precisely in the postauricular fold. These subcutaneous tissues were dissected down to the periosteum and the periosteum was divided sharply and retracted.

Bleeders were controlled by electrocoagulation. The mastoid cortex was entered at the spine of Henle with a cutting bur and as the cells were reached, they were found to be filled with mucoid fluid. Granulations were also noted in the mastoid. The antrum was reached. Exenteration of all of the mastoid cells was done with a cutting bur. The tip cells were removed. The sino-dural angle was cleaned. A small dural exposure occurred there. Trautmann's triangle was cleaned and the posterior bony canal wall was thinned down. All cells showed evidence of inflammation of a rather active degree with granulation. There was no evidence of cholesteatoma.

The aditus region was widened until the thickened lining of the incus came into view. This was not disturbed. The entire mastoidectomy was performed using the operating microscope to assure good exenteration of all cells. Under high power magnification, the posterior superior and superior lining of the bony external auditory meatus was now elevated. The tympanic membrane together with the annular ligament were lifted out of the annulus and the middle ear was thus opened. It was immediately apparent that there was an adhesion between the head of the stapes and the tympanic membrane. There had been a necrosis of the long process of the incus. There was no connection between the long process of the incus and the head and neck of the stapes. The stapes appeared to be mobile and intact. Gentle rocking movements were applied and a good round window reflex could be seen.

Working in the middle ear was considerably hindered by intense capillary bleeding. The chorda tympani was now elevated in a downward direction and could be placed in such a position that it filled the gap between the head of the stapes and the remaining long process of the incus. Prior to this, the tympanic membrane was carefully dissected free from the capitulum of the stapes. A small tear in the tympanic membrane from this dissection was repaired by using a free fascia graft obtained by sharp dissection through a postauricular incision.

After proper realignment of the ossicular chain, a small piece of Teflon sheeting was placed over the long process of the incus to prevent adhesions between it and the inner surface of the tympanic membrane. Achromycin-Hydrocortisone Ophthalmic Ointment was injected into the middle ear cavity. The tympanomeatal flap was replaced. The external auditory canal was cleaned and inspected.

A myringotomy incision was made in the tympanic membrane and a Shea polyethylene drainage tube was inserted through the incision to provide adequate drainage. The mastoid cavity was filled with Achromycin-Hydrocortisone Ointment. A small polyethylene drain was inserted into the mastoid cavity and brought out through a postauricular incision.

The incision was closed with 0000 dermalon sutures. A routine mastoid dressing was applied.

Revision of Type III Tympanoplasty with Insertion of 4.5 x 0.6 mm. Stainless Steel Malleal Foot-plate Piston

With the patient in the supine position and the head turned to the right, the left ear was sterilely prepared, draped and injected with 1% Xylocaine with adrenalin.

A vein was taken from the left antecubital area which was closed in the usual manner.

A Lempert endaural incision was made and hemostasis obtained by clamping and ligating or electrocoagulation. As the graft cholesteatoma appeared to extend outward on the posterior canal wall, a canal wall flap was not made. The cholesteatomatous portion of the old graft was outlined by sharp incision and this was carefully dissected from the drum and ossicles as well as the attic area. The drum inferiorly was noted to be normally intact and on removing the graft, it was found that the fibrous middle layer and the mucosal layer left gave an intact drum. However, there was a skin pocket in the attic which extended inferiorly behind the body of the incus. It was later noted that this pocket which contained some cholesteatoma debris had destroyed the greater portion of the incus leaving only a portion of the long process and a small portion of the ossicular surface with the malleus. The skin pocket was then dissected from behind the ossicles and a small amount of skin was removed from behind the head of the malleus. However, this area was felt to be skin free prior to grafting. The middle ear space was entered by a standard tympanomeatal flap and the chorda tympani nerve was sacrificed. The distal portion of the incus was thin and fibrotic and did not transmit motion of the incus to the stapes.

The incudostapedial joint was therefore divided as was the malleoincudal joint and the remnant of the incus was then removed. This was insufficient for a columella and was discarded.

The stapes appeared to be fully intact and the mucosal layer over the mid-portion of the malleal handle was incised and elevated from the malleus.

A 4.5 x 0.6 mm. stainless steel piston which was angled posteriorly and inferiorly was then inserted to contact the stapes foot-plate and was crimped over the malleus. Motion was transmitted well through this columella.

A small amount of bone was taken down from the atticotomy posteriorly; however, only slightly swollen mucosa was noted in this area and further mastoid work was not done. The atticotomy was obliterated with Gelfoam and soft tissue and two strips of vein were laid in to cover the raw outer surface of the upper one half of the tympanic membrane as well as the attic space.

The usual packing of rayon strips and Cortisporin soaked cotton was inserted after which the endaural incision was closed in the usual manner.

The patient tolerated the procedure well and left the operating room in good condition, after a head dressing had been applied.

Tympanoplasty Type IV — Using Fascia, Skin Grafts and Teflon Prosthesis

After surgical preparation and draping, the left mastoid cavity was exposed through a Lempert's endaural incision. A previous musculoplasty had been done and the muscle, as expected, had been replaced by dense connective tissue which served to fill in the mastoid cavity. The skin was carefully peeled off this mass and the middle ear was exposed.

The middle ear was filled with granulation tissue and scar tissue. This was carefully removed to peel the back from the medial wall of the tympanic cavity. The eustachian tube was probed and found to be patent. The foot-plate of the stapes remained and this was mobile. A Teflon umbrella prosthesis was fitted onto the foot-plate and held in place by packing around it with Gelfoam soaked in Achromycin-Hydrocortisone Ointment.

A very thin portion of skin graft from along the posterior wall of the external auditory canal was cut out. A graft obtained from the left arm was used to replace it. The fascia obtained from the left Temporalis muscle was placed over the Teflon umbrella prosthesis and fitted underneath the previous existing graft in the tympanic cavity. Skin was placed over this fascia. The skin graft and fascia graft were held in place with Gelfoam packing reinforced with Iodoform gauze packing.

All incisions were closed with white nylon subcutaneously and 00000 dermalon for the skin. A mastoid bandage was applied. At the conclusion of surgery, when the patient reacted, it was noted that the facial nerve function was normal.

Tympanoplasty Type V — Fenestration from Vestibule and Insertion of Stainless Steel Wire Prosthesis

The left ear was sterilely prepared and draped in the usual manner. After injection of 1% Xylocaine with epinephrine at the usual points, a Heerman incision was made following the outline of the old incision.

A small eye retractor was inserted splitting the external auditory canal in its membranous portion. A tympanomeatal flap was outlined with the usual incisions and elevated. The tympanic membrane was lifted out of its sulcus together with the annular ligament. A flap was reflected forward and the middle ear was exposed. It was immediately apparent that the previously placed wire had slipped off the long process of the incus and was not in contact with the incus or oval window region any more. It was attached by adhesions to the undersurface of the tympanic membrane. It was carefully removed by sharp dissection using high power magnification. Following this, the oval window region was reinspected. There was still a small puncture opening. Proceeding from this area, a wide opening was made into the vestibule of the inner ear. This was technically difficult because thick bone had to be removed piecemeal with small foot-plate hooks. No drill was used in order to avoid injury to the inner ear structure. The facial nerve was clearly visualized and appeared to be completely exposed in its course through the middle ear. There was a very marked overhang of the facial nerve.

An attempt was made to place a wire piston prosthesis into the newly created opening into the vestibule. This proved impossible because of the continuous contact of the piston with the exposed facial nerve. Therefore a House wire of suitable size was selected and placed on the long process of the incus with its proximal end into the open vestibule. It was crimped in place tightly. The excess opening was covered up with compressed Gelfoam. The middle ear was now filled with Achromycin-Hydrocortisone Ointment.

The tympanomeatal flap was reflected into its original position where it was gently packed in place with a gauze strip smeared with the same ointment. The endaural incision was closed with interrupted 00000 dermalon sutures. A mastoid dressing was applied.

Myringotomy With Insertion of Polyethylene Collar Buttons, Bilaterally

The Zeiss operating microscope was brought into position and the tympanic membrane was well visualized.

An incision was made in the posterior inferior quadrant of the tympanic membrane. The middle ear was aspirated. Following this, a polyethylene collar button was inserted with a tympanoplastic alligator forceps and a pick through the myringotomy incision. The same procedure was carried out on the opposite ear.

Musculoplasty With Skin Grafting

After surgical preparation and draping, the left mastoid was exposed through a Lempert endaural incision.

The mastoid cavity was found to be filled with granulation tissue. There were two or three areas of definite cholesteatoma. These were all removed. The mastoid cavity had been operated on previously but many pockets of bone and overhangs remained. These were drilled out completely.

Musculoplasty was performed by rotating a free muscle pedicle graft from the left Temporalis muscle into the mastoid cavity. A postauricular skin graft was obtained and sutured in place. The skin was also held in place by packing which consisted of Gelfoam and Iodoform gauze.

Modified Radical Mastoidectomy

Under general anesthesia employing an endotracheal tube, the area of the right ear was prepared with pHisoHex and draped sterilely.

A Lempert endaural incision was made and carried down to the periosteum of the mastoid process. The periosteum was reflected anteriorly and posteriorly with a periosteal elevator after fashioning a conchal flap. A self-retaining endaural retractor was inserted. Using a Jordan-Day drill and cutting bur, the mastoid antrum was approached using Henle's spine as a landmark.

Upon approaching the mastoid antrum it became evident that a considerable amount of granulation tissue filled the antrum and extended posteriorly and inferiorly towards the mastoid tip. The granulation tissue was removed. The mastoid was quite sclerotic. The mastoid was not well pneumatized and the mastoid cells were few. The dura was quite low and the sigmoid sinus was situated quite far anteriorly. After removing the granulation tissue from what few mastoid cells there were, the dissection was carried anteriorly.

The lateral wall of the epitympanum was then removed and the bony bridge was also removed. At this point it became evident that the entire attic was filled with cholesteatoma. This was meticulously removed. The cholesteatoma had imbedded in the incus and head of the malleus and had extended into the sinus tympanicus. It was therefore necessary to remove the incus and to amputate the head of the malleus following which, the cholesteatoma matrix was carefully removed from the remaining portion of the malleus and undersurface of the tympanic membrane. It was also removed from the sinus tympanicus. The middle ear appeared normal, otherwise.

At one point the dura was exposed; however, the dura was not penetrated. The meatal flap was laid over the facial ridge which had previously been taken down. All of the diseased tissue appeared to have been removed.

Sulfadiazine powder was sprinkled into the cavity. The cavity was then packed with vaseline gauze. Additional Sulfadiazine powder was then placed externally into the meatus.

The postauricular incision was sutured in two layers using 0000 plain and 00000 dermalon sutures for the skin. A small Penrose drain was left in the inferior aspect of the posterior auricular incision and a mastoid type dressing was applied. The facial nerve function was normal at the conclusion of the procedure.

THE STAPES

The stapes is one of the three small bones of the middle ear. It is shaped like a stirrup and can be replaced by a prosthesis to restore continuity to the ossicular chain. Commonly used techniques are listed as follows:

STAPEDECTOMY TECHNICS:

Guilford
Hough
House

Schuknecht
Shea

Left Stapedectomy With Piston Prosthesis

The left ear was sterilely prepared and draped in the usual manner. Local anesthesia was obtained by injection of 2% Xylocaine with adrenalin.

A Heerman incision was made splitting the membranous portion of the external auditory canal at 12 o'clock. A semicircular incision was now made about 4 to 5 mm. external to the annulus tympanicus around the posterior circumference of the bony external auditory canal. The tympanomeatal flap was elevated. The tympanic membrane was lifted out of its sulcus together with the annular ligament without perforation. The tympanomeatal flap was reflected anteriorly, thus exposing the middle ear. A fair amount of bone was curetted away from the posterior superior aspect of the annulus, thus exposing the long process of the incus, stapes and oval window niche.

The stapes showed whitish otosclerotic bone anteriorly and a complete anterior fixation. The posterior portion of the foot-plate was blue. The niche was very deep with an overhanging facial nerve.

A small hole was made in the blue portion of the foot-plate with a fine stapes pick. Following this, the incudostapedial joint was separated sharply. The Stapedius tendon was cut, the crura fractured and the superstructure of the stapes removed. Using fine stapes hooks, the posterior part of the foot-plate was now removed.

The wire piston prosthesis was manipulated over the long process of the incus and hooked onto its long process with the piston part of the wire prosthesis protruding into the opening in the oval window. The wire was crimped down to assure a good fit. The hearing of the patient improved immediately on the operating table.

The tympanomeatal flap was replaced in its original position. The external canal was filled with Achromycin-Hydrocortisone Ointment and a small gauze wick with the same ointment was inserted.

The Heerman incision was closed with interrupted 00000 dermalon sutures and a routine mastoid dressing was applied.

Stapedectomy With Stainless Steel Prosthesis and Gelfoam

After surgical preparation and draping, 1% Xylocaine with adrenalin was infiltrated into the external auditory canal.

An incision was made in the posterior wall of the external auditory canal about 5 mm. external to the tympanic membrane. The tympanomeatal flap was elevated. The posterior portion of the bony annulus was removed extensively with a curet. The stapes was found to be fixed. The incudostapedial joint was dislocated. The stapedial tendon was cut and the superstructure of the stapes was removed. A very thick foot-plate was removed with some difficulty using picks and fistula hooks.

Gelfoam was placed over the open oval window and a 4½ mm. preformed House stainless steel prosthesis was fitted. The proximal end laid on the Gelfoam and oval window. The distal end was crimped around the long process of the incus. A good round window reflex was obtained and the patient's response to gross testing was satisfactory.

The middle ear was cleansed of blood. Achromycin-Hydrocortisone Ointment was instilled. The tip of the meatal flap was replaced. The entire ear canal was filled with Achromycin-Hydrocortisone Ointment.

Fenestration of Right Lateral Semicircular Canal

The right ear was sterilely prepared and draped in the usual manner. A Shambaugh endaural incision for fenestration was made. The anterior portion of the conchal cartilage was removed in a semilunar fashion and the subcutaneous tissue was excised. The entire operation was performed using a Zeiss operating microscope.

The canal incisions were made in the usual fashion at about 12 and 6 o'clock, respectively. The membranous canal was dissected free in its posterior circumference. For a short distance, the bony canal was separated from its periosteal membranous lining. Using cutting burs, the bony part of the canal was widened. A few superficial mastoid cells were drilled away and the exenteration of mastoid air cells was continued to the antrum. Following this, the middle ear was explored under high power magnification. There were no new findings. There was no evidence of any oval window reflex present. The facial nerve was identified superiorly, above the oval window. The lateral wall of the attic was now removed, partly with Diamond burs, partly with curets and partly with cutting burs. This exposed the short process of the incus and the body of the incus, as well as the long process of the incus. The incus was malformed and was fused to the head of the malleus. The head of the malleus and the incus were now removed. The surgical dome of the vestibule, consisting of the anterior part of the lateral semicircular canal, was now clearly in view as was the facial nerve.

The middle ear was again inspected and a round window niche was visualized, but we could not be certain that there was a round window membrane. The cavity was smoothed out. All bleeding was controlled with a Diamond bur. A flap was then fashioned until a perfect fit had been obtained and the flap fitted well over the surgical dome of the latera ends of the semicircular canal. Following this, the entire cavity was thoroughly irrigated and all bone dust removed. Bleeders were again carefully and meticulously controlled.

The next step consisted of the creation of a fenestra into the lateral semicircular canal. This was done with a Diamond bur under continuous irrigation with Ringer's solution. The surgical dome of the semicircular canal was first encumberalized after the blue line was visualized. The remainder of the fenestra was completed by a cupula technique. An opening in the labyrinth was made after the cupula had been completed with a small pick. The bone was completely removed from the fenestra. A good, clean fenestra was obtained under high power magnification. The membranous part of the semicircular canal was clearly visible.

No remarkable bleeding occurred during this procedure. There was no large accumulation of blood in the vestibule. The tympanomeatal flap was now placed over the broken fenestra and secured with a cotton pack smeared with Achromycin-Hydrocortisone Ointment. The flap was then packed in place with gauze smeared with the same ointment. The outer part of the cavity was packed with the same material. The upper portion of the endaural incision was approximated with a 00000 dermalon suture and a routine mastoid dressing was applied.

The patient moved the right side of his face indicating that the facial nerve was unimpaired.

DISEASES OF THE MIDDLE EAR
(and tympanic membrane)

Absence of ossicles
Adenocarcinoma of the ear
Adenoma of the ear
Ankylosis of incudostapedial joint
Basal cell carcinoma of the ear
Cholesteatoma
Chondroma of the ear
Deafness, congenital
Deformity of the ossicles
Diverticulum of eustachian tube
Epidermoid carcinoma of the ear
Fibroma of the ear
Fibrosarcoma of the ear
Fistula of the mastoid
Foreign body in mastoid
Fracture of petrous pyramid
   and mastoid
Fusion of ossicles
Glomangioma of the ear
Granulations in middle ear
Granuloma of the middle ear
Hemangioma
Lipoma
Lymphangioma of auricle
Mastoiditis
   acute
   chronic
   coalescent
   hemorrhagic
   necrotic
Mucous polyp of middle ear
Myringitis
Necrosis of ossicles
Neurofibroma of auricle
Osteoma of mastoid
Otalgia
Otitis media
Panotitis
Papilloma of
Perforation of pars tensa
Perforation of Shrapnell's
   membrane
Persistence of arteria stapedia
Petrositis
Pigmented nevus of
Pseudocholesteatoma
Reflex otalgia
Rupture of tympanic membrane
Salpingitis, eustachian
Sarcoma of ear
Stricture of eustachian tube
Supernumerary ossicles
Syphilis of ear
Tinnitus
Tuberculosis of ear

OPERATIONS ON THE MIDDLE EAR

Drainage of petrous pyramid air cells
Exenteration of air cells of petrous
   pyramid
Exploration of petrous pyramid air
   cells
Mastoid antrotomy
Mastoidectomy
   simple
   radical
Myringotomy
Ossiculectomy
Plicotomy
Stapedectomy
Tympanoplasty
Tympanotomy

THE LARYNX

The larynx is a musculocartilaginous structure which has the shape of an inverted triangle. This pyramidal tube, situated above the trachea in the neck, is regarded chiefly as the organ of speech. When excision of the larynx *(laryngectomy)* becomes necessary due to carcinoma or other grave condition, the patient is fitted with an artificial larynx and rehabilitated until he can communicate distinctly enough to be understood.

Examination and biopsy of the larynx is performed endoscopically by a procedure called a *laryngoscopy,* using an instrument called a *laryngoscope.* Some of the other commonly used laryngeal instruments have been listed here to further familiarize the secretary with the armamentarium of the otolaryngologist.

ANATOMIC FEATURES OF THE LARYNX

Anterior commissure
Arch
Articular capsule
Aryepiglottic fold
Arytenoid cartilage
Cartilages of Santorini
Cartilages of Wrisberg
Conus elasticus
Cords
Corniculate cartilage (Santorini)
Cornu
Cornua
Cricoarytenoid ligament
Cricoid cartilage
Cricotracheal ligament
Crista arcuata
Cuneiform cartilage (Wrisberg)
Cuneiform tubercle
Esophageal introitus
Epiglottis
False cords
Foveae

Fusiform fossa
Glossoepiglottic folds
Hyoepiglottic ligament
Hyothyroid ligament
Hyothyroid membrane
Inferior laryngeal nerve
Intrathyroid cartilage
Lamina
Laryngeal prominence (Adam's apple)
Mucous membrane
Pyriform sinus
Rima glottidis
Superior laryngeal nerve
Thyroid cartilage
Thyroid notch
Thyroepiglottic ligament
True cords
Valleculae
Ventricular bands
Vestibule
Vocal cords
Vocal process

MUSCLES OF THE LARYNX

Arytenoideus (interarytenoid)
Cricoarytenoideus
Cricothyroid
Interarytenoid (Arytenoideus)

Internal thyro-arytenoid
Lateral crico-arytenoid
Posterior crico-arytenoid
Thyroarytenoideus

LARYNGEAL INSTRUMENTS

Abraham laryngeal cannula
Abraham laryngeal syringe
Andrews chest support
Artificial larynx
Carabelli mirror cannula
Cordes-New laryngeal punch
Dean laryngeal applicator
Erich laryngeal biopsy forceps
Fauvel forceps
Ferguson-Metzenbaum scissors
Fraenkel forceps
Haslinger head rest
Holinger cannula
Holinger laryngeal dissector
Jackson core mold
Jesberg laryngectomy clamp
Jurasz laryngeal forceps
Killian suspension gallows
Krause laryngeal snare
LeJuene laryngofissure scissors
Lewy laryngoscope holder
Lukens laryngeal syringe
Lynch knife
McKenzie laryngeal forceps
Myerson laryngectomy saw
New's speaking tube
Record laryngeal syringe
Roberts vocal cord fixer
Sawtell laryngeal applicator
Tobold-Fauvel forceps
Vasconcelos-Barretto clamp
Yankauer-Little tube forceps

LARYNGEAL TUBES

Chevalier Jackson
Clerf
Holinger
Lewis
Martin
Schell

LARYNGOSCOPES

Adult reverse bevel
Albert Andrews modified Jackson
Anterior commissure
Atkins-Tucker shadow free
Bizzarri-Giuffrida
Broyles anterior commissure
Broyles optical
Broyles wasp waist
Chevalier Jackson
Clerf
Dual distal lighted
E.S.I.
Fink
Flagg
Foregger
Guedel
Haslinger
Holinger anterior commissure
 hour-glass
Holinger anterior commissure
 slotted
Holinger modified Jackson
Hook-on folding
Jackson
Lewy
Lundy
Lynch suspension
McIntosh
Miller
Multipurpose
Polio
Roberts self-retaining
Rotating
Sam Roberts
Sanders intubation
Siker mirror
Standard
Tucker anterior commissure
Welch-Allyn
Wis-Foregger
Wis-Hipple
Yankauer

Laryngopharyngeal Region

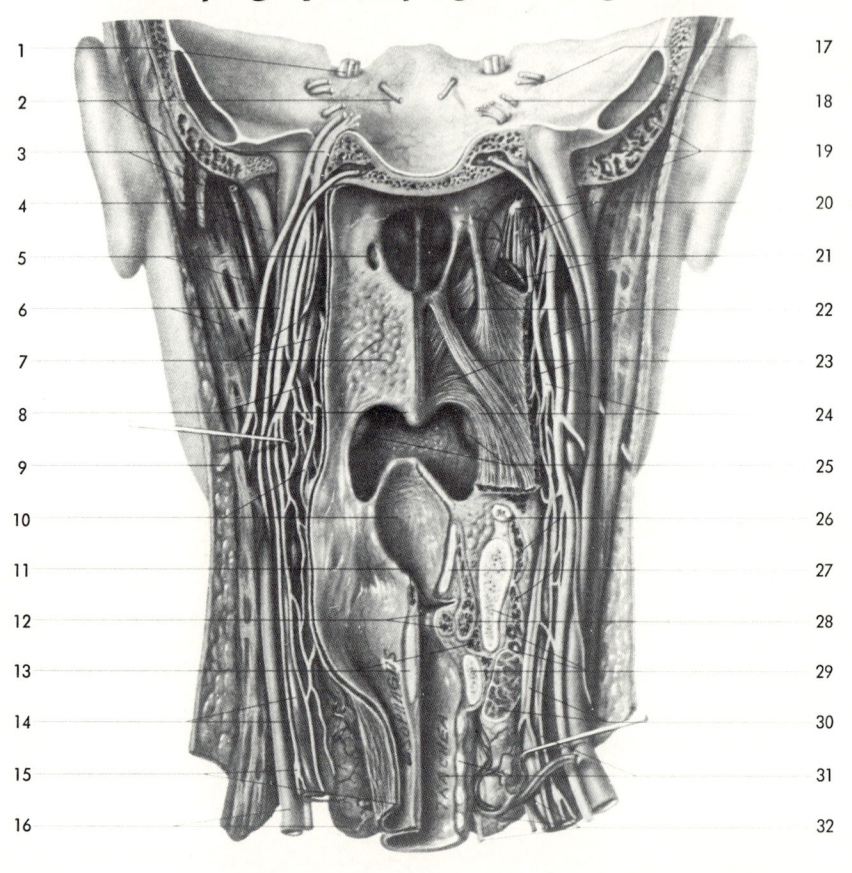

1 Trigeminal nerve
2 Splenius capitis muscle; abducens nerve
3 Longissimus capitis muscle; intracranial ganglion of vagus nerve
4 Occipital artery; styloid process
5 Digastric muscle; pharyngeal opening of auditory tube
6 Sternocleidomastoid muscle; hypoglossal nerve
7 Internal carotid artery and nerve; mucous glands of pharynx
8 Superior laryngeal nerve; palatine uvula
9 Accessory nerve
10 Pharyngeal branch of vagus nerve; epiglottis
11 Arytenoid muscle; ventricular fold
12 Vocal fold; vocalis muscle
13 Cricoid cartilage; lateral cricoarytenoid muscle
14 Sympathetic trunk; common carotid artery
15 Middle cervical ganglion; esophagus
16 Internal jugular vein; thyroid gland
17 Facial and acoustic nerves
18 Glossopharyngeal nerve; sigmoid portion of transverse sinus
19 Mastoid cells; internal jugular vein
20 Otic ganglion; ascending pharyngeal artery
21 Salpingopharyngeus muscle; nodose ganglion
22 Levatorveli patatini muscle; vagus nerve
23 Pharyngopalatinus muscle; superior laryngeal nerve
24 Stylopharyngeus muscle; superior cervical ganglion
25 Palatine tonsils
26 Greater cornu of hyoid bone; thyrohyoid muscle
27 Quadrangular membrane; sternothyroid muscle
28 Thyroarytenoid muscle; thyroid cartilage
29 Cricoid cartilage; superior thyroid artery and vein
30 Thyroid gland (cut); superior cardiac nerve
31 Trachea and tracheal cartilage; sympathetic trunk
32 Inferior thyroid artery and vein; recurrent laryngeal nerve

Figure 87 Laryngopharyngeal region
Courtesy Lederle Laboratories

DISEASES OF THE LARYNX

Abscess of larynx
Absence of larynx
Adenocarcinoma
Adenoma
Ankylosis of cricoarytenoid
    articulation
Aphthous ulcer of larynx
Arthritis of cricoarytenoid
    articulation
Atresia
Calcification
Chondroma
Constriction
Cricoid cartilage union
    with thyroid cartilage
Cyst of epiglottis
Cyst of larynx
Defect of larynx
Elongation of petiolus
Epidermoid carcinoma
Epiglottitis
Fibroma of larynx
Fissure of epiglottis
Fistula of larynx
Herpes simplex
Hypertrophy of vocal cords
Hypoplasia of epiglottis
Laryngeal struma
Laryngitis
Laryngoptosis
Laryngotracheitis
Lipoma
Malformation of larynx
Mucous polyp of larynx
Mucous polyp of vocal cord
Obstruction of larynx
Papilloma of larynx
Perichondritis
Prolapse of laryngeal ventricle
Spasm of glottis
Stenosis, laryngeal
Stricture of larynx
Subglottic laryngitis
Syphilis of larynx
Tuberculosis of larynx
Varix of vocal cord
Ventral cleft of thyroid cartilage
Ventricular laryngocele
Ventricular sacculation,
    intralaryngeal
Web of larynx

OPERATIONS ON THE LARYNX

Arytenoidectomy
Arytenoidopexy
Biopsy of the larynx
Cordopexy
Epiglottidectomy
Hemilaryngectomy
Incision and drainage
Intercricothyrotomy
Intubation of larynx
Laryngectomy
    partial (hemilaryngectomy)
    total
Laryngopharyngectomy
Laryngofissure
Laryngoscopy
    with biopsy
    with dilation
    with division of adhesions
    with drainage
    with exploration
    with insertion of radioactive
        material
Laryngoplasty
Laryngostomy
Laryngotomy
Local excision of lesion
Punch resection of vocal cords
Puncture of larynx
Thyrochondrotomy
Thyrocricotomy
Thyrotomy
Ventriculocordectomy

Direct Laryngoscopy With Stripping of Cord

Under general anesthesia, using an endotracheal tube in the posterior commissure, a Jackson anterior commissure laryngoscope was inserted and held in the operative position with a Luer retractor.

There was a marked irregularity of the left and right vocal cord, particularly at the anterior third. Numerous biopsies were taken from both cords. The mucosal lining was stripped from the right cord. No other areas of tumefaction, ulceration or bleeding were noted. The scope was withdrawn and the biopsy specimens submitted to the pathologist for histopathologic examination.

Total Laryngectomy — with radical neck dissection

General anesthesia was administered via endotracheal tube. The right neck and part of the chest were prepared and draped in a sterile manner.

A double Y-incision was made and the upper limb of the incision extended from the symphysis of the mandible anteriorly, to the mastoid process posteriorly. This was joined by the vertical limb which extended into the inferior limb, stretching from the suprasternal notch to the posterior triangle of the neck. Skin flaps were dissected by blunt and sharp dissection and a radical neck dissection was carried out.

Following the neck dissection, the hyoid bone was freed from the suprahyoid musculature which was detached by sharp dissection. Midline dissection was then continued and the thyroid cartilage was identified. The thyroid isthmus was ligated.

Attention was then turned to the right upper area of dissection and the superior cornu of the hyoid bone was retracted. The thyrohyoid membrane was identified. Superior laryngeal vessels consisting of the superior laryngeal artery, vein and laryngeal nerve were ligated. The superior thyroid artery was previously ligated during the neck dissection. A similar procedure was repeated on the left side. The superior laryngeal blood vessels and nerves on the left were also sectioned. The dissection was continued downward. The left lobe of the thyroid gland was left intact. The attachments of the inferior constrictor muscles to the thyroid cartilage were sectioned and the ribbon muscles were sectioned inferiorly. The larynx became quite mobile and was retracted with ease to the right side. The trachea was then sectioned at the level between the second and third tracheal rings. The endotracheal tube was then removed and a new tube was placed in the tracheal stump. The dissection continued from the lower aspect of the trachea. The superior stump of the trachea and larynx were separated from the esophagus, bluntly. The superior cornu of the right thyroid cartilage was then identified and the pharynx was entered at this area.

There was a large lesion involving the right pyriform sinus, right side of the epiglottis and base of the tongue. The pharyngeal mucosa was then cut approximately 2 cm. away from the lesion obtaining free healthy margins. The specimen consisting of the right sternocleidomastoid muscle, jugular vein, submandibular gland, thyroid gland, larynx and hyoid bone was removed in toto. This necessitated a ligation of the inferior thyroid arteries on both sides. Bleeding was minimal.

The pharynx was closed with 0000 continuous catgut sutures and closed over with 000 silk sutures. The closure was quite adequate. A feeding tube was inserted prior to the closure. The tracheal stump was then mobilized and a button hole was made in the suprasternal notch. The tracheal stump was brought to the outer surface and sutured to the skin with 000 silk sutures. Anesthesia was then administered via the tracheal stump. The skin flaps were attached to the underlying tissues by catgut sutures and the skin was closed with interrupted 0000 dermalon. Pressure dressing was applied. Only 500 cc. of whole blood was given during the operation.

Laryngoplasty With Insertion of Teflon Mold and Right Arytenoidectomy; Tracheotomy

The neck was sterilely prepared and draped in the usual manner. The tracheotomy was performed under local anesthesia, using 1% Xylocaine. An incision was made in the old tracheotomy scar which was dissected away. A longitudinal incision was made in the trachea at the level of the previous tracheotomy and a #8 tracheotomy tube was inserted. An anesthetist's endotracheal tube was then inserted into the tracheotomy tube and general anesthesia was administered.

The neck was entered through a previous arytenoidectomy incision on the right side. Dissection was carried through heavy scar tissue to the site of the previously removed thyroid cartilage. Dissection was carried deeper in order to find the arytenoid cartilage. It was located but it was noted that there was very extensive cicatrization of the endolarynx.

The incision was widened and the upper portion of the trachea and the entire larynx in its right lateral aspect were freed. It was now apparent that this was an extensive crushing injury of the larynx with much scar tissue formation and that this was the cause of the patient's airway obstruction, rather than the recurrent laryngeal nerve paralysis.

The arytenoid cartilage was freed by sharp dissection with much difficulty through heavy scar tissue and lateral pull was again exerted on it while the larynx was inspected through an anterior commissure laryngoscope. The lateral pull did not give an adequate airway and it was therefore decided to split the larynx, excise the scar tissue and do an arytenoidectomy. It was further decided to split the anterior larynx with an endolaryngeal mold in order to assure a good airway later.

A vertical midline incision was then made from the tracheotomy incision to the hyoid region. The strap muscles were divided in the midline and the framework of the larynx was exposed. The thyroid cartilage was split in the midline. The endolaryngeal tissues were divided by sharp dissection, a short distance right of the anterior commissure, in order not to injure the anterior commissure. The lumen of the larynx was thus entered.

The entire dissection had to be carried through very heavy scar tissue. Arytenoidectomy was completed with removal of the right arytenoid cartilage. Endolaryngeal scar tissue was dissected free and removed.

Teflon sheeting was now used and a suitable sized triangular shape mold was made. This was inserted into the laryngeal lumen extending from the cricoid region in a superior direction, to about the arytenoid region. The laryngeal mold was sutured in place with #30 wire sutures being brought out on both sides of the neck lateral to the midline incision. One #30 wire suture was then used to reapproximate the thyroid cartilage. The muscle and fascial layers were closed with interrupted 0000 chromic catgut and the skin was closed with interrupted 0000 white nylons and 00000 dermalon.

The lateral incision was closed in a similar fashion and a small Penrose drain was inserted deep into the incision. A pressure dressing was applied to the neck.

Bleeding was quite heavy during the operation and very hard to control; however, this was done by clamping and electrocoagulation. The patient received 50 cc.'s of whole blood in addition to 1000 cc.'s of 5% glucose in water intravenously.

Tonsillectomy and Adenoidectomy (T & A)

The patient was taken to the operating room where general anesth was administered employing an intratracheal tube. A Jennings mo gag was inserted.

The tonsils were removed by sharp dissection and a tonsil snare. It was necessary to insert one 00 chromic suture in the superior pole of both tonsillar fossae to secure hemostasis.

The adenoids were removed with adenoid curettes and St. Clair-Thompson forceps. The fossa of Rosenmuller was cleaned with St. Clair-Thompson forceps and a Meltzer punch.

After the procedure was completed, both tonsillar fossae were injected with a mixture of Depo-Medrol, Depo-Cer-O-Cillin and 2% Xylocaine.

Tonsillectomy

Under local anesthesia, the patient was prepared and draped in a reclining position.

A retractor was applied to the hypertrophied tonsil and the anterior pillar was pulled forward. The entire mass of the tonsil was grasped with a forceps and the handles were closed. A curved elevator was used to lift the anterior pillar away from the tonsil after being inserted at the upper attachment of the pillar. The snare wire was drawn into the cannula, removing the tonsil. As the stylet of the snare impinged upon the tonsillar tissue, the handle of the instrument was directed outward.

The remaining defect was packed with a sponge to control bleeding. The mouth and throat were suctioned. After a few minutes, the sponge was removed. Further bleeding was controlled with 00 double catgut sutures.

THE NOSE AND PARANASAL SINUSES

Surgery on the inner nose and paranasal sinuses is performed by the otolaryngologist. This phase of ENT surgery is called *rhinology* and should not be confused with plastic surgery although these specialties overlap in this area. The plastic surgeon often performs a submucous resection, Weir operation, turbinate crushing, etc. in the course of a rhinoplasty.

Examples of operative procedures performed on the nose, other than those listed in Chapter 14 are presented here with descriptions of procedures performed on the accessory sinuses.

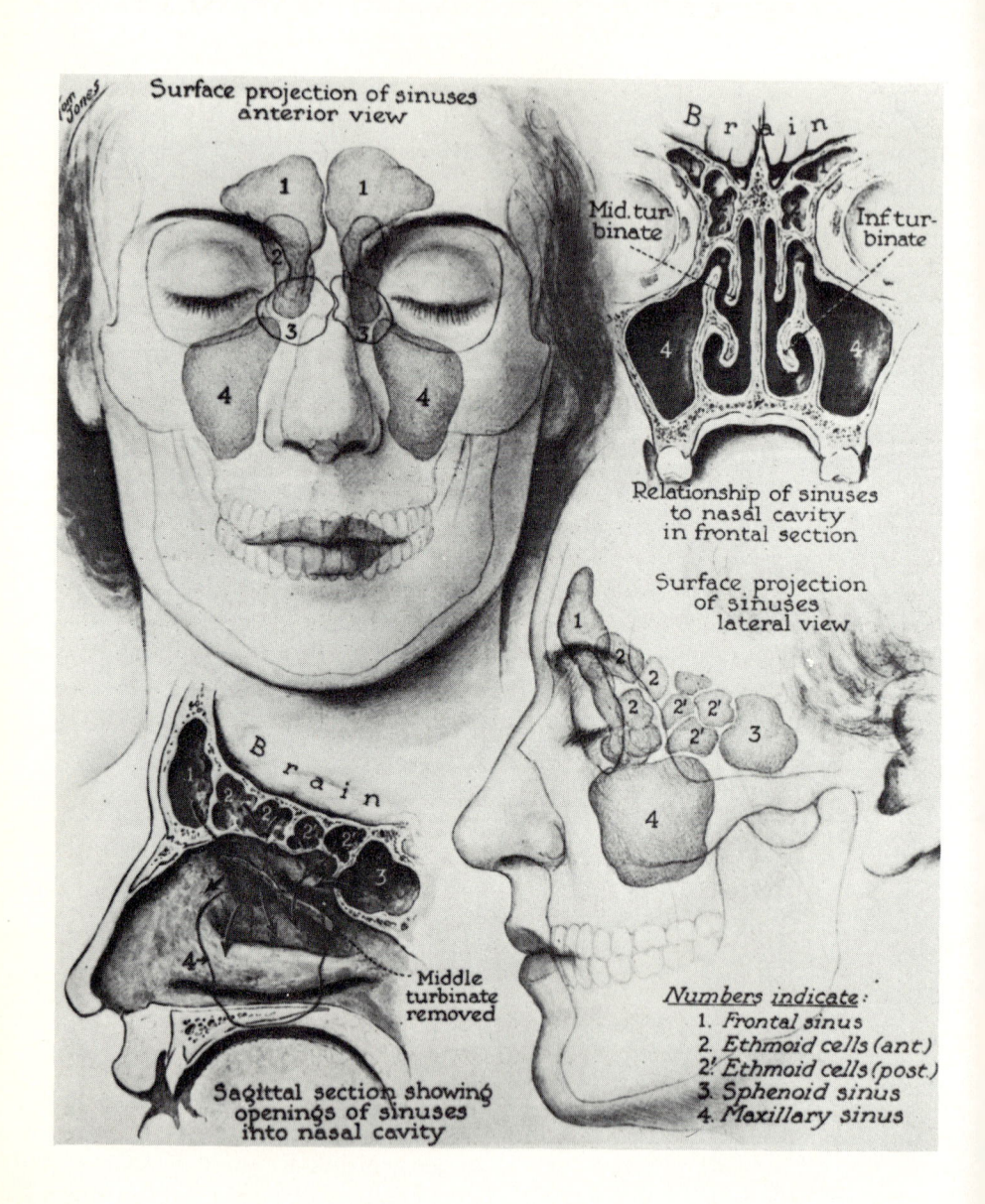

Figure 88   The paranasal sinuses
Courtesy S. H. Camp Company

ANATOMIC STRUCTURES OF THE NOSE AND PARANASAL SINUSES

Ala (pl. alae)
Alanasi
Alar cartilages
Aponeurosis
Atrium
Bridge
Bulla ethmoidalis
Cartilaginous septum
Cartilaginous vault
Choana (pl. choanae)
Clinoid process
Columella
Columna
Concha (pl. conchae)
Cribriform plate of ethmoid
Crista galli
Crura
Crus laterale
Crus mediale
Dorsum nasi
Ethmoidal air cells
Frontal processes of maxillae
Greater alar cartilage
Hamular process
Hiatus semilunaris
Hypophyseal fossa
Inferior meatus
Infundibulum
Kiesselbach's plexus
Lateral crus
Lateral wall
Lesser alar cartilage
Medial crus
Middle meatus
Mucoperichondrium
Mucous membrane
Nares
Nasal bones
Nasal conchae
Nasal crest
Nasal spine
Nasion
Nasolabial junction
Nasopalatine recess
Nostrils
Ostium maxillare
Palatine bone
Perpendicular plate of ethmoid
Piriform opening
Plica nasi
Rostrum of sphenoid
Septum
Septum mobile nasi
Sesamoid cartilages
Sinus groove
Spheno-ethmoidal recess
Sphenoidal process
Superior meatus
Turbinates
Uncinate process
Vestibule
Vomer
Vomeronasal cartilage
Vomeronasal organ of Jacobson

PARANASAL SINUSES

Ethmoidal
Frontal
Maxillary
Sphenoidal

ARTERIES OF THE NOSE

Alar br. of ext. maxillary
Alveolar br. of int. maxillary
Ant. ethmoidal br. of ophthalmic
Dorsal nasal br. of ophthalmic
Infraorbital br. of int. maxillary
Pharyngeal br. of int. maxillary
Post. ethmoidal br. of ophthalmic
Septal br. of ext. maxillary
Septal br. of superior labial
Sphenopalatine br. of int. maxillary

DISEASES OF THE PARANASAL SINUSES

Actinomycosis of sinus
Aspergillosis
Cystic degeneration
Fistula
Granuloma
Mucocele
Myiasis
Pansinusitis
Polypoid degeneration
Rhinolith

Sinusitis
   acute purulent
   chronic nonpurulent
      ethmoid
      frontal
      maxillary
      sphenoid
Syphilis of sinuses
Tuberculosis of sinuses
Vacuum of sinus

OPERATIONS ON THE PARANASAL SINUSES

Antrum window operation
Aspiration of sinuses
Biopsy
Caldwell-Luc window operation
Closure of oral fistula
Ethmoidectomy
   complete
   partial
   external
Ethmoidotomy
Excision of lesion
Frontal sinusotomy, intranasal simple

Frontal sinusotomy, external simple
Frontal sinusotomy, external radical
Irrigation of sinuses
Maxillary antrotomy, radical
Maxillary sinusotomy, simple
Maxillary sinusotomy, radical
Sphenoidotomy
Sphenoid sinusotomy
   intranasal
   external
Window operation

NERVES OF THE NOSE

Ant. alveolar br. of maxillary
Anterior ethmoidal
Anterior palatine
External nasal
Facial
Infraorbital of maxillary
Infratrochlear br. of ophthalmic
Nasal br. of sphenopalatine ganglion
Nasociliary br. of ophthalmic
Nasopalatine
Nerve of pterygoid canal
Olfactory

Nasal Polypectomy and Caldwell-Luc

The right side of the nose was packed with 10% cocaine. The area over the canine fossa on the right side was injected with 1% Xylocaine and epinephrine.

A ½ inch horizontal incision was made over the fossa, through the mucosa and submucosal tissues and periosteum. An elevator was used to fracture the lateral wall of the right antrum. Bone biting forceps were used to enlarge the opening.

The mucosa of the antrum was very edematous and polypoid. The \trum was scraped clean and bleeding was minimal. The ostium appeared to be markedly enlarged.

The pack was removed from the nose and some small polypi were removed from the middle meatus. A large polyp remained and this had to be removed from behind the soft palate, through the mouth. The ostium was further enlarged. When bleeding was controlled the antrum was packed with two Cod liver oil soaked strips. The two ends of the strips were brought out into the nasal cavity. The incision was closed with two 000 silk sutures. There was no evidence of bleeding in the posterior nasopharynx.

Submucous Resection (Also: Septectomy or SMR)

Under local anesthesia, a curvilinear incision was made on the convex side of the septum with a Freer knife. Particular care was taken not to enter the mucous membrane or perichondrium. The mucoperichondrium and mucoperiosteum were raised intact. The mucoperichondrium and cartilage of the opposite side were separated utilizing an elevator. The cartilage was exposed and the mucous membrane retracted on each side of the nasal septum. The cartilage was trimmed with a Ballenger swivel knife and removed as a single piece with forceps.

Using a Foster-Ballenger forceps, we grasped the portion of the perpendicular plate of the ethmoid to be removed and snipped it away piecemeal. Hurd's reversible septal ridge forceps were introduced into the incision and the deflected portion of the vomer was bitten away. Hajek's chisel was further utilized in this procedure. All bleeding was controlled. The wound was left open to permit drainage.

Bilateral Intranasal Ethmoidectomy, Transnasal Sphenoidotomy and Caldwell-Luc

An infraorbital block was accomplished with 1% Xylocaine with epinephrine. The septum and anterior ethmoid region were infiltrated. Using cocaine flakes on applicators, a bilateral sphenopalatine block and anterior ethmoid block were carried out.

There was a marked spur of the anterior septum on the right. An incision was made in the right mucocutaneous junction. Bilateral mucoperiosteal elevation was carried out. The spur was removed using a chisel and mallet.

A thorough exenteration of all accessible ethmoid cells was carried out through the nose under direct vision. Much polypoid tissue was also noted in both sphenoid sinuses. The sphenoid sinuses were also exenterated. The sphenoid and ethmoid sinuses on both sides were packed off with Tincture of Benzoin gauze.

An incision was made in the right canine fossa and carried through submucosal tissue and periosteum. The periosteum was elevated and the right maxillary sinus was entered through the canine fossa. It was noted to be completely filled with polypoid tissue and polypoid degeneration of the lining. The entire lining of the maxillary sinus was removed. A large window was made at the level of the inferior nasal meatus. An inferior pedicle mucosal flap was developed from the nasal mucosa of the inferior meatus and folded into the maxillary sinus. The maxillary sinus was then packed with Compound Tincture of Benzoin gauze. This was repeated on the opposite side. The incision was closed with interrupted 0000 chromic catgut sutures. The nose was packed with finger cots smeared with Achromycin-Hydrocortisone Ointment after closing the septal incision with 0000 chromic catgut sutures.

Blood loss was estimated at 500 cc.'s because of copious bleeding during the operation. Transfusion was not deemed necessary.

14 { Plastic Surgery

Plastic surgery is a surgical specialty concerned with repair and reconstruction of congenital, developmental and traumatic deformities of the external body for the purpose of restoring function and providing the individual with a more acceptable physical image of himself. Numerous techniques are employed to achieve this end including tissue grafts, foreign implants, tattoo, dermabrasion, repair and reconstruction.

Some of the most interesting and impressive advances in surgery have been made in the use of tissue transplants. Genetic compatibility between the host and the transplant has been established as one of the most important factors in success with certain tissues, notably the skin. Whenever possible, the patient acts as his own donor; however, avascular tissues such as the cornea, cartilage and epidermis may be transplanted from one human to another.

Tissue transplants are classified into three main types based on the donor source.

AUTOGRAFTS – (autogenous transplants) In these grafts, tissue is transplanted from one site to another on the same individual. The tissues used most successfully include split skin, cornea, bone and cartilage.

HOMOGRAFTS — (isografts, homogenous transplants) These grafts consist of tissues transplanted from one human to another and include those composed of avascular tissue such as cornea, cartilage and epidermis. Tissues are exchanged between single ovum twins, but grafts utilizing tissues other than the avascular types mentioned have not been used successfully. Skin homografts, at the present time, are used primarily as biologic dressings over severe burn areas to prevent loss of body fluids. They are also utilized as temporary coverings in reconstructive surgery where defects have been created in donor sites. Such skin grafts are usually rejected by the host between the ninth and fifteenth day after transplantation although the survival time of the graft can be prolonged by using a closely related individual as the donor.

ZOOGRAFTS – (animal tissue) Transplant of tissues from animals to man was regarded as an experimental curiosity a few years ago. Today, successful use is made of bovine fascia, ox bone as well as calf bone and cartilage.

ALLOTRANSPLANTATION – transplants from the body of one individual in a species to that of another in the same species.

XENOTRANSPLANTATION – transplant from one species to another.

THE IMMUNE RESPONSE

At this stage in our understanding of physiologic processes within the body which result in the immune response, we are not yet able to isolate and identify antigen-antibody reactions involved in homograft (tissue graft from one man to another) rejection. Although the causative factors are still hidden from understanding, their effect, the impending failure or destruction of a homograft, are easily recognized.

The theory that circulating conventional antibodies are responsible for rejection in homografts is no longer popularly held. It is believed rather that the rejective process is an actively acquired immunity reaction. This belief is supported by the observation that a second homograft imposed on a donor who has rejected the first homograft is rejected at an increased rate.

Modern transplant surgery involving homografts attempts to inhibit the tissue rejection by the use of immuno-suppressive treatments consisting of (1) drugs including anti-folics such as A-methopterin; DNA base analogues such as 6-mercaptopurines or agents liberating this substance; alkylating agents such as cyclophosphamides; antibiotics influencing cellular synthesis such as the actinomycins; and, corticosteroids such as prednisone, (2) anti-lymphocytic sera, and (3) whole body irradiation. None of these treatments have been refined to a point where they are specific in their reaction toward either the antigenic phenomena or the homograft. The drugs are used primarily to interfere with metabolic processes in a general way.

The most potent immuno-suppressive agent recognized to date is the anti-lymphocytic sera. One of its effects is the destruction of lymphocytes; however, its value is not believed to be limited to this result alone. The full scope of its influences is not completely understood. It is commonly held that the lymphocytes are a prime mover in the homograft rejection, that is, the cell which recognizes and initiates the reaction against the foreign antigens. In the laboratory lymphoid cells have been demonstrated to surround and destroy a donor target cell in tissue culture.

Avascular tissues (without blood vessels) such as the cornea, cartilage and epidermis are freely transplanted from one individual to another without threat of rejection.

An understanding of the physiologic mechanisms responsible for homograft rejection is still a part of the future of medicine. When we fully comprehend the factors responsible for rejection, the mechanics of the rejective process and the means by which these processes may be suppressed, we will have opened up a dramatic era of organ transplant with all of the promises which attend such a realization.

SKIN GRAFTS

In the light of our present knowledge, it is the patient who serves as his own donor for skin grafts when a lasting result is desired. Such grafts assume the form of free grafts or pedicle grafts.

The *free graft* is removed entirely from one area and implanted into another area. The *pedicle graft,* as distinguished from the free graft, is raised from its bed except for one or more points at which it remains attached. These points of attachment are called pedicles and serve to provide the flap with an adequate blood supply until a circulation can develop at the recipient site. This graft remains attached to both the donor and recipient sites. It is severed at a later date when viability and a satisfactory vascular supply have been assured at the site of implantation.

A particular type of pedicle graft frequently used is the *tube pedicle*. In this method of skin transfer, the skin is formed into a tube and advanced by descriptive techniques known as caterpillaring, waltzing or conveyance. One of the extremities is used as the carrier in the latter method.

When skin grafts are referred to by the physician they are usually designated as being of full thickness or split thickness. These terms are defined below with two less often used grafts.

FULL THICKNESS (Wolfe graft)   Whole thicknesses of skin ranging in thickness from .030 to .050 inches are used for replacing large areas of tissue loss. This type of graft is frequently used for the face.

SPLIT THICKNESS   These grafts range in thickness from 0.010 to 0.020 inches and are used for repair of skin defects on the face. They also serve the purpose of epithelial inlays.

CHESSBOARD (Gabarro)   Small split thickness grafts cut into 5 to 10 mm. squares from a large sheet of skin are placed on a wound 1 cm. apart.

PINCH GRAFT (Reverdin)   Rounded bits of skin are used to cover the granulating surface of a wound such as that which follows a burn. This technique is seldom used today. These grafts often resulted in cobblestone-like scarring.

Skin Graft Techniques — By Eponymic Title

BLAIR-BROWN .... Split thickness graft of medium thickness.
BRAUN .... Thick skin graft.
BRAUN-WANGENSTEEN Smaller implanted skin grafts obtained from a larger graft.
DOUGLAS .... A mesh-like graft.
DRAGSTEDT .... A corrugated type graft.
ESSER (Stent) .... A full thickness graft applied over a resin plastic (stent material) with which the graft is fitted into the recipient site.
GILLIES .... A rope-like graft.
KONIG .... A composite graft from the ear (skin and cartilage).
KRAUSE-WOLFE .... A full thickness graft.
OLLIER-THIERSCH ...... A thin epidermal graft with some dermis present.
REVERDIN .... A pinch graft.
THIERSCH .... A very thin epidermal graft.
VAN MILLINGEN .... A lip graft.
WOLFE .... Full thickness graft.

SKIN FLAPS

Skin flap techniques are used when a thick graft with subcutaneous fat is desired. This method of tissue transfer has already been discussed in the opening of this chapter and therefore we will confine ourselves here to distinguishing between the various procedures through which this method is applied.

Types of Flaps

Bilobed .... A two lobed flap on a single pedicle.
Compound .... Addition of bone or cartilage to the flap before transfer.
Compound lined .... A flap with a lining and covering of epithelium between which bone or cartilage are inserted.
Delayed .... A flap raised from its bed except for a pedicle attachment. It is replaced to promote dependence on its pedicle and is transferred at a later operation.

Double pedicle ...... A flap with two vascular attachments.
French (sliding) ..... A flap with one pedicle which is advanced by sliding it over from an adjacent area.
Indian (rotation) ... A flap taken from a site near enough to the recipient site to permit transfer by simple turning or rotation.
Italian (distant) ..... A distant donor site made possible by bringing the donor and recipient sites together. An arm may be brought to the forehead, etc.
Jump .... A chest or abdominal flap lined with a hinge flap turned down from the forearm.
Marsupial .... An abdominal flap is folded on itself to provide a lining and in stages is attached to the forearm and then the forearm freed from the abdomen.
Tumbler .... A hinge or folding flap.

In addition to skin, other tissues are used successfully in grafting including avascular animal tissues. Some of these tissues include the following:

Bone

The most common site from which bone grafts are taken is the ilium of the hip. This bone has a large surface area which consists of compact as well as cancellous elements. The ribs afford another source of bone graft material. Bone is preferred to cartilage by many surgeons because of its ability to replace lost bone in function as well as in structure.

Cartilage

Cartilage grafts are usually obtained from the septum, auricle of the ear and costal cartilages. Such grafts are used to fill in contour defects resulting from loss of bone. Some of the sites in which cartilage is used include the malar bone (cheek), nose and chin. It is interesting to note that autogenous cartilage need not be placed in contact with host cartilage in order to survive. In this respect cartilage differs from bone which becomes one with its host.

Cornea

Corneal grafts are classified as either penetrating (deep) or lamellar (superficial). The penetrating graft requires a fresh and transparent cornea which should have been enucleated not more than 5 hours after death and transplanted not more than 12 hours after enucleation. Eye donors are preferred in the age range between 12 and 45 years; however, occasionally an older donor with good eyes will be accepted. Preserved specimens can be used for lamellar grafts.

Fascia

Autogenous fascia lata and bovine fascia are being successfully used.

Hair Bearing

Grafts must be taken from hair bearing areas such as the scalp or eyebrows to replace tissue in hair bearing areas. New hope is being offered to men who regard their baldness as a cosmetic detriment.

Mucous Membrane

Mucous membrane may be taken from the lower lip, inner cheek, upper eyelid or vaginal mucosa to replace conjunctiva of the eye or vermilion border of the lip.

Nerve

Autogenous nerve grafts are the only ones which survive.

Tendon

Autogenous free tendon grafts are used successfully and grow with the recipient site.

TISSUE BANKS

The INTERNATIONAL EYE BANK (MEDICO, a service of CARE), a non-governmental, non-sectarian, non-profit organization, financed by contributions of citizens, has its headquarters and laboratory at the Washington Hospital Center in Washington, D.C. This agency receives eye donations from eye banks all over the U.S.A. and ships them, free of charge, to foreign countries all over the world, where eye banks do not exist.

A great need for eye donors exists. All persons associated with the field of medicine should be made aware of this need to recruit prospective donors. Eye donors are preferred in the age range between 12 and 45 years but an older donor may be considered. Where demise is anticipated within this age span, arrangements should be made through the nearest large city hospital eye department or the International Eye Bank for donation of the eyes. Preliminary registration of the donor is necessary in order that the next of kin be properly instructed in the procedure to be followed in assuring satisfactory specimens.

A TISSUE BANK is located in the U.S. Naval Hospital at Bethesda, Maryland, just outside Washington, D.C., from which tissues may be obtained free of charges other than those necessary for shipping. Tissues stored in the bank are obtained by sterile autopsy from donors who arranged for the removal of salvageable tissues prior to death.

The following surgical reports have been included in this chapter to further familiarize the secretary with the terminology of plastic surgery.

Split Thickness Skin Graft To Right Posterior Auricular Surface and Sulcus

With the patient in the supine position, under excellent general endotracheal anesthesia, the left leg and head were prepared and draped in the customary manner.

A split thickness skin graft of 10/1000 of an inch in thickness was taken from the left thigh with a Brown dermatome and preserved in saline moistened gauze.

The right auricle was then released from the scar tissue binding it down by sharp dissection. The dissection was continued along the posterior aspect of the auricle until the entire right ear lobe was freed to the sulcus. Hemostasis was well controlled with electrocautery.

An Esser inlay stent graft was then made by suturing the split thickness graft to the posterior aspect of the right auricle and to the posterior auricular skin. The graft was sutured in the sulcus with a continuous suture of 0000 chromic catgut. After a small saline moistened gauze stent was placed behind the ear, the auricle was sutured down to the skin with the skin graft using a continuous suture of 00000 monofilament nylon.

A moderate pressure dressing was applied. One piece of Adaptic was placed over the donor site and this was then covered with several saline moistened gauze flats. The wound was dressed with a 4 inch Kerlix bandage.

Excision of Scar and Old Graft
(Closure by means of interpolated nasolabial full flap)

The operative area was prepared with pHisoHex and water and draped in the usual manner. General anesthesia was used with oral endotracheal intubation.

Six months prior to admission, a full thickness postauricular graft was used to cover a defect on the left side of the nose. The resulting scar and deformity in the area caused some blockage of the airway. Patient readmitted for a more definitive plastic repair.

The scar and old graft were removed from the left side of the nose leaving a defect approximately 1 inch in diameter. A flap was designed from the left nasolabial fold area superiorly in order to fit into the defect with better coverage and a more satisfactory cosmetic result. The flap was developed by means of sharp dissection. All bleeding points were clamped and tied with 00000 plain surgical catgut free ties. The skin edges of the nasolabial area were undermined and the subcuticular tissue approximated by means of interrupted 00000 white nylon sutures. Skin edges were approximated by interrupted 00000 blue nylon suture.

The flap was shaped to conform to the defect and was sutured in place by means of interrupted 00000 nylon sutures. Dry sterile dressing was applied.

Fascia Lata Graft (For residual Bell's Palsy of right face)

The upper left thigh was completely prepared with soap and water as was the entire face, following anesthesia. General anesthesia was supplemented with 1% Xylocaine.

The first approach was to obtain fascia lata from the left thigh. This was done through a four inch incision over the greater trochanter. With our fascia stripper, we removed three long pieces of fascia about $\frac{1}{4}$ of an inch in width by about 8 inches in length. The wound on the hip was closed with 0000 plain and 00000 nylon. A drain was left in place. A pressure dressing was applied along the entire leg.

Attention was turned to the face. An attempt is being made here to support the entire right side of the face and the right lower eyelid. First, a piece of fascia lata was inserted which extended from the left side of the lower lid, beyond the midline to the angle of the mouth, and up to the Temporalis muscle. The second strip extended from the upper lid, beyond the midline, through the left side (the good side), up to the corner of the mouth and to the temporalis region of the right side. The third strip of fascia extended from the left Frontalis muscle, which is good, down to the inner canthus along the lower eyelid margin and up to the Temporalis muscle. An incision made over the left Temporalis muscle was used to expose the fascia and the muscle. The three strips of fascia were then drawn up tightly to overcorrect the deformity. The fascia was sutured to the muscle with 0000 plain nylon.

The wound in the face was closed with 000000 nylon and in the scalp with 00000 nylon. All suturing of the fascia to the muscle on the face and Frontalis was done with 0000 nylon. A pressure dressing was applied to the face.

THE EXTERNAL EARS

The operation for plastic repair and reconstruction of the external ear is termed an otoplasty. A variety of techniques are used to correct deformities of the external ear which result from congenital errors in shape, size and position or traumatic deformities with loss of substance. Corrective surgery may range from alteration of the shape of the ear to complete reconstruction. By reconstruction of the external ear, it must not be construed that the surgeon can perfectly duplicate the intricate design of the external ear when total reconstruction is necessary.

Anatomic terms encountered in otoplasty reports, a listing of some of the more popular techniques and representative operative dictations follow to assist the secretary with this phase of terminology peculiar to plastic surgery.

ANATOMIC STRUCTURES OF THE EXTERNAL EAR

Antihelix
Antitragus
Auricle
Auricular tubercle of Darwin
Cauda helicis
Cavum conchae
Cephalo-auricular angle
Concha (pl. conchae)
Conchal fossa
Conchal mastoid angle
Crus of the helix
Cymba conchae
Eminentia conchae
Eminentia triangularis
External acoustic meatus
Fissure antitragohelicina
Fossa of the antihelix
Fossa triangularis
Helix
Incisura intertragica
Inferior crus of the antihelix
Intertragic notch
Lobule
Ponticulus
Retro-auricular sulcus
Scapha
Scaphoconchal angle
Scaphoid fossa
Sulcus antihelicis transversus
Superior crus
Tragus
Tympanic sulcus

SOME TECHNIQUES FOR OTOPLASTY

Adams
Alexander
Barsky
Becker
Binnie
Converse
Davis and Kitlowski
Demel and Ruttin
Dieffenbach
Eckstein-Kleinschmidt
Eitner
Erich
Fomon
Gavello
Gersuny
Holmes
Joseph
Kitlowski
Kolle-Lexer
Lexer
Luckett
Monks

SOME TECHNIQUES FOR OTOPLASTY (Continued)

Morestin
Nelaton
Ombredanne
Parkhill
Straith

Swenson
Szymanowski
Vogel
Young

Otoplasty, Bilateral

The patient presented bilateral protrusion of the ears with absence of the posterior crus of the antihelix and a poorly formed antihelix on each side.

Under adequate preoperative sedation, the operative area was prepared with pHisoHex and draped. The ear was blocked by means of 1% Xylocaine which was infiltrated anteriorly and posteriorly to the ear.

An elliptical piece of skin was excised from the posterior aspect of the ear following the curve of the antihelix. This ellipse extended the full length of the ear and was approximately 6 mm. in width. By means of Keith needles, which were inserted from the anterior to the posterior aspect of the ear, the new posterior crus of the antihelix and the new antihelix itself were marked.

An incision was made through the cartilage to form the new posterior crus and antihelix. The excess cartilage was trimmed, as needed, in order to restore the ear to its correct position. The cartilage was approximated by means of a continuous suture of 00000 multiple filament white nylon. The skin was then closed by means of a subcuticular suture of 0000 monofilament nylon with interrupted sutures of this material where necessary.

The same procedure was carried out on the other side. A modified compression dressing consisting of a moist 4 x 4 Kerlix and 2 inch roller bandage was applied.

THE EYELIDS

Plastic repair of defects of the eyelid is termed a *blepharoplasty*. There are many variations of the blepharoplasty, performed for a wide variety of anomalies, ranging from congenital defects to traumatic deformities. Ptosis of the eyelid (blepharoptosis) is one of the most prevalent defects. The popular techniques for correcting this condition have been listed separately in this section.

ANATOMIC FEATURES OF THE EYELID

Aponeurosis
Canthus
Caruncula
Ciliary margins
Conjunctiva
Fibers of Orbicularis oculi
Fornix
Inferior tarsus
Lacrimal ducts
Lacrimal sac
Lacus lacrimalis
Lamina
Lateral canthus
Levator palpebrae superioris
Medial palpebral ligament
Meibomian glands
Mueller's muscle
Nasojugal
Nasolacrimal duct
Orbital margins
Orbital septum
Palpebral fissure
Palpebral furrow
Palpebral raphe
Palpebrarum
Plica semilunaris
Posterior lamina
Riolan's muscle
Superior fornix
Superior tarsus
Tarsal glands
Tarsal muscles
Tarsal plate
Tarsus (pl. tarsi)
Tarsus orbital septum
Tunica conjunctiva

TECHNIQUES FOR EYELID REPAIR

Alsus-Knapp
Arlt
Beard-Cutler
Blair
Blaskovics
Burow
Cutler
Derby
Duke-Elder
Dupuy-Dutemps
Essers
Everbusch
Fox
Fricke's
Gaillard
Gifford
Hess
Hotz
Hughes
Jaesche
Jones
Krönlein
Kuhnt-Szymanowski
Lagleyze
Langenbeck
Lexer
Malbec
Minsky
Motais
Mueller
Panas
Reese
Sayoc's
Smith
Snellen
Spaeth
Stallard
Straith
Szymanowski
Tripier
Truc
Ulloa
Van Millingen
Verhoeff
Verweys
von Blaskovics-Doyen
Wheeler
Wicherkiewicz
Wiener
Wies lid fracturing

PTOSIS CORRECTION TECHNIQUES

Allport	Machek
Alvis	Magnus
Angelucci	Malbran
Berke	Motais
Berke-Motais	Mules
Blair	Pagenstecher
Blaskovics	Panus
Crawford	Reese
Elschnig	Rosenburg
Fergus	Savin
Friedenwald-Guyton	Schimek
Gayet	Snellen
Gifford	Sourdille
Grimsdale	Spaeth
Guyton	Tansley
Harman	Trainor-Nida
Iliff	Wiener
Johnson	Wolff
Lancaster	Worth
Leahey	Wright
Lexer	Young

ANESTHETICS USED IN LID SURGERY

Carbocaine	O'Brien Akinesia
Cocaine hydrochloride	Pontocaine
Hyaluronidase (adjunct drug)	Procaine with epinephrine
Lidocaine	Tetracaine
Mepivacaine 2%	Van Lint Akinesia

DRESSINGS

Cikloid	Telfa
Collodion	Telfa plastic film
Fluffed gauze	Tie-over
Pressure	Wet

Blepharoplasty, Upper and Lower

The excess skin of the upper eyelid was picked up at the inner and outer portion of the lid by means of thumb forceps. This produced a bridge of tissue which was clamped with a Hunt clamp. A few drops of 1% Xylocaine with ½ cc. of adrenalin to the ounce was infiltrated into the lid for anesthesia.

By means of a #11 Bard-Parker blade the upper lid tissue, which was held in a Hunt clamp, was incised. The clamp was then removed and at the inner and outer angle of the lid the skin was further trimmed so that the whole excision was moderately fusiform in shape. After it had been determined that sufficient excess skin had been excised, the skin of the lid was reapproximated by means of a subcuticular suture of 00000 dermalon.

Bleeding throughout the procedure was controlled by means of cautery. The same procedure was repeated on the opposite eye.

Terramycin Ophthalmic Ointment was placed in the eye and a modified pressure dressing applied.

The skin of the lower lid was then infiltrated with 1% Xylocaine containing adrenalin as was the lateral canthal region. A curvilinear line was carefully made along the lower lid approximately 3 cm. inferior to the tarsal plate edge. Undercutting was then carried out of the entire lower flap of skin from this incision. The lateral end of this incision was then extended in an oblique angle parallel to a line of crowfeeting. This skin was completely raised from the underlying muscle. The fat pads were then easily isolated through the Orbicularis oculi muscle fibers. The assistant applied moderate pressure to the eyeball so that this fat would herniate. The excess was carefully estimated and removed. Several 00000 white nylon stitches were used to reapproximate the muscle fibers.

A lower skin flap was then carefully smoothed in position so that no wrinkles remained in the lower lid. An excess could then be determined where it overlapped the upper skin edge. This was carefully removed.

Closure was accomplished by one subcuticular stitch of white nylon through both edges of the incision at the outer canthus of the eye angle. A 00000 dermalon subcuticular stitch completed both closures. A similar procedure was performed on the opposite eye.

A moderate pressure bandage was then built up over both eyes.

THE LIPS

An operation designed to correct a deformity of the lip (s) is called a *cheiloplasty*. A number of various type operations are performed to correct defects and deformities of the lip.

Some of the more frequently seen lip deformities are listed here with a listing of the more commonly used methods of cheiloplasty. Anatomic structures involved in cheiloplasty procedures are also given to assist the secretary with transcriptions.

Deformities of the Lip

CLEFT LIP	— A congenital fissure of the lip; also called a harelip.
DOUBLE LIP	— Hypertrophy (enlargement), usually of the upper lip with a longitudinal groove running parallel with the lip giving the appearance of a double lip.
ECTROPION	— Turning out of the lip.
ENTROPION	— Inward curling of the lip.
FLAT LIP	— Flatness of the upper lip.
MACROCHEILIA	— Abnormal enlargement of the lip.
MACROSTOMIA	— An abnormally large mouth.
MICROSTOMIA	— Abnormally short lips and small mouth.

ANATOMIC STRUCTURES OF THE LIP

Areolar tissue
Buccal mucosa
Frenulum
Frenum labiorum
Gingivolabial sulci
Labial

Mucocutaneous border
Orbicularis oris muscle
Philtrum
Sphincter oris
Vermilion border

ARTERIES SUPPLYING THE LIP

Lower lip:
  inferior labial
  mental
  submental

Upper lip:
  infra-orbital
  superior labial (coronary)

CHEILOPLASTY TECHNIQUES

Abbe I & II stage
Bell
Brauer
Brown-Blair
Cronin
Esmarch
Gillies
Giralde
Hagedorn
Hagedorn-LeMesurier
Hagerty
Joseph
Kilner cleft lip
Kowalzig
LeMesurier
Lexer
Marcks
McCash-Randall
McDowell

Millard
Mirault
Mirault-Brown-Blair
Owens
Pfeifer
Pierce-O'Connor
Randall
Rose
Schuchardt-Pfeifer
Simon
Teale
Tennison
Thompson
Veau
Veau-Axhausen
von Langenbeck
Webster
Wolfe

Tennison Harelip Repair

1% Xylocaine with adrenalin was infiltrated about the mouth, in the upper lip and base of the nose region.

The edges of the cleft were freshened by removing the mucous membrane and excess skin at the lower end of the incision on the medial cleft. A 1/8 inch incision was made into the lip from the mucous membrane border. This allowed the cupid's bow to rotate downward leaving a triangular defect with the apex in the center of the lip. The opposite mucous membrane was pared and trimmed. A small flap with its base laterally and inferiorly was rotated into the triangular defect.

Three sutures were inserted using a 0000 nylon figure-of-eight and were tied in the mucous membrane. The excess mucous membrane was then excised and approximated with 000000 silk. A subcuticular 00000 nylon suture was used to approximate the skin edges. Interrupted nylon sutures were used to close the floor of the nostril and reshape the nostril and ala.

A Logan Bow was applied. A wet Streptomycin dressing was placed over the skin edge.

THE NOSE AND PARANASAL SINUSES

Some of the more commonly used anatomic terms encountered in operative dictations describing procedures performed on the nose and accessory sinuses are listed here to assist the secretary with her transcription.

ANATOMIC STRUCTURES
Nose and Paranasal Sinuses

Ala (pl. alae)
Alanasi
Alar cartilages
Aponeurosis
Atrium
Bridge
Bulla ethmoidalis
Cartilaginous septum
Cartilaginous vault
Choana (pl. choanae)
Clinoid process
Columella
Columna

Concha (pl. conchae)-(turbinates)
Cribriform plate of ethmoid
Crista galli
Crura
Crus laterale
Crus mediale
Dorsum nasi
Ethmoidal air cells
Frontal processes of maxillae
Greater alar cartilage
Hamular process
Hiatus semilunaris
Hypophyseal fossa

ANATOMIC STRUCTURES—Nose and Paranasal Sinuses (Cont.)

Inferior meatus
Infundibulum
Kiesselbach's plexus
Lateral crus
Lateral wall
Lesser alar cartilage
Medial crus
Middle meatus
Mucoperichondrium
Mucous membrane
Nares
Nasal bones
Nasal conchae
Nasal crest
Nasal spine
Nasion
Nasolabial junction
Nasopalatine recess
Nostrils

Ostium maxillare
Palatine bone
Perpendicular plate of ethmoid
Piriform opening
Plica nasi
Rostrum of sphenoid
Septum
Septum mobile nasi
Sesamoid cartilages
Sinus groove
Sphenoethmoidal recess
Sphenoidal process
Superior meatus
Turbinates
Uncinate process
Vestibule
Vomer
Vomeronasal cartilage
Vomeronasal organ of Jacobson

PARANASAL SINUSES

Ethmoidal
Frontal

Maxillary
Sphenoidal

ARTERIES OF THE NOSE

Alar branches of ext. maxillary
Alveolar br. of int. maxillary
Anterior ethmoidal br. of ophthalmic
Dorsal nasal br. of ophthalmic
Infraorbital br. of int. maxillary

Pharyngeal br. of int. maxillary
Posterior ethmoidal br. of ophthalmic
Septal br. of ext. maxillary
Septal br. of superior labial
Sphenopalatine br. of int. maxillary

NERVES OF THE NOSE

Ant. alveolar br. of maxillary
Anterior ethmoidal
Anterior palatine
External nasal
Facial
Infraorbital of maxillary
Infratrochlear branch of ophthalmic

Nasal branches of sphenopalatine ganglion
Nasociliary branches of ophthalmic
Nasopalatine
Nerve of pterygoid canal
Olfactory

Rhinoplasty and Submucous Resection

Under adequate preoperative sedation, the face was prepared and draped in the usual manner. Under local infiltration and bilateral infraorbital block anesthesia, the usual intercartilaginous incision was made bilaterally and the skin of the nose was elevated by sharp dissection. After the intended nasal bridge had been measured with a profilometer, the saw was inserted through the incision and the nasal bone sawed through according to the measurements. This was repeated on the opposite side. The knife was inserted through the saw cut and the septum was cut through and separated from above, downward at the same level as the bone cut. The bony hump was removed. Irregularities were removed with a rasp.

The upper lateral cartilages on both sides were then cut free from the septum from below, upward and were lowered. The upper lateral cartilages were then shortened bilaterally.

By use of the scalpel, the septum was shortened by excising a wedge of septum and mucous membrane from the lower end of the septum, the base of the wedge being upward.

The lower lateral cartilages were then trimmed and a small amount of cartilage removed from the superior edge of each. A 1/32 of an inch saw was inserted into the intercartilaginous incision and a vertical saw cut was made on each side of the septum.

Bilateral osteotomies of the nasal processes over the maxillary bones were done extending from the lower limits of the maxillary bone to the region of the medial canthus of the eye. The bones were infractured.

The mucous membrane of the nose was anesthetized as required. A curved vertical incision was made through the mucous membrane and 1 cm. from the anterior end of the septum the cartilage was cut through to the opposite side. The mucoperichondrium on each side was elevated by means of a sharp and blunt dissector. The cartilage of the septum was then cut through with scissors leaving a 1 cm. dorsal strut to support the nasal bridge. Intervening cartilage was removed with a rongeur. The mucoperichondrial flap was then approximated with interrupted sutures of 0000 chromic.

* * * * * *

The following procedure is sometimes performed in conjunction with a rhinoplasty.

Bilateral Weir

The ala on each side was cut free from its attachment to the face. A piece of wedge-shaped tissue approximately 3/16th of an inch in width was excised. The base of the ala of the nose on each side was resutured by means of two figure-of-eight sutures using 00000 dermalon. The dog-ears of the upper extremity of the incisions were excised. The skin was approximated with a subcuticular suture using 00000 dermalon. Occasional twists were put in for more accurate approximation of the edges.

THE PALATE

The roof of the mouth consists of a structure called the palate. The anterior portion of this covering is designated as the *hard palate* in contradistinction to the posterior portion which is called the *soft palate*. Both the hard and soft palates sometimes exhibit a congenital defect referred to as a *cleft palate*, where proper fusion of the palate has failed to occur. This deformity is sometimes associated with a cleft lip or a cleft velum. Investigators believe that heredity is an important factor concluding that cleft palate alone may be attributed to a simple dominant gene with sex limitation to the female.

Repair of defects of the palate is termed a *palatoplasty* and may include pharyngeal flaps and pharyngoplasty. The techniques for repair which have received popular acceptance are listed here with anatomic terms used in reporting surgery of the palate and pharynx.

ANATOMIC FEATURES OF THE PALATE AND PHARNYX

Alveolar arches
Alveolar ridge
Alveolus
Aponeurosis of the velum
Foramina of Scarpa
Fossa(e) of Rosenmüller
Greater palatine foramen
Gums
Hamulus
Hard palate
Incisive canal
Incisive foramen
Incisive papilla
Isthmus faucium
Lesser palatine foramina
Linear raphe
Major palatine artery
Maxilla (pl. maxillae)
Maxillary tubercles
Medial pterygoid plate
Median raphe
Mucoperiosteum
Muscles of the palate
   Glossopalatinius
   Levator veli palatini
   Musculus uvulae
   Pharyngopalatinus
   Tensor veli palatini

Nasopharyngeal area
Neurovascular bundle
Oral mucosa
Palatal shelves
Palates, primary and secondary
Palatine aponeurosis
Palatine arches
Palatine bones
Palatine process
Palatine tonsil
Palatine uvula
Palatine velum
Palatum durum
Palatum mole
Passavant's cushion
Periosteum
Pharyngeal aperture
Pharyngeal bursa
Pharyngeal hemisphincter
Pharyngeal ostium
Pharyngeal recess
   (fossae of Rosenmüller)
Pharyngeal tonsil
Pillars of fauces
Posterior pharynx
Pterygoid plate
Pterygomandibular raphe
Pterygopalatine canal

ANATOMIC FEATURES OF THE PALATE AND PHARYNX (Cont.)

Salpingopalatine fold
Salpingopharyngeal fold
Salpingopharyngeus muscle
Soft palate (velum)
Sphenopalatine artery
Sphenopalatine nerve

Superior constrictor muscle
Torus (cushion)
Transverse mucosal rugae
Uvula
Velopharynx
Velum

CLEFT PALATE INSTRUMENTS

Also: See Chapter 5

Austin dental knife
Barsky double-end elevator
Brophy bistoury
Dott mouth gag
Freer elevator

Kilner suture carrier
Latrobe soft palate retractor
MacKenty cleft palate knife
McIndoe hawk's-beak elevator
Reverdin needles
Sluder palate retractor
Veau elevator

PALATE REPAIR TECHNIQUES

Barsky pharyngoplasty
Brown's push-back
Dieffenbach-Warren
Dorrance push-back
Gillies-Fry
Palatoplasty
Pharyngeal flap
Schuchardt-Pfeifer

Staphylorrhaphy
Uranoplasty
V-Y operation
Veau
Veau-Axhausen
von Langenbeck
W-Y retroposition
Wardill-Kilner four flap

Modified von Langenbeck Repair of Cleft Palate

The patient presented a Veau Type II cleft of the palate which included all of the soft palate and approximately ¾ths of the hard palate. The palate was separated approximately 1 cm. at its widest part.

Under nasal endotracheal anesthesia, the skin of the face was prepared and draped. A Dott mouth gag was inserted after the mouth and throat had been packed with gauze which contained 5% cocaine and adrenalin. This pack was allowed to remain in place for 15 minutes. 1% Xylocaine with ¼ cc. of adrenalin to the ounce was injected along the edges of the defect in the soft and hard palate and around the point of exit of the anterior palatine artery. By means of a Veau elevator, the mucoperiosteum was elevated from each side and the front of the underlying palatine bone. The palatine aponeurosis was cut by means of scissors and the soft palate elevated. The edges of the mucoperiosteum of the hard palate, soft palate and uvula were trimmed on each side by means of a #11 Bard-Parker blade.

An incision was made through the mucous membrane of the posterior tonsillar pillar approximately 1/8 of an inch from the anterior surface of the pillar. This mucous membrane was then split for a distance of approximately 1/4 inch. At this time Brophy plates were inserted on each side of the soft palate just anterior to the uvula and were held in place by means of silver wires. The plates were not tied down tightly at this time.

The mucoperiosteum was approximated by means of interrupted vertical mattress sutures of 0000 black silk. The soft palate was approximated in the same manner. The anterior and posterior surfaces of the uvula were approximated by means of plain interrupted sutures of 0000 black silk. The posterior tonsillar pillars were approximated for a distance of about 2 1/2 cm. by means of interrupted vertical mattress sutures of 0000 black silk. At this time the Brophy plates were set into position and held there by means of hemostats and the wires tightened. Care was taken not to wire the plates down too tightly. The excess wire was cut off and the ends bent in order that they not stick into the tongue.

Wardill Repair of Cleft Palate

Adequate anesthesia was obtained with oral endotracheal intubation. The patient was prepared with pHisoHex and water to the skin and Aqueous Zephiran intraorally. The patient was then surgically draped and a nasopharyngeal pack applied to catch any bloody drainage. Some local infiltration with 2% Xylocaine with epinephrine was performed along the course of incision of the palate.

The mucoperiosteal flap was raised on the right side after the method of Wardill. The dissection was carried down to the greater palatine neurovascular bundle. Care was taken not to disturb the neurovascular bundle in this area. The posterior lip of the pterygoid canal in this area was removed by means of an osteotome. The hamular process was fractured. This mobilized the right side of the flap sufficiently so it could be brought across the midline. The same procedure was carried out on the left side of the palate.

The edges of the cleft were freshened by means of a # 11 Bard-Parker blade, removing a portion of the edge down to normal tissue. After this had been performed, the nasal septum which was evident was split down its center. Repair of the nasal portion of the mucous membrane was carried out to the mucosa of the nasal septum by means of interrupted 0000 chromic catgut sutures. This also required repair of the soft palate by means of interrupted 0000 chromic catgut suture down to the uvula. The oral surface of the mucosa of the soft palate was repaired by means of interrupted 000 chromic catgut vertical mattress sutures.

A push-back procedure was performed by repairing the edge of the Y closure with interrupted 000 chromic catguts with the Y-suture being used to tack the upper portion of the flap down to the nasal septum in that area.

RESTORATION BY FOREIGN MATERIALS

Over the years a variety of synthetic materials have been tried in different body sites to fill defects and restore a more normal contour to the area. These have included the use of paraffin, rubber, plastics, polyvinyl sponges and others which, for numerous reasons, were eventually discarded. A new material called silastic is being used currently in the form of implants and liquid with satisfactory results. The following two operative reports illustrate two examples of popular application.

Silastic Injection into Area of Malar Bone Deficiency

The patient presented a Treacher-Collins syndrome. Attention was focused this time on the deficiency of the malar bones.

An incision was made at the supra-auricular hairline and through this incision the dissection was deepened, separating the fibers of the temporal muscle. The temporal bone was then exposed.

Using periosteal elevators, the zygomatic arch was followed. The malar bone was freed from its underlying soft tissues which were elevated. Into this pocket a liquid silastic with a catalyst was injected. The material gradually filled up the deficiency of bone to the lower rim of the orbit and to the malar bone.

Closure of the wound was accomplished using a white nylon interrupted suture to reapproximate the temporal muscle fibers. Three interrupted white nylon sutures were placed subcuticularly. A running 00000 dermalon suture was placed intracuticularly. Interrupted sutures for the skin were placed as needed.

Eye patches and a moderately compressive pressure dressing were applied to the operative area.

Augmentation Mammoplasty, Bilateral

The patient presented small, shrunken, atrophic breasts, the left slightly larger than the right.

After adequate sedation with the patient under general endotracheal anesthesia, the anterior chest was prepared and draped in the usual manner. A very long strand of 000 Zytor suture was stitched to the skin at the midportion of the suprasternal notch. This was used for measuring the breast position of both nipples. A slightly curved incision was marked in the line of the submammary sulcus. An incision was made through the dermis and subcutaneous tissue and deepened to the fascia of the Serratus anterior. It was carried upwards until the border of the Pectoralis major was encountered. The deep muscle fascia was opened and lifted forward along with the breast and skin. Care was taken not to expose breast tissue. Final dissection was completed by inserting two index fingers and working them against one another in order to bluntly enlarge the pocket.

Careful hemostasis was obtained by packing the pocket with several 4 x 4 sponges and by use of electrocoagulation.

The larger size silastic implant was inserted into the pocket on the right with a twisting motion and carefully placed to lie against the Pectoralis major muscle. An antibiotic solution was applied over this implant.

The wound was closed in layers using 00000 white nylon stitches to approximate the implant to the fascial layers. The skin was approximated with interrupted 00000 white nylon subcutaneously and running 00000 Ethicons for subcuticulars. Antibiotic solution containing Bacitracin was injected into the pocket containing the implant. Careful pressure dressing was applied to the breast by using Kerlix and Ace bandages.

The operation was repeated on the opposite breast.

OPERATIONS ON THE FACIAL SKIN

In addition to reconstructive and repair operations performed on the face, a number of other procedures are employed for the purpose of improving the cosmetic image. Such operations include dermabrasion of acne scarred complexions, tattoo of discolored areas of the skin, rhytidectomy for the removal of wrinkles, revision of scars, etc.

Operative reports to illustrate several of these procedures appear below.

Total Facial Dermabrasion

The patient presented severe pitting and scarring of the cheeks and chin with a few superficial pits on the forehead. There was a very large amount of inspissated sebaceous material present throughout the entire face. Pressure was used to remove as much of this material as possible from the pores.

Under general nasal endotracheal anesthesia, the skin of the face was cleansed with pHisoHex and draped.

By means of an Iverson dermabrader, the entire face was sanded deeply. Bleeding was controlled by means of wet sponges containing saline and adrenalin. After completion of the sanding, the face was covered with fine mesh gauze soaked in saline and adrenalin. This was covered with moist 4 x 4's and a 2 inch roller bandage.

Face Lift

The skin of the face and scalp were prepared with pHisoHex and Aqueous Zephiran.

The frontal scalp, on the right, was locally infiltrated with $\frac{1}{2}\%$ Xylocaine containing 8 drops of adrenalin to the ounce. This subcutaneous infiltration was carried down in front of the ear and behind the ear, throughout the upper neck region, and across the entire anterior portion of the face and forehead. A one inch swath of hair had previously been shaved across the frontoparietal area extending from approximately one inch lateral to the midline down to the supra-auricular area.

An incision was carried along the posterior margin of this shaved area down to the supra-auricular area and then carried preauricularly down the cheek to the inferior pole of the attachment to the ear. The incision was then carried posteriorly just within this hairline to a position approximately $3\frac{1}{2}$ inches behind the ear. The forehead and the entire right cheek were elevated by means of sharp and blunt dissection, care being taken to remain in as superficial a plane as possible to guard against injury to the branches of the 7th nerve. Subcutaneous elevation was similarly carried out inferiorly throughout the upper two-thirds of the cervical region on the right side.

The skin of the forehead and face were then drawn up to a position of new snugness and contour, where it was secured by means of two 00 monofilament dermalon sutures placed in a pulley mattress fashion in a position just above the ear.

Closure was performed throughout the hair bearing areas with interrupted 0000 black silk braided sutures placed in central and vertical mattress fashion after removal of a small dog-ear triangle at the superiormost position of the scalp excision defect. In the preauricular region and in the retroauricular region the closure was carried out with buried white nylon and subcuticular 0000 dermalon with twists as needed.

The exact procedure was carried out on the left side. Following completion of the operation, a large pressure dressing was applied to the entire scalp, face and neck, leaving only the mouth exposed.

Hemostasis was obtained by means of clamping and white nylon ties. Blood loss was considered minimal for this type of operation.

REPAIR OF HYPOSPADIAS

A congenital abnormality sometimes occurs in the male in which the urethra opens on the underside of the penis or on the perineum. Such an anomalous opening is called a *hypospadias*. The counterpart of this condition in the female consists of an anomalous opening of the urethra into the vagina.

Hypospadias in the male is often associated with a condition known as *chordee* in which there is a downward bowing of the penis. A hooded prepuce often is seen with hypospadias

The techniques proposed for the repair of this condition are legion. Only some of the more frequently used methods are listed here.

REPAIR TECHNIQUES FOR HYPOSPADIAS

Blair-Byars	Horton's one stage
Broadbent	Humby
Cecil	Marion-Perard
Cloutier	Marshall-Spellman
Culp	McCormack
Davis	McIndoe
Denis Browne	Memmelaar
DesPrez	Mustarde
Devine	Nesbit
Dieffenbach-Duplay	Nove-Josserand
Duplay I and II	Ombredanne
Farmer	Thiersch-Byars
Havens	Wehrbein
Heineke-Mikulicz	Young-Benjamin

Second Stage Cecil Procedure for Hypospadias

The patient already has had an operation for correction of chordee and a first stage Cecil procedure for correction of the hypospadias.

Under general anesthesia the scrotum and lower abdomen as well as the upper thighs were cleansed with pHisoderm and then draped.

A traction suture of 5 monofilament nylon was placed through the glans penis. A # 12 French catheter was inserted into the bladder. By means of a # 15 Bard-Parker blade an incision was made releasing the penis from the scrotum. Care was taken to leave sufficient tissue so that the reconstructed urethra would not be entered. After the penis was released, there were two raw areas, one on the posterior aspect of the penis and another on the anterior surface of the scrotum. Bleeding was controlled by means of cautery.

The skin was reapproximated with a subcuticular suture of 0000 chromic catgut with twists of the same material where necessary.

A small incision was made into the glans penis. Bleeding was controlled by means of cautery. An attempt was made to transplant the meatus into the glans penis. The meatus was sutured into position in the glans with interrupted sutures of 0000 chromic catgut. The incisional line was covered with Achromycin gauze and a modified compression dressing consisting of fluffs and Elastoplast was applied. The French catheter was left in the bladder.

15 | Thoracic Surgery

CHEST

The specialty of thoracic surgery is concerned with diseases of the thorax involving the tracheobronchial tree, lungs, and mediastinum. Expert roentgenography, physical examination and bronchoscopy are the principal diagnostic procedures in this specialty.

Radiologic examinations of particular value in thoracic disease include fluoroscopy, roentgenography, bronchography, tomography, magnification, angiography, cineradiography, roentgenkymography, photofluorography and radioactive isotopes.

Laboratory examinations constitute an important adjunct to the diagnostic work-up when these findings are correlated with the clinical evaluation. Pulmonary secretions are obtained by sputum collection, tracheal, bronchoscopic and gastric lavage and by laryngeal swabs. These specimens are examined for acid-fast bacilli and malignant cells. Gram stains are performed on the sputum along with cultures, guinea pig inoculations and microscopic examinations. Serologic tests, important in confirming thoracic diseases, include the Youman's-Parlett serologic test for tuberculosis, tests for coccidioidomycosis, syphilis and viral diseases. The aspiration of secretions and lavage of the bronchi for the purpose of obtaining specimens is most effectively accomplished by bronchoscopy. Malignant cells can often be detected in specimens obtained bronchoscopically when such cells are not observed in expectorated sputum studies.

Scalene lymph node biopsy also represents another valuable diagnostic aid. Diseases of the mediastinum and lungs that can be transmitted by way of the lymph channels tend to involve the lymph nodes of the supraclavicular fossa from which the scalene node biopsy is taken. This procedure is of value in discovering sarcoidosis, diffuse pulmonary disease and undifferentiated types of bronchogenic carcinoma.

Bronchoscopy is one of the most important and frequently employed diagnostic procedures performed by the thoracic surgeon. Endoscopic examination of the bronchus may also be performed by trained internists and surgeons, but is usually referred to a thoracic surgeon because of his special understanding and experience with thoracic diseases.

Bronchoscopic examination enables the physician to examine the entire tracheobronchial tree, from the larynx to the orifices of the segmental bronchi. Most of the observed lesions are accessible for biopsy with the possible exception of those situated distal to the orifice of the upper lobe bronchi. Angled-vision lens systems are used to visualize these more remotely situated areas. The right-angle telescope is particularly useful in examining the upper lobe segmental orifices.

The secretary should be acquainted with the nomenclature for the tracheobronchial tree and the standard numbering system used to designate the segmental bronchi. There is a growing preference among radiologists and thoracic surgeons to refer to the segmental bronchi by number rather than by name.

RIGHT BRONCHIAL TREE	LEFT BRONCHIAL TREE
Right Upper Lobe Bronchus	Left Upper Lobe Bronchus
Apical	Apical posterior 1, 2
Posterior	Anterior 3
Anterior	Superior lingular 4
Middle Lobe Bronchus	Inferior lingular 5
Lateral	
Medial	(no middle lobe on the left)
Right Lower Lobe Bronchus	Left Lower Lobe Bronchus
Superior (apical)	Superior (apical) 6
Medial basal	Anteromedial basal 7, 8
Anterior basal	Lateral basal 9
Lateral basal	Posterior basal 10
Posterior basal	

The American terminology for the segmental bronchi is identical to that of the British except that they refer to the superior segments of the lower lobes as apical segments.

ANATOMY OF THE TRACHEA, BRONCHI AND LUNGS

The oral cavity continues at the back of the mouth as the oral pharynx or upper throat. At a level just below the chin this passageway divides into two passages, the esophagus serving the digestive tube, and the opening to the larynx of the respiratory system.

THORACIC SURGERY

Thoracic surgery is concerned anatomically with the trachea, bronchi, lungs and mediastinum. The larynx belongs to the domain of the otolaryngologist.

The Trachea

The trachea (windpipe) is a cartilaginous and membranous tube which extends from the lower larynx to the level of the fifth thoracic vertebra where it divides into the right and left bronchus leading to the right and left lung, respectively. The bifurcation point at the bottom of the trachea, between the right and left bronchus, is called the carina.

The Bronchi

The right bronchus enters the right lung at about the level of the fifth thoracic vertebra. It branches into three bronchi, one leading to each lobe of the right lung. These are designated as the right upper lobe bronchus, middle lobe bronchus and right lower lobe bronchus. These bronchi in turn branch again into segmental bronchi deep within the lung.

The left bronchus divides into two branches, one for each lobe of the left lung which has only two lobes. These bronchi are designated as the left upper lobe bronchus and the left lower lobe bronchus. These bronchi each branch into four segmental bronchi.

Viewing the bifurcation of the bronchi at the bottom of the trachea through a bronchoscope one observes that the right bronchus is more in line with the trachea than is the left bronchus which diverges at a sharper angle. The right bronchus also has a larger lumen or opening than has the left bronchus. For these reasons foreign bodies which enter the trachea usually drop into the right bronchus.

Ingested materials are diverted to the esophagus and prevented from entering the respiratory tube by a forward movement of the arytenoid cartilages toward the cushion of the epiglottis. Certain actions such as laughing, hasty eating, etc. sometimes permit food, liquids and foreign bodies to find their way into the air passages. The foreign bodies are most commonly nuts, hardware, pins, needles, dental material, safety pins and bone. The reaction may range from a severe bout of coughing to wheezing, cyanosis and death due to suffocation. A large bolus of food trapped in the trachea can result in asphyxia and death. Suffocation will also result if both bronchi are completely occluded.

Conditions manifested by nausea and vomiting are always attended by the possibility of aspiration. Deaths as a result of this occurrence were more common when general anesthetics were customary. Where general anesthetics are used food and water are withheld preoperatively. It is also

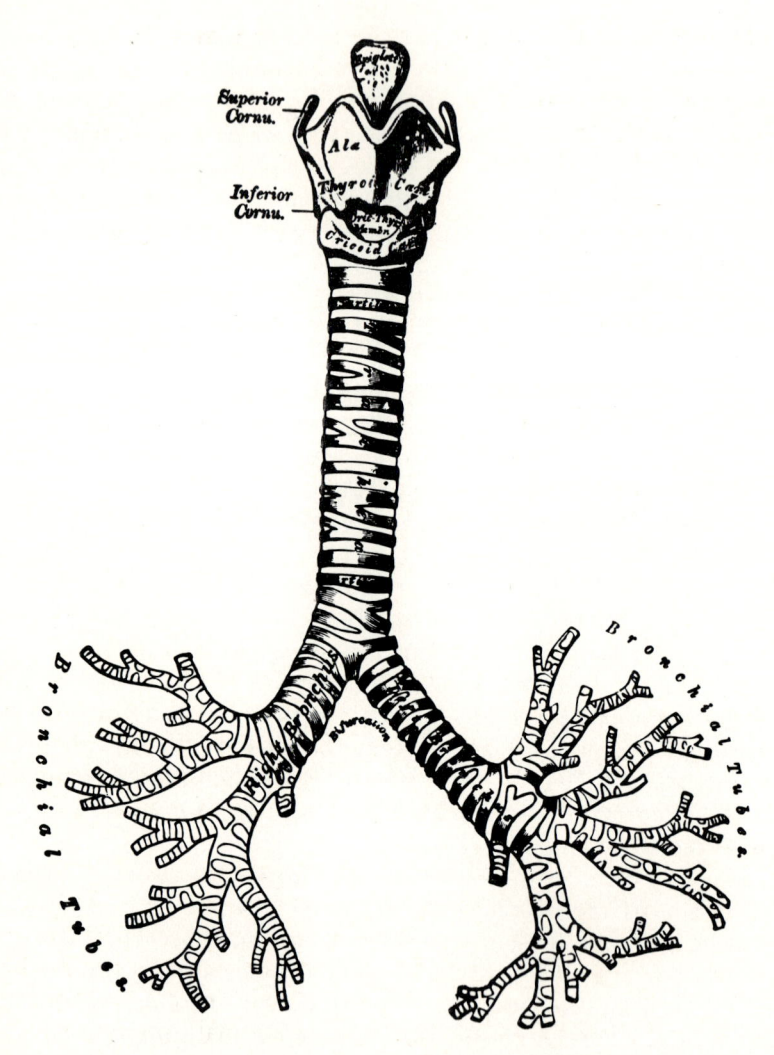

Figure 89 Front view of cartilages of larynx, trachea and bronchi as well as bronchial tubes
From Gray's Anatomy courtesy Lea & Febiger Publishers.

a routine practice to question all obstetrical patients who will be receiving a general anesthetic regarding the time and amount of their last meal.

When obstruction of the air passages by foreign materials does occur, emergency measures must be employed immediately. In high occlusions emergency tracheotomy is performed to establish an airway. See Fig. 90. In lower obstructions bronchoscopy with removal of the foreign material is necessary. Unfortunately, when complete obstruction of the trachea or both bronchi occurs and cannot be relieved by coughing, wheezing or percussion, suffocation generally results before surgical intervention can be arranged.

Partial obstruction of the bronchus results in expiratory trapping of air and distal emphysema. Complete occlusion leads to collapse of the lung and eventually to drowned lung. Sometimes the foreign body progresses to a lobar or segmental bronchus where, after a bout of coughing, it may become symptomless for days or weeks. These patients usually develop asthma-like symptoms due to a lung abscess or bronchiectasis which has developed as a result of the foreign body. Treatment is surgical consisting of bronchoscopy with removal of the foreign material.

The Lungs

The lungs are two in number, one on either side of the chest. The left lung is divided into two lobes, a superior lobe and an inferior lobe. The right lung is divided into a superior, inferior and middle lobe. The right lung weighs more than the left, its average weight being about 625 Gm. as compared to 567 Gm. for the left. The lungs are heavier in the male than in the female.

One of the laboratory examinations performed on the lungs is a measurement of vital capacity. It is a determination of the amount of air that can be exhaled by the strongest expiration following the deepest inspiration the patient can perform. Results vary with the individual. The average for an adult man is 3700 cc. Tidal air, noted in the examination, is the amount of air exhaled or inhaled during normal respiration. The average volume for an adult man is 500 cc.

The arterial circulation to the lungs consists of the pulmonary artery and the bronchial arteries. The pulmonary artery carries blood from the heart to the lungs for oxygenation before recirculation. This blood is returned to the left atrium of the heart by the pulmonary veins which usually number two for each lung. The other arterial supply consists of the bronchial arteries, one to the right lung and two to the left lung. Their function is nutrition of the lungs.

The Pleura

The pleurae consist of two serous membranes lining the thoracic cavity and investing the lungs. That portion of the membrane which covers the surface of the lung and extends into the depressions between the lobes is called the **pulmonary pleura.** The remainder of the membrane lines the inside of the chest wall and diaphragm and is called the **parietal pleura.** The parietal pleura is more specifically designated depending upon its location as: the costal pleura (lining inner surface of ribs and Intercostales), cervical pleura or cupula of the pleura (portion which extends into the neck), diaphragmatic pleura (covering the diaphragm), mediastinal pleura (covering the lateral surface of the mediastinum) and the pericardial pleura (covering the pericardium which invests the heart).

The parietal and pulmonary pleurae are continuous with one another around and below the root of the lung. In other areas of the lung they are in contact with one another. There exists a potential space between them known as the **pleural cavity.** As a result of conditions such as lung collapse, pneumothorax (air in pleural cavity), hemothorax (blood in pleural cavity), hydrothorax (watery fluid in pleural cavity), etc. the actual pleural cavity becomes apparent. The right and left pleural sacs are separate from each other. The space between the two sacs is called the mediastinum.

The Mediastinum (septum mediastinale)

The space in the midline of the thoracic cavity dividing the pleural sacs of the right and left lung is the mediastinum. It contains the heart and its great vessels, the trachea, esophagus, thymus and lymph nodes. It is protected from the front by the sternum and from the back by the thoracic vertebrae.

THORACIC DISEASES

Symptoms which call attention to possible pulmonary disease consist of dyspnea (shortness of breath), persistent cough with or without hemoptysis (coughing up blood or bloody sputum), and chest pain. Although these symptoms may also indicate cardiovascular disease, they are the most representative symptoms of pulmonary disease.

Common medical conditions of the trachea, bronchi and lungs include conditions resulting from inflammation, infection, inhalation of foreign substances, etc. such as pneumonia, tuberculosis, asthma, emphysema, mycotic infections, pneumoconiosis, etc. Surgical diseases include lung abscess, bronchiectasis (dilatation of the bronchi or bronchioles), atelectasis (collapse of the lung), bronchial obstruction, broncholithiasis (concretions in the tracheobronchial tree), cystic disease of the lungs, foreign bodies in the air passages, hemothorax, pneumothorax as well as benign and malignant tumors.

Statistics of the American Cancer Society disclose that in 1968, a total of 55,000 persons died of lung cancer, 46,000 of whom were men and 9,000 of whom were women. These deaths were largely preventable and primarily caused by cigarette smoking. Cancer of the lung now leads as the cause of cancer deaths in men. The death rate is spiraling with the increase in cigarette smoking. It is currently fifteen times higher than it was 35 years ago. It has been established that a man who smokes two packs of cigarettes a day has one chance in ten of developing lung cancer while a nonsmoker has only one chance in 270. Heavy smokers as well as light smokers expose themselves to possible lung cancer. It is unfortunate that in spite of a concerted effort by oncologists and health authorities to educate smokers, 55,000 of these persons die unnecessarily each year.

Most lung cancers have their origin in the bronchus. Early invasion of the lymphatics and vascular channels is a consistent feature of this disease. The earliest symptoms are often due to metastases to the mediastinum, supraclavicular lymph nodes, bone, brain, liver and adrenal cortex. When the tumor encroaches on the bronchus to the point of obstruction there is atelectasis, distal bronchiectasis, hemoptysis, recurrent pneumonitis, and in some cases, lung abscess. The earliest symptoms of the disease consist of cough with or without hemoptysis and chest pain.

Treatment consists of radical pneumonectomy in patients who can tolerate this procedure. Patients with local or distant metastases are usually rejected for surgery. This amounts to about 50 per cent of symptomatic patients who present themselves for treatment. About one third of the remaining 50 per cent of symptomatic patients prove to have resectable lesions. The five year survival rate is only about five per cent in these operable cases. In older patients less extensive operations such as lobectomy (removal of one lobe of the lung) or partial pneumonectomy (resection of the lung) with plastic reconstruction of the bronchus are performed. Irradiation and chemotherapeutic agents such as nitrogen mustard are used for palliation purposes.

Oncologists contend that the only hope of reversing the ever increasing number of lung cancer deaths rests in early detection through periodic chest X-rays. Survival is much greater in patients who are operated upon when the X-ray findings are limited to a "coin lesion" or "solitary nodule."

THE TRACHEA

The trachea (windpipe) is a membranocartilaginous tube-like structure which extends for about 4½ inches from the larynx down into the thorax where it bifurcates into the right and left bronchus. The tracheal tube consists of a series of segments composed of semicircular rings which do not close on the back surface of the tube. Their continuity is provided by muscle fibers and fibrous tissue. By placing the fingers to the throat, one can feel these ring-like segments.

Incision into the trachea (*tracheotomy*) is often employed as a life saving measure to establish an airway. This is usually followed by introduction of a tube to maintain an open airway.

TRACHEAL INSTRUMENTS

Bernay tracheal retractor
Brewster retractor
Flexible shaft retractor
Jackson laryngofissure retractor
Jackson perichondrial elevator
Jackson tracheal bistoury
Jackson tracheal scalpel
Jackson tracheal scissors
Jackson tracheal tenaculum
Jackson-Trousseau dilator

Laborde tracheal dilator
Lukens thymus retractor
Moore tracheostomy buttons
Rockey cannula
Rockey trachea forceps
Rockey mediastinal cannula
Rockey fenestration scope
Rockey vascular clamp
Salvatore-Maloney tracheotome

TRACHEAL TUBES

Atkins-Cannard
Chevalier Jackson
Gabriel Tucker
Holinger
Jackson
Jackson cane-shaped
Jackson extra long
Jackson short length
Kistner plastic

Lepley-Ernst
Lore-Lawrence
Luer
Martin
Mosher life-saving
Pilling
Pilling duralite
Polisar-Lyons
Tucker suction

Tracheotomy

Under local anesthesia, a skin incision was made 2 fingerbreadths above the sternoclavicular junction. The Platysma was incised. Bleeders were clamped and ligated with 000 intestinal sutures. The midline between the strap muscles was grasped and the fascia was incised. Using blunt and sharp dissection, the trachea was exposed. An orbicular ring was cut from the anterior surface. A #8 tracheostomy tube was placed. Interrupted 000 chromic sutures were used to close the subcutaneous tissue and cotton was used to close the skin.

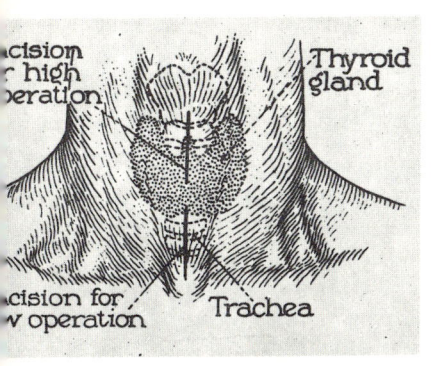

THORACIC SURGERY 565

1. Surface anatomy showing relationship of high and low incisions to underlying structures.

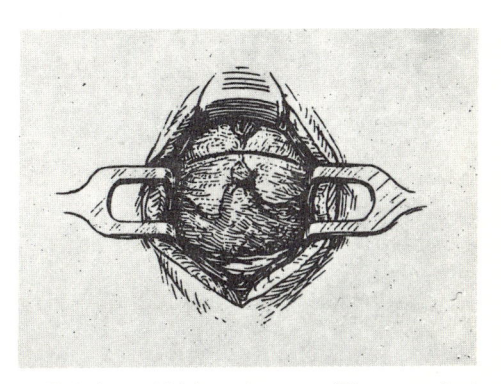

2. Technique of high tracheotomy. The pretracheal fascia is incised at the level of the cricoid cartilage.

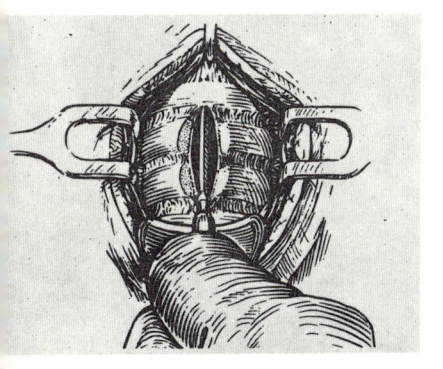

3. Cricoid cartilage retracted to steady trachea. First, second, and third cartilaginous rings incised.

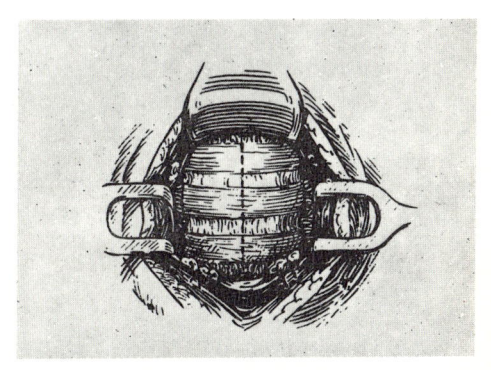

4. Technique of low tracheotomy. Dotted line indicates incision. Low site is inadvisable in children.

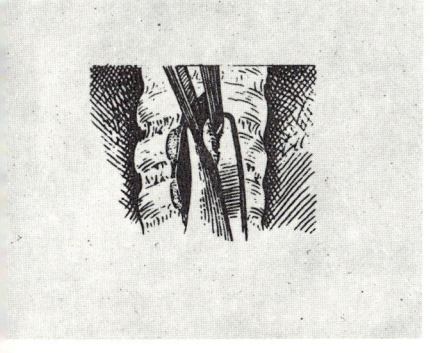

5. Method of trimming edges of tracheal incision in order to establish an oval-shaped opening (Digby).

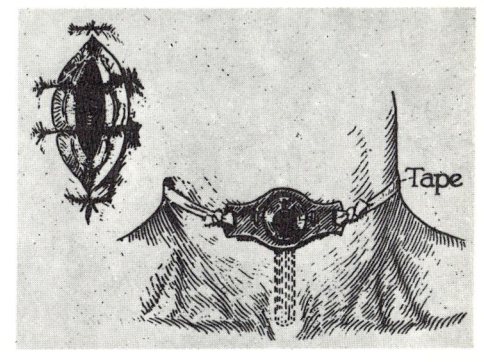

6. Method of fixing trachea by through and through sutures. Method for holding tracheal tube by tape.

Figure 90 Tracheotomy to establish airway
Courtesy Ethicon, Inc.

DISEASES OF THE TRACHEA

Absence of
Adenoma of
Arrested development of tracheal rings
Calcification of
Chondroma
Defect of tracheal rings
Diverticulum of
Epidermoid carcinoma
Fistula of
Foreign body in
Fracture of trachea
Incomplete separation of tracheal rings

Lipoma of trachea
Malformation of tracheal rings
Papilloma of trachea
Stenosis of trachea
Stenosis of tracheotomy wound
Syphilis of trachea
Tracheocele
Tracheo-esophageal fistula
Tuberculosis of trachea
Ulceration of trachea
Varix of trachea

OPERATIONS ON THE TRACHEA

Biopsy of the trachea
Closure of tracheal fistula
Cricotracheotomy
Excision of lesion of trachea
Laryngotracheotomy
  with biopsy
  with exploration
  with removal
Tracheoplasty
Tracheorrhaphy
Tracheoscopy

  with biopsy
  with dilation
  with excision
  with instillation
  with irrigation
Tracheostomy
Tracheotomy
  with biopsy
  with excision
  with exploration
  with removal

BRONCHOSCOPIC EXAMINATIONS

Bronchoscopy is an endoscopic examination in which a scope (bronchoscope) is introduced beyond the larynx and into the bronchus for the purpose of examination, biopsy and/or aspiration of secretions for cell study.

BRONCHOSCOPES

Broyles telescopes
Bruening
Chevalier Jackson
Davis
Double channel irrigating
Emerson
Foregger
Haslinger
Holinger
Holinger-Jackson
Hook-on
Jackson full lumen

Jackson standard
Jesberg
Kernan-Jackson coagulating
Michelson infant
Moersch
Negus
Pilling
Safar ventilation
Staple
Tucker
Yankauer

Bronchoscopy

The pharynx, larynx and trachea were anesthetized with 5% cocaine. The larynx was inspected first by means of a laryngeal mirror. The cords were found to move normally and the intrinsic larynx appeared entirely normal. Direct inspection of the larynx was also made with a laryngoscope. The arytenoids were normal except for moderate hyperemia. The ventricular bands were entirely normal in appearance. The cords were normal and appeared to approximate well on phonation. There was no evidence of disease in the intrinsic larynx. The laryngoscope was removed.

A 7 x 40 Chevalier Jackson bronchoscope was passed through a normal appearing larynx and trachea. The carina was sharp and freely movable in the midline. There was no evidence of subcarinal lymphadenopathy. There was normal flexibility of the bronchial tree. The mucosa of the trachea appeared essentially normal throughout, having been inspected from the carina to immediately under the glottis.

The bronchial trees were examined to their secondary divisions. The right upper lobe (RUL) bronchial orifice was normally patent as was the orifice of the middle lobe and of the right lower lobe on this side. There was no evidence of endobronchial tumor. The left stem bronchus was also examined. There was mild hyperemia. The upper lobe bronchial orifice and the orifices of the lower lobe and its divisions were visualized and found to be normal.

Secretions were collected for cell block and histologic examination. Cytologic studies were ordered.

Conclusion: This is an essentially normal tracheal tree and entirely normal intrinsic larynx. There is no evidence of endotracheal or endobronchial tumor. There is no evidence of laryngeal tumor. No evidence was found of any extrinsic pressure encroaching upon the trachea.

Left Thoracotomy — Mediastinal Tumor Excision

The patient was placed in the lateral position with the left uppermost. A curved periscapular incision was made and deepened. The periosteum overlying the fifth rib was incised and stripped away and a long segment of the fifth rib was removed. The pleural cavity was then entered.

There were no adhesions except at the left upper lobe where it was adherent to the chest wall. As this was dissected free, a degenerated tissue gushed forth. Specimens of this tissue were sent to the laboratory for frozen section. It was the feeling that this might possibly represent a fibrin ball which had been encapsulated between the lung and the chest wall. After all of this tissue had been evacuated and a rather granulomatous lining had been dissected free from the posterior aspect of the left upper lobe and chest wall, there was no evidence of any residual tissue which appeared abnormal.

The pathologist reported that the lesion was quite cellular and could possibly be a lymphoma, but more likely, was a neurofibroma or neurolemoma. He felt that no further distinction could be made until the permanent sections were obtained.

If this were truly a malignant tumor, it would require a left upper lobectomy and excision of a portion of the chest wall. Since it was believed that this was actually a benign process, the operation was discontinued. Hemostasis was obtained.

An intercostal tube was placed posteriorly just above the diaphragm and connected to a water-seal drainage bottle.

The intercostal muscles, extracostal bundles, subcutaneous tissues and skin were closed with interrupted silk. Dry sterile dressings were applied.

Left Lower Lobectomy of the Lung

After satisfactory positioning of the patient in the right lateral position with the arm extended anteriorly and upward, the patient is sterilely prepared and draped. Artificial scoliosis is created by placing a sandbag under the right chest for support. Just prior to draping, the course of the 7th rib is marked.

A skin incision, extending from the spine to the cartilage, is made along the upper edge of the 7th rib. The incision is deepened through the musculature. The fascia of the sacrospinalis muscle is likewise incised. The 7th rib is removed from the cartilage to the costal angle. The pleura is opened and adhesions between the visceral pleura and the parietal pleura are separated by blunt and sharp dissection. A rib spreader is inserted and the thoracotomy wound is gently widened. Hemostasis is accomplished with the use of silver clips.

The interlobar fissures are opened in their entirety. The phrenic nerve is crushed. The hilar vessels are exposed as is the bronchus. The visceral pleura is then incised for about 5 cm. The three branches of the great artery supplying the basal segment are ligated with No. 1 silk after the placing of clamps. The inferior pulmonary vein is then ligated after having been identified by transillumination. The lower lobe is retracted anteriorly. A single ligature is placed around the main trunk of the vein and a second suture around each of the three branches. The vessel is cut between clamps. Shenstone's tourniquet is used to temporarily clamp off the bronchus and the bronchial artery. Two centimeters distal to this, heavy clamps are applied. A small piece of lung tissue is left with which to cover the bronchial suture. The lumen of the bronchial artery is clamped and cut. The bronchus is closed with 000 chromic catgut mattress sutures and the suture line covered with the pedicle of lung tissue. The 7th intercostal nerve is then resected.

100,000 units of penicillin in 20 cc. of saline is introduced into the pleural cavity. A drain is placed through a separate stab wound in the 9th intercostal space in the posterior axillary line. The lung is inflated and the thoracotomy wound closed with approximation of the ribs adjacent to the incision by pericostal sutures. The intercostal drain is clamped and the wound closed in anatomic layers. The tube is then connected to underwater drainage and the clamp released.

Pneumonectomy, Right

After the patient had been sterilely prepared and draped in the supine position, an incision was made anteriorly in the third interspace. A self-retaining retractor was introduced to spread the 3rd and 4th ribs apart. The mediastinal pleura was incised. The right pulmonary artery and the right superior pulmonary vein were exposed. The azygos vein was identified at the level of the bifurcation of the trachea. Just below the azygos vein, the right primary bronchus was noted.

The right azygos vein was doubly ligated and then sectioned. The mediastinal pleura was then incised at its transition into the visceral pleura and it was reflected medially. Retraction of the vena cava was then carried out. Careful dissection of the areolar tissues overlying the hilar structures was accomplished and using fine curved dissectors the artery was freed. Two silk threads were placed around the artery but not tied yet.

The superior pulmonary vein was isolated and cut between ligatures, utilizing two proximal ligatures and one at the distal end of each branch. The caudal branches of the artery were then identified and ligated. Better exposure was obtained of the pulmonary vein which was identified at the upper end of the divided pulmonary ligament. The pulmonary vein was ligated and transected. A transfixion ligature was placed over the central stumps of the doubly ligated artery and veins.

Attention was then turned to the bronchus where a pair of light Kocher forceps were applied below the clamps. Several interrupted fine silk sutures were inserted and the closure completed using a running suture of chromic catgut.

Sulfa was powdered over the raw area and the pleural edges approximated over the divided hilar structures with continuous catgut sutures. The stump of the bronchus was covered with a pad of viable tissue. A small opening was left at the upper and lower angles of the mediastinal suture to permit escape of air should the bronchial stump separate. The wound was carefully rechecked and hemostasis secured. The incision was closed anatomically.

Decortication of Right Lung

The patient was placed in the recumbent position before anesthesia as administered. With the electrocardiograph running, it was noted that he patient had a pulsus bigeminus. This was corrected. The patient was hen anesthetized. An endotracheal tube was inserted and the patient was turned in the lateral position with the right side uppermost. The pulse continued at a normal rate and the blood pressure remained stabilized.

The thoracic area was sterilely prepared and draped. A curved periscapular incision was made and deepened. The periosteum overlying the sixth rib was incised and stripped away. A long segment of the sixth rib was removed. The pleural cavity was entered. There was a copious gush of purulent fluid encountered. This was aspirated. Cultures were taken and sent to the laboratory. Palpation then revealed that there were numerous pockets of pus and a thick visceral peel. Considerable difficulty was encountered in removing the peel. The process consumed about three hours. During this procedure, at least six large separate pockets of pus had been evacuated. The visceral peel overlying all of these areas had been removed. The lung was capable of full expansion.

No underlying disease was palpable in any segment of the lung or in the mediastinum. No bronchopleural fistula was found.

Copious flushing with saline and aspiration were then carried out. Bleeding points were coagulated. Oxycel gauze was used over areas which were bleeding diffusely. An intercostal tube was placed posterolaterally just above the diaphragm and an intercostal catheter was placed in the midaxillary line at the third interspace. Both were connected to water seal drainage bottles. Intercostal bundles were approximated with interrupted silk sutures. The extracostal muscles and subcutaneous tissues were approximated with interrupted cotton sutures. The skin was closed with interrupted silk sutures. Dry, sterile dressing was applied.

Thoracotomy and Cardiac Massage

The patient was given a spinal anesthetic and during the preparation the anesthesiologist announced that there was no blood pressure or pulse.

The surgeon struck a sharp blow to the precordial region with no effect. Two external cardiac compression maneuvers were performed with no reaction.

An incision was made in the left chest through the fourth interspace. The heart was found to be greatly dilated and in diastole. By means of massage the heart was reduced to normal size and effective carotid pulse was obtained by massage. A total of 10 cc. of calcium gluconate was then introduced into the right ventricle. A normal heart beat was then obtained. It was felt that an effective pulse rate was obtained in approximately three minutes from the time that arrest was noted. The chest was left open and the heart observed for approximately 15 minutes. It continued to beat normally. The thoracotomy wound was therefore closed using 00 silk.

The patient gradually began to regain consciousness to a semiconscious level. There was considerable difficulty with secretions at this point. The patient was quite excited. It was noted that there were choreic athetoid movements of the right arm.

A tracheostomy was performed following the usual skin preparation. It was felt that the patient was having convulsions and therefore I.V. Pentothal was given.

A midline skin incision was made over the base of the neck overlying the trachea. By means of sharp and blunt dissection the trachea was reached. A segment of the third ring was excised. A #6 tracheostomy tube was inserted and the patient thoroughly suctioned.

A left cephalic vein cutdown as well as a left greater saphenous vein cutdown were performed during the course of treatment.

The patient's level of consciousness never reached that of normal in the three hours of treatment and observation in the operating room. Following stabilization of the blood pressure and pulse the patient was sent to the recovery room.

Esophagectomy (Cor Carcinoma of the Esophagus)

The patient was prepared and draped in the right lateral position with the left arm pulled upward above the head.

A skin incision was made at the level of the third spinous process and extended down parallel to the spine to the seventh intercostal space. The incision was carried around the lower angle of the scapula to the midaxillary line. The chest muscles were opened and retracted and the thorax opened in the 6th intercostal space. Bites of the 5th, 6th and 7th ribs were taken close to the spine proper. Intercostal vessels were ligated and the 4th, 5th and 6th intercostal nerves cut. Rib spreaders were used to enlarge the wound. The pleura was opened. Upon separation of the leaves of the mediastinal pleura the esophagus was exposed.

The tumor in the esophagus was identified. A strip of rubber tubing was gently placed above and below the tumor. There were no structures outside the esophagus intimately adherent to the tumor mass. Arteries branching off the aorta were ligated between silver clips. The portion of the right pleura involved in the tumor was resected. The defect was closed by suturing the edges of the right lung over it with fine interrupted silk sutures.

The esophagus was cut between two heavy silk ligatures. The stump was carbolized. The cardiac stump was inverted into the stomach using a few silk sutures. The hiatus was likewise closed with the same type sutures. The remaining stump of the esophagus was covered by a firmly tied rubber finger.

Dissection of the esophagus was continued until the jugular notch could be felt. The wound in the chest was then closed and the patient repositioned on his back with the head and neck in an extended position.

After a complete change of drapes, gown and instruments, an incision was made along the anterior margin of the sternocleidomastoid muscle. The tumorous portion of the esophagus was gently brought into view. A tunnel was created subcutaneously extending from the lower cervical incision down to the second rib. A transverse incision about 3 cm. in length was made at the end of the tunnel. A forceps was passed up through this incision to the lower part of the cervical incision where the lower end of the esophagus projected. The esophagus was pulled down through the tunnel. At the point of the transverse incision it was attached to the skin edges of the incision using fine silk sutures. The approximation was rechecked to assure an airtight closure. The skin incision was closed and the patient repositioned on his right side. The temporary closure of the thoracic wound was reopened. The mediastinal pleura was closed. A catheter was introduced through the 9th intercostal space at the posterior axillary line. The chest was closed in anatomic layers. The intercostal tube was connected to a suction machine with underwater-seal drainage.

DISEASES OF THE THORACIC RESPIRATORY SYSTEM
(trachea, bronchi, lungs, pleurae)

Abscess of lung
Adenocarcinoma of lung
Adenoma of lung
Adenoma of trachea
Adhesions of pleura
Asbestosis
Asthma
Atelectasis
Atypical pneumonia
Bronchiectasis
Bronchiolar carcinoma of lung
Bronchiolectasis
Bronchiolitis
Bronchitis
Bronchocutaneous fistula
Broncholithiasis
Bronchopleural fistula
Bronchopneumonia
Calcification of lung
Calcification of pleura
Calcification of trachea
Chondroma of lung
Chondroma of trachea
Chylothorax
Collapse of lung
Deformation of bronchus
Diabetic gangrene of lung
Diverticulum of bronchus
Diverticulum of trachea
Edema, pulmonary
Embolism, pulmonary
Empyema
   interlobar
   sacculated
Emphysema
   compensatory
   interstitial
   obstructive
Epidermoid carcinoma of lung
Epidermoid carcinoma of the trachea
Fibroma of lung
Fibrosis of lung
Fistula of trachea
Foreign body in bronchus
Foreign body in lung
Foreign body in trachea

Fracture of trachea
Gangrene of lung
Glanders of lung
Hamartoma of lung
Hemopneumothorax
Hemothorax
Hernia of lung
Hydropneumothorax
Hydrops of pleura
Hypostatic congestion of lung
Infarction of lung
   due to embolism
   due to thrombosis
Injury of bronchus
Injury of lung
Interstitial pneumonia
Laceration of lung
Laceration of pleura
Lipoma of trachea
Lobar pneumonia
Loeffler's syndrome (eosinophilic
   pneumonitis)
Mesothelioma of pleura
Neurofibroma of pleura
Oleothorax
Papilloma of trachea
Passive congestion of lung
Pleural shock
Pleurisy
   diaphragmatic
   fibrinous
   interlobar
   plastic
   serous
Pleurodynia, epidemic
Pneumonitis
Pneumothorax
Pulmonary fibrosis
Pulmonary granulomatosis
Pulmonary hemorrhage secondary
   to mitral valvular disease
Pyopneumothorax
Sarcoma of pleura
Senile atrophy of lung
Silicosis
Silicotuberculosis

DISEASES OF THE THORACIC RESPIRATORY SYSTEM (continued)

Spontaneous pneumothorax
Stenosis of bronchus
Stenosis of trachea
Subpleural bleb
Tracheal bronchus
Tracheitis
Tracheocele
Tracheoesophageal fistula
Tuberculoma of lung
Tuberculoma of pleura
Tuberculosis of lung
Ulceration of bronchus
Ulceration of trachea
Varix of trachea
Virus bronchopneumonia

OPERATIONS ON THE TRACHEA, BRONCHI AND LUNGS

Apicolysis
  extrafascial
  extrapleural
Biopsy of the bronchus
Biopsy of the pleura
Biopsy of the trachea
Bronchoplasty
Bronchoscopy
  with aspiration
  with biopsy
  with dilatation
  with drainage
  with insertion
  with irrigation
  with removal
Bronchostomy
Bronchotomy
  with biopsy
  with exploration
  with removal
Closure of bronchocutaneous fistula
Closure of bronchopleural fistula
Crushing of phrenic nerve
  (phrenicotripsy)
Decortication of lung
Lobectomy
  complete
  partial
Phrenicectomy
Phrenicoexeresis
Phrenicotomy
Phrenicotripsy
Pleurectomy
Pneumonectomy
  complete or total
  partial
Pneumonolysis
  extraperitoneal
  intrapleural
    closed
    open
Pneumonotomy
Pneumothorax
Ransohoff operation (cruciate
  incision of scar on visceral pleura)
Resection of parietal pleura
Scalenectomy
Scalenotomy
Thoracentesis
Thoracoplasty
  complete
  partial
    anterior
    anterolateral
    apical
    paravertebral
    posterolateral
  with replacement of
  inverted ribs (Overholt's operation)
Thoracoscopy
  with biopsy
  with excision
  with removal
Thoracotomy (opening of chest)
  with closed drainage
  with open drainage
  with exploration
  with removal
Tracheoplasty
Tracheorrhaphy

OPERATIONS ON THE TRACHEA, BRONCHI AND LUNGS (cont.)

Tracheoscopy
  with biopsy
  with dilation
  with excision
  with insertion
  with irrigation
  with removal

Tracheostomy
Tracheotomy
  with biopsy
  with excision
  with exploration
  with removal

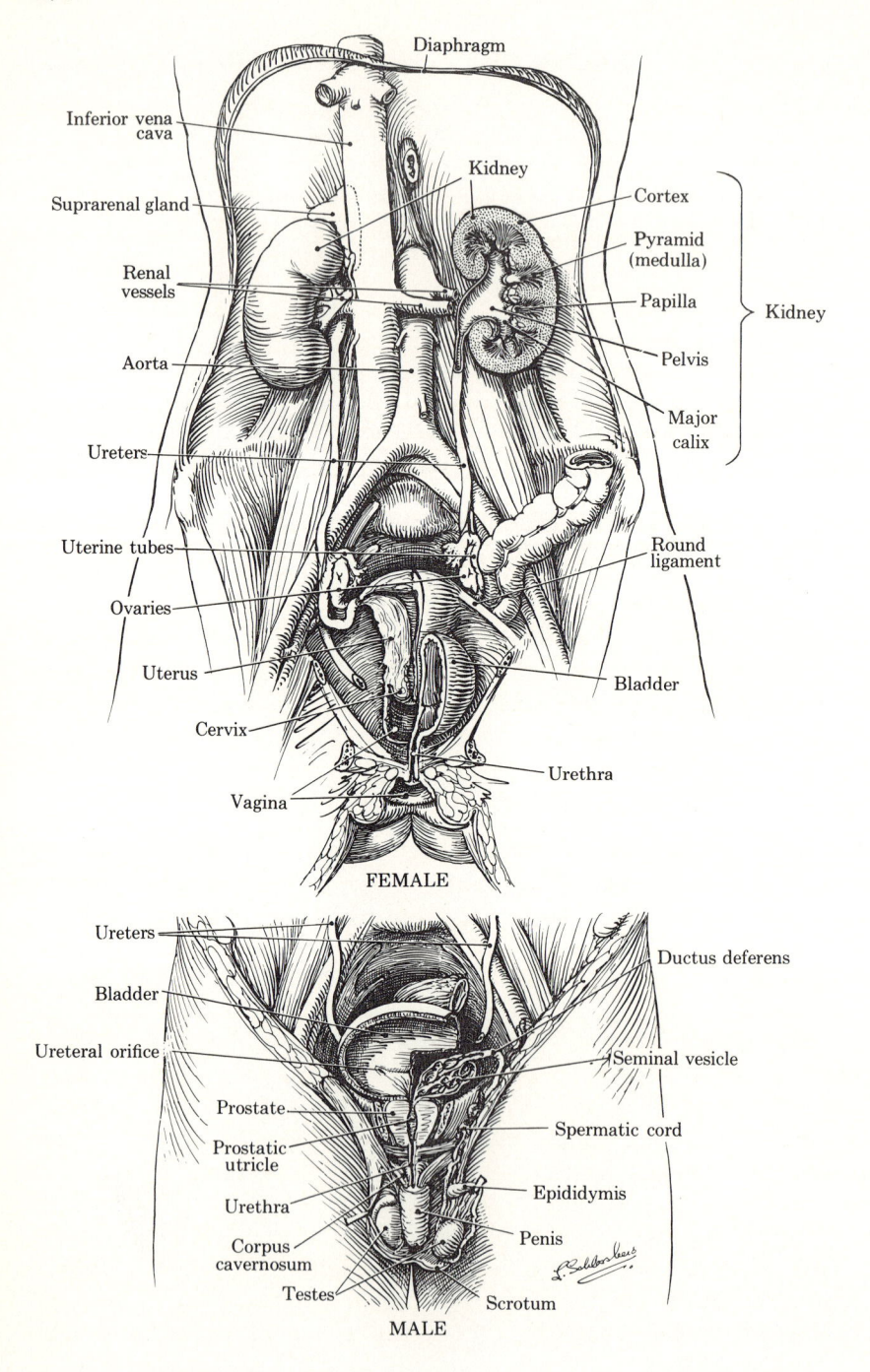

Figure 91 Urogenital System, Male and Female
*From Dorland's Illustrated Medical Dictionary
Courtesy W. B. Saunders Company*

16 } *Urology*

Urology is a surgical specialty concerned with inflammatory and surgical lesions of the urinary tract in the male and female. It also extends to include diseases of the male genitalia. Diseases of the female genital system are managed by the gynecologist rather than the urologist. In both sexes the major anatomic structures of the urinary tract are comprised of the kidneys, renal pelves, ureters, urethra and urinary bladder.

The major male genital organs consist of the testes, epididymis, spermatic cord, vas deferens, seminal vesicles, prostate and the external genitalia consisting of the penis and scrotum.

In this chapter features of the urinary system and of the male genital system will be described, anatomic terms listed and representative operative reports presented to thoroughly familiarize the secretary with this phase of surgical terminology.

THE KIDNEYS AND URETERS

The kidneys are two in number, situated behind the peritoneum on either side of the spinal column, between the level of the third lumbar vertebra and the twelfth thoracic vertebra. The kidney and its vessels are situated in a fatty cushion referred to as the *adipose capsule* or *perirenal fat* which together with the kidney is enclosed in the *renal fascia*. The kidneys are not rigid structures but move freely with the diaphragm during respiration. They are maintained in their anatomic position by the renal fascia which attaches to the fascia of surrounding structures such as the diaphragm, Psoas major muscle and Quadratus lumborum muscle. The kidneys might be described as bean shaped with a cleft or depression in their mid-portion, facing the spinal column. This area is called the *hilum* (hilus) and serves as the point at which the ureter, blood vessels, nerves and lymphatic channels enter and leave the kidney. The hilus expands into a cavity called the *renal sinus* which contains the branched *calyces* and the upper part of the *renal pelvis*. The renal pelvis is a fanned out structure within the kidney which diminishes in caliber and continues as the ureter. The average length of the ureter, which extends from the kidney to the bladder, varies from 28 to 34 cm.

Diseases which cause irreversible major damage to the kidney resulting in a nonfunctioning, septic, toxic or malignant organ provide indications for its removal. Such an operation is termed a *nephrectomy*. Excision of the ureter is referred to as *ureterectomy*.

In dealing with terminology referable to the kidney, the secretary should keep in mind the Latin term for kidney (ren pl. renes). Structures pertaining to the kidney use the term ren-; e.g., renal pelvis, renal capsule, etc.

ANATOMIC STRUCTURES OF THE KIDNEYS, URETERS AND RELATED AREAS

Adipose capsule of the kidney
Arcuate arteries
Arcuate veins
Bowman's capsule
Bröedel's line
Calyx (pl. calyces)
Cortex of the kidney
Costovertebral angle
Diaphragm
Exsanguinated zone of Hyrtl
Fascia renalis
Genitocrural area
Genitofemoral area
Gerota's capsule
Glomeruli
Hilum
Hilus
Hypogastric artery
Iliocostal space
Iliohypogastric
Ilio-inguinal
Inferior vena cava
Inferior vesical artery
Infundibulum
Intercostal nerves
Interlobar arteries
Interlobar veins
Interlobular arteries
Internal spermatic vessels
Lamella
Medulla
Obturatorius internus muscle
Paranephric fat body
Pararenal fat
Parenchyma of the kidney
Pedicle
Pelvis
Perinephritic areolar tissue
Perirenal fat
Pole of the kidney
Psoas major muscle
Pyramids
Quadratus lumborum muscle
Renal artery
Renal fascia
Renal papillae
Renal pedicle
Renal pelvis (pl. pelves)
Renal plexus
Renal pouch
Renal sinus
Renal vein
Retroperitoneal space
Sacral plexus
Subserous fascia
Suprarenal area
Suprarenal glands
Transversus abdominis muscle
Ureter
Ureteropelvic junction
Vas deferens
Vesical artery

Malignant Tumors of the Kidney

Malignant tumors of the kidney account for two per cent of all cancer deaths reports the American Cancer Society. The most common adult form is hypernephroma, a tumor seen more often in men than in women. The first symptom is usually painless intermittent hematuria. Another symptom is obscure fever in the absence of any apparent infection. About two-thirds of the patients demonstrate a classic triad of symptoms consisting of hematuria, flank pain and an abdominal mass. It is not unusual for the disease to progress to an advanced stage before evidence of tumor becomes apparent. The treatment of choice is radical nephrectomy often followed up with radiotherapy. Hypertension, present in some of these cases, is not relieved by the nephrectomy. Five year survival rate is approximately 45 per cent, with about 25 per cent of patients surviving for ten or more years. Metastases after five years are not unusual.

Another malignant tumor of the kidney is Wilms' tumor, an embryonal carcinosarcoma which develops in early childhood. This tumor accounts for approximately 25 per cent of all malignancies in children and is seen before the age of seven in about 90 per cent of the cases. It is a rapidly growing tumor which may attain an enormous size. It is detected as a result of the unusual abdominal swelling it produces. The treatment favored is nephrectomy followed by irradiation therapy immediately after surgery. Irradiation is sometimes employed preoperatively to reduce the size of the tumor and lessen the hazard of surgery. It is the only renal tumor associated in a large number of cases with hypertension. The five year survival rate is approximately 30 per cent. When metastases to the lungs are present, nitrogen mustard and actinomycin sometimes benefit these children.

Papillary neoplasms of the renal pelvis are frequently seen in association with similar tumors of the urinary bladder and ureter. They often coexist with calculi and infection. Hematuria is likewise a salient symptom in this renal malignancy. The prognosis for carcinoma of the renal pelvis is worse than that for hypernephroma.

KIDNEY TRANSPLANTS

Kidney transplants have been performed for more than ten years now with varying degrees of success. As with all other vascular organ transplants, the foremost problem is that of immediate or late rejection of the graft by the recipient's body. Chemotherapeutic and X-ray immunosuppressive measures developed in recent years have prolonged the success of numerous transplants but not without introducing additional problems into the clinical picture. Whole body irradiation in sublethal doses used by early investigators proved lethal to some patients. Blood dyscrasias and fatal bone marrow aplasia has resulted from the use of certain drugs. The use of cortisone steroids (adrenocorticals) has enhanced early infections, caused bleeding gastrointestinal ulcers and contributed a variety of other complications. Antibiotics are not used in transplant patients unless there is a specific indication for them because patients receiving immunosuppressive therapy, which includes Imuran and corticosteroids, develop a strong vulnerability to overwhelming infection with unusual organisms, particularly fungal and viral ones.

In selecting a kidney donor, an individual is sought who is not hypertensive or does not have another general disease which might imperil the success of the graft. His ABO blood type must be compatible with that of the recipient and his renal function should be excellent bilaterally.

Renal transplants between identical and nonidentical twins have not been as successful as might be expected. There are, however, identical twin transplants reported in the literature alive after ten and a half years and nonidentical transplants alive seven and a half years after transplantation. Parental and sibling donors constitute the next best organ source. Other blood relatives are roughly comparable to sibling and parental transplants. Results obtained in a large series of unrelated living donors have been disappointing to the point where some surgeons are abandoning this donor source. Transplants from animals to man have failed to survive.

A cadaver donor is selected from patients dying with head injuries or following heart operations. Absence of respiration and heart beat in addition to a flat electrocardiogram and electroencephalogram are used as indices of death. Both kidneys are removed shortly after death, one for each of two waiting recipients. The kidneys are perfused and cooled and may be kept for three or four hours and yet function immediately after transplantation despite the prolonged period of anoxia.

Cadaver homografts are not as successful as those from related living donors; however, the difference is not as great as was previously supposed. Generally, a donor is sought who is not older than 65. It has been observed that transplants from young cadavers have been more successful than those from older ones. Kidneys may be grafted from old subjects to young and from young subjects to old. Interracial grafts to date have done as well as intraracial ones.

Kidney recipients below the age of 14 have responded better than older patients. Fifty years is currently accepted as the age limit of prospective recipients.

Rejection

Rejection of the grafted kidney may occur minutes after completion of the anastomosis, while the patient is still on the operating table, or hours or even days after surgery. When failure is recognized in the operating room, the kidney is removed. This is classified as acute rejection. Patients who experience such acute rejection within the first week following surgery are less likely to have a successful result with a second transplant than if the rejection had proceeded more slowly.

Rejection is most likely to occur within the first four months postoperatively. This guarded postoperative period is extended, however, when a cadaver kidney is used.

The classical signs of rejection include fever, swelling and tenderness of the transplant, mild loss of appetite and decreased urination. The most commonly used indices in the daily observation for rejection consist of decreased urinary output (oliguria) with elevation of the blood urea nitrogen, occurring with or without fever. Symptoms which suggest threatened rejection occur in about 75 per cent of cases where a living related donor was used and in about 95 per cent of cases where there was a cadaver donor. Such developments are usually controlled with immunosuppressive drugs consisting of prednisone and actinomycin C and sometimes with local irradiation of the transplant.

Patients in whom the first renal transplant fails are offered another kidney approximately forty or more days after removal of the rejected organ. This is estimated to approximate the time required for high levels of antibody titer to subside following removal of the first transplant. Patients are offered second and third transplants with good results after experiencing failure with their first graft.

Complications

Rejection does not represent the only major postoperative problem. It has been shown that diseases may be transmitted to the recipient by the transplanted kidney. Six cases have been reported in the literature where cancer was transmitted to the recipient by a kidney removed from a donor with cancer. Two kidney recipients have died of cancer metastases acquired from the transplanted kidney. Other transmitted diseases reported in the literature include infectious hepatitis, thrombocytopenic purpura, histoplasmosis and delayed hypersensitivities.

The possible hazards which attend renal homotransplantation are many. They may arise from immunosuppressive therapy, rejection responses, operative problems, sepsis (infection) and a number of other causes.

It is encouraging that as the operative series grows and our knowledge of the rejection phenomenon unfolds, longer survivals are being obtained. Donor sources will continue to be a problem. It is believed by many that the ultimate answer lies not in tissue transplant, but in substitution of an implantable mechanical kidney for the diseased organ.

NEPHRECTOMY INSTRUMENTS

Also: See listings in Chapter 5

Blake stone forceps
Bozeman dressing forceps
Deaver retractor
Desjardin stone forceps
Guyon-Pean vessel clamp
Herrick pedicle clamp
Metzenbaum scissors

Moynihan probe
Moynihan scoop
Ochsner spiral probe
Ochsner trocar
Ockerblad kidney clamp
Randall stone grasping forceps
Rochester-Pean forceps
Walther kidney pedicle clamp
Young renal pedicle clamp

INCISIONS USED IN KIDNEY SURGERY

Bardenheuer (trap door)
Bergman-Israel (oblique)
Langenbeck
Lateral flank

Pararectus
Pean
Simon
Vertical

TECHNIQUES FOR NEPHRECTOMY

Abdominal
Israel's method
Lowsley ribbon gut method
Lumbar

Morcellement operation (piece-meal removal of the kidney)
Transperitoneal
Tuffier Morcellement

Nephrectomy

Under endotracheal general anesthesia, the patient was placed on the table in the decubitus position with the right flank elevated. The skin of the abdomen, flank and back was sterilely prepared and draped.

A right subcostal incision was made beginning at the costovertebral angle, extending downward onto the abdomen for a distance of approximately 12 cm. This incision was carried down through the subcutaneous tissue, extending through the external oblique, internal oblique and transversalis muscles. Gerota's fascia was identified and opened posteriorly.

Dissection revealed a markedly scarred, shriveled right kidney with the presence of pus within the upper collecting system. The upper ureter was obstructed by several calculi.

The kidney was freed with considerable difficulty owing to inflammatory adhesions. The vascular pedicle was freed, doubly clamped and divided. The stump of the pedicle was individually ligated with ties of No. 1 chromic catgut. The ureter was traced down with some difficulty for about half its length beyond which it became incased in impassable scar tissue. The ureter was exposed and freed to the extent possible. At the greatest possible depth of this dissection, it was doubly clamped, transected and its stump ligated with 0 chromic catgut. The wound was examined for hemostasis. This was satisfactory.

Two Penrose drains were placed into the wound, one in the renal fossa and the other in the ureteral area. These were brought out through the posterior angle of the wound.

The wound was closed in layers using interrupted 0 chromic catgut suture on individual layers. The subcutaneous tissues were closed with interrupted 00 plain catgut and the skin with interrupted 00 silk. A sterile dressing was applied.

TECHNIQUES FOR NEPHROPEXY (Suspension of the Kidney)

Deming's hammock method	Narath's method
Edebohl's	O'Conor operation
Hugh H. Young	Stanischeff operation
Kelly modification of Dodson	Vogel's method
Lowsley method with ribbon gut	Young technique

Nephropexy

After sterile preparation and draping, with the patient in the kidney position on his left side, a subcostal flank incision was made. The muscles were divided. The fatty capsule of the kidney was opened and retracted. An oblique incision, 1.5 cm. in length and parallel to the long axis of the kidney, was made on its posterior surface in the upper pole region. It penetrated the fibrous capsule to the parenchyma of the kidney. A similar incision was made through the fibrous capsule to the parenchyma, parallel to it, near the lateral border of the organ. Using a Kocher director, a connection was created between these two incisions. The 12th rib was insinuated through this tunnel. A few sutures were placed to attach the kidney to the periosteum of the rib. As a precaution against slipping, the 12th rib was fractured about 4 cm. from its end. After being reflected upward, it was attached to the periosteum of the contiguous rib with catgut sutures.

The fatty capsule was resutured over the kidney and the fractured rib. The adipose capsule was attached to the lumbar musculature with a few sutures.

The wound was closed in layers without drainage.

OTHER KIDNEY OPERATIONS

A variety of conditions may indicate the establishment of a temporary or permanent urinary opening from the kidney. Such a procedure is called a *nephrostomy*. It is a lifesaving procedure when the ureters are accidentally severed during surgery. It is a palliative procedure where malignancy or other disease process has obstructed the ureters. A temporary type nephrostomy is sometimes required preliminary to reconstructive surgery on the ureters.

This operation consists of the introduction of a nephrostomy tube into the kidney for purposes of drainage.

In order to familiarize the secretary with the terminology used in reporting this procedure, the following description of the operative proceedings is presented.

Nephrostomy

With the patient under general anesthesia, in the right decubitus position, and the kidney rest elevated, the operative field was prepared and draped.

A lateral flank incision was made just below the 12th rib. The muscles were divided. The transversalis fascia was divided. The kidney which had been palpated was freed of its perinephritic fat. It was brought into view. It measured approximately three times its normal size. Numerous adhesions binding it inferiorly, laterally and medially were lysed.

The first portion of the ureter was brought into view. It was freed by blunt dissection. Blunt dissection was carried upward until a small intrapelvic kidney pelvis was isolated. After the kidney was exposed, a pyelotomy incision was made between stay sutures of fine plain catgut. A curved clamp was then passed through this pyelotomy incision, into the lower calyx and through the parenchyma. The clamp was then used to grasp the end of the nephrostomy tube and bring it into the pelvis. Bleeding was controlled by placing a Halsted type of mattress suture of plain catgut through the renal parenchyma around the drain.

The pyelotomy wound was loosely approximated and the kidney replaced in the renal fossa. The nephrostomy tube was allowed to extend in a direct line from the wound. The lateral flank wound was closed in layers and a Penrose drain placed behind the kidney and brought out through a separate stab wound.

Nephrolithotomy and Pyelolithotomy (Removal of calculus from kidney and kidney pelvis)

After satisfactory general anesthesia, the patient was placed in the lateral decubitus position with the left side elevated by a kidney rest.

A 12 cm. curvilinear incision was made in the left subcostal area extending onto the anterior abdomen. The incision was deepened through the subcutaneous tissues and the Latissimus dorsi, external oblique, internal oblique and transversalis muscles. The lumbodorsal fascia was opened posteriorly and the retroperitoneal space entered. Gerota's capsule was identified and opened posteriorly. The left kidney was freed and exposed by blunt dissection.

Examination of the kidney revealed a healthy appearing organ except for a readily palpable stone in the lower pole and a suggestion of a second calculus in the infundibulum. A 2 cm. incision was made longitudinally over the left renal pelvis after appropriate freeing and exposure of this area. Using stone forceps, the infundibular calculus was grasped and removed. The calyceal stone could not be reached through the renal pelvis and therefore, a radial nephrotomy was performed over the palpable calyx. The stone was removed. Bleeding was controlled.

The incised renal parenchyma was closed with interrupted mattress sutures of 00 chromic catgut which controlled bleeding. The pyelotomy incision was loosely closed with interrupted 0000 chromic catgut.

One unit of blood was started during the procedure. A Penrose drain was placed into the perirenal space and the kidney was replaced in its usual anatomic position.

The wound was closed in layers using interrupted 0 chromic catgut sutures on the muscle layers, interrupted 00 plain on the subcutaneous tissues and interrupted 00 silk sutures for the skin. The drain was brought out posteriorly.

THE URINARY BLADDER

The urinary tract structures above the level of the urinary bladder are situated bilaterally in the body in a normal anatomic situation. Urine is secreted in the kidneys from whence it passes into the branched calyces, renal pelves and ureters into the urinary bladder. The bladder, a musculo-membranous sac, receives urine via both ureters and acts as a reservoir and medium by which the urine is eventually discharged from the body.

The urinary bladder is subject to many defects; congenital, developmental, and acquired. Fortunately, it is not an organ which is essential to life. Its removal in part or in toto is sometimes necessary. Such an operation is designated as a *cystectomy,* total or subtotal. In cases where complete cystectomy is indicated, urinary diversion by reimplantation of the ureters into the sigmoid (ureterosigmoidostomy), ileum (ureteroileostomy) or skin (cutaneous ureterostomy) is performed preliminary to the bladder excision.

Other operations on the bladder include incisions into the urinary bladder (cystotomy) for removal of lesions which cannot be successfully managed endoscopically; incision into the bladder for purposes of drainage (cystotomy); and the frequently performed endoscopic examination *cystoscopy,* which is used for bladder exploration, biopsy, fulguration and removal of calculi, foreign bodies and various lesions.

The Latin (B.N.A.) term for the bladder is vesica urinaria. It is from this designation that the use of "vesical" is derived in reference to bladder structures; e.g., vesical neck, perivesical fascia, etc. It should not be confused with the word "vesicle".

Malignant Tumors of the Urinary Bladder

The urinary bladder may be the site of a variety of malignant tumors of which the very low grade tumors or papillomas have an excellent prognosis. The earliest symptoms of bladder cancer include hematuria, frequency and painful urination. Late symptoms consist of pain, obstruction and renal disease. Death may result from metastases or from ureteral obstruction with uremia and sepsis.

Bladder evaluation is carried out through urinalysis for detection of red blood cells, Papanicolaou study of cells, endoscopic biopsy by way of cystoscopy and intravenous and/or retrograde pyelograms.

Treatment of these lesions may consist of radon seed implantation plus external irradiation. If the tumor is believed to be localized it is excised through cystoscopic electrocautery. Once the tumor has penetrated the muscular wall of the bladder, the prognosis becomes less favorable. In some cases segmental resection of that portion of the bladder containing the tumor is performed via an abdominal route (cystectomy). In certain cases with extensive disease a total bladder resection may be performed with or without the surrounding tissues. In these cases it is necessary to reimplant the ureters either into the small bowel, large bowel or onto the skin.

Inoperable bladder malignancies are treated by supravoltage rotational irradiation therapy.

ANATOMIC FEATURES OF THE URINARY BLADDER AND URETHRA

Anterior abdominal wall
Bas-fond
Bladder reflection
Bladder wall
Bulbourethral
Cavernous portion of urethra
Cavum Retzii
Cellules
Detrusor urinae muscle
Dome of the bladder
Ductus deferens (deferentes)
External urethral orifice
False ligaments of bladder
Fossa navicularis urethrae
Fundus
Hypogastric arteries
Hypogastric plexus
Inferior fascia
Internal urethral orifice
Interureteric ridge
Intravesical space
Lacuna magna
Lacuna (pl. lacunae)
Lateral false ligaments
Lateral puboprostatic ligaments
Lateral umbilical folds
Medial puboprostatic ligaments
Membranous urethra
Middle umbilical fold
Middle umbilical ligament
Mucous membrane
Obliterated hypogastric arteries
Paraurethral glands
Paravesical fossa
Peritoneal reflection
Peritoneum (peritoneal)
Posterior false ligaments
Preperitoneal space
Prevesical space
Prostate
Prostatic area
Pubovesical ligaments
Pubovesicalis muscle
Rectovesical fascia
Rectovesical fold of peritoneum
Rectovesical pouch
Rectovesicalis muscle
Retzius space
Sacrogenital folds
Seminal vesicles
Skene glands
Space of Retzius
Sphincter vesicae
Summit
Torus uretericus
Trabeculations
Trigone
Trigonum vesicae
Urachus
Ureteral orifice(s)
Ureteric ridge
Urethra
Urethral crest
Urethral orifice(s)
Urogenital diaphragm
Uvula vesicae
Vas deferens
Vertex
Verumontanum
Vesical
Vesicouterine excavation
Viscus

BLADDER ARTERIES

Inferior gluteal	Middle vesical
Inferior vesical	Obturator
Internal iliac	Superior vesical

Operative reports, typical of those the surgeon's secretary will be required to transcribe, are presented here for the purpose of affording the secretary a reference of terms used in contextual form. This is intended to promote familiarity with the words and their usage.

CYSTOSCOPY

One of the most frequently performed urologic examinations is the cystoscopy. It consists of the examination of the urinary bladder by means of an instrument called a cystoscope or foroblique pan-endoscope, a type of cystoscope. By means of a lens system the interior of the urinary bladder can be examined. Attachments permit use of the cystoscope for: crushing and removal of bladder stones (litholapaxy); removal of new growths and biopsy specimens, evacuation of blood clots and debris; control of bleeding; irrigation of the bladder, renal pelves and ureters; instillation of diagnostic media; dilation of stenotic areas; collection of split urines and instillation of x-ray contrast media into the renal pelves by way of the ureters for retrograde pyelography studies. Very frequently the retrograde pyelogram is done with the cystoscopy. Pyelographic roentgen studies may also be done by injecting the contrast solution intravenously, through the arm, with study of the kidneys, ureters and renal pelves after these structures have been filled with the injected contrast material.

TYPES OF CYSTOSCOPES

Braasch direct catheterizing	McCarthy-Campbell **miniature**
Brown-Buerger	McCarthy foroblique **pan-endoscope**
Butterfield	McCarthy miniature
Kelly	National **general purpose**
Lowsley-Peterson	Nesbit
McCarthy-Peterson	Ravich convertible

Cystoscopy With Retrograde Pyelogram

After satisfactory general anesthesia with intravenous Surital, the patient was placed on the cystoscopy table in the lithotomy position. The skin of the perineum and genitalia was sterilely prepared and draped.

A #24 McCarthy Pan-Endoscope was introduced. Examination of the urethra revealed generalized chronic inflammatory change. No definite urethral polyps were noted. There was no evidence of vesical neck contracture.

The bladder was then surveyed with a #21 Brown-Buerger Cystoscope. A mild chronic inflammatory mucosal change was observed. No stones, foreign bodies or neoplastic growths were noted. The air bubble was in the midline situated at the dome of the bladder. There was a good bladder light reflex. No diverticulum of the bladder was seen. There were many large and small interlacing trabeculations with considerable cellule formation.

The ureteral orifices were well seen. There was a clear urinary spurt on the right. No definite urine reflux was seen on the left. No. 5 ureteral catheters were passed bilaterally with ease. There was no drainage from the left catheter.

Indigo carmine was given intravenously and excreted in +++ concentration in four minutes on the right. There was no demonstrable excretion on the left. Retrograde pyelography was done demonstrating a staghorn calculus on the left.

Endoscopic Bladder Litholapaxy (Crushing and Removal of Bladder Calculi)

The patient was prepared and draped in the dorsal decubitus position. Under local anesthesia of 5 cc. of 1:500 Nupercaine Solution with equal parts instilled into the posterior and anterior urethra, a lithotrite was introduced into the bladder. The instrument passed smoothly along the trigone to the base of the bladder. Following this, the instrument was unlocked and the male blades opened. The blades were closed over the stone which had been visualized through the lens at the beak of the instrument. The lithotrite was then locked and raised slightly off the base of the bladder. The male blade was screwed home thus crushing the stone. The lithotrite was unlocked and used again in a similar manner until all of the stones were crushed. The blades were then closed securely and the instrument withdrawn. The tiny fragments were evacuated from the bladder along with other debris by irrigation and an Ellik Evacuator.

Cystoscopy; Urethroscopy with Dilation and Transurethral Biopsy of Bladder and Urethra

After satisfactory spinal anesthesia was obtained, the patient was placed in the lithotomy position on the operating table. The skin of the perineum and genitalia was prepared and draped.

A #20 McCarthy Pan-Endoscope was passed but some obstruction was encountered in the bulbomembranous area of the urethra. Urethral dilation was carried out with metal sounds to 22 French caliber without difficulty. The pan-endoscope was reinserted without further obstruction.

The posterior urethra revealed evidence of mild urethral stricture in the obstructed area. The prostate was moderately enlarged and partially obstructing. There was a moderate bladder neck contracture. The remainder of the urethra was normal.

The urinary bladder was examined with a No. 21 Brown-Buerger Cystoscope. Examination disclosed a chronic inflammatory change throughout the vesical mucosa, most marked about the bladder floor. There were four or five slightly elevated lesions about the trigone and vesical neck. These raised areas were approximately 1-1.5 cm. in their greatest diameter and were pale in appearance as contrasted with the surrounding mucosa. Using an Iglesias Resectoscope, biopsies were taken of the urethra and the bladder lesions.

#20 Foley catheter was left indwelling.

URETHROPLASTY

Urethroplasty

Complete destruction of the urethra is a rare occurrence. Partial defects are more commonly encountered which have developed as a result of obstetrical injury, radiation necrosis or operative damage. When the distal portion of the urethra is involved there may be no urinary incontinence. Plastic repair of these defects is termed urethroplasty.

URETHROPLASTY AND ACCESSORY OPERATIVE TECHNICS

Bevan-Rochet	Martius "bolster" operation
Cystourethropexy	Martius-Harris
Everett-TeLinde	Mays
Interposition operation	Sling operation
Kelly-Stoeckel plication of bladder neck and urethra	

Suprapubic approach may be:

    1. extraperitoneal transvesical
* 2. extraperitoneal extravesical
    3. intraperitoneal intravesical
* 4. intraperitoneal extravesical

* Techniques 2 and 4 are the most important.

THE MALE GENITAL SYSTEM

Urology also encompasses the male genital system comprised of a pair of testes with paired seminal ducts, seminal vesicles, ejaculatory ducts and bulbourethral glands (Cowper's glands). The single structures in this system include the urethra, penis, scrotum and prostate gland.

In the fetus the two testes are contained in the abdominal cavity. Prior to birth they descend into the scrotum with a portion of their spermatic cord. Failure of this process to occur, either bilaterally or unilaterally, is known as *cryptorchism* (undescended testis). A corrective operation termed an *orchiopexy* (suspension of the testis) is performed in these cases. Spermatogenesis and testosterone production take place within the testes. In an undescended testis, body temperatures reduce and finally completely suppress spermatogenesis.

In a normal anatomic situation, the testes and a portion of their spermatic cords are suspended in a cutaneous pouch known as the *scrotum*. The testes consist internally of communicating chambers which contain the seminiferous tubules. These tubules unite and continue outside the testis as a tortuous tubule called the *epididymis*. This structure connects the testis with the *seminal duct* (ductus deferens; vas deferens) which is the excretory duct of the testis. The seminal duct follows a winding course to the base of the prostate where its caliber diminishes and it is joined by the duct of the seminal vesicle to form the *ejaculatory duct*. The ejaculatory duct opens into the prostatic area of the urethra near the orifice of the prostatic utricle. This is a bilateral process.

The seminal vesicles are two in number situated between the fundus of the bladder and the rectum. They secrete a fluid substance which is excreted into the seminal stream at the base of the prostate, where the two seminal vesicles converge, each uniting with its respective seminal duct to produce the ejaculatory duct. The ejaculatory ducts are two in number and extend to the urethra, into which they discharge their secretions.

The external male genitalia consist of the penis and scrotum. The penis serves as the copulatory organ of the male through which spermatozoa are injected into the vagina. The penis also contains the greatest portion of the urethra through which urine as well as semen are discharged to the outside of the body.

The penile shaft consists of three bundles of cavernous tissue. The lateral two masses are called the *corpora cavernosa penis* and the medial portion, containing the urethra, is known as the *corpus cavernosum urethrae*. The end of the corpus cavernosum consists of a cap-like structure which covers the tip of the penis. This is called the *glans penis*.

The penis is a flaccid organ attached at the front and sides of the pubic arch, just above the scrotum. In response to stimulation or sexual excitement, the venous spaces in the cavernous tissue become distended with blood causing the penis to become erect and rigid.

The prostate gland is surgically important because of its location. It is situated just below the internal urethral orifice and around the urethra in a doughnut shape. Since the urethra is surrounded by this gland, any enlargement of the prostate diminishes the urethral caliber. This often occurs in older men and ranges from narrowing of the urethra to complete obstruction with retention of urine. Enlargement of the prostate is termed *hypertrophy of the prostate* and although it is usually a benign process, malignancy must be ruled out because of the incidence of carcinoma in the prostate gland. Hypertrophy of the prostate is relieved by an operation known as a *prostatectomy* which can be performed from below as a transurethral resection of the prostate (TUR) with a resectoscope or through the abdominal route as a suprapubic prostatectomy.

The prostate secretes a fluid which further facilitates the flow of the spermatozoa.

Two additional glands of the male genital system consist of the *bulbourethral glands* (Cowper's). They are two pea-sized bodies located at either side of the membranous portion of the urethra, just below the prostate gland. Each of these glands secretes a fluid which is carried by an excretory duct emanating from each gland to the cavernous portion of the urethra, just before the urogenital diaphragm.

SURGERY OF THE PENIS

The circumcision (excision of redundant foreskin) is the most common surgical procedure performed on the penis and for this reason an operative report describing the operation is included here. Anatomic structures of the penis and related anatomy have been listed below in addition to those terms one might expect to use in a circumcision report.

ANATOMIC FEATURES OF THE PENIS AND RELATED STRUCTURES

Arcuate pubic ligament
Arteries:
   dorsal
   helicine
   internal pudendal
Buck's fascia

Meatus
Median raphe
Muscles:
   Bulbocavernosus
   Ischiocavernosus
   Transversus perinei superficialis

UROLOGY

Bulb	Neck of penis
Bulbus urethrae	Prepuce
Colle's fascia	Preputial glands (Tyson)
Corona glandis	Preputial space
Corpora cavernosa penis	Pubis (pl. pubes)
Corpus cavernosa urethrae	Pudendal nerve
Corpus spongiosum	Retroglandular sulcus
Crura	Scarpa's fascia
Crus penis	Scrotum
Dartos tunic	Septum of penis
Deep dorsal vein	Septum pectiniforme
External perineal fascia	Smegma (sebaceous material)
Foreskin	Superficial fascia
Frenulum	Suspensory ligament of penis
Glans penis	Urethra
Ischiopubic rami	Urethral mucous membrane
Lamina	Urogenital diaphragm
Ligamentum fundiforme penis	

Circumcision

Using an infiltration anesthetic of 2% Novocain and filling the preputial sac with a 4% solution of Novocain for five minutes, the area was prepared for surgery.

An artery forceps was used to engage the prepuce. A grooved director was passed beneath the prepuce over the head of the penis. A Gomco clamp was applied, the prepuce cut away and the clamp removed.

One blade of a scissors was passed between the glans penis and the inner layer of the mucous membrane which was divided back as far as the margin of the corona glandis. A cuff of mucous membrane was turned back. The mucosa was trimmed. The edges of the mucous membrane were united to the integumental border with interrupted catgut sutures. Coaptation was satisfactory.

SURGERY OF THE TESTES

Orchiopexy (suspension of an undescended testis) and orchiectomy (removal of the testis) are probably the most common operations performed on the testes.

Diseases and operations pertaining to the testes assume the prefix "orchi-" from the Greek term for the testes, "orchis." Inflammation of the testis is known as orchitis, pain in the testis is called orchialgia, etc.

Anatomic terms pertaining to the testes, their investing tissues and related structures have been listed below with several operative reports exemplifying procedures performed on these organs.

Anatomy of the Male Genitalia

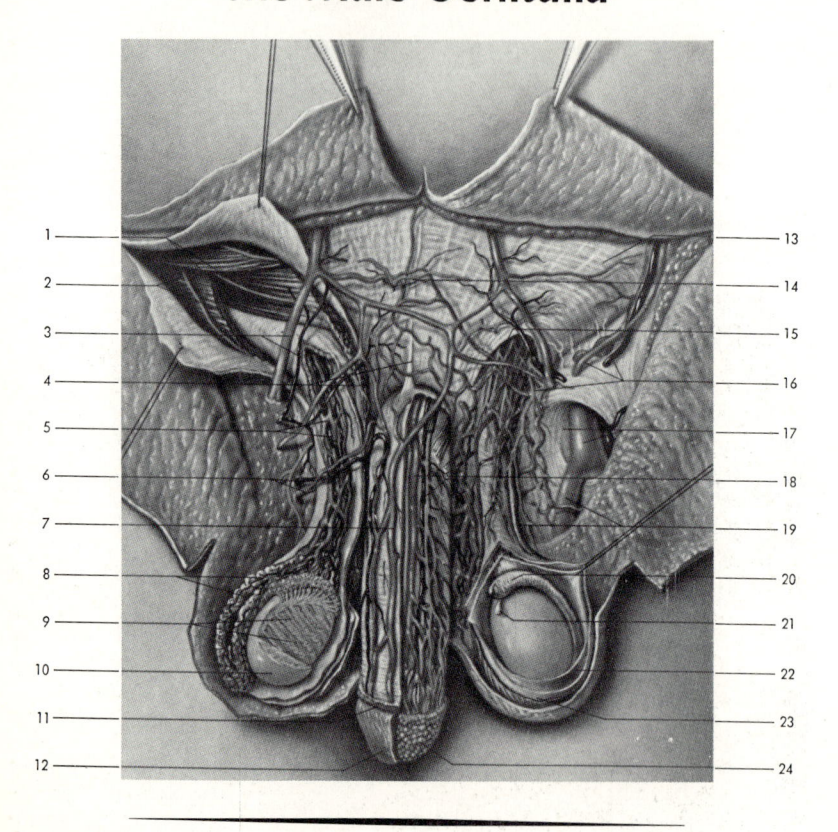

1 Transversus abdominis muscle and iliohypogastric nerve
2 Obliquus abdominis internus muscle and ilioinguinal nerve
3 Superficial epigastric artery and vein
4 Genital branch of genitofemoral nerve and suspensory ligament of penis
5 Internal spermatic artery and pampiniform plexus
6 External pudendal artery and vein
7 Superficial dorsal vein of penis
8 Vas deferens and deferential artery
9 Lobules of testis
10 Testis (covered by visceral tunica vaginalis)
11 Prepuce
12 Glans penis
13 Abdominal aponeurosis
14 Anterior cutaneous branch of subcostal nerve
15 Subcutaneous inguinal ring
16 Ilioinguinal nerve and superficial iliac circumflex artery and vein
17 Fossa ovalis and femoral artery and vein
18 Dorsal artery and nerve, and deep dorsal vein, of penis
19 Cremaster muscle and great saphenous vein
20 Head of epididymis
21 Appendix of testis
22 Parietal layer of tunica vaginalis
23 Infundibuliform fascia
24 Plexus cavernosus

Figure 92   Anatomy of the male genitalia
Courtesy Lederle Laboratories

UROLOGY

The Male Pelvic Organs

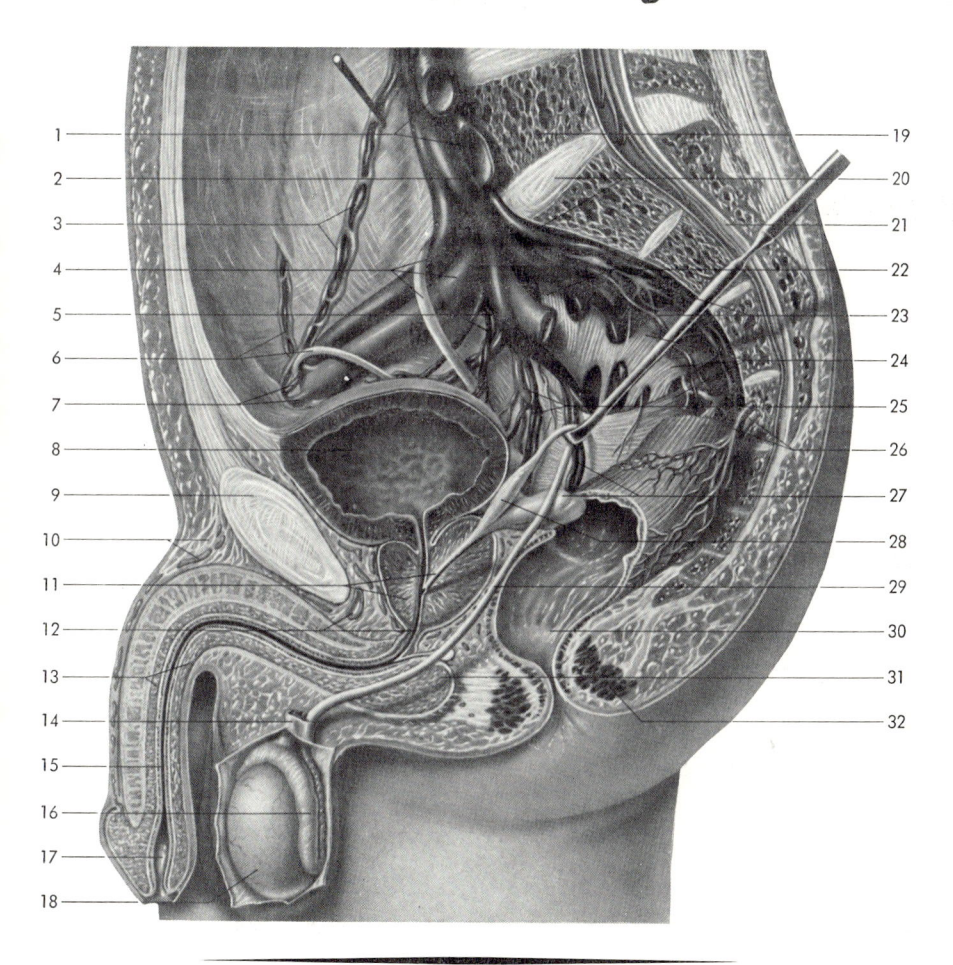

1 Common iliac artery and vein
2 Internal iliac (hypogastric) artery
3 Spermatic artery and vein
4 Ureter; external iliac artery and vein
5 Superior vesical artery and vein
6 Deep iliac circumflex artery and vein; right ductus deferens
7 Inferior epigastric artery and vein
8 Urinary bladder
9 Symphysis pubis
10 Fundiform ligament of penis; superficial dorsal vein of penis
11 Prostate gland; ejaculatory duct
12 Deep dorsal vein of penis; prostatic urethra
13 Corpus cavernosum
14 Spermatic cord (cut)
15 Cavernous urethra
16 Epididymis
17 Navicular fossa
18 Testis
19 Fifth lumbar vertebra
20 Middle sacral artery; intervertebral fibrocartilage
21 Vertebral canal
22 Lumbosacral trunk; superior gluteal artery
23 Lateral sacral artery; sympathetic trunk ganglion
24 Sacral nerves; coccygeus muscle
25 Inferior vesical artery and vein
26 Superior hemorrhoidal artery and vein
27 Seminal vesicles; middle hemorrhoidal artery and vein
28 Ampulla of ductus deferens
29 Left ductus deferens
30 Rectum
31 Bulb of urethra
32 Sphincter ani externus muscle

Figure 93   The male pelvic organs
Courtesy Lederle Laboratories

Malignant Tumors of the Testes

Cancer of the testes is not a common malignancy, accounting for less than one per cent of cancer deaths in men. The incidence is more common in the undescended testicle (1 in 2,000) than in the normal testicle (1 in 100,000). Testicular cancer is found primarily in young men between the ages of 20 and 35.

The various malignant tumors which involve the testes, in their order of frequency are: seminoma (germinoma), teratocarcinoma, embryonal carcinoma (includes chorioepithelioma) and teratoma. The incidence of seminoma rises with age.

One year survival is rare for embryonal carcinomas and chorioepitheliomas, not unusual for teratomas and teratocarcinomas, and the usual for seminomas.

The first symptoms of testicular cancer consist of painless enlargement of the testis with a sensation of heaviness and aching in the perineum. Metastases may occur while the tumor is still small. This has been observed to occur in a regular manner, first involving the lumbar group of lymph nodes about the renal vein and then up the paraortic lymph nodes to the mediastinal nodes. The liver and lungs are also common sites of metastases.

Treatment, in the absence of apparent metastases, consists of simple orchiectomy. This is followed by postoperative irradiation of the lumbar lymph nodes. In the seminoma type testicular tumor, such combined therapy yields 80 per cent five year survival rates. Because of the radiosensitivity of seminoma, irradiation of the abdomen, even in cases of generalized metastases, produces a more favorable survival rate. In malignant teratoma where the metastases may not be particularly radiosensitive, radical retroperitoneal node dissection is sometimes performed. The chorioepitheliomas have been shown to be extremely sensitive to antimetabolic agents such as Methotrexate.

ANATOMIC FEATURES OF THE TESTES AND RELATED STRUCTURES

Ampulla	Cremasteric fascia
Appendix of epididymis	Cremasteric layer
Areolar tissue	Dartos tunic
Arteries:	Ductulus aberrans inferior
cremasteric	Ductulus aberrans superior
deep external pudendal	Ductus deferens
int. & ext. spermatics	Ductus deferentes
superficial perineal	Ejaculatory duct

ANATOMIC FEATURES OF THE TESTES AND RELATED STRUCTURES (Continued)

Epididymis
  head (globus major)
  tail (globus minor)
External spermatic fascia
Fascia innominata of Gallaudet
Gubernaculum chorda
Infundibuloform fascia
Integument
Internal spermatic fascia
Mediastinum testis (corpus Highmori)
Paradidymis (organ of Giraldes)
Parietal lamina
Plexus pampiniformis
Prostate gland
Raphe
Rete testis
Rugae

Scrotum
Seminal duct
Seminal vesicles
Spermatic cord
Spermatic veins
Testicle
Testicular
Testis (pl. testes)
Trabeculae
Transversalis fascia
Tunica albuginea
Tunica Dartos
Tunica vaginalis
Tunica vasculosa
Vas aberrans of Haller
Vas deferens
Visceral lamina

Hydrocelectomy (Andrews Bottle Operation)

With the patient in the supine position on the operating table, the external genitalia were sterilely prepared and draped.

The tunica vaginalis was opened at its upper pole and its fluid contents expressed. The testicle was brought out of the scrotum, extruding it through the opening in the sac. The sac was everted without a suture. The blood supply to the testis was adequate. The testis and everted tunica vaginalis were reposited into the scrotum. The wound was closed without drainage.

Bilateral Orchiectomy (Removal of Testes)

The patient was prepared and draped in the supine position. A 6 cm. vertical midline scrotal incision was made. Dissection was then carried into the right scrotal compartment, through the various testicular tunics, to expose the testes and epididymis as well as the lower spermatic cord on the right. The lower cord was transected and its proximal stump doubly ligated with 00 chromic catgut. The testes, epididymis and lower cord were then removed. A similar procedure was carried out on the opposite side.

A Penrose drain was drawn through the wound and brought out through the lower corner. The incision was closed in two layers, using interrupted 00 chromic catgut. A sterile dressing was applied.

Orchiopexy (Torek Operation) First Stage

The patient was prepared and draped in the supine position. An incision was made in the inguinal canal providing good exposure. The testis was liberated from the cremaster muscle, gubernaculum and surrounding tissues. The spermatic cord was likewise stripped of its investments; however, the vas deferens and spermatic vessels were allowed to remain intact. Dissection of the vessels was carried out to the level of the transversalis fascia.

The liberated testis was laid on the thigh to the extent that it would reach. A point above this level was selected for the incision. A transverse incision was made, long enough to accommodate the length of the testis, and carried to the fascia of the thigh. Using two fingers, a pocket was created extending from the lower end of the inguinal incision to the bottom of the scrotum. An opening in the pocket was then made by an incision matching the incision in the thigh, in length as well as in direction. A strip of gauze was passed through the tunnel thus created.

The upper end of the wound of the thigh was approximated to the identical wound in the scrotum, passing the suture from surface to depth and from depth to surface. The knot was brought to lie on the skin surface. Interrupted sutures were used. The cut posterior lip of the scrotal wound was then approximated with the corresponding edge of the thigh wound using catgut sutures. The testis, which had been replaced in the inguinal wound, was delivered through the channel created. Two fine sutures of chromicized catgut were placed through the tunica albuginea and fascia of the thigh. Particular care was exercised to avoid the saphenous and femoral veins.

Fine silk was used to approximate the anterior lip of the scrotal wound to the lower lip of the wound in the thigh. Closure of the wound was carried out uniting the internal oblique and transversus muscle to Poupart's ligament. The aponeurosis of the external oblique was also approximated. Following this, the skin was closed and a strip of gauze drawn through the canal in the skin between the scrotum and thigh.

A second operation will be performed in three months to free the testis from the thigh and bury it in the scrotum.

SURGERY OF THE PROSTATE

One of the most frequently encountered surgical conditions of the prostate is benign prostatic hypertrophy. The prostate is also a common site of malignancy and when detected early enough can be eradicated by surgery.

Resection of the prostate is referred to as a *prostatectomy*. It may be perineal, radical, retropubic, suprapubic (transvesical) or transurethral in type. The transurethral method is referred to in the vernacular as a TUR and is performed with a resectoscope passed endoscopically through the urethra. The suprapubic and transurethral methods are employed more often than the other approaches mentioned.

Malignant Tumors of the Prostate Gland

Hypertrophy (enlargement) of the prostate gland is a condition which plagues the majority of elderly males in a benign form. American Cancer Society statistics reveal that cancer of this gland is the third most common malignancy in men when we exclude skin cancer. Malignant prostatic tumors are rare before the age of forty, however, the incidence rises sharply with age. Approximately 15 per cent of men in their fifth decade will develop prostatic carcinoma while as many as 40 per cent will manifest the disease in their eighth decade. Only about one-fourth of the tumors become clinically symptomatic prior to death.

About three-fourths of prostatic carcinomas arise in the posterior prostatic lobe and can be readily palpated on rectal examination. Early symptoms simulate those of benign prostatic hypertrophy, i.e., frequent and painful urination with difficulty in starting and stopping the urinary stream. Low back or sacral pain is another common symptom. Punch biopsy of the prostate through the perineum is used to confirm a diagnosis of prostatic cancer.

Radical prostatectomy is performed in the treatment af carcinomas confined to the prostate. The five year survival rate is about 48 per cent. When the disease has progressed beyond the gland, symptomatic relief is sometimes provided by a transurethral resection of the prostate through a cystoscope. Metastatic tumors are treated by decreasing the androgens through orchidectomy and adrenalectomy and by the administration of female sex hormones.

ANATOMIC FEATURES OF THE PROSTATE AND ASSOCIATED STRUCTURES

Arteries:
  inferior vesical
  internal pudendal
  middle hemorrhoidal
Apex of prostate
Base of prostate
Bladder mucosa
Bladder neck
Capsule
Central tendon
Denonvillier's fascia
Ejaculatory ducts
External urethral sphincter
Internal urethral orifice
Isthmus
Lateral fossae
Lateral lobes of prostate
Levator ani muscles
Levatores prostatae
Median furrow
Membranous urethra
Middle lobe of prostate
Mucosal cuff
Paravesical spaces
Plexus of Santorini
Prostatic cavity
Prostatic fossa
Prostatovesicular junction
Puboprostatic ligaments
Rectourethralis muscle
Subtrigonal spheroids
Suprapubic sinus
Transverse perinei muscles
Trigone
Urethra
Urogenital diaphragm
Verumontanum
Vesical orifice

Suprapubic Prostatectomy

The patient was prepared and draped in a supine position. A transverse incision was made midway between the umbilicus and the symphysis pubis and carried through the subcutaneous tissues. A small Gelpi vaginal retractor was inserted. The anterior rectus sheath was incised transversely and the underlying rectus muscles separated in the midline and retracted laterally with a Farr retractor. Using moist gauze manipulation, the peritoneum was reflected upward from the dome of the bladder. The retropubic space was exposed.

The clamp on the urethral catheter was released by an assistant permitting the previously instilled sterile water to flow out of the urinary bladder. The catheter was removed from the bladder.

A transverse incision was made in the bladder wall 2 cm. above the prostatovesicular junction for approximately 4 cm. in length. A traction suture of 0 chromic was inserted through the bladder wall on both sides. A Judd retractor was then introduced into the bladder and inspection carried out under direct vision. No diverticuli, calculi or neoplastic growths were noted. Using a sharp scalpel, circumcision of the mucosa around the vesical neck was performed. The dissecting finger was steadied by two left fingers in the rectum which also pushed the prostate forward toward the suprapubic opening. The gland was shelled out en masse.

The prostatic cavity was tightly packed with three-inch gauze. Direct inspection was carried out of the bladder neck and floor. Bleeders were coagulated. Hemostasis was satisfactory. A No. 22 Foley bag was placed and inflated to 60 cc. at the vesical neck. A No. 32 right angle de Pezzer catheter was placed through a stab wound in the bladder and the bladder closed in two layers with 0 chromic catgut. Prior to closure of the muscle layers a split rubber drain was placed leading from the prevesical space.

DISEASES OF THE URINARY SYSTEM

Abscess of bladder wall
Abscess of bulbourethral gland
    (Cowper's gland)
Abscess of kidney
Abscess, periurethral
Abscess, perivesical
Abscess of urachus
Abscess of urethral gland
Absence of urinary bladder
    congenital
    postoperative
Absence of kidney, one or both
    congenital
    postoperative
Absence of ureter, one or both
    congenital
    postoperative
Absence of urethra
    congenital
    postoperative
Accessory blood vessels of kidney
Adenitis of bulbourethral gland
    (Cowper's gland)
Adenitis of Skene's glands
Adenocarcinoma of the urinary
    bladder
Adenocarcinoma of bulbourethral
    gland
Adenocarcinoma of kidney
Adenocarcinoma of ureter
Adenocarcinoma of urethra
Adenoma of the kidney
Adhesions, perirenal
Adhesions, perivesical
Adhesions of prostatic urethra
Albuminuria
Amebiasis of the bladder
Amyloid disease of kidney
Amyloidosis of bladder
Aneurysm of renal artery
Angulation of ureter
Anomalous origin of renal vessels
Anomalous implantation of ureter
Arteriolar nephrosclerosis
Atony of bladder
Atresia of urethra

Atrophy of kidney
Basal cell carcinoma of kidney
Bifurcation of renal pelvis
Bifurcation of ureter
Calcification of kidney
Calcification of ureter
Calculus in calyx
Calculus of kidney
Calculus in pelvis of kidney
Calculus in ureter
Calculus in urethra
Carcinoma of kidney
Carcinosarcoma of kidney
Caruncle of urethra
Chancre of urethra
Chancroid of urethra
Chondrosarcoma of bladder
Colliculitis
Construction of ureter
Contracted kidney
Contracture of bladder
Contracture of bladder neck
Contracture, vesicourethral orifice
Cortical necrosis of kidney
Crossed ectopia of kidney
Cyst of bladder
Cyst of kidney
Cyst at ureterovesical orifice
Cyst of urethral gland
Cyst of utriculus masculinus
Cyst of verumontanum
Cystitis
    acute
    allergic
    chemical
    chronic
    cystica
    exudative
    follicularis
    gangrenous
    glandularis
    hemorrhagic
    interstitial
Cystocele
Deformity of urethra
Dietl's crisis (kinking ureter)

UROLOGY

DISEASES OF THE URINARY SYSTEM (continued)

Dilatation of bladder
Dilatation of calyx
Dilatation of ureter
Dilatation of urethra
Displacement of bladder
Displacement of kidney
Diverticulitis of bladder
Diverticulum of bladder
Diverticulum of calyx
Diverticulum of ureter
Diverticulum, ureterovesical orifice
Diverticulum of urethra
Double bladder
Double kidney with double renal pelvis
Double meatus urinarius
Double pelvis with double ureter
Double ureter
Double urethra
Ectopic bladder
Ectopic kidney
Electric burn of urethra
Embolism of bladder
Embolism of renal artery
Endometriosis of kidney
Epidermoid carcinoma of bladder
Epidermoid carcinoma of renal pelvis
Epidermoid carcinoma of ureter
Epidermoid carcinoma of urethra
Epispadias
Exotrophy of bladder
Extravasation of urine
Fibroma of bladder
Fibroma of kidney
Fibroma of ureter
Fibroma of urethra
Fibrosarcoma of kidney
Fistula of bladder
Fistula of kidney
Fistula of penis
Fistula of ureter
Fistula, ureteroduodenal
Fistula, ureterorectal
Fistula, ureterosigmoid
Fistula, ureterovaginal

Fistula of urethra
Foreign body in bladder
Foreign body in kidney
Foreign body in ureter
Fused kidney
Giant kidney
Glomerulonephritis
Gumma of ureter
Hemangioma of bladder
Hemangioma of kidney
Hemangioma of urethra
Hemangiosarcoma of ureter
Hematoma, perirenal
Hemorrhage of bladder
Hemorrhage of kidney
Hemorrhage of urethra
Hernia of bladder
Herniation of kidney
Herpes zoster of bladder
Horseshoe kidney
Hydronephrosis
Hypospadias
Hydroureter
Hyperplasia of kidney
Hypertrophy of kidney
Hypertrophy of interureteric ridge
Hypertrophy of verumontanum
Hypoplasia of kidney
Incomplete fusion of kidney
Infarction of kidney
  due to embolism
  due to thrombosis
Infection of utriculus masculinus
Injury of ureter
  during surgery
  traumatic
Intercapillary glomerulosclerosis
Intussusception of ureter
Inversion of bladder
Laceration of urethra
Leiomyoma of bladder
Leiomyoma of kidney
Leiomyosarcoma of bladder
Leiomyosarcoma of kidney
Leiomyosarcoma of ureter

DISEASES OF THE URINARY SYSTEM (continued)

Leukoplakia of bladder
Leukoplakia of pelvis of kidney
Leukoplakia of urethra
Lichen planus of bladder
Lipoma of bladder
Lipoma of hilus
Lipoma, perirenal
Liposarcoma, perirenal
Liposarcoma of ureter
Lobulation of kidney
Lower nephron nephrosis
Luxation of kidney
Lymphangioma of bladder
Lymphangiosarcoma of bladder
Lymphangiosarcoma of ureter
Malacoplakia of the bladder
Malacoplakia of the urethra
Malignant nephrosclerosis
Melanoma of the urethra
Mesenchymal mixed tumor of bladder
Mesothelioma of bladder
Mucinous carcinoma of bladder
Myoma of kidney pelvis
Myxoma of bladder
Myxoma of hilus
Myxosarcoma of bladder
Myxosarcoma of hilus
Nephritis
  acute hemorrhagic
  congenital
  interstitial
Nephroblastoma
Nephroptosis
Nephrosis
  of alkalosis
  due to diabetes
Nephrotic syndrome
Neurofibroma of ureter
Obstruction of ureter
Osteoma of bladder
Papillary carcinoma of bladder
Papillary carcinoma of kidney pelvis
Papillary carcinoma of ureter
Papillary carcinoma of urethra
Papilloma of bladder
Papilloma of renal pelvis
Papilloma of Skene's gland
Papilloma of urethra
Paralysis of bladder
  flaccid
  postpartum
  spastic
Paralysis of external sphincter
Paralysis of internal sphincter
Paramedial vesicourethral orifice
Parasitic infection of bladder
Paresis of bladder, tabetic
Patent urachus
Penile fistula
Periarteritis nodosa of kidney
Pericystitis
Perinephritis
Periurethral abscess
Periurethral cellulitis
Perivesical hernia
Polycystic kidney
Polyp of bladder
Polyp of ureter
Polyp of urethra
Prolapse of bladder
Prolapse of mucosa of bladder
Prolapse of ureter
Prolapse of urethra
Ptosis of kidney
Puncture of bladder
  during surgery
  posttraumatic
Pyelitis
Pyelitis cystica
Pyonephrosis
Pyoureter
Redundancy of ureter
Renal glycosuria
Renal hematuria
Renmobilis
Retrocaval ureter
Rhabdomyoma of bladder
Rhabdomyosarcoma of bladder
Rupture of abscess into bladder
Rupture of bladder
Rupture of kidney

UROLOGY

DISEASES OF THE URINARY SYSTEM (continued)

Rupture of urethra
Sacculation of bladder
Sarcoma of bladder
Sarcoma of kidney
Sarcoma of ureter
Sarcoma of urethra
Serous papillary cystic tumor
Shield kidney
Strangulation of bladder
Stricture of meatus urinarius
Stricture of ureter
Stricture at ureteropelvic junction
Stricture of ureterovesical orifice
Stricture of urethra
Stricture of vesicourethral orifice
Squamous cell papilloma of ureter
Squamous cell papilloma of urethra
Strangulation of bladder
Stress incontinence
Supernumerary kidney
Syphilis of bladder
Teratoma of bladder
Teratoma of kidney
Teratoma of ureter
Teratoma of urethra
Thrombosis of renal artery
Torsion of pedicle of kidney
Transitional cell carcinoma
   of bladder
   of renal calyx
   of ureter
Trichomonas infection of bladder
Trigonitis
Triple kidneys
Triplication of ureter
Tuberculosis
   of bladder
   of Cowper's gland
   of kidney
   of ureter
   of urethra
Ulcer of bladder
Ulcer of meatus urinarius
Ureteritis
Ureteritis cystica
Ureterocele
Ureteroduodenal fistula
Urethral caruncle
Urethral fever and chill
Urethral meatitis
Urethral stricture
Urethritis
   acute
   chronic
   granular
   polypoid
   posterior
Urethroperineal fistula
Urethrocele
Urethrorectal fistula
Urethrovaginal fistula
Valve formation in ureter
Valve formation at ureteropelvic junction
Valve formation at ureterovesical orifice
Valve formation of urethra
Varicosis of urethra
Varix of bladder
Varix of renal papilla
Vesical fistula
Vesicoabdominal fistula
Vesicoenteric fistula
Vesicoperineal fistula
Vesicoureteral fistula
Vesicouterine fistula
Vesicovaginal fistula
Wandering kidney

OPERATIONS ON THE URINARY SYSTEM

Biopsy of the bladder
Biopsy of the kidney
Biopsy of the ureter
Closure of fistula of ureter
Closure of fistula of urethra
Closure of nephrostomy
Closure of ureterovaginal fistula
Closure of urethrorectal fistula

OPERATIONS ON THE URINARY SYSTEM (continued)

Closure of urethrovaginal fistula
Cystectomy
  complete
  partial
Cystoplasty
Cystorrhaphy
Cystoscopy
  with biopsy
  with dilation
  with division of bladder neck
  with drainage
  with excision
  with instillation
  with irrigation
Cystotomy
  with drainage (cystostomy)
  with exploration
  with removal of calculus
    (cystolithotomy)
Decapsulation of kidney
Dilation of urethra
  with metal sound
Division of aberrant renal vessels
Drainage of bulbourethral gland
Drainage of kidney
Drainage of perirenal tissues
Drainage of periurethral tissues
Ligation of urachus
Litholapaxy (crushing & removal
  of calculus)
Lithotripsy (crushing of calculus)
Meatotomy
Nephrectomy
  complete
  partial
Nephrolysis
Nephropexy
Nephrorrhaphy
Nephrotomy
  with drainage (nephrostomy)
  with exploration
  with removal of calculus
    (nephrolithotomy)
Pyeloplasty
Pyelotomy
  with drainage (pyelostomy)
  with exploration
  with removal of calculus
    (pyelolithotomy)
Removal of foreign body, perirenal
Ureterectomy
  complete
  partial
Ureterocolostomy
Ureterocystostomy
Ureterolysis
Ureteroplasty
Ureteropyelostomy
Ureterorrhaphy
Ureterosigmoidostomy
Ureterostomy
Ureterotomy
  with drainage (ureterostomy)
  with exploration
  with removal of calculus
    (ureterolithotomy)
Ureteroureterostomy
Urethroplasty
Urethroscopy
  with biopsy
  with dilation
  with drainage
  with excision
Urethrorrhaphy
Urethrotomy
  with drainage
  with exploration
  with removal

17 Vascular Surgery

VASCULAR SURGERY

The surgical specialty of vascular surgery concerns itself with the diagnosis, repair and reconstruction of heart and blood vessel defects. The more representative operations are being performed in large teaching university affiliated hospitals where skilled operating teams and facilities may be developed to accommodate the needs of this specialty.

Beginning with the work of Crafoord and Gross in 1939, some of the most dramatic advances in surgery have occurred in the vascular field. Their work in ligation of patent ductus defects was followed by techniques for enlargement of the narrowed mitral valve, a residual of rheumatic fever, in an operation called commissurotomy. Shunting operations developed by Blalock and by Potts further spearheaded the assault on heart defects. Studying the heart and its hemodynamics in analogy to a pump, vascular surgeons have since developed numerous mechanical replacements for diseased vascular tissue. Mechanical heart valves are replacing useless ones, plastic patches are being used to obliterate abnormal openings between chambers of the heart, segments of the aorta and blood vessels are being replaced by prosthetic grafts and pacemakers are being inserted into the heart for control of heart block. One of the goals in heart surgery has been realized with the replacement of a diseased human heart by a human donor heart. The operation, which represents one of the great milestones of medicine, was performed on December 3, 1967, by Dr. Christian Barnard of Capetown, South Africa. The goals of surgeons is now to insure the survival of such transplants and ultimately, to replace the human heart by a mechanical pump. Such an achievement would solve the donor shortage which currently hampers surgeons.

Heart donors are selected from among persons dying as a result of injuries or from persons in whom brain death has occurred but the heart still beats. In the latter instance, the patient is dead for all practical considerations and the remaining heart beat, likewise destined to cease, can only be regarded as compatible with life in the most aesthetic context. When death is imminent, the donor's heart is kept alive and nourished by maintenance of the circulation until the recipient's heart has been removed and the patient made ready for the transplant.

The mortality rate in such a new operation is understandably high. Much remains to be learned from those patients who have survived. The problems which continue to confront the surgeon after a mechanically successful operation are those which concern the delicate physiologic balance which ultimately determines acceptance or rejection of the transplanted tissue. Although a new area of understanding is evolving relative to the immune response, much remains to be learned about the body processes which must be altered to insure success of the transplant, and the consequences of such altered physiology.

Transplant surgeons generally agree that the early drugs designed to suppress the body's immune reaction with tissue rejection were poor from the standpoint that they indiscriminately blocked disease-fighting antibody formation. This left the patient vulnerable to overwhelming infection by organisms which are common in all of us.

The newest means of controlling tissue rejection is through use of anti-lymphocyte serum or globulin. The serum is produced by injecting human white blood cells into horses, which produce antibodies against them. The antibody content is extracted from the animal's serum and injected into the transplant patient where it interferes with the capacity of his own white blood cells to produce antibodies against the transplanted tissue. The serum, abbreviated as ALG is regarded as a stopgap measure until more successful methods are devised. Its disadvantage lies in the fact that transplant patients can never be weaned of it and some patients develop severe allergic reactions to it.

Experiments to develop a substance which will successfully control transplanted tissue rejection are being directed against transplant antigens, tiny protein molecules which are so minute that they cannot be seen with the electron microscope. They are believed to exist on the outer surface of the cell where they readily trigger an antibody reaction and rejection process when the cells are transplanted, in the form of an organ, into another individual. The lack of compatibility between host and donor tissue is explained on the basis that these antibodies are different in size and composition from one person to another, except possibly in identical twins. The successful vaccine or drug which will evolve from research on this subject will either nullify or selectively destroy the hostile antibody activity responsible for the rejection phenomenon. The body possesses a remarkable capacity for developing increasing tolerance to medications to the point where their effect is gradually lost. This is a factor which must be considered in using any substance on a continuing basis which is simply designed to suppress the rejection process.

Organ transplant is still so new that surgeons, physiologists and biochemists cannot predict all of the eventualities in such surgery. Knowl-

VASCULAR SURGERY

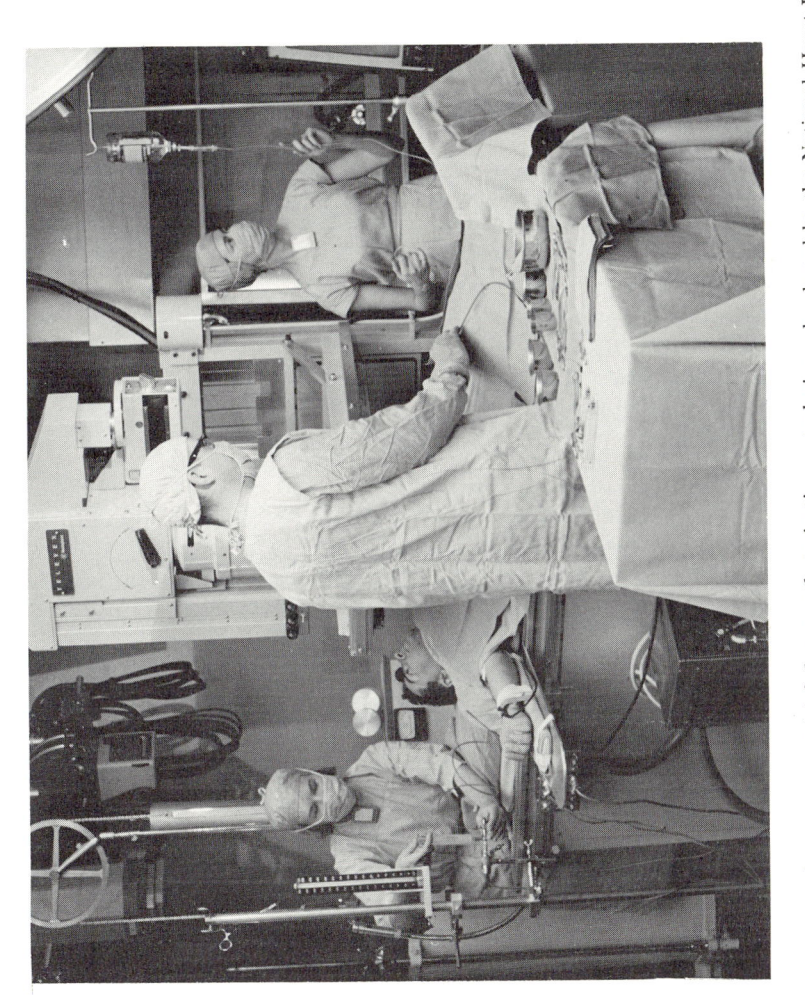

Figure 94 Preparation of a patient for a transseptal left heart catheterization, a technique developed by the National Heart Institute as an aid in diagnosing heart defects. The procedure is performed using fluoroscopy projected on a television screen. The surgeon is guided by the television image (fluoroscopic image) of the catheter as it is threaded through a leg vein into the left chamber of the heart.

Photo courtesy National Institute of Health

edge which remains to be discovered will surely be among the most fascinating in the annals of medicine.

DIAGNOSTIC EXAMINATIONS OF THE HEART

Surgical correction is available today for numerous heart conditions for which, only a few years ago, there was little to offer the patient other than a diagnosis. This is not to say that every patient with a particular surgical cardiac lesion is a candidate for surgery. Every patient is an individual consideration.

Congenital as well as acquired heart defects often exist in combination with other heart abnormalities. Their very existence in many cases produces secondary problems which militate against surgical intervention. Other considerations include the general condition of the patient and his ability to withstand surgery, the possible presence of other pathology within the body which might hazard operative results, as well as the secondary problems which might be created for the patient as a result of surgery. It is for these reasons that patients presenting surgical heart lesions are carefully evaluated with the aid of special examinations designed to provide the surgeon with the necessary information to formulate a complete diagnosis. A description of the examinations usually performed follows.

ROENTGENOGRAPHY—Fluoroscopic examination is usually carried out on patients suspected of having a cardiac malformation. Full size chest films in the posteroanterior and oblique positions, with barium in the esophagus, are also obtained. The position and size of the great vessels and heart chambers, the pulsations observed during fluoroscopy and the vascularity of the lung fields are important factors in establishing the diagnosis.

ANGIOCARDIOGRAPHY—This examination is often performed in conjunction with cardiac catheterization. Anatomic deformities are evaluated radiographically after injection of radiopaque material into a specific site or chamber.

Right angiocardiography is used to define the relative sizes of the great vessels coming off the heart and their relationship to one another. The dye is useful in outlining the main pulmonary artery which in severe tetralogy may be hypoplastic or absent (truncus).

Left-sided angiocardiography is used to define acquired valvular lesions or coronary artery disease.

CARDIAC CATHETERIZATION—Nobel prize recognition was accorded Cournand and Richards for this contribution to medicine. It is an examination employed in evaluating patients for cardiac surgery or medical management. Right cardiac catherization is sometimes used to assess congenital heart defects. A catheter is threaded into the right heart to measure intracardiac pressures, pressure curves and gradients and to obtain blood samples for gas analysis. Catheterization of the left heart is most often used to evaluate acquired defects of the aortic or mitral valves. In congenital heart disease, a right and left catherization is sometimes carried out to localize left-to-right shunts and to estimate pulmonary vascular resistance.

The risk to life attending this procedure is small, being estimated at about 0.05 per cent. Most fatalities are severely ill patients with pulmonary hypertension and cyanosis.

CINERADIOGRAPHY (cine)—This is a motion picture record of successive images appearing on a fluoroscopic screen. It provides a continuous record of the passage of contrast medium and may demonstrate details not readily appreciated in a single film.

ELECTROCARDIOGRAPHY—This is a method of evaluating the action of the heart muscle through study of a graphic tracing of the electric current produced by contraction of that muscle.

In congenital heart disease this examination is more sensitive than roentgenography in determining specific ventricular hypertrophy. Right ventricular hypertrophy and enlargement are common with many types of congenital cardiac malformations.

PHONOCARDIOGRAPHY—This is an examination which consists of a recording of the chest wall vibrations produced by the heart. It is used to assist in the interpretation of auscultation examinations, particularly when precise timing of an extra heart sound or the duration of a murmur is in question.

The format for recording these examinations should include the complete title of the procedure, the indication for it, a description of what was done, a report of any eventful occurrences during the examination and an immediate interpretation of the films, in addition to information completely identifying the patient by name, age, case number, room number and name of the attending physician.

The following examples demonstrate the format and context of typical reports exclusive of patient identification.

CONTRAST MATERIALS USED FOR VASCULAR X-RAY EXAMINATIONS

Angio-Conray
Conray
Conray-400
Hypaque 20%

Hypaque 50%
Hypaque-M 75%
Hypaque-M 90%

Right Subclavian Arteriogram

Indications: Evaluation of arterial supply of the right arm in a patient with Buerger's Disease and gangrene.

Procedure:

The patient was placed on the x-ray table in the supine position. The skin over the right neck in the supraclavicular region was prepared and draped in the usual manner. The skin over the pulsating right subclavian artery was anesthetized with 1% Xylocaine.

A short 17 gauge needle was introduced into the right subclavian artery. Good backflow was obtained. A routine injection consisting of 20 cc. of 50% Hypaque was administered. The patient experienced minimal discomfort. These films were not satisfactory and it was felt to be partially due to insufficient contrast material. A second injection of 50% Hypaque was given with good film results. Pressure was maintained over the puncture site and hemostasis appeared to be satisfactory. This was followed by PA and lateral chest films.

Immediate Interpretation of Films:

1. Distal small artery disease with occlusion of the ulnar artery below the brachial artery bifurcation and the radial artery proximal to the level of the wrist.

Right Femoral Arteriogram

Indications: Right popliteal aneurysm

Procedure:

The patient was placed in the supine position. The right groin was prepared with Merthiolate and draped in the usual fashion. Using a special needle of the Rochester type, the femoral artery was entered. The metal stylet was withdrawn and a plastic catheter was then left in the right common femoral. One injection was made utilizing 20 cc. of Angio-Conray. Films were obtained in the AP position. A second run was then made with the leg in the lateral position using the same quantity of dye and again films were obtained at the usual rate.

Immediate Interpretation of Films:
1. Popliteal aneurysm with thrombosis of the wall; the aneurysm measuring approximately 1 inch in length.
2. Arteries normal with good outflow.

Aortogram

Indications: This 70 year old white male stepped on a nail 4 weeks ago, subsequent to which he developed an ulcer of the left foot followed by gangrene of the left first toe. Popliteal pulse on left diminished as compared with the right. Pedal pulses on the left very faint.

Procedure:

The patient was placed in the prone position and the lumbar area prepared and draped. 1% Xylocaine was infiltrated locally. A 17 gauge needle was introduced at a level below the renal arteries in the aorta with good backflow in all four quadrants. Two test films at two second intervals were obtained after injection of 10 cc. of Conray-400. The usual run of eight films at two second intervals after 25 cc. of Angio-Conray was obtained. The films were of good quality. The needle was withdrawn.

The distal arteries of the left extremity were not entirely visualized and a left femoral arteriogram was done.

Left Femoral Arteriogram

With the patient in the supine position, the groin area was prepared with Merthiolate and 1% Xylocaine was infiltrated locally. A 17 gauge needle was introduced into the left common femoral artery with good backflow in all four quadrants. Eight films at two second intervals were taken after injection of 25 cc. of Angio-Conray. The films were of good quality. The needle was withdrawn.

Immediate Interpretation of Films:
1. Patent femoral system on left
2. High bifurcation of popliteal with takeoff of peroneal artery from left anterior tibial artery
3. Stenosis of the left posterior tibial and peroneal arteries
4. Low femoral (common) bifurcation on the left

Translumbar Aortogram

Indication: Postoperative aortic bilateral external iliac dacron bypass

Procedure:

With the patient in the prone position the back was prepared and draped in the usual manner. 1% Xylocaine was used to anesthetize the back area. A 17 gauge needle was then inserted into the aorta. A good backflow was demonstrated. A test dose of 8 cc. of Angio-Conray showed the needle to be in good position. A final run was then made using 20 cc. of Angio-Conray. A total of three runs were made, each using 20 cc. of Angio-Conray.

Immediate Interpretation of Films:
1. Patent aorto-iliac bypass

Right Open Transbrachial Arch Aortogram

Indications: Possible thoracic aneurysm on routine chest x-ray

Procedure:

The patient was placed on the aortogram table in the supine position. The skin of the right arm and shoulder was prepared and draped in the usual manner. The skin and subcutaneous tissues over the lower third of the right brachial artery were anesthetized with 1% Xylocaine.

A 4 cm. longitudinal incision was made and carried through the skin and subcutaneous tissues. The brachial artery was easily exposed. Bleeding points were clamped and ligated with 0000 Tevdek as encountered. The brachial artery was isolated for a distance of 2½ cm. and slung with cord tapes proximally and distally. It was necessary to clamp and ligate only a small arterial branch and this was done with 0000 Tevdek. The brachial artery was clamped proximally and 20 cc. of ½ mg. per cc. Heparin was injected into the distal arterial tree. The distal cord tape was tightened and an arteriotomy incision was made.

A No. 8 NIH catheter was passed into the ascending aorta under fluoroscopy using 50 cc. of 50% Hypaque. A test film was taken using 20 cc. of 50% Hypaque and this film was found to be of satisfactory quality. A routine injection with the patient in the oblique position was then made, the patient receiving 40 cc. of 90% Hypaque at a pressure of 600 lbs. per square inch. A second set of films was then taken with the patient in the straight PA position, using the same quantity of dye under the same injection technique. The catheter was withdrawn and the proximal and distal arterial tree flushed.

The arteriotomy incision was closed with a running suture of 000000 Mersilene with satisfactory hemostasis. The fascia and subcutaneous tissues were closed with interrupted 0000 Tevdek. The skin was closed with interrupted deep mattress sutures of the same material.

A dry sterile dressing was applied and the patient returned to his room in good condition with an easily palpable full right radial pulse.

Immediate Interpretation of Films:
1. Presence of thoracic aortic aneurysm noted

OPERATIONS ON THE AORTA AND VESSELS

A considerable amount of investigation has been carried out on autogenous vein grafts particularly to bypass occluded portions of the peripheral arteries; however, because of the high incidence of postoperative aneurysm or thrombosis eventuating in failures, surgeons prefer synthetic vascular implants or arterial homografts. Because homologous arterial transplants (segments of artery taken from one individual and transplanted into another) do not act as true grafts, artificial prosthesis may be used just as well. Heterologous arterial transplants (vascular segments used from another species) were used successfully by Carrel in 1907; however, some authorities believe that they do not function as well as homologous transplants and are therefore unsatisfactory as vascular transplants. Experimental work is being done with bovine arterial segments in the hope that methods of preparation and preservation can be developed to permit successful use of this material.

The lack of readily available transplants for vascular grafts has long prompted investigators to seek suitable substitutes. Rigid materials were used initially but soon abandoned in favor of pliable tubes. The first successful use of such tubes for arterial replacement was introduced in 1952 by Voorhees, Jaretski, and Blakemore, using vinyon-N cloth. In the years which have followed, a variety of different materials have been tried experimentally. Dacron, Teflon and Terylene cloth are some of the more popular materials used today. The actual success of these vascular transplants can only be tested by time. The techniques for replacement and use of these fabrics will be better appreciated in a few years when studies can be based on significant survival rates.

Another factor being carefully observed by scientific investigators is the carcinogenic (cancer causing) potential of these foreign implants in the body. Experiments have demonstrated carcinomatous growths in mice at the site of implantation of some of these materials but it does not follow that an identical response will occur in man. Numerous substances exist which are carcinogenic in experimental animals and innocuous in man. Time holds the answer to this question also.

Some of the materials, types of prostheses and sutures used in vascular surgery have been listed here with typical operative dictations to acquaint the secretary with the terminology characteristic of this specialty.

VASCULAR PROTHESES

Cartwright
Crimped dacron tube
#25 dacron bifurcation
DeBakey
Edwards seamless bifurcated
Frozen arterial homograft
Gott low profile hinged leaflet
Helanca seamless tubes
Hufnagel low profile discoid valve
Kay-Suzuki disc valve
Knitted

4 A Magovern valve
Magovern-Cromie sutureless ball valve
Nylon
Orlon
M 2 Starr-Edwards valve
SCDT valve
Teflon tri-leaflet
Terylene cloth
Wada hingeless valve
Woven tube

SUTURES AND TECHNIQUES

Carrel method interrupted Lembert
Dacron
Deknatel silk
Halsted mattress
Mersilene

Metal bands
Silk
Tevdek
Transfixion silk

AORTIC VALVE PROSTHESES (total replacement)

Silastic bicuspid valve with compressed Ivalon rim
Silastic flap valve with compressed Ivalon base
Silastic impregnated Teflon felt three-cusp valve

For a complete listing of arteries and veins the secretary is referred to chapter 6.

Left Femoropopliteal Bypass and Autogenous Vein Graft

Indications: Patient is a 64 year old colored male with rest pain in his left foot secondary to superficial femoral artery (probably malignant) and small artery disease. Femoral arteriography revealed a patent popliteal stump of poor quality.

Technique:

With the patient on the operating table in the supine position, the entire left leg and groin were prepared and draped for surgery.

A groin incision was made over the fossa ovalis exposing the saphenous vein. Hemostasis was obtained throughout with fine Tevdek. The saphenous vein was isolated at one point, retained with a rubber band and by meticulous dissection, both distally and proximally, was freed from surrounding tissue. Its tributaries were ligated with 000 Tevdek and divided. The saphenous vein was of good quality although somewhat narrow. A satisfactory link was obtained from the fossa ovalis to below the knee. The skin did not need to be undermined to obtain the vein.

The popliteal artery was exposed in the customary fashion without cutting the pes anserinus. The popliteal artery was of poor quality and the bifurcation was therefore exposed revealing a discrete plaque at the branching of the anterior tibial and posterior tibial arteries. When a satisfactory link of artery had been obtained, a Pott's clamp was placed proximally and the artery was opened with a longitudinal incision. This incision was carried down to the bifurcation previously mentioned. Backflow was poor and therefore an endarterectomy was performed. The resulting backflow was improved to a sufficient degree to warrant grafting.

The lower portion of the incision was closed with a running 00000 Tevdek suture. A catheter was threaded down this artery and the distal limbs heparinized through this catheter. A Pott's clamp was placed across the artery where it had been sewn, isolating the area for anastomosis.

The vein was prepared, distended and irrigated. The proximal portion was prepared for anastomosis. This was performed in the usual manner with 000 Tevdek using an end-to-side anastomosis. The vein was passed up the thigh behind the Sartorius muscle, care being taken not to twist it. The distal part of the vein was prepared for proximal anastomosis. The common femoral artery was isolated including its bifurcation. Pott's clamps were placed across all of the major arteries. The distal limbs were heparinized. A longitudinal incision was made in the anterior portion of the common femoral artery. The artery was of excellent quality at this level. An anastomosis was carried out in an end-to-side manner. All clamps were removed. Flow was established and an excellent pulse was palpable in the distal popliteal artery, including its branches. One portion of the vein above the lower anastomosis ballooned out, weakened by removal of its adventitial layer. This was imbricated with a 0000 patching suture.

The anastomosis was checked and found to be leakproof. The wound was closed in layers with 000 and 0000 Tevdek on the deep fascia and 0000 Tevdek on the skin. A cotton dressing was applied.

Intimectomy of Right Common Femoral and Deep Femoral Arteries With Autogenous Vein Bypass From Right Common Femoral to Right Popliteal Artery

Indications:

Patient is a known diabetic with severe claudication and rest pain involving the right foot. Angiographic studies revealed complete occlusion of the superficial femoral and the deep femoral artery on the right side with a very narrow popliteal artery with no outflow noted. The operation was a desperate attempt to save the limb.

Technique:

The patient was placed in the supine position and the right leg was prepared and draped in the usual fashion using vi-drape and Tincture of Zephiran. An incision was made along the medial aspect of the lower leg posterior to the tibial ridge. The incision was extended downward until the saphenous vein was identified. It was in good condition. Dissection was carried down further through the crural fascia until the Gastrocnemius was identified and retracted posteriorly. Dissection was carried in the popliteal space where the popliteal vein and artery were identified. Dissection of the popliteal artery was carried out both upward and downward. The anterior tibial artery was noted to be occluded; however, the popliteal artery was thought to be in fairly good condition. The distal outflow tree was thought to be in rather poor condition. There was noted to be some slight amount of backflow through the popliteal artery after a clamp had been placed proximal to a needle injection in the distal popliteal. Attempts at irrigation and suctioning of the distal arterial tree were performed in an attempt to open up thrombosed channels.

The right groin was explored. The right common femoral was identified as well as the saphenous vein. The deep femoral artery and superficial arteries were isolated and slung individually. The incision was carried along the medial aspect of the leg in order to facilitate the dissection of the long saphenous vein. This was removed and its branches clamped and tied with a 0000 Tevdek suture. The vein was found to be in relatively good condition. It was removed and prepared in the usual fashion. Dissection of the groin was completed.

An incision was then made in the right common femoral which was found to be markedly involved with arteriosclerosis. The common femoral was endarterectomized and the deep femoral was identified. The wall of the deep femoral was incised and a large intimal plaque was removed from it. The deep femoral incision was then reconstructed. The saphenous vein was then approximated to the popliteal artery using 00000 Tevdek suture in an end-to-side fashion. After completion of the anastomosis, release of the clamps revealed a watertight anastomosis. The distal arterial tree had been previously heparinized.

A McDonald clamp was then applied to the saphenous vein after it had been flushed with Heparin. The vein was then passed beneath the crural fascia, beneath the tibial plateau, upward into the leg and into the right groin. The vein was then anastomosed to the right common femoral artery in an end-to-side fashion using 00000 Tevdek suture. The remaining incised portion of the common femoral was closed in a longitudinal manner. Distal and proximal clamps were all removed and hemostasis in the proximal anastomosis as well as the distal anastomosis was found to be hemostatic. The blood pulsation in the popliteal flow was quite evident.

The crural fascia was closed throughout its entirety using 000 Tevdek suture. The subcutaneous tissue was closed using interrupted 0000 Tevdek suture. The skin was then closed using an interrupted vertical mattress 00000 Tevdek suture. The groin was closed in a similar fashion.

A dry sterile dressing was applied. The leg was then wrapped in a bulky dressing and Ace bandage.

Crafoord Operation for Coarctation of the Aorta

The patient was placed on the operating table on his right side and sterilely prepared and draped. The left arm was used to raise the scapula anteriorly and upward. A blood transfusion was started.

An incision was made at the level of the 2nd rib and extended to the posterior axillary line, encircling the inferior scapular angle. The incision was deepened through the muscles. The scapula was transected and lifted. The 3rd rib was resected between the midaxillary line and the paravertebral portion. A small paravertebral bite was taken from the 2nd and 4th ribs. The intercostal nerves were resected and the intercostal vessels ligated.

A rib spreader was introduced to separate the ribs. The lung was collapsed and retracted downwards with wet pads.

The mediastinal pleura was incised over the aortic arch exposing the stenosed area. Further ligation of vessels leading to the esophagus and intercostal spaces was carried out. The aorta 4 cm. above and below the stenosis was then clamped with Kochers and the stenosed area resected. The stumps of the aorta were then aligned with the use of the clamps. The lumina of the stumps were washed out. Intima was approximated to intima. The anterior wall was sutured first. Two holding sutures were placed followed by interrupted mattress sutures. The Kochers were then rotated 180 degrees to bring the posterior wall into view. This was likewise sutured. A pressure packing was placed around the suture line and the Kochers released. After a few minutes the packing was removed and the anastomosis checked for leakage. None was found. The pleura was closed with a continuous suture and the wound closed in anatomic layers. A catheter was inserted at the 9th intercostal space just prior to closure of the chest.

Arteriotomy with Removal of Emboli

The operation was begun under 1% Xylocaine. The femoral vessels were exposed through a longitudinal incision. The profunda femoris at the junction with the common femoral artery was identified. There was no pulsation at this point of the artery. The artery did not appear to be in spasm. Its wall was soft and pliable. It was therefore decided that the embolus was higher in the common femoral area, possibly at the bifurcation of the aorta.

The patient was repositioned and spinal anesthesia administered. After redraping the operative field, the incision was carried superiorly, coursing through the inguinal area with division of the fascia and muscles until the retroperitoneal space was reached. The iliac artery was then identified and noted to be pulsating to the point of junction with the hypogastric artery on the right side. At this site, a small induration, thought to represent an embolus, was found. After isolating the artery and freeing it with tape, the artery was clamped with bulldogs. An arteriotomy was done immediately above the bulge at the junction. A 1 X 2 cm. clot was extruded. The inferior clamp was then removed but reconstitution was unobtainable. There was good reconstitution from the hypogastric artery. By gently milking the femoral artery, two small clots were evacuated through the arteriotomy wound. The reconstitution of blood was brisk. The clamps were reapplied and the artery was irrigated with Heparin solution.

The arteriotomy was closed longitudinally with a continuous running 00000 silk suture. There were no leaks through this closure after the clamps were removed. The femoral pulses became readily palpable at the termination of the procedure. The wound was closed in layers with interrupted chromic. The skin was reapproximated with interrupted cotton.

Intimectomy for Leriche's Syndrome

Under spinal anesthesia the patient was prepared and draped in the supine position.

A right pararectus incision was made. The skin was incised from the xiphoid to the pubis. The anterior rectus sheath was incised and the rectus muscle was retracted. The posterior sheath was opened. The aorta was exposed.

Upon palpation of the aorta there was an impulse present approximately 3 inches below the renal artery and distal to that point. The colon and small bowel were grasped and herniated out of the abdomen and retracted superiorly.

An incision along the peritoneum of the aorta and the iliac arteries bilaterally was made with the reflection of the peritoneum away from the vessels. An incision through the anterior portion of the external and internal iliacs was then made in three places bilaterally. One was just proximal to the femoral canal; the other was in the mid-portion of the external iliac; and the other was just proximal to the bifurcation of the iliacs. Following the incisions, the intimectomy knife was used to remove the large calcified plaques present in the center of these vessels. It was noted that pulsations were present in both of the iliacs to the level of the femoral canal after removal of the intima and plaques.

The small and large bowels were packed back into the abdomen. The posterior sheath and peritoneum were closed with 00 continuous lock stitch anteriorly, No. 30 wire double loop suture for the anterior rectus sheath, and 00 chromic interrupted for the subcutaneous tissues. The skin was closed with 000 cotton mattress suture.

Saphenous Vein Ligation and Stripping

Under spinal anesthesia with the patient in a supine position, the lower extremities were prepared and sterilely draped.

A subinguinal incision was made over the fossa ovalis. By blunt and sharp dissection the greater saphenous vein was isolated and its tributaries transected and ligated with 000 silk to the edge of the foramen ovale. The saphenous vein was transected and tied with one 000 cotton. A stick tie of 000 cotton was placed over its base. Beginning at the medial aspect of the ankle, the saphenous vein was unroofed and stripped in a retrograde fashion.

In the area of the knee of the left leg two incisional areas were used to tie off the perforating branches. On the right leg one incision on the medial aspect was made to tie off the perforating branch. Minimal bleeding was encountered.

The fossa ovalis was closed with a purse-string of 000 silk. The subcutaneous tissues were closed with 000 intestinal chromic and the skin was closed with a mattress 000 chromic suture.

Ligation of the External Carotid Artery

The area of the neck was prepared and draped in a sterile manner. It was decided to ligate the external carotid artery between the lingual and the superficial temporal branches of the artery, just below the digastric muscle.

A three inch incision parallel to the course of the artery along the anterior border of the sternocleidomastoid muscle was made. The center of the incision was at the level of the hyoid bone.

Identification was carried out of the hypoglossal nerve and the posterior belly of the digastric muscle. The apex of the great cornu of the hyoid bone was exposed under which the sheath of the artery was incised. The superior laryngeal nerve was identified and avoided immediately below the artery. The external jugular vein and its anastomosis with the facial was likewise identified and avoided. The sternocleidomastoid muscle was identified as was the stylomandibular ligament. After all structures were identified with certainty, a ligature was placed around the external carotid artery and tied.

The wound was closed in layers.

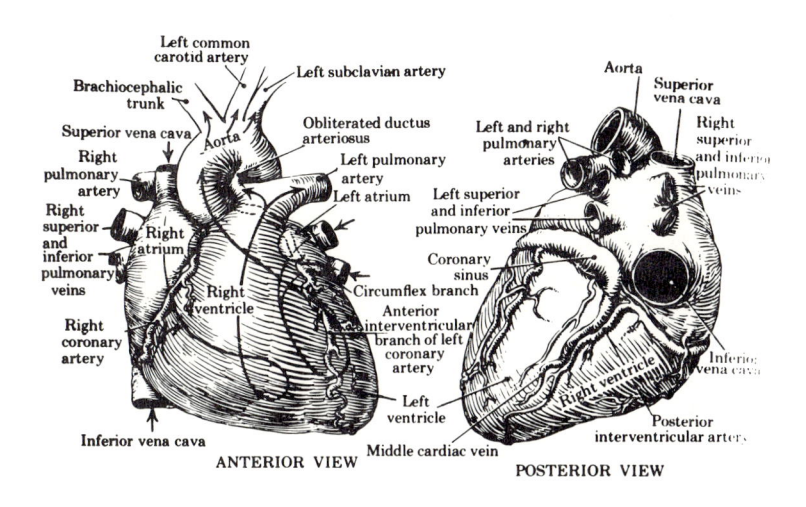

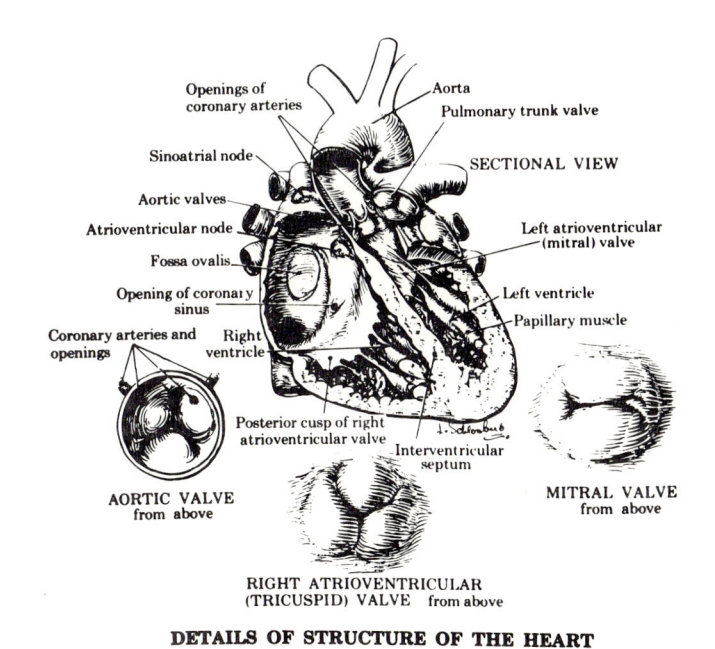

Figure 95 Details of structure of the heart

From Dorland's Illustrated Medical Dictionary Courtesy W. B. Saunders Company

OPERATIONS ON THE HEART

Heart diseases for which surgical treatment is currently available constitute only about two per cent of all heart diseases. They include abnormal openings in the atrial or ventricular septa (septal defects), valve defects resulting in stenosis and insufficiency, as well as vessel disease. Surgical treatment consists of closure of anomalous septal openings by suture closure or prosthetic patch; resection of defective segments of vessels with reanastomosis as in aortic coarctation; closure of an abnormal passage such as that seen in patent ductus arteriosus; enlargement of a scarred valve (commissurotomy) as occurs in mitral stenosis (rheumatic heart disease); correction of various valvular defects with the aid of mechanical prostheses or partial plastic closure; rerouting of intake and output vessels in cases of transposition of the great vessels; and, most recently, actual heart transplants.

Heart Lungs By-Pass

Introduction of the heart lungs by-pass machine (see photo on opposite page) has enabled vascular surgeons to perform longer and more exact procedures on the heart than was possible by former techniques. The machine takes over the function of the patient's heart and lungs, pumping blood through the systemic circulation with exchange of oxygen and carbon dioxide between the blood and tissues. The first successful open heart operation using by-pass of the heart and lungs was performed in 1953 by Dr. John H. Gibbon, Philadelphia, Pennsylvania.

Large amounts of blood are required in open heart surgery for purposes of priming the extracorporeal circuit (outside the body). Most machines in use today require between 1500 and 3000 ml. of blood. The machines requiring larger blood volumes sometimes use a mixture of blood and a blood substitute such as Ringer's lactate solution. Fresh heparinized blood is preferred; however, in cases where the patient has a rare blood type, citrated blood must be used. For an average perfusion in an adult, approximately 1500 ml. of citrated blood and 1500 ml. of Ringer's lactate solution are used to prime the machine. Heparin is added to prevent clotting. Sodium bicarbonate is added to the oxygenator to offset the acidity of ACD blood (citrated). About five minutes before cannulation, 2 mg. of heparin per kg. of body weight is given I.V. to the patient to prevent clotting. The patient is also given a priming dose of 25 Gm. of mannitol. After this, a 10 per cent solution of mannitol in 0.3% NaCl (sodium chloride) solution is dripped I.V. at a rate sufficient to produce a urinary output of 5 ml. per minute throughout the perfusion. The machine is tapped into the patient at the vena cava by means of inert

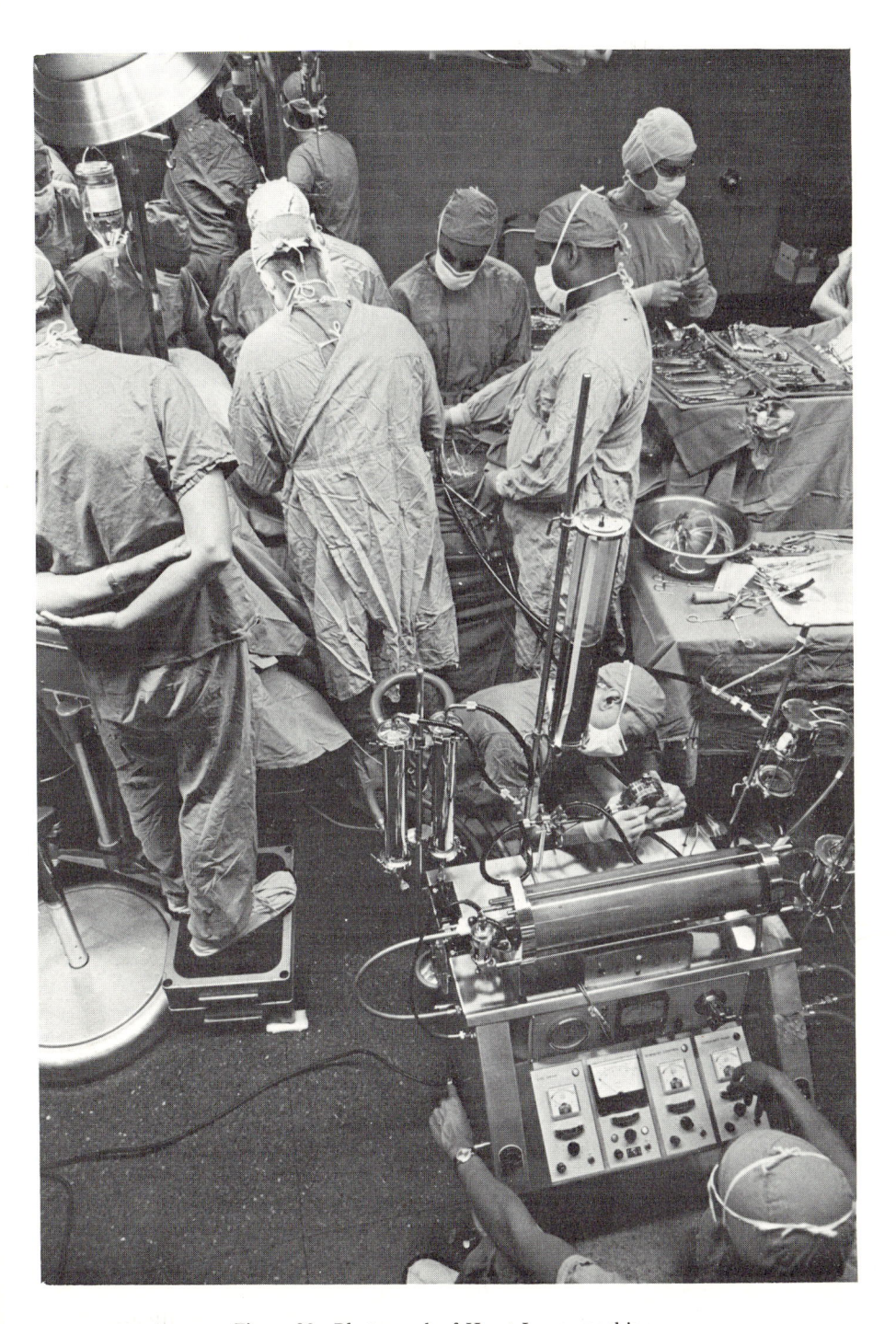

Figure 96 Photograph of Heart-Lungs machine

plastic tubing. The patient's venous blood is thus introduced into the machine where it is circulated and oxygenated as it would be in its course through the lungs. The oxygenated blood is returned to the patient's body by way of a catheter in either the femoral or subclavian artery. Prior to being placed on by-pass, the operative field is flooded with gaseous carbon dioxide. Since this gas is heavier than air it will displace air from the depths of the thorax. Any gas trapped within the heart at the conclusion of the operation (cardiotomy) will be carbon dioxide which is readily absorbed from the blood stream.

The advantage in use of this equipment is that with the heart in a state of arrest the surgeon is able to operate under direct vision with greater thoroughness and precision. At the conclusion of the operation, the connections to the machine are disconnected, the vessels repaired at the catheter insertion points, heparin (clot prevention drug) in the patient's circulation neutralized with a drug such as protamine to restore normal clotting, and the chest closed. The patient's own heart and lungs take over again.

Coronary Artery Perfusion

In aortic valvular disease perfusion of both the left and right coronary arteries is important. When the aortotomy (incision into the aorta) is to be closed, the cannulae supplying blood are withdrawn with resulting anoxic arrest. During the 10 minutes when the sutures are being placed the heart is surrounded by saline slush. After completion of the aortic suture line, the aorta is unclamped. The resulting ventricular fibrillation is corrected by electrical defibrillation.

Hypothermia

Open heart operations may also be performed under conditions of hypothermia (lowering body temperature from 36.8° C. to 20-30° C.) produced by circulating the blood through a heat exchanger, wrapping the patient in a refrigerating blanket or immersing the anesthetized patient in a bath of ice cold water. The lowered metabolism reduces the body's oxygen requirements. This method of circulation stoppage limits the surgeon's working time to about 5 to 15 minutes. One distinct advantage of the cardiopulmonary by-pass (heart lungs machine) is that it relieves the surgeon of the pressure of working against time.

Anatomy of the Heart

A brief review of the anatomy of the heart will assist the reader in developing a better comprehension of the surgical defects of this organ and their secondary manifestations. The heart may be thought of as a pumping station consisting of two pumps with two chambers and two valves in each pump. Prior to birth, when the lungs are not yet functional in the fetus, two openings exist, (1) the foramen ovale in the atrial septum, and, (2) the ductus arteriosus between the pulmonary artery and the aorta. These communications usually close after birth. Ideally, the blood flows in one direction with the right side of the heart (right atrium and ventricle) pumping blood through the lungs for oxygenation, and the left side of the heart (left atrium and ventricle) pumping blood through the systemic circulation. Blood is returned to the heart by the venous circulation. It enters the heart at the right atrium from whence it flows into the right ventricle. It is pumped into the pulmonary artery and capillaries to the lungs where it is oxygenated. It then enters the pulmonary veins for transportation back to the heart. It enters the heart at the left atrium and proceeds to the left ventricle which pumps it out into the aorta and out into the systemic circulation by way of the arteries. After circulating through the body, it begins its return to the heart by passing into the venous system (veins) and then into the vena cavae, entering the heart at the right atrium to begin another cycle. Defects in the walls between the chambers of the heart such as holes or abnormal passages, defective valves which permit backflow of blood or fail to function by opening and closing properly, or strictures in the major vessels constitute the most common varieties of lesions amenable to surgery. When these defects are present at birth they are spoken of as congenital heart defects. When they are developed later as a result of infection or other disease process, they are classified as acquired heart disease.

The more commonly encountered cardiac conditions for which surgical treatment is available are described in the following pages.

Atrial septal defect—This is a common congenital heart defect where an opening exists in the septum (wall) between the right and left atrium permitting oxygenated blood from the left atrium to pass into the right atrium rather than out into the systemic circulation. Ideally each atrium is a separate chamber and the flow of blood is from the right atrium to the right ventricle and from the left atrium to the left ventricle. When the flow of blood is short-circuited through a hole in the atrial septum there develops an increase in the load of the pulmonary circulation and right side of the pump.

Atrial septal defects are classified into two types: persistent ostium primum and persistent ostium secundum. The primum is located low in the atrial septum and frequently involves the atrioventricular valves. It is regarded as the more serious and difficult to repair of the two types.

Death due to heart failure represents the greatest threat with repair usually carried out in childhood. Surgery is performed by the open heart method using cardiopulmonary by-pass.

Aortic insufficiency—This is an acquired heart defect which may be secondary to rheumatic heart disease, dissection of the aorta, subacute bacterial endocarditis (SBE), syphilis or valvular damage. Valve replacement is performed in suitable candidates.

Aortic stenosis—This is an acquired heart disease which results from rheumatic valvular heart disease and is manifested by a constriction at the aortic, and often at the tricuspid and mitral valves. The defective valve interferes with the flow of blood from the left ventricle, resulting in left ventricular hypertrophy. Suitable candidates for surgery undergo replacement of the defective valve by a prosthetic valve such as the Starr-Edwards ball-and-cage type. These patients must thereafter be maintained on anticoagulants for the remainder of their lives to prevent blood clot formation.

Coarctation of the aorta—A congenital vascular disease with narrowing of the aorta at about the level of the ductus arteriosum. Rare cases have been encountered with coarctation in the midthoracic aorta, at the diaphragm and even in the abdomen. Obstruction of the aorta causes decreased blood pressure and flow to the lower portion of the body and increased pressure and flow to the head, neck, upper chest and arms. Infants with coarctation usually develop collateral circulation (side branching of blood vessels which develop to carry the blood when a major artery becomes obstructed). Symptoms do not usually appear until late childhood or adulthood. These patients often develop cardiac failure, cerebral accidents, rupture of the aorta and other complications of hypertension. Approximately 51% of these patients die before their fortieth year if their condition is not corrected surgically. Surgery is usually performed between the ages of 8 and 20, consisting of resection of the obstructed area with reanastomosis of the vessel. In some cases a graft is required for bridging the defect.

Mitral insufficiency—An acquired heart disease usually resulting from rheumatic valvular heart disease. The condition may be of congenital origin in association with a low interatrial or high interventricular septal defect. Coronary disease may also be a cause. Symptoms are caused by a deformity of valve leaflets, scarring of the chordae tendineae and papillary muscles, and a widened annulus. The incompetent valve may be repaired with open heart surgery and use of the by-pass pump; however, such surgery is still hazardous. Valve replacement is usually performed using a mechanical prosthesis in preference to plastic procedures on the defects.

Mitral stenosis—This condition is almost always the result of rheumatic fever. Such patients are regarded as having rheumatic heart disease. There is often attending mitral insufficiency. The valve leaflets are inadequate due to scarring and deformity. The mitral opening is often severely constricted, blocking flow of blood from the left atrium. This eventuates in atrial hypertrophy and dilatation as well as pulmonary circuit congestion and hypertension. Gratifying results are obtained by opening the commissures with a dilator or finger, breaking up the scarring constriction either with finger fracture of use of a scalpel blade attached to the end of the finger. Such surgery is usually performed after the age of 30 when the likelihood of recurrent rheumatic fever is lessened.

Patent ductus arteriosus—This is a congenital defect manifested by a persistent opening between the pulmonary artery and aorta. Under normal circumstances, this opening closes in the first few weeks after birth. When the anomalous connection persists, oxygenated blood intended for circulation throughout the body finds its way into the pulmonary circulation. There follows excessive flow to the pulmonary circulation and inadequate flow to the systemic circulation. Surgery consists of ligation and division of the persistent ductus arteriosus. The heart-lung by-pass machine is not used in this operation.

Pulmonic stenosis—This is usually a congenital defect. It manifests itself as an acquired defect in malignant carcinoid and liver metastases. It is rarely due to rheumatic fever. Septal defects are often encountered in conjunction with this condition. The stenosis may be relieved surgically. The heart-lungs by-pass machine is used.

Tetralogy of Fallot—This condition accounts for about 20% of congenital heart defects. The tetrad consists of ventricular septal defect, pulmonary stenosis, right ventricular hypertrophy and straddling aorta. Unoxygenated blood from the right heart intended for the lungs is routed into the systemic circulation with resulting hypoxia and cyanosis. The stenosed pulmonary artery resists flow of blood through it resulting in right ventricular hypertrophy. Very few patients survive beyond the age of thirty. The Blalock-Taussig operation provides increased blood flow to the lungs through an artificial ductus. Best results are obtained by enlargement of the pulmonary stenosis and closure of the septal defect using open heart surgery and the heart-lungs by-pass machine. Potts's operation (side-to-side anastomosis of the aorta and pulmonary artery) is sometimes used in poor risk patients.

Tricuspid stenosis—This is an acquired heart defect which occurs in about 4 per cent of cases with mitral stenosis. When both lesions occur in the same patient, both valves are usually widened at the same operation. There is obstruction to the flow of blood as a result of the stenotic tricuspid valve with resulting overwork of the right atrium. The defect is repaired with open heart surgery using the heart-lungs by-pass.

Ventricular septal defect—This is a congenital heart defect with an abnormal communication either high in the membranous septum or low in the muscular septum, the latter being of lesser physiological significance. In this condition there is shortcircuiting of oxygenated blood into the right ventricle rather than into the left atrium, left ventricle and systemic circulation. Defects may range from small communications in the membranous septum which exists between the right and left ventricles of the heart to complete absence of the septum resulting in a one ventricle heart. In high septal defects, the oxygenated blood goes almost directly into the pulmonary artery with increased blood flow to the lungs. The late stage of high ventricular septal defect is called Eisenmenger's complex. The hazards attending surgery for this condition are higher than those for atrial septal defects. Repair is accomplished with open heart surgery using the heart-lungs by-pass.

The following operative dictations are designed to illustrate some of the vascular operations and the language used in describing these procedures.

Pott's Shunt for Transposition of the Great Vessels and Pulmonary Stenosis

The patient was anesthetized with general endotracheal anesthesia and positioned on the operating room table in the right lateral decubitus position. The left chest was prepared and draped.

The left hemithorax was entered through a posterolateral thoracotomy incision going through the 4th intercostal space. Bleeding vessels were controlled by electrocoagulation.

The pulmonary artery was identified. The main left pulmonary artery and its distal branches were dissected free using a combination of blunt and sharp dissection. Ligatures of silk were looped around the distal branches of the pulmonary artery and a large silk ligature was looped around the left pulmonary artery proximally. Following this, the pleura over the thoracic aorta distal to the subclavian artery was incised. This portion of the thoracic aorta was dissected free using a combination of sharp and blunt dissection. A right angle clamp could be passed around the thoracic aorta easily. The ligature was looped around the proximal portion of the pulmonary artery and was passed posterior and medial to the thoracic aorta. The left pulmonary artery and thoracic aorta were approximated by tension on this ligature. A partially occluding clamp

VASCULAR SURGERY

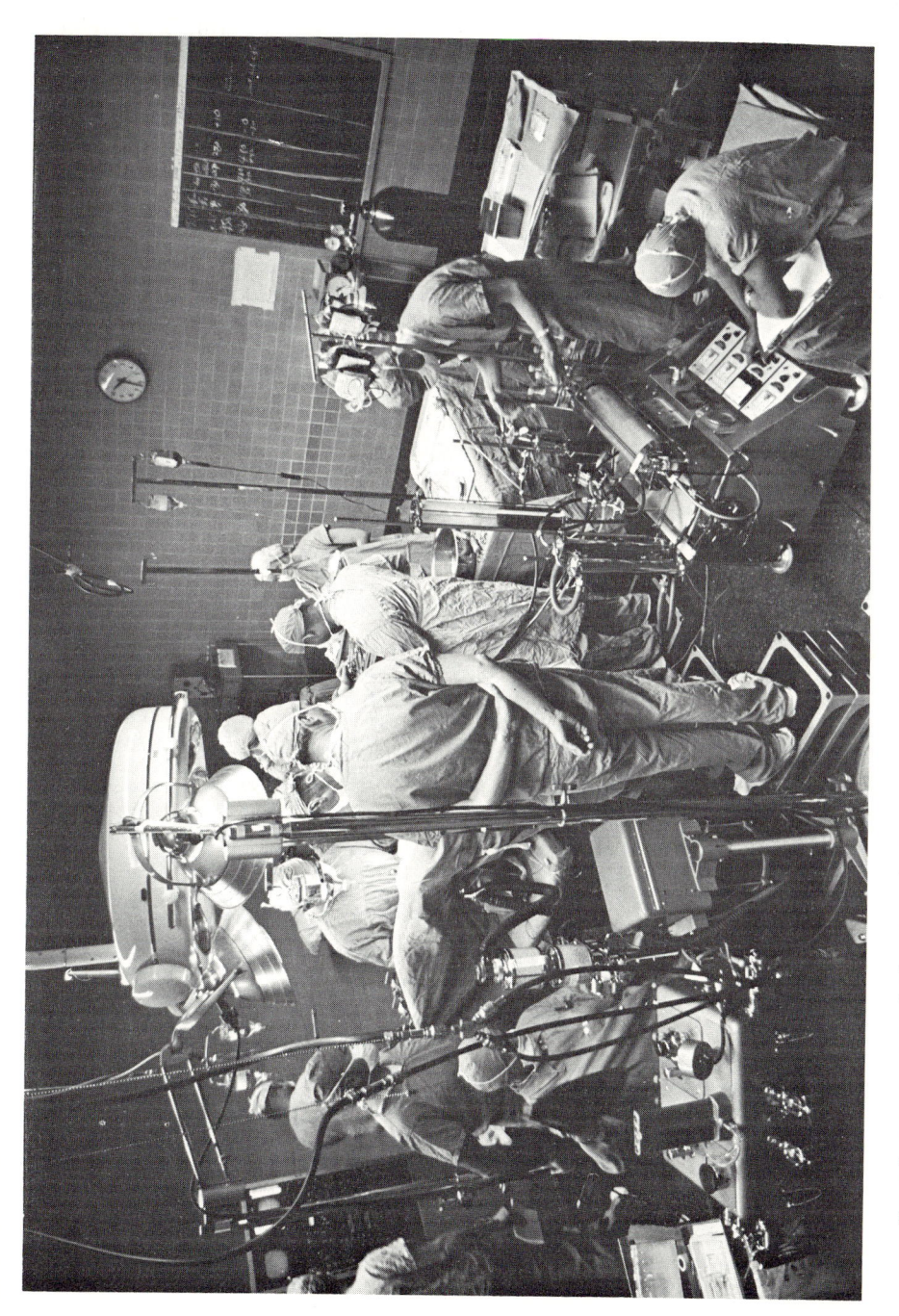

Operating room scene during open heart surgery at the Montefiore Hospital and Medical Center, New York City. Note modern heart and lung machine in right foreground.

was placed on the anterior aspect of the thoracic aorta which was adjacent to the pulmonary artery. The clamp was applied in a longitudinal fashion. An incision approximately 3 mm. in length was then made in this occluded portion of the thoracic aorta, and a transverse incision approximately 2 mm. in length was made transversely in the pulmonary artery which was adjacent to the incision in the thoracic aorta. A stoma was then created between the thoracic aorta and the left pulmonary artery by approximating these two incisions. The anastomosis was completed with a continuous 5-0 silk everting mattress type suture. After completion of the suture, the clamps were removed as well as the loops around the vessels. There was no leak.

The incision was closed in layers using continuous chromic sutures. The skin was approximated with continuous 4-0 nylon suture. The estimated blood loss was 250 cc's.

Ligation of Patent Ductus Arteriosus

After the induction of general endotracheal anesthesia, the patient was positioned on the operating table in the right lateral decubitus position. The left chest was prepared and draped in the usual manner.

The left pleural cavity was entered through a posterolateral thoracotomy incision going through the 5th intercostal space. The pleura over the ductus arteriosus, proximal aorta and subclavian artery was then incised. The vagus and recurrent laryngeal nerves were then identified. The ductus arteriosus was exposed using blunt and sharp dissection. This was approximately 9 mm. in diameter and approximately 1 cm. in length. It was ligated at either end with a 00 silk ligature. A 5-0 silk suture ligature was then placed in the middle of the ductus arteriosus.

All bleeding was controlled by electrocoagulation or ligation using ligatures of silk. A French catheter was placed into the chest and brought out through the 7th intercostal space in the midaxillary line. It was attached to water seal drainage with suction.

The incision was closed in layers using continuous and interrupted chromic sutures throughout. The skin was approximated with continuous 5-0 nylon suture. The patient tolerated the procedure well and was sent to PAR in good condition.

Patch Closure of Interatrial Septal Defect Using Cardiopulmonary By-pass. Correction of Anomalous Venous Drainage

The patient was anesthetized with general endotracheal anesthesia. She was positioned on the operating table in the dorsal decubitus position with the right side elevated at an angle of 45 degrees. The right anterior chest and right groin were prepared and draped in the usual fashion.

The right pleural cavity was entered through an anterior thoracotomy incision going through the 4th intercostal space. The 5th costal cartilage was transected and the 5th rib was displaced. The pleural cavity was entered. The lung was retracted and the pericardial sac was exposed. The pericardium was incised in a longitudinal fashion, anterior to the phrenic nerve. The heart and the great vessels were exposed. A vertical incision was made over the right common femoral artery which was exposed by blunt and sharp dissection. A metal cannula was introduced into the femoral artery after intravenous administration of heparin 2 mg/kg. The metal cannula was then attached to the pump oxygenator. Following this, the inferior and superior vena cava were cannulated through the right atrium. The venous cannula was similarly attached to the pump oxygenator. The entire operative field was flooded with carbon dioxide. Following this, the patient was placed on total cardiopulmonary by-pass.

A longitudinal atriotomy was made in the wall of the right atrium. The incision was extended over the proximal portion of the superior vena cava. An atrial septal defect of the secundum type was found which measured approximately 2½ x 2 cm. The pulmonary vein of the right upper lobe was also found to drain into the proximal portion of the superior vena cava. A Teflon patch was fashioned and sewn into the interatrial septum so as to deflect the pulmonary venous drainage into the left atrium and to cover the interatrial septal defect. The patch measured 2½ x 3½ cm. It was sutured in place using continuous and interrupted 00 silk sutures throughout. The right antriotomy was closed with continuous 00 silk using mattress type sutures. This suture line was similarly sewn with a continuous 4-0 silk suture. The cardiopulmonary by-pass was gradually discontinued. The venous cannula was removed and the incision into the right atrium was closed with 00 silk pursestring suture. The metal cannula was then removed from the femoral artery and the femoral artery was closed with interrupted 5-0 silk sutures. The pericardium was closed with three sutures of 00 silk.

A #24 French chest tube was placed in the right pleural cavity and was brought out through a stab wound in the 7th intercostal space and attached to water seal drainage.

The incision was closed in layers using continuous and interrupted chromic sutures throughout. The skin was approximated with a continuous 4-0 suture of nylon. All bleeding was controlled by electrocoagulation. Blood loss was estimated at 1,000 cc.'s. The patient received 1,000 cc. of blood during the operation. She tolerated the procedure well and was sent to the PAR in good condition.

Closure of Ventricular Septal Defect

The patient was anesthetized using a general endotracheal anesthesia. The anterior chest wall and both groins and thighs were prepared and draped in the usual fashion.

The pericardial sac was exposed through a mediasternotomy incision. The pericardium was then incised in the middle to expose the heart and the great vessels. Extensive adhesions were encountered between the parietal and visceral pericardium. These adhesions were lysed using blunt and sharp dissection. The pulmonary artery was palpated and the thrill could be felt over the pulmonary muscle tracts. The superior and inferior vena cava were then cannulated with a plastic cannula inserted through the wall of the right atrium. The right common femoral artery was then exposed through a semicircular incision in the right groin. It was dissected out using a combination of blunt and sharp dissection. It was cannulated with a metal cannula. The venous and arterial cannulas were connected to the pump oxygenator and the patient was placed on cardiopulmonary by-pass. A drain was placed in the left ventricle through the wall of the left atrium. The operative field was flooded with one atmosphere of carbon dioxide.

A transverse incision was made in the anterior aspect of the right ventricle between the branches of the coronary artery and the ventricular septum was exposed. Upon examination of the ventricular septum, a high ventricular septal defect which measured approximately $2 \times 2\frac{1}{2}$ cm. was found. A Teflon patch was then tailored to cover the defect and the defect was closed by suturing the Teflon patch in place with interrupted silk sutures.

The ventricular incision was then closed with a continuous 00 silk suture. The suture line was over end with a continuous 4-0 silk suture. Throughout the procedure the heart maintained a regular beat. The cardiopulmonary by-pass was gradually discontinued. The venous cannula was then removed and the incision in the right atrial wall was closed with a 00 silk pursestring suture. The pump was also removed from the left ventricle and the incision in the left atrium was also closed with a 00 silk pursestring suture. The arterial cannula was removed and the femoral artery was reapproximated with interrupted 5-0 silk everting mattress type sutures.

A pacemaker electrode was implanted in the wall of the right ventricle and was brought out through the skin externally. A similar electrode was also implanted in the subcutaneous tissue of the mediasternotomy incision and it was likewise brought out externally. A #22 French catheter was placed between the pericardium and sternum and a #24 French catheter was placed in the pericardial sac. Both of these catheters were brought out through external stab wounds and one attached to suction.

The sternum was approximated with interrupted sutures of 00 Tevdek. The remainder of the incisions were closed with continuous chromic sutures. The skin was approximated with continuous 4-0 nylon suture. All bleeding points were controlled by electrocoagulation.

The patient tolerated the procedure well and was sent to PAR in good condition.

Heart Transplant
(Technique of Dr. Denton A. Cooley, Houston, Texas)

FINDINGS: This patient had severe coronary artery disease with chronic congestive failure and severe angina. After removing the heart it was noted that there was a left ventricular aneurysm with paper thin wall and a laminated clot on the inside measuring approximately 5 cm. in diameter.

PROCEDURE: With the patient in the supine position and under adequate general anesthesia, the abdomen, groins and chest were prepared and draped in routine fashion.

The chest was opened through a midline sternotomy. Hemostasis was obtained with bone wax and Bovie. A vertical incision was made in the pericardium with a tube on either side, near the base. The right groin was then opened with a vertical incision over the femoral artery and vein. Tapes were passed around the artery and vein and the vein was cannulated with a #28 Argyle chest catheter which was advanced up to just beneath the diaphragm. The artery was cannulated for arterial perfusion. The superior cava was then cannulated with a #24 catheter after placing a purse-string below the atrial appendage. At this point, total cardiopulmonary by-pass was instituted.

An incision was made in the right atrium and the auricular appendage with the right atrium portion was excised. Following this the left atrium was excised. The aorta and pulmonary arteries were then transected and the heart removed.

The donor heart was then brought into the room, trimmed and a suture begun on the back wall of the left atrium using an over-and-over continuous suture of 000 Tycron. The left atrium and the right atrium were sutured together following which the pulmonary artery was anastomosed in the aorta. After completing these anastomoses and confirming hemostasis, the clamp across the aorta was removed. Air was aspirated from the aorta before the clamp was removed and more air removed after the clamp was released. Several aspirations of air were also carried out at the apex of the heart.

The heart resumed spontaneous sinus rhythm with a good blood pressure. Complete by-pass was discontinued and the superior caval catheter was removed. The incision was closed with 000 silk. The femoral catheter was then clamped and removed. The femoral vein was anastomosed with a running 5-0 Tycron suture. A #32 Argyle chest catheter was then placed in the right chest. A catheter was brought into the mediastinum just below the incision.

The pericardium was approximated with 00 silk. The sternum was approximated with #22 stainless steel wire. The midline fascia was closed with #1 Mersilene in an interrupted suture with buried knots. The subcutaneous fascia was closed with 00 chromic catgut. The skin was closed with running 000 silk.

The femoral incision was closed with a 00 chromic catgut in a running and interrupted suture. Interrupted 000 silk was used to close the skin.

The patient tolerated the procedure well. He received 500 cc. of blood. There were no complications and the patient left the operating room in satisfactory condition with a blood pressure of 130 and a sinus rhythm.

CARDIAC PACEMAKERS

The concept of pacemaking is not new. Man has known for hundreds of years that electrical stimulation of the heart provides an effective treatment for cardiac arrhythmias. However, it was not until 1960, that the first pacemaker unit was inserted into a human subject. Since that time more than 25,000 such implantations have been performed in patients ranging from six months to 94 years of age. The pacemaker provides stimuli for ventricular contraction and may be used to increase the heart rate, slow the rate or increase myocardial contractility.

The heart beats approximately seventy times per minute, one hundred thousand times per day and thirty seven million times per year. The average rate of 70 per minute is lessened during sleep and increased with activity. The tiny nerve which pulses the heart muscle and sets the pace for the heartbeat sometimes is damaged or destroyed, causing the heart to slow down or stop completely. The slow down is called **heart block** and the stoppage called **Adams-Stokes disease.** The latter condition was an inevitably fatal one before introduction of the cardiac pacemaker.

External pacemaker units are employed in emergency situations for resuscitation in cardiac arrest and in cardiac arrhythmia or heart block until the heart rhythm has returned to normal or an implantable pacemaker has been attached to the heart. The external unit provides stimuli for ventricular contraction of the heart through external electrodes applied to the skin.

The internal pacemaker consists of a small case housing a battery generator to which two insulated wires with electrode tips are attached. The electrode tips are implanted in the heart while the generator is placed in a subcutaneous pouch created in the axilla or abdominal wall for accessibility.

Implantable (internal) pacemakers are of three types. The most commonly used model has a fixed rate which is independent of the atrial or ventricular heart rates. The second type, called synchronous, responds to atrial rate and rhythm. The third type is a stand-by pacer which stimulates contraction only when the spontaneous A-V conduction delay is so long that it falls below a predetermined minimum such as 70/minute.

Indications for use of the pacemaker include the following conditions when they fail to respond to drug therapy: Adams-Stokes disease, shortness of breath, refractory congestive failure, easy fatigability and/or precordial pain at rest or upon slight exertion.

A slowed heart rate of 60/minute or less is called **bradycardia.** In certain cases of heart block there is a danger of this rate falling to dangerously low levels and even complete standstill with a threat to life. Changes in heart rate influence coronary flow and cardiac output.

An increased heart rate of more than 100/minute is called **tachycardia.** This rate may likewise become exaggerated to levels above 160/minute with danger of heart failure and myocardial infarction. The pacemaker is designed to assist the heart in maintaining a rhythm within normal limits.

Implantable Pacemaker Units

Cordis Atricor	Medtronic 5860
Demand	Medtronic 5870
Electrodyne TR 14	Transvenous
General Electric A 2065 (dual or single-pass)	

A variety of surgical techniques have been devised for implantation of pacemaker units. For the insertion of myocardial electrodes, a left anterior thoracotomy under general anesthesia is necessary to expose the heart. The electrodes are inserted into the wall of the left ventricle near the apex in an avascular area. A separate transverse incision is made in the left upper quadrant of the abdomen forming a subcutaneous pouch to accommodate the pulse generator. The generator and electrodes are connected by a subcutaneous tunnel through which the electrodes are passed from the abdominal pocket to the chest.

The newest and preferred method of implantation dispenses with the thoracotomy. A transvenous catheter-type electrode is inserted under local anesthesia through a small incision in the cephalic vein below the clavicle or in the external jugular vein. The electrode tip is advanced to the apex of the right ventricle under fluoroscopic control. It is fixed in position at the point where it enters the vein. A subcutaneous pocket is then formed in the subclavicular or axillary region to accommodate the pulse generator. The minute electrical pulses from the generator are transmitted through the blood to the heart muscle to stimulate a regular heartbeat. After closure of the wounds the unit functions without attention from the patient. A daily pulse record is kept by the patient. The generators must be changed when the batteries approach the end of their serviceable life which is about 24 months. This requires a new incision into the subcutaneous pocket, exposure of the generator and removal with connection of a new unit to the electrodes. General Electric has developed a threshold analyzer which is used to evaluate the implanted

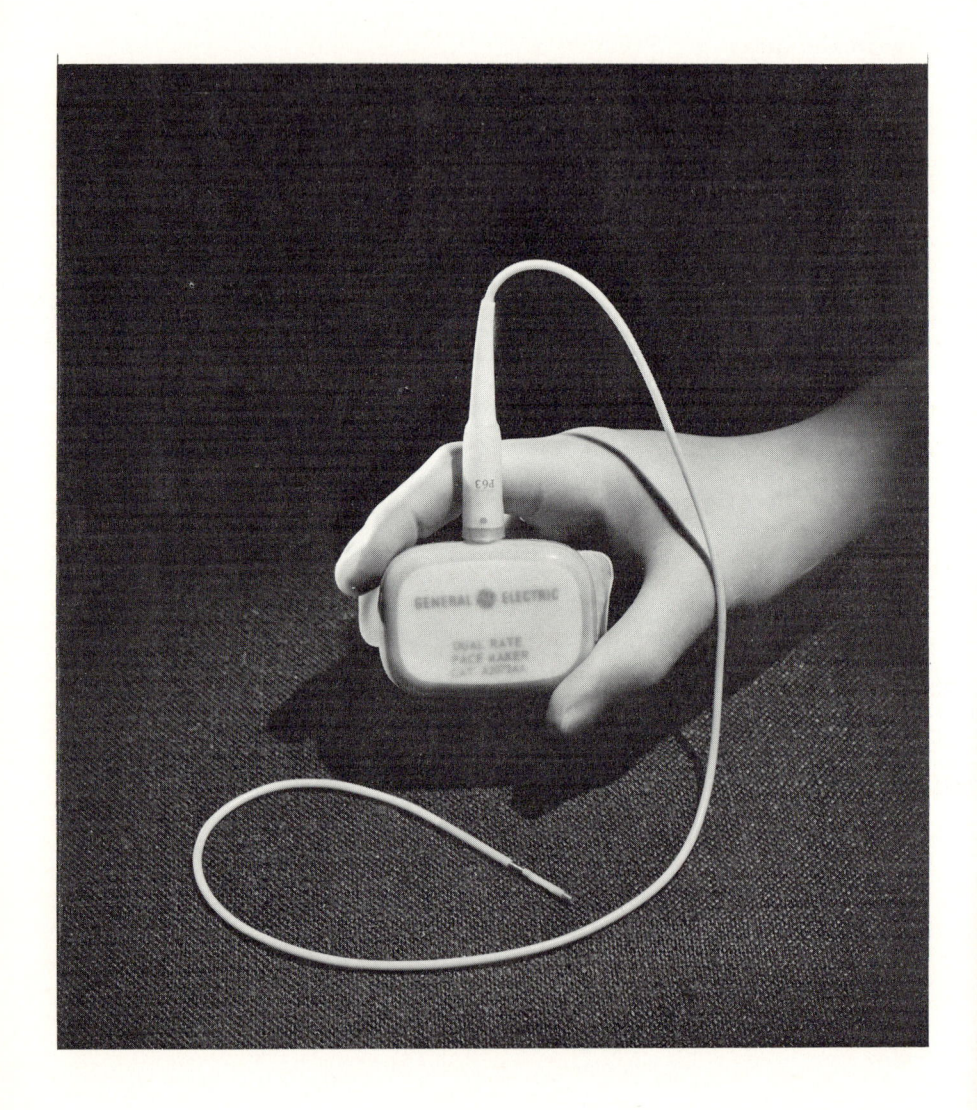

Figure 97 This is a dual rate implantable pacemaker generator with attached intracardiac catheter electrode. Thoracotomy is not required. The catheter tip is threaded into the apex of the right ventricle through the superior vena cava, usually from the right external jugular vein. It is connected to the generator box buried under the pectoralis muscle of the chest.

Courtesy of General Electric

pacemaker and predict the end of battery life. No surgery or disrobing is required. Determinations are made by the placement of a small detector coil near the implanted pacemaker.

Researchers believe that the pacemaker principle may eventually be utilized for the control of hypertension, diabetes and gallbladder disease.

Heart Block due to Pacemaker Battery Failure

Indications:

> This young white male approximately two years ago sustained repair of an intra-atrial septal defect following which he developed a heart block. Subsequently, a myocardial pacemaker was inserted with the battery located in the left axilla. The battery is dead and needs to be changed.

Technique:

Under general anesthesia a transverse incision was made over the battery. The fascial lining of the battery sac was incised and opened. The General Electric battery was changed without difficulty.

The pace was being maintained at a heart rate of approximately 82/minute.

The wound was irrigated with saline and closed in two layers of running chromic catgut sutures. The patient tolerated the procedure well.

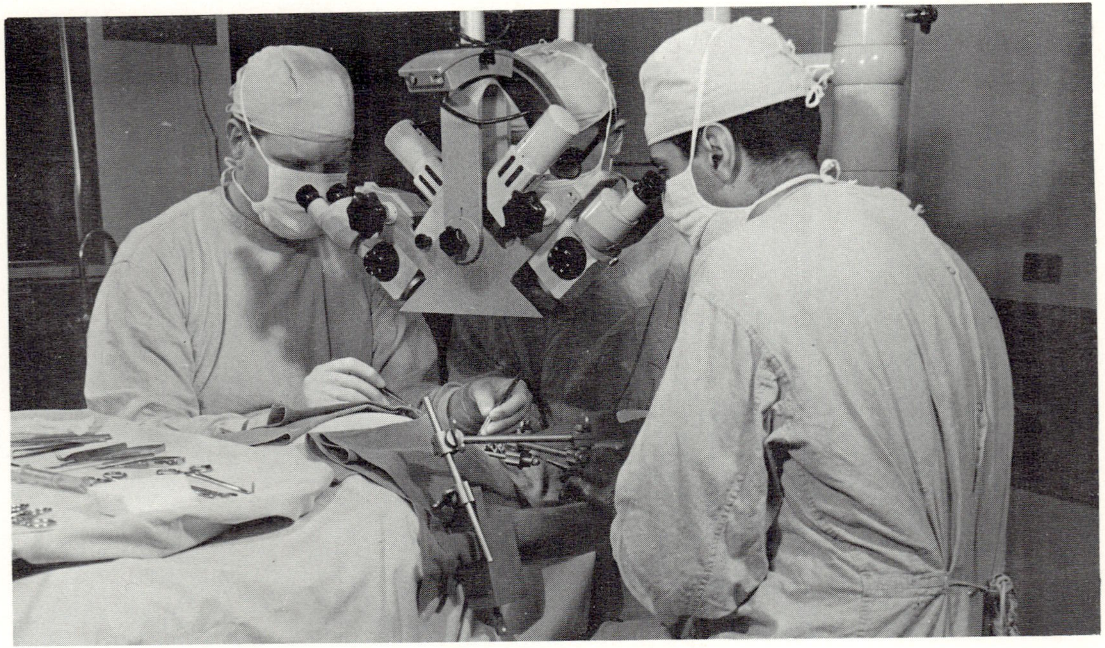

Figure 98 Using a double binocular microscope surgeons perform new microsurgery techniques they have developed to remove fatty deposits or blood clots from vessels as small as 0.8 to 4.0 millimeters in diameter. The dissecting microscope is capable of 6- to 40- power magnification enabling the surgeon to see and operate on vessels previously considered inoperable. A special clamp stabilizes the minute vessel while the surgeon operates with instruments containing miniaturized tips and sutures thinner than human hair. The microsurgery techniques were developed by Drs. J. H. Jacobson and E. L. Suarez at Mt. Sinai Hospital, New York City.

Photo courtesy National Institute of Health

18 | The Language of Medicine

Fluency with a language requires lifelong study and dedicated effort. Thousands of words are being added to the dictionary annually. Advances in the sciences have contributed significantly to this growth with medicine figuring prominently in the development.

Medicine has a language of its own. It is a highly technical and extremely specialized mode of communication. Knowledge of one phase of this language does not assure comprehension of its other subdivisions. How many M.D.'s or D.O.'s would have any suspicion of what a doctor of veterinary medicine might be referring to when he declared that an animal was "fardel-bound with a distended omasum and inflamed abomasum."?

There is a fundamental division of terminology which constitutes the foundation basic to all divisions of medicine. This level of the language includes terms relative to anatomic position, direction and location in addition to commonly used combining forms, prefixes and suffixes. From this beginning it is possible to build a vocabulary of more particularized terms.

Initial exposure to medical terminology might prove discouraging to the student until an orderly system is introduced into the plan of study. The degree of application necessary to develop any proficiency with the language requires the same interest and determination necessary for the study of a foreign language. The element of "want to" must prevail over the element of "have to" in the student's approach to the subject. With continued study, an intelligent curiosity about unfamiliar words and liberal use of the dictionary, the language of medicine eventually becomes comprehensible.

After the student has mastered the rudiments of terminology presented in the following pages, the next step consists of learning human anatomy and physiology. The application of anatomic terms has been demonstrated in the preceding pages. Several excellent textbooks on the subject of anatomy and physiology are available. One of the most popular of such references is ANATOMY AND PHYSIOLOGY by Kimber, Gray, Stackpole and Leavell. Following a study of anatomy, the student will have sufficient background and orientation to develop her vocabulary further in terms of the technical information presented in this book.

In the space allotted here, it is impossible to do more than introduce the student to terminology and recommend steps toward further development of this knowledge. The extent to which her vocabulary will grow depends largely upon the effort and energy expended to this end.

Anatomic Position

The anatomic position consists of the body erect, facing us, with the arms at the sides and palms turned toward us. The soles of the feet are comparable anatomically to the palms of the hand and we must therefore imagine the soles of the feet turned upward facing us as are the palms. The aspect of the foot we look down on from above is actually the back of the foot although it is continuous with the front of the body. The front view of the body is regarded as the anterior or ventral aspect and yet the view of the foot continuous with it is the dorsum of the foot rather than the ventral aspect. A stationary uniform position is necessary for the development of references indicating position, direction and aspect.

The suffix -ad is used to indicate direction toward; e.g., caudad, cephalad, anteriad, posteriad, etc.

Basic to the knowledge of medical terminology is proper orientation relative to position and direction. Some of the more frequently used references are listed here with their antitheses.

POSITION REFERENCES

Anterior	Front view of the body; same as ventral view or face surface.		
Posterior	Back view of the body; same as hind or dorsal aspect.		
Inferior	Located or directed below a point of reference.		
Superior	Located or directed above a point of reference.		
Medial (mesial)	Middle or toward the middle.		
Lateral	Away from the middle, toward the outside aspect.		
Distal	Furthest point from a point of reference.		
Proximal	Nearest point to a point of reference.		
Caudal	Direction away from the head; caudad.		
Cranial	Toward the head or in the region of the head; craniad.		
Dorsal	Back or hind aspect.		
Ventral	Front or face aspect.		
Internal	Inside	**Supine**	Lying face up
External	Outside	**Prone**	Lying face down

In addition to the terms listed above, various compounded combinations of these words may be used by dropping the ending of the first word, adding the combining -i or -o and attaching the second word; e.g., mediolateral (median lateral), anterolateral (anterior lateral), posteromedial (posterior medial), dorsoposterior (dorsal posterior), etc.

Elements of Terminology

Medical terms may be analyzed into their component parts consisting of roots, stems, prefixes, infixes, suffixes, combining forms and inflectional endings. In order to build a medical vocabulary the student need not make a study of philology or even etymology, but recognition of the divisions in word structure can do much to promote facility with usage of the language.

Roots constitute the basic word element from which words are derived by one or more extensions comprised of prefixes, suffixes or inflectional changes. The stem is that portion of the word which remains unchanged throughout a given inflection. The root and stem are sometimes identical, although the stem is more often derived from the root with some formative suffix. With the aid of such suffixes, word endings are changed to indicate distinctions of case, gender, mood, person, tense, etc. These changes are called inflectional endings.

Combining forms are used so extensively throughout medical terminology that familiarity with them can assist the student immeasurably in understanding new terms. They consist of a word or word element combined with another word or word element to form a compound. These compounds may assume the form of a simple union between two words; e.g., eyebrow, workman, earache, etc. Compound words may also consist of word unions where o or i have been added to Greek or Latin stems; e.g., abdomino-anterior, abdominohysterectomy, uterosacral, etc.

Prefixes consist of one or more letters placed at the beginning of a word to modify its meaning. Infixes are inserted within the word and suffixes are placed at the end of the word to provide an inflectional, derivative or formative function.

A knowledge of commonly used prefixes and suffixes is basic to the understanding of medical terminology. Those which should prove most helpful have been listed below with some of the more important combining forms.

PREFIXES AND COMBINING FORMS	MEANING	EXAMPLE
a-, an-	negative	avascular (without vessels)
a-, ab-, abs-	away from	abstain
ad-	toward	adduct (bring toward)
aer-	air	aeremia
alb-	white	albino (without pigment)
alge-	pain	algesia (pain sensitivity)
all-	other	allaxis (exchange)
amb-	both	ambidextrous
amph-	all around	amphibious
an-, ana-	up; increase	anabolism (build up)
angio-	blood vessels	angiospasm (vessel spasm)
ante-	before	antepartum (before birth)
anti-	against	antibiotic
apo-	from	aponeurosis (expansion from tendon)
auto-	self	automatic
bi-, bis-	two; double	bistratal (in two layers)
brachy-	short	brachybasia (short steps)
brady-	slow	bradycardia (slow heartbeat)
cardi-	heart	cardiogram (heart test)
cat-, cata-	down	catabolism (breakdown)
cephal-	pert. to head	cephalalgia (headache)
chole-	gallbladder	cholecystitis (inflamed gallbladder)
chrom-	color	chromogenic (producing color)
circum-	around	circumcision
co-, com-, con-	together	combine
contra-	against	contraindicate (warn against)
cyst-	bladder	cystocele
dacry-	tears	dacryocystitis (inflamed tear sac)
dactyl-	fingers	dactyledema (edema of fingers or toes)
de-	from	deduce
demi-	half	demigauntlet (half bandage)
dent-	pert. to teeth	dentist
derma-	skin	dermatology
di-	double; in two forms	dimorphous (two forms)
dia-	between	diaphragm
diplo-	double	diplopia (seeing double)
dis-	negative; double	disjoint
dys-	difficult	dystocia (difficult childbirth)

THE LANGUAGE OF MEDICINE

PREFIXES AND COMBINING FORMS	MEANING	EXAMPLE
en-	in	encapsulated (in a capsule)
endo-	within	endoceliac (within the abdomen)
entero-	intestine	enterocolitis (inflamed intestine)
epi-	upon	epineural (upon neural arch)
eu-	well	euphoria (well-being)
ex-	out	exophthalmos (bulging eyes)
extra-	beyond; outside	extraocular (outside the eye)
fore-	in front of	foreskin
galact-	milk	galactocele (cyst of milk gland)
gastro-	stomach	gastrotomy (stomach incision)
glosso-	tongue	glossoplegia (tongue paralysis)
hemato-	pert. to blood	hematology (study of blood)
hemi-	half	hemiplegia (paralysis on one side)
hepa-	liver	hepatitis (liver infection)
hetero-	dissimilar	heterogenous
holo-	all; entire	holocephalic (entire head)
homo-	same	homogenous
hydro-	water	hydrocephalus (fluid in head)
hyper-	over; above	hypertension (elevated blood pressure)
hypo-	under; below	hypothyroidism (decreased thyroid)
idio-	peculiar to one	idiosyncrasy
ileo-	pert. to ileum	ileocecal
in-	in; into	internal
infra-	beneath	infraorbital (below orbit)
inter-	between	intermittent
intra-	within	intra-abdominal
iso-	equal	isotonic
juxta-	close by	juxtaposition
kera-	hard	keratosis (horny growth)
laryng-	larynx	laryngoscope
latero-	side	laterodeviation
leuko-	white	leukorrhea (white discharge)
lith-	stone	lithiasis
macro-	large; long	macrostomia (large mouth)
mal-	poor; inadequate	malabsorption

PREFIXES AND COMBINING FORMS	MEANING	EXAMPLE
medi-	middle	medicommissure
mega-	large	megacolon (enlarged colon)
melan-	black	melanoma (black neoplasm)
meso-	middle	mesocardia (heart in midline)
meta-	beyond	metaphysics
micro-	small	microscope
mono-	single	monograph
multi-	many	multilobular (many lobed)
myo-	muscle	myositis (inflamed muscle)
myelo-	marrow	myelocystocele
neo-	new	neonate (newly born)
nephro-	kidney	nephrolithiasis (kidney stone)
neuro-	nerve	neurosurgery
non-	not	nonunion
ob-	closing	obstruction
oculo-	eye	oculopathy (eye disease)
odont-	teeth	odontology
omo-	shoulder	omodynia (shoulder pain)
oophoro-	ovary	oophorocystectomy (excision of ovarian cyst)
orchi-	testicle	orchitis (inflamed testis)
ortho-	straight	orthopedics
os-	mouth	ostium (a mouth)
oss-	bone	osseous (bony)
osteo-	bone	osteomyelitis (bone infection)
pan-	all; entire	panhysterectomy (total removal of uterus)
para-	beyond; beside	parahepatic (beside the liver)
path-	disease	pathology
pend-	hang down	pendulous
per-	through	percussion (through tapping)
peri-	around	periosteum (bone covering)
phleb-	vein	phlebothrombosis (vein clot)
pneu-	air	pneumothorax (air in chest)
poly-	many	polychromatic (multicolored)
post-	after	postpartum (after childbirth)
pre-	before	prenatal (before delivery)
pro-	before	prophylactic (preventive)
proct-	anus	proctoscope
pseudo-	false	pseudocyesis (false pregnancy)

THE LANGUAGE OF MEDICINE

PREFIXES AND COMBINING FORMS	MEANING	EXAMPLE
psych-	mind	psychiatry
pyo-	pus	pyosalpinx (pus tubes)
re-	again; back	regain
ren-	kidneys	renal
retro-	backward	retrograde
rhino-	nose	rhinoplasty (nose repair)
sacro-	sacrum	sacrolumbar
salpingo-	tube	salpingitis (inflamed tubes)
sclero-	hard	sclerosis
semi-	half	semilunar (half moon)
sub-	under	subcutaneous (under skin)
super-; supra-	above	superficial
tact-	touch	tactile
thyro-	thyroid	thyrocele (thyroid cyst)
tox-	poison	toxicology
trans-	across	transverse
tri-	three	trilobar (three lobed)
trich-	hair	trichopathic (hair disease)
uni-	one	unilateral (one side)
uro-	urine	urogenital
vaso-	vessel	vasoconstrictor
vesic-	bladder	vesicotomy (bladder incision)
xanth-	yellow	xanthochromic (yellow colored)

SUFFIXES

The prefixes frequently indicate the site of the disease process, operation or point of reference. The suffixes more often indicate the pathology, type of operation or phenomena occurring at the site.

-algesia	pain	analgesia (loss of pain)
-cele	cyst; hernia	cystocele (hernia of bladder wall)
-cide	to kill	germicide
-cyte	cell	lymphocyte
-dynia	pain	coccygodynia (pain in coccyx)
-ectomy	cutting out	splenectomy (cutting out spleen)

-emesis	vomiting	hyperemesis (excessive vomiting)
-emia	blood	uremia (urinary elements in blood)
-esthesia	feeling	anesthesia (without feeling)
-flect	divert	reflect
-form	form	malformed
-fuge	flee; repel	centrifuge
-genetic	form; originate	cytogenic (producing cells)
-gogue	to flow	hemagogue (favoring discharge of blood)
-gram	tracing; graph	electrocardiogram
-iasis	pathologic	amebiasis (amebic infection)
-ism	condition	alcoholism
-itis	inflammation	glossitis (inflamed tongue)
-ize	to treat	adrenalectomize (to remove adrenals)
-kinesis	motion	hyperkinesia (increased mobility)
-lith	stone	cholelith
-logy	study of	hematology (study of blood)
-lysis	separation	enterolysis (separating intestines)
-megaly	very large	acromegaly (enlarged bones)
-meter	measure	centimeter (unit of measure)
-oid	shape	scaphoid (boat-shaped)
-oma	tumor; neoplasm	hepatoma (liver tumor)
-osis	disease	sclerosis
-ostomy	incision into	gastrostomy (stomach incision) with drainage
-otomy	cutting into	ileotomy (incision into ileum)
-pellent	drive	repellent
-penia	deficiency	pancytopenia (deficiency of cell components of the blood)
-phobia	fear	agoraphobia (fear of wide open areas)
-phylaxis	protection	prophylaxis
-plasty	restoration	cineplasty (muscle restoration)
-plegia	stroke; paralysis	hemiplegia (paralysis on one side)
-rhagia	flow	hemorrhage; menorrhagia
-rhaphy	repair	herniorrhaphy
-rhea	discharge	rhinorrhea (nasal discharge)
-sclerosis	hardness	arteriosclerosis
-scopy	to view	cystoscopy (viewing of bladder)
-stomosis	form a mouth	anastomosis
-tomy	cutting	vagotomy (cutting vagus nerves)
-uria	urine	hematuria (blood in urine)

THE LANGUAGE OF MEDICINE

COMMONLY USED MEDICAL ABBREVIATIONS AND SYMBOLS

A_2	aortic second sound
abort.	abortion
a.c.	before meals
AJ	ankle jerk
A-P	anteroposterior
A-P & Lat	anteroposterior and lateral
A-V	arteriovenous
abd	abdomen
accom.	accommodation
acid p'tase	acid phosphatase
ad. lib	at pleasure
alk. p'tase	alkaline phosphatase
adm.	admission
alb	albumin
amp	ampule
ant. ax line	anterior axillary line
aort. regurg	aortic regurgitation
aort. sten	aortic stenosis
aur. fib.	auricular fibrillation
b.i.d.	twice a day
bis	twice
BM	bowel movement
BMR	basal metabolic rate
BP	blood pressure
BRP	bathroom privileges
BSP	bromsulphalein
BUN	blood urea nitrogen
baso	basophile
bili	bilirubin
bl. cult.	blood culture
br. sounds	breath sounds
c	with
CC.	chief complaint
cc.	cubic centimeter
cap.	capsule
CA	carcinoma
ca	calcium
cath.	catheter
CHO	carbohydrate
chol.	cholesterol
chol. est.	cholesterol esters
Cl	chloride
cldy	cloudy
cm.	centimeter (2.5 cm = 1 inch)

COMMONLY USED MEDICAL ABBREVIATIONS AND SYMBOLS

cmpd	compound
cont	continued
cta	catamenia
D & C	dilation & curettage
DL	danger list
DIE	died in Emergency Rm.
DOA	dead on arrival
decr	decreased
DERM	dermatology
diag	diagnosis
dil	dilute
dim	one half (ss)
disch	discharge
div	divide
dr.	dram
EKG	electrocardiogram
EDC	estimated date of confinement
EEG	electroencephalogram
ENT	ears, nose and throat or **Ear, Nose & Throat** specialty
EOM	extraocular movement
emul	emulsion
epith	epithelium
expir.	expiration; expiratory
F	Fahrenheit temperature
FH	family history
FB	foreign body
fract.	fracture
F.U.O.	fever of undetermined **origin**

Fetal Position & Presentation:

LOA	left occiput anterior
LOT	left occiput transverse
LOP	left occiput posterior
ROA	right occiput anterior
ROT	right occiput transverse
ROP	right occiput posterior
LSA(RSA)	left sacrum anterior (rt.)
LST(RST)	left sacrum transverse (rt.)
LSP(RSP)	left sacrum posterior (rt.)
LFA(RFA)	left fronto-anterior (right)
LFT(RFT)	left frontotransverse (rt.)
LFP(RFP)	left frontoposterior (rt.)
LMA(RMA)	left mento-anterior (right)
LMT(RMT)	left mentotransverse (right)
LMP(RMP)	left mentoposterior (right)

THE LANGUAGE OF MEDICINE

COMMONLY USED MEDICAL ABBREVIATIONS AND SYMBOLS

GBS	gallbladder series
G.I.	gastrointestinal
G.U.	genito-urinary
Gm.	gram
gr	grain
Grav. I	pregnancy one
gtt.	drops
Gyn.	Gynecology
(H)	per hypo
Hct	hematocrit
Hgb	hemoglobin
hpf	per high powered field
h.s.	at bedtime
I^{131}	radioactive iodine
I & D	incision and drainage
IM	intramuscular
I Q	intelligence quotient
IV	intravenously
IVP	intravenous pyelogram
incr.	increase
inspir	inspiration
K	potassium
KJ	knee jerk
KUB	kidney, ureter & bladder (X-ray =plain film of the abdomen)
Kg.	kilogram
L	left
LLL	left lower lobe (lung)
LUL	left upper lobe (lung)
LLQ	left lower quadrant of the abdomen
LUQ	left upper quadrant of the abdomen
LMP	last menstrual period
LNMP	last normal menstrual period
lot	lotion
LP	lumbar puncture
l & w	living and well
lab	laboratory
lat	lateral
lb	pound
lymphs	lymphocytes
M_1	mitral first
mEq	milliequivalents
mg	milligram

COMMONLY USED MEDICAL ABBREVIATIONS AND SYMBOLS

med	medicine
Mg	magnesium
mg%	milligrams per 100 milliliters
mitt	send
ml	milliliter
mm.	millimeter
Mn	manganese
mono	monocyte
Na	sodium
NB	newborn
NB:	note well
NPN	nonprotein nitrogen
NPO	nothing by mouth
NS	Neurosurgery
noct	nocturnal
OB	Obstetrics
O_2	oxygen
O_2 cap.	oxygen capacity
O_2 sat.	oxygen saturation
O.D.	right eye
OR	operating room
O.S.	left eye
OT	old tuberculin
O.U.	both eyes
Ortho.	Orthopedics
P	phosphorus
P_2	pulmonic second heart sound
P-A	postero-anterior
PBI	protein bound iodine
pc	after meals
PE	physical examination
PH	past history
pH	hydrogen ion concentration—pH 7.00 = neutral; pH below 7.00 is acid and above is alkaline
PI	present illness
p.o.	by mouth
p.r.	per rectum
prn	as often as necessary
Para I	woman with one child
Ped	Pediatrics
P & A	percussion & auscultation
P.T.	Physical Therapy

COMMONLY USED MEDICAL ABBREVIATIONS AND SYMBOLS

polys .... polymorphonuclear leucocytes
prep. .... preparation
prot .... protein
pro. time .... prothrombin time
pt. .... patient
Pelvic Measurements (pelvimetry)

> DC .... diagonal conjugate
> OC .... obstetrical conjugate
> bisp .... bispinous diameter (interspinous diameter)
> IT .... intertuberous
> Ant. Sag .... anterior sagittal diameter
> Post. Sag .... posterior sagittal diameter
> A-P D .... anteroposterior diameter
> Trans D .... transverse diameter

PSP .... phenolsulfonphthalein

q .... every
q AM .... every morning
q d .... every day
q.i.d. .... four times daily
q.n. .... every night
q.s. .... as much as suffices
q.n.s. .... quantity not sufficient
q 2 h .... every two hours
q 3 h .... every three hours
quant. .... quantity

rbc .... red blood cell
RBC .... red blood count
Rh .... Rhesus blood factor
RRE .... round, regular and equal
Rx .... therapy
R/O .... rule out

s .... without
SB .... stillborn
SC .... subcutaneous
SH .... social history
sol .... solution
s.o.s. .... repeat once if urgent need exists
SR .... review of systems
ss enema .... soap suds enema
sed. rate .... erythrocyte sedimentation rate

COMMONLY USED MEDICAL ABBREVIATIONS AND SYMBOLS

sp. gr	specific gravity
spec	specimen
Staph	Staphylococcus
stat	immediately
Strep	Streptococcus
subling	under the tongue
SURG	Surgery; surgical
sympt	symptoms
tab	tablet
T & A	tonsillectomy and adenoidectomy
t.i.d.	three times per day
TPR	temp, pulse & resp.
TBC	tuberculosis
URI	upper respiratory infection
Urol.	Urology
vag	vaginal
VD	venereal disease
WD, WN	well developed and well nourished
wbc	white blood cell
WBC	white blood count
wt	weight

MEDICAL SYMBOLS

ℨ	dram
℥	ounce
>	greater than
<	less than
♀	female
♂	male

19 } *Style Guide*

Some of the most perplexing problems which beset the secretary have to do with three items classified in the category of style. These include punctuation, capitalization and hyphenization. Many rules have been set down by many authorities with listings of exceptions which always outnumber the rules. There is no universal concurrence on the subject of style. Seldom do two authorities agree completely in all respects. Usage has a great nullifying effect on rules. The degree to which usage is recognized as an important enough factor to warrant exception to a rule likewise varies with authorities.

Those rules which most readily apply to common transcription problems have been listed here.

Formation of Plurals

Numerous situations exist in medical terminology where irregular plural endings are used. The singular and plural endings are given here with medical terms which illustrate these endings.

SINGULAR ENDING	PLURAL ENDING	EXAMPLES (SINGULAR AND PLURAL FORMS)
a	ae	aorta-aortae; verruca-verrucae ampulla-ampullae; pleura-pleurae vertebra-vertebrae; intima-intimae
ax	aces	thorax-thoraces
en	ina	foramen-foramina; lumen-lumina tegmen-tegmina; flumen-flumina
ex	ices	cortex-cortices; vertex-vertices
is	es	anastomosis-anastomoses; testis-testes pubis-pubes; unguis-ungues

SINGULAR ENDING	PLURAL ENDING	EXAMPLES (SINGULAR AND PLURAL FORMS)
is	ides	iris-irides; epulis-epulides
ix	ices	appendix-appendices; varix-varices
on	a	phenomenon-phenomena
u	ua	cornu-cornua; genu-genua
um	a	dorsum-dorsa; curriculum-curricula frenulum-frenula; medium-media infundibulum-infundibula
ur	ora	femur-femora
us	i	annulus-annuli; meniscus-menisci; embolus-emboli; fundus-fundi; alveus-alvei; fungus-fungi; (but: crus-crura)
x	ces	calyx-calyces; falx-falces
y	ies	anomaly-anomalies; biopsy-biopsies; deformity-deformities

Capitalization

We cannot attempt to list rules to cover every conceivable situation where a question regarding the use of a capital letter might arise; however, a list has been prepared to cover the usual instances where problems develop.

Capitalize the First Letter of:

1. Proper nouns (name of a particular person, place or thing) and proper adjectives in English and Latin.
2. Trade-mark names; e.g., Pyrex tube, Ethicon sutures, Teflon, and trade names of drugs.
3. Scientific Latin names but not their English derivatives; e.g., Obliquus abdominis internus (but: internal oblique muscle).
4. Names of genera but not of species; e.g., Escherichia coli, Aerobacter aerogenes, Staphylococcus pyogenes.
5. Derivatives of proper names; e.g., Foley catheter; Jurasz laryngeal forceps; Cantor tube.
6. Abbreviated forms of proper names and titles of tests; e.g., NPN, PBI, IVP, VDRL.

Do Not Capitalize:

1. A common noun or adjective standing in the place of a proper noun; e.g., acid-fast bacilli
2. Words derived from proper nouns which have developed specialized meanings; e.g., platonic, cesarean section, pasteurize, bunsen burner, fallopian tube
3. Usage sanctions the lowercasing of some proper names. When in doubt, consult the dictionary.
4. Units of measurement; e.g., centimeter (cc); ounce (oz.)

Hyphenation

Use of the hyphen is another phase of style which often proves perplexing to the secretary. In recent years the tendency has been away from hyphenation, to the extent possible, but there remain instances when it must be used to prevent misunderstanding or difficulties with pronunciation.

Rules designed to guide the secretary with the use of hyphens in medical and scientific terminology follow.

The Hyphen Is Used:

1. When the first part of the word is a capital letter.

   X-ray   Y-incision   Z-plasty
   T-tube   U-shaped   S-flap

2. Between three word segments.

   cul-de-sac   end-to-end   back-to-back
   felo-de-sac   side-to-side   Roux-en-Y

3. To avoid tripling a consonant or doubling a vowel.

   grill-like   anti-insulin   intra-abdominal
   shell-less   supra-axillary   infra-auricular

4. Between word elements in which the first ends in a vowel and the second begins with a vowel, except the combination of *iu*.

   intero-inferiorly
   para-umbilical   (but: periumbilical)

5. In compound numerals *under 100* when written out.

   forty-five
   six-and-thirty   (but: one hundred and five)

6. Between words expressing fractions when used as adjective modifiers.

   one-half size   one-quarter section

7. With two or more compounds having a common base and used in sequence. The hyphen may be used and the base omitted except for the last word.

   pre- and postoperative   in- and outpatients

The Hyphen Is Not Used:

1. After some prefixes unless followed by a proper noun or proper adjective.

bi-	non-	re-
co-	over-	sub-
ex-	post-	super-
in-	pre-	un-
inter-	pro-	under-

   EXAMPLE: international   BUT: inter-American

2. In chemical terms used as adjectives.

   sodium chloride solution
   hydrochloric acid test

3. In diagnoses or operative titles except as indicated under rules governing use of hyphens.

gastroenterostomy	NOT:	gastro-enterostomy
panhysterectomy	NOT:	pan-hysterectomy

   BUT: salpingo-oophorectomy
               Roux-en-Y anastomosis
               Z-plasty

Problems which cannot be solved with the use of these rules may be resolved with the aid of a dictionary. There are a number of sanctioned uses of hyphenation which are not covered by any of the rules. The occurrence of unwieldy word combinations should alert the secretary to the possibility of hyphenation.

GLOSSARY OF OPERATIVE TITLES

ABBE FLAP—Technique for repair of the lip.

ABDOMINAL PARACENTESIS—Direct drainage of the abdominal cavity with the aid of a trocar and cannula. Technique used to withdraw ascitic fluid accumulating in the abdomen as a result of diseases such as cirrhosis of the liver and carcinoma of the ovary.

ADENOIDECTOMY—Excision of adenoidal tissue from the nasopharynx.

ADRENALECTOMY—Removal of the adrenal gland(s).

ALBEE—Technique for spinal fusion.

ALVEOLECTOMY—Removal of the dental alveolus (tooth socket).

AMPUTATION—Removal of a projecting part of the body such as a limb, penis, breast, fingers or toes.

ANASTOMOSIS—Restoration of continuity to a passage or tube by suturing it in an end-to-side, end-to-end, or side-to-side manner.

ANEURYSMECTOMY—Surgical removal of a sac-like defect from the wall of a blood vessel.

ANEURYSMORRHAPHY—Surgical closure of the sac of an aneurysm.

ANGIECTOMY—Excision of a portion of a blood vessel.

ANGIOPLASTY—Repair and reconstruction of a blood vessel.

ANGIORRHAPHY—Suture of a blood vessel.

ANGIOTOMY—Incision into a blood vessel.

ANOPLASTY—A plastic repair of the anus.

ANOSCOPY—Examination of the anus with a proctoscopic speculum (anoscope).

ANTROTOMY—Incision through the wall of a cavity (antrum)

AORTOTOMY—Incision into the aorta.

APICECTOMY—Excision of the apex of a tooth root.

APICOLYSIS—Artificial collapse of the upper portion of the lung by divesting it of its parietal pleura.

APPENDECTOMY—Removal of the vermiform appendix situated at the distal tip of the cecum.

APPENDICOSTOMY—Incision into the intestine via the vermiform appendix for the purpose of emptying the cecum.

ARGYLL ROBERTSON—Strap operation for ectropion of the eyelid.

GLOSSARY OF OPERATIVE TITLES (Continued)

ARLT—Operation on the eyelid for symblepharon and internal tarsorrhaphy.

ARTERIECTOMY—Excision of segment of an artery.

ARTERIOPLASTY—Repair of an artery.

ARTERIOTOMY—Incision into an artery.

ARTHRECTOMY—Excision of a joint.

ARTHROCENTESIS—Incision into a joint and insertion of a needle for withdrawal of fluid.

ARTHRODESIS—Surgical immobilization of a joint.

ARTHROPLASTY—Repair and reconstruction of a joint.

ARTHROSTOMY—Temporary opening made in a joint.

ARTHROTOMY—Incision into a joint.

ARYTENOIDECTOMY—Excision of arytenoid cartilage of the larynx.

ARYTENOIDOPEXY—Surgical fixation of arytenoid cartilage.

ASPIRATION—Withdrawal of fluid, purulent matter, etc.

ASTRAGALECTOMY—Removal of astragalus (bone of ankle joint).

BAFFES—Inferior vena cava and right pulmonary vein transplant.

BALANOPLASTY—Plastic operation on the glans penis.

BANCROFT-PLENK—Operation for peptic ulcer.

BANKART—Corrective procedure for chronic shoulder dislocation.

BASIOTRIPSY—Crushing operation on the skull of a fetus for delivery when a live infant is impossible.

BASSINI—Technique for inguinal herniorrhaphy.

BAUDELOCQUE—Cutting into posterior cul-de-sac of the vagina for the purpose of removing an ovum in ectopic pregnancy.

BECK—Cardiopericardiopexy.

BECK-JIANU—Gastrostomy for stomach carcinoma.

BEER—Cataract flap operation.

BELFIELD—Cutting into deferent duct.

BERGENHEM—Implantation of ureter into rectum.

BERKE—Ptosis operation on the eyelid.

GLOSSARY OF OPERATIVE TITLES (Continued)

BILLROTH I—Resection of the pylorus with end-to-end anastomosis of the duodenum and stomach.

BILLROTH II—Resection of the pylorus and most of the lesser curvature of the stomach; closure of open ends of stomach and duodenum with a posterior gastrojejunostomy.

BIOPSY—Removal of a sample of tissue for pathologic examination.

BISCHOFF'S—Abdominal removal of a pregnant uterus.

BLAIR-BROWN—Intermediate skin graft.

BLALOCK (Blalock-Taussig)—Anastomosis of carotid artery, right or left subclavian or innominate artery to the pulmonary artery to increase pulmonary circulation in certain congenital cardiovascular conditions.

BLEPHARECTOMY—Resection of the eyelid.

BLEPHAROPLASTY—Plastic repair or reconstruction of the eyelid.

BLEPHARORRHAPHY—Repair or suturing of an eyelid; (tarsorrhaphy).

BLEPHAROTOMY—Incision into an eyelid.

BLOODGOOD—Technique for inguinal herniorrhaphy.

BONNET—Enucleation of the eyeball.

BORTHEN—Stretching operation of the iris.

BOUILLY—Partial excision of the mucous membrane of the cervix uteri.

BOWMAN—Double needle operation on a cataract, making an opening through the lens at its center and separating the membrane into two halves. Also: slitting of canaliculus of the eye.

BOZEMAN—Operation for uterovaginal fistula.

BRAILEY—Stretching of supratrochlear nerve.

BRAUN—Pinch graft technique.

BRAUER—Breaking up adhesions of the pericardium around the heart.

BRENNER—Inguinal herniorrhaphy technique utilizing the cremaster muscle for support.

BRETT—Osteoperiosteal iliac bone graft.

BROCK—Transventricular valvotomy.

BRONCHOPLASTY—Plastic repair of the bronchus.

BRONCHORRHAPHY—Repair of the bronchus.

BRONCHOSCOPY—Endoscopic examination of the bronchus utilizing a bronchoscope (viewing instrument).

GLOSSARY OF OPERATIVE TITLES (Continued)

BRONCHOSTOMY—Incision into the bronchus with aspiration or removal of contents.

BRONCHOTOMY—Incision into the bronchus.

BROWN-BLAIR—Intermediate split skin graft.

BRUNSCHWIG—Pancreatoduodenectomy; excision of pancreas and a portion of the duodenum adjacent to it.

BUROW—Flap operation used to cover a lip defect.

BURSECTOMY—Excision of a bursa.

CALDWELL-LUC—Window operation; opening made in the canine fossa for removal of contents from maxillary antrum.

CANTHOPLASTY—Plastic repair of the canthus which is the angle where the lids meet on either side of the eye.

CANTHORRHAPHY—Repair of the canthus.

CANTHOTOMY—Splitting operation of the canthus used for lengthening the palpebral fissure (opening between the upper and lower eyelids).

CAPSULECTOMY—Excision of a capsule such as that found on the lens or around the kidney. This also applies to the joint capsule.

CAPSULORRHAPHY—Repair of a capsule, especially a joint capsule.

CAPSULOTOMY—Incision into a capsule.

CARDIOCENTESIS—Surgical puncture of the heart.

CARDIOPLASTY—Repair or plastic reconstruction of the cardiac portion of the stomach; esophagogastroplasty.

CARDIORRHAPHY—Suture repair of the heart muscle.

CARDIOTOMY—Incision into the heart. Incision into the cardia of the stomach.

CARPECTOMY—Excision of carpal bones of the wrist.

CASTRATION—Removal of the testicles in the male or ovaries in the female resulting in sterility.

CATHETERIZATION—Insertion of a narrow tube into a cavity for drainage.

CATTELL—Method of reconstruction in pancreaticoduodenectomy.

CAVERNOSTOMY—Opening made in a cavity to promote drainage. (speleostomy)

CECECTOMY—Resection of the cecum; typhlectomy.

GLOSSARY OF OPERATIVE TITLES (Continued)

CECOCOLOSTOMY—Creation of a communication between the cecum and colon.

CECO-ILEOSTOMY—Creation of a communication between the cecum and ileum.

CECOPEXY—Fixation or securing operation of the cecum.

CECOSIGMOIDOSTOMY—Creation of a connection between the cecum and sigmoid.

CECOSTOMY—Creation of a fistula in the cecum.

CECOTOMY—Incision into the cecum.

CELIOTOMY—Exploratory laparotomy.

CELSUS—Lithotomy operation by cutting of the stone; amputation operation performed with a single circular maneuver of the knife.

CERVICECTOMY—Amputation of the cervix; also called a trachelectomy.

CESAREAN SECTION—Removal of fetus through an abdominal incision and direct incision into the uterus.

CHEILOPLASTY—Plastic repair of the lip.

CHOLECYSTECTOMY—Excision of the gallbladder.

CHOLECYSTODUODENOSTOMY—Creation of a direct connection between the gallbladder and duodenum.

CHOLECYSTOGASTROSTOMY—Creation of a connection between the gallbladder and stomach.

CHOLECYSTORRHAPHY—Repair or suture of the gallbladder.

CHOLECYSTOSTOMY—Incision and drainage of the gallbladder.

CHOLECYSTOTOMY—Incision into the gallbladder, usually for removal of a calculus.

CHOLEDOCHECTOMY—Surgical excision of a portion of the common bile duct.

CHOLEDOCHODUODENOSTOMY—Creation of a communication between the duodenum and common bile duct.

CHOLEDOCHOENTEROSTOMY—Creation of a communication between the common bile duct and a part of the intestine.

CHOLEDOCHOLITHOTOMY—Cutting into the common bile duct for removal of a calculus.

GLOSSARY OF OPERATIVE TITLES (Continued)

CHOLEDOCHOPLASTY—Plastic repair on the common bile duct.

CHOLEDOCHORRHAPHY—Repair of the common bile duct.

CHOLEDOCHOSTOMY—Incision into the common bile duct, usually for drainage.

CHOLEDOCHOTOMY—Incision into the common bile duct for exploration and/or removal of calculus.

CHONDRECTOMY—Excision of a cartilage.

CHOPART—Amputation of the foot through the midtarsal bones.

CHORDOTOMY—Transection of a cord nerve tract for relief of pain.

CIRCUMCISION—Male: Excision of foreskin or prepuce of glans penis. Female: Clitoridotomy.

CLARK—Technique used with subscleral implant for scleral buckling in cases of retinal detachment.

CLAVICOTOMY—Surgical division of the clavicle (collar bone).

CLEIDOTOMY—Separation of the collar bones of the fetus to facilitate delivery.

CLITORIDECTOMY—Excision of the clitoris in the female.

CLITORIDOTOMY—Female circumcision.

CLOSED REDUCTION—Reduction of a fracture or dislocation without incision.

COAKLEY—Frontal sinus operation with scraping of the mucous membrane.

COCCYGECTOMY—Excision of the coccyx (tail bone).

CODIVILLA—Use of tibial osteoperiosteal grafts for insertion around a pseudarthrosis.

COLECTOMY—Resection of the large bowel.

COLOCOLOSTOMY—Surgical formation of a continuity between two anatomically noncontinuous portions of the colon.

COLOPROCTOSTOMY—Creation of a continuity between the rectum and a section of colon not continuous with the rectum anatomically; colorectostomy.

COLOSIGMOIDOSTOMY—Formation of a connection between a portion of the colon and sigmoid.

COLOSTOMY—Formation of an artificial anus by making an opening in the colon and bringing it up through the abdominal wall.

GLOSSARY OF OPERATIVE TITLES (Continued)

COLOTOMY—Incision into the colon.

COLPECTOMY—Excision of the vagina; vaginectomy.

COLPOCLEISIS—Obliteration of the vaginal canal.

COLPOPERINEOPLASTY—Repair of the perineum and vaginal wall.

COLPOPERINEORRHAPHY—Reconstruction of the perineum and vaginal wall.

COLPOPEXY—Suspension of a prolapsed vagina by attachment to the abdominal wall.

COLPOPLASTY—Plastic repair of the vagina; elytroplasty.

COLPORRHAPHY—Tightening of a relaxed vaginal wall and excision of redundant tissue performed as an anterior repair for a cystocele and a posterior repair for a rectocele.

COLPOTOMY—Incision into the vagina; elytotomy.

COMMISSUROTOMY—Surgical division of a fibrous band.
  Mitral—Division of scar tissue around the mitral orifice by insertion of a finger with an attached scalpel blade into the mitral orifice.

CONDYLECTOMY—Excision of a condyle (rounded prominence at the articular surface of the bone).

CONJUNCTIVOPLASTY—Plastic repair of the mucous membrane which covers the anterior surface of the eyeball.

CORDOPEXY—Fixation to a side of one or both vocal cords for the relief of laryngeal stenosis.

COREOPLASTY—Plastic repair of a deformed pupil.

COTTING—Excision of tissue on either side of a persistent ingrowing toenail.

COSTECTOMY—Excision of a rib.

COSTOTRANSVERSECTOMY—Excision of the transverse process of a vertebra with its adjacent rib.

CRANIECTOMY—Excision of a section of the skull (cranium).

CRANIOCLASIS—Crushing of the fetal skull to facilitate removal of the dead fetus from the uterus.

CRANIOPLASTY—Plastic repair of a defect of the cranium (skull).

CRANIOTOMY—(Trephination). Boring of a hole in the skull for purposes of decompression, biopsy, aspiration of the brain, etc.

GLOSSARY OF OPERATIVE TITLES (Continued)

CRICOTRACHEOTOMY—Incision separating the cricoid cartilage and the upper rings of the trachea for emergency respiratory relief because of occlusion of the glottis.

CRITCHETT—Resection of anterior eyeball.

CROSBY-COONEY—Drainage of ascites (fluid accumulation) in the abdomen by means of a glass tube.

CURETTAGE—A scraping operation performed within a cavity for purposes of cleaning, debriding or biopsy.

CYCLODIALYSIS—Formation of a connection between the anterior chamber of the eye and the suprachoroidal space to relieve pressure within the eye.

CYCLODIATHERMY—Electrocoagulation of the ciliary body of the eye by use of heat produced by a high frequency current.

CYSTECTOMY—Resection of the bladder, usually the urinary bladder; (gallbladder removal—cholecystectomy); removal of a cyst.

CYSTOLITHOTOMY—Endoscopic removal of a calculus with a cystoscope.

CYSTOPLASTY—Surgical repair of a bladder defect.

CYSTORRHAPHY—Bladder repair.

CYSTOSCOPY—Endoscopic (viewing instrument with lighted tip) examination of the urinary bladder. With various attachments the cystoscope may be used for biopsy, crushing of calculi, fulguration of tumor, etc.

CYSTOSTOMY—Surgical opening made into a bladder for purposes of drainage through an abdominal incision.

CYSTOTOMY—Incision into the bladder, usually suprapubic, through the abdominal wall.

CZERNY—Radical herniorrhaphy.

DACRYOADENECTOMY—Excision of the lacrimal gland.

DACRYOCYSTECTOMY—Excision of the lacrimal sac.

DACRYOCYSTORHINOSTOMY—Formation of a communication between the lacrimal sac and nasal cavity to facilitate drainage.

DACRYOCYSTOSTOMY—Drainage of the lacrimal sac.

DACRYOCYSTOTOMY—Incision into the lacrimal sac.

DANA—Resection of the posterior spinal nerve roots for alleviation of pain.

DAVIEL—Incision into the capsule of the lens for removal of a cataract.

GLOSSARY OF OPERATIVE TITLES (Continued)

DAVIS GRAFT—Thick pinch graft of skin.

DEBRIDEMENT—Freshening and cleansing of a wound by removal of all friable, necrotic and nonviable tissue.

DECOMPRESSION—Relief of pressure.

DECORTICATION—Removal of the outer layer of an organ, usually the lung.

DEPAGE-JANEWAY—Gastrostomy for carcinoma of the stomach.

DESMOTOMY—Incisional division of a ligament.

DIAPHYSECTOMY—Partial removal of a bone, particularly the shaft of a long bone.

DICKEY—Operation for ptosis of the eyelid.

DIEFFENBACH-WARREN—Technique for palatoplasty.

DILATION—Enlargement of a canal by stretching with the aid of a dilator. Also: dilatation.

DISARTICULATION—Removal of a limb through a joint without incision through a bone.

DISCISSION—Needling as a destructive procedure, usually used in soft cataract over the lens.

DIVERTICULECTOMY—Excision of a diverticulum (abnormal pouch) in the contour of an organ such as the intestine or bladder.

DOUGLAS GRAFT—Full thickness sieve skin graft.

DRAGSTEDT—Accordion skin graft.

DRUMMOND-MORISON—Operation for the formation of anastomosis between portal venous and systemic circulation to relieve ascites.

DUDLEY—A splitting operation on the cervix uteri; suspension operation on the uterus with shortening of the round ligaments.

DÜHRSSEN INCISION—Three surgical incisions into the cervix at 2, 6 and 10 o'clock for purposes of rapid dilation to facilitate delivery of the infant.

DÜHRSSEN'S OPERATION—Fixation of the uterus to the vagina.

DUODENECTOMY—Resection of the duodenum (first portion of small intestine).

DUODENOCHOLEDOCHOTOMY—Cutting into the common bile duct and proximal duodenum.

GLOSSARY OF OPERATIVE TITLES (Continued)

DUODENOCHOLEDOCHOSTOMY—Formation of a communication between the common bile duct and the duodenum.

DUODENODUODENOSTOMY—Formation of a communication between two noncontinuous portions of the duodenum.

DUODENOENTEROSTOMY—Formation of a communication between the duodenum and another portion of the intestine such as the jejunum, ileum, duodenum, etc.

DUODENORRHAPHY—Repair of the duodenum following perforation or tear.

DUODENOSTOMY—Incision into the duodenum, usually for drainage.

DUODENOTOMY—Cutting into the duodenum, usually for exploration.

DUPUY-DUTEMPS—Technique of dacryocystorhinostomy.

DURAPLASTY—Plastic repair of the outer layer (dura mater) enveloping the brain.

ECK'S—End-to-end anastomosis between portal vein and inferior vena cava.

EDEBOHLS—Stripping of kidney capsule to promote better vascular supply.

ELECTROCOAGULATION—Passage of high frequency current through tissue producing coagulation of tissue cells and also destruction of tissue.

ELLIOT—Trephination of the eyeball for relief of tension as associated with glaucoma.

ELLIS—Bilateral vagotomy plus procedure for excision of esophageal stricture and esophagogastric junction with resection of distal end of stomach with antrum and reconstruction of continuity by esophagogastrostomy and gastroduodenostomy of Schoemaker, Billroth I type.

EMBOLECTOMY—Incision into a blood vessel for removal of an embolus (plug usually made up of portion of a blood clot which has broken off a thrombus).

EMMETT—Operation for suture of the cervix.

ENDOSCOPY—Examination of a body cavity by introduction of a scope with a lighted tip; includes specific examinations such as bronchoscopy, laryngoscopy, cystoscopy, proctoscopy, etc.

ENTERECTOMY—General term for resection of a portion of the intestine (enteron); specifically it may be a duodenectomy, jejunectomy, ileectomy, etc.

ENTEROENTEROSTOMY—General term for an anastomosis formed surgically between two noncontinuous sections of the intestine; more specifically, it may be a duodenoduodenostomy, jejunojejunostomy, etc.

GLOSSARY OF OPERATIVE TITLES (Continued)

ENTEROLYSIS—Division of adhesions between intestines.

ENTEROPEXY—Suspension or attachment, for purposes of fixation, of a portion of intestine to the abdominal wall.

ENTERORRHAPHY—Suturing of an intestine for closure purposes.

ENTEROSTOMY—Formation of an orifice for excretion of feces through the abdominal wall by bringing the intestine up through the wall and making an opening; specifically, called a colostomy, ileostomy, etc.

ENTEROTOMY—Incision into an intestine.

ENUCLEATION—Shelling out of an organ, cyst or tumor in toto.

EPIDIDYMECTOMY—Removal of the epididymis (portion of the excretory duct of the testes).

EPIDIDYMOTOMY—Incision into the epididymis.

EPIDIDYMOVASOSTOMY—Formation of a communication between the epididymis and vas deferens when obstruction occurs in the ductus deferens leading from the epididymis to the prostatic urethra.

EPIGASTRIC HERNIORRHAPHY—Repair of a defect in the wall of the middle upper region of the abdomen.

EPIGLOTTIDECTOMY—Excision of the epiglottis (cartilaginous plate which closes over the windpipe opening in the process of swallowing).

EPILATION—Extraction of hair from the eyelid, face etc. (depilation)

EPIPLOECTOMY—Excision of omentum (epiploon).

EPIPLOPEXY—Suturing of the omentum to the abdominal wall.

EPIPLORRHAPHY—Suturing of the omentum.

EPISIOTOMY—Incision of the vulva prior to delivery to facilitate delivery and prevent laceration.

ESOPHAGECTOMY—Resection of the esophagus.

ESOPHAGODUODENOSTOMY—Surgical formation of a continuity between the esophagus and the duodenum.

ESOPHAGOGASTROSTOMY—Surgical formation of a communication between the stomach and esophagus.

ESOPHAGOPLASTY—Plastic repair of the esophagus.

ESOPHAGOSCOPY—Endoscopic (use of scope) examination of the esophagus.

ESOPHAGOTOMY—An incision into the esophagus.

GLOSSARY OF OPERATIVE TITLES (Continued)

ESSER—Operation for epithelial inlay.

ESTES—Therapeutic operation for sterility consisting of implantation of an ovary into a uterine cornu.

ESTLANDERS—Operation performed for empyema (accumulation of pus in pleural cavity) in which ribs and involved pleura are excised to permit collapse of the abnormal cavity.

ETHMOIDECTOMY—Resection operation of the ethmoid sinuses.

EVERBUSCH—Procedure for correcting ptosis of the eyelid.

EXCISION—Cutting out; surgical incisional removal.

EXENTERATION—Surgical removal of the contents (anatomic) of an organ or cavity; procedure for bringing the bowel up through the abdominal wall.

EXPLORATORY—Procedure performed in search for pathology; exploratory laparotomy of the abdomen.

EXTERIORIZATION—Temporary exposure of a viable organ by bringing it outside the body cavity, e.g., exteriorization of bowel.

EXTIRPATION—Removal of a structure or mass in toto.

EXTRACTION—Process of removal by drawing or pulling out.

FALK-SHUKURIS—Hysterectomy with cornual excision by means of a transverse fundal incision.

FARABEUF—Surgical division of the ischiopubic ramus and ascending ramus of the pubes.

FASCIECTOMY—Excision of fascia.

FASCIODESIS—Suturing of fascia to a skeletal attachment.

FEHLING—Operation on the anterior vaginal wall for prolapse of the uterus.

FEMORAL HERNIORRHAPHY—Repair of a femorocele or bulging defect in the crural or upper thigh region.

FENESTRATION—Formation of a window or opening; operation to improve hearing in cases of otosclerosis by making an opening into the labyrinth.

FERGUSON REPAIR—Technique for repair of an inguinal hernia.

FERGUSSON—Excision of the upper jaw bone (maxilla).

FINNEY—Formation of an enlarged opening between the stomach and duodenum. Finney modification of von Haberer-Billroth I.

GLOSSARY OF OPERATIVE TITLES (Continued)

FINOCHIETTO—Method of Billroth I.

FINSTERER—Modification of Billroth II.

FINSTERER-HOFMEISTER—Gastric resection in gastric carcinoma or duodenal ulcer.

FISTULECTOMY—Excision of a fistula (abnormal communication between two cavities or a hollow organ and the abdominal wall).

FISTULOTOMY—Incision into a fistula.

FOERSTER—Operation performed in locomotor ataxia which involves transsection intradurally of the 7th, 8th and 9th dorsal nerve roots.

FOERSTER-PENFIELD—Removal of scar tissue from the brain in an attempt to treat traumatic epilepsy.

FOLEY—Procedure for relief of ureteropelvic junction stricture consisting of a Y-plasty operation.

FOTHERGILL—Suspension of the cardinal ligaments for relief of uterine prolapse. Manchester operation.

FOWLER—Decortication of the lung in pulmonary empyema.

FOX—Operation for senile entropion.

FRANCO—Incision into the urinary bladder via an abdominal route.

FRANK—Gastrostomy with formation of a communication of the stomach and chest wall through which a tube is inserted.

FRANKE'S—Removal of intercostal nerves in cases of tabes.

FREDET-RAMSTEDT—Pyloroplasty consisting of a longitudinal incision of the thickened serosa and muscularis in cases of pyloric stenosis.

FREUND'S—Total removal of the uterus for cancer; surgical division of cartilage in funnel chest deformity.

FREYER'S—Suprapubic enucleation of prostate.

FRIEDRICH'S—In cases of unilateral tuberculosis, removal of ribs on one side of chest to cause collapse of the lung. Pleuropneumonolysis.

FROMMEL'S—Operation for correcting the retrodisplacement of the uterus by shortening the uterosacral ligaments.

FROST-LANG—Insertion of a gold ball prosthesis for cosmetic purposes following enucleation of the eyeball.

FUCH'S—Technique for tarsorrhaphy.

FUKALA—Lens removal in severe nearsightedness.

GLOSSARY OF OPERATIVE TITLES (Continued)

FULGURATION—Utilization of sparks from a d'Arsonval current for destruction of tissue.

FUSION—Operation for uniting two structures as in spinal fusion where an immobilization of two segments of the bony spine is formed.

GALBIATI'S—Bilateral ischiopubiotomy performed on a fetus to facilitate delivery in contracted pelvis.

GANGLIONECTOMY—Excision of a ganglion which may be a collection of nerve cells or may manifest the form of a cystic tumor of a tendon sheath.

GANT'S—Division of the shaft of the long thigh bone below the lesser trochanter to cause ankylosis of the hip joint.

GASTRECTOMY—Resection of the stomach.

GASTRODUODENOSTOMY—Surgical formation of a communication between the stomach and the duodenum.

GASTROGASTROSTOMY—Communication formed surgically between the pylorus and cardiac portion of the stomach.

GASTROJEJUNOSTOMY—Formation of a communication between the stomach and the jejunum.

GASTROMYOTOMY—Incision through the muscular wall of the stomach (pylorus).

GASTRORRHAPHY—Repair of a stomach wound.

GASTROSCOPY—Examination of the interior stomach by means of a scope inserted via the mouth and esophagus.

GAUNTLET FLAP—A plastic procedure using a piece of tissue connected at one end to its original site. Used to cover a defect of the hand and fingers.

GENYPLASTY—Plastic operation on the cheek (of the face).

GERSUNY—Operation performed on the rectum for incontinence of feces; performed also on female urethra for urinary incontinence.

GIFFORD—Incision into the cornea.

GIFFORD-PUNTENNY—Procedure for correcting ptosis of the eyelid.

GIGLI—Sectioning of the os pubis with a Gigli chain saw to facilitate delivery of the fetus.

GILL—Insertion of a wedge of bone to limit plantar flexion in cases of foot drop (paralysis of dorsiflexor muscles of foot causing toes to drag in walking).

GILLIES GRAFT—A tube graft.

GLOSSARY OF OPERATIVE TITLES (Continued)

GILLIAM—Operation on the round ligaments for suspension of the uterus in cases of uterine retroversion.

GILLIES OPERATION—Use of an epithelial flap to form skin of the eyelid in ectropion of the eyelid.

GINGIVECTOMY—Excision of a section of the gums of the mouth.

GOEBEL-STOECKEL—Suspension of the uterus.

GLOSSECTOMY—Resection of the tongue.

GOFFE—Operation for correction of cystocele (defect in anterior vaginal wall).

GONIN—In cases of retinal detachment, closure of the laceration by electrocautery.

GONIOTOMY—Operation performed in certain cases of glaucoma consisting of the opening of Schlemm's canal under direct vision.

GOTTSCHALK—Shortening of uterosacral ligaments suspending uterus via the vaginal route.

GRABER-DUVERNAY—Boring holes leading to the center of the femoral head for the purpose of promoting circulation.

GRAFT—Implantation of skin, bone, tissue, etc. for the purpose of correcting a defect.

GRANT'S—Operation for excision of tumor of the lip and reapproximating the lip edges cosmetically.

GRATTAGE—Removal of diseased tissue by scraping or abrasion.

GRITTI-STOKES—Supracondylar amputation of the femur with preservation of the patella.

GROSSMAN—Operation for treatment of retinal detachment by withdrawal of subretinal fluid and injection of warm salt solution into the vitreous.

GUSSENBAUER—Cutting through an esophageal stricture from an esophagotomy made above the obstruction.

GUYON—Amputation of the foot.

HAGNER—Epididymotomy for purposes of drainage.

HAHN—Gastrotomy with correction of gastric stenosis.

HALPIN—Operation for removal of lacrimal gland in toto.

HALSTED—Technique for inguinal herniorrhaphy.

HANCOCK—Amputation of the foot at the ankle joint.

GLOSSARY OF OPERATIVE TITLES (Continued)

HANDYSIDE—Ovariotomy.

HARTLEY-KRAUSE—Removal of gasserian ganglion and its roots.

HAYNES—Drainage of cisterna magna in meningitis.

HEATH—An operation performed in the mouth with division of the ascending rami of the lower jaw for ankylosis.

HEATON—Technique for inguinal herniorrhaphy.

HEGAR—Technique for perineorrhaphy.

HEINE—Operation for relieving pressure in glaucoma. (cyclodialysis)

HEINEKE—Operation for cancer of the rectum.

HEINEKE-MIKULICZ—Technique for pyloroplasty.

HEISRATH—Operation for trachoma of conjunctiva and cornea by excision of the tarsal folds.

HELLER—Esophagocardiomyotomy.

HEMIGLOSSECTOMY—Resection of half of the tongue.

HEMILAMINECTOMY—Resection of laminae of the vertebra of one side only.

HEMILARYNGECTOMY—Resection of a half of the larynx.

HEMINEPHRECTOMY—Resection of a part of the kidney.

HEMITHYROIDECTOMY—Subtotal resection of the thyroid.

HEMORRHOIDECTOMY—Excision of infected rectal varices.

HEPATECTOMY—Resection of a portion of the liver.

HEPATICODUODENOSTOMY—Formation of a communication between the hepatic duct and the duodenum.

HEPATICOGASTROSTOMY—Formation of a communication between the hepatic duct and the stomach.

HEPATICOLITHOTOMY—Cutting into the hepatic duct for the purpose of removing calculi.

HEPATICOSTOMY—Opening made into the hepatic duct.

HEPATORRHAPHY—Repair of the liver.

HERBERT—Formation of a filtering cicatrix in glaucoma using a displaced wedge-shaped portion of sclera.

GLOSSARY OF OPERATIVE TITLES (Continued)

HERNIORRHAPHY—Repair of a weakened body wall which has permitted bulging of cavity contents.

HERNIOTOMY—Operation for repair of hernia; kelotomy, celotomy.

HEWETT—Ligation of the oviduct in three sections for the purpose of producing sterility.

HEY—Foot amputation with the incision made just before the tarsometatarsal joint.

HIBBS—Operation performed for stabilizing the spine or hip. Hibbs spinal fusion; Hibbs arthrodesis of the hip.

HOCHENEGGE—Rectal operation for carcinoma.

HOFFA (Hoffa-Lorenz)—Operation for congenital dislocation of the hip.

HOFMEISTER-FINSTERER—Gastric resection with gastrojejunostomy.

HOFMEISTER-POLYA—Antecolic gastrojejunostomy.

HOLMES—Operation for excision of the os calcis.

HOLTH—Punch operation for removal of sclera of the eye.

HORSLEY—Method of Billroth I and pyloroplasty.

HOTCHKISS—Plastic repair of facial defect in the cheek region.

HOTZ-ANAGNOSTAKIS—Procedure for correcting entropion of the eyelid.

HUGGINS—Castration operation performed for carcinoma of the prostate.

HUGHES—Operation for lower lid repair.

HUGIER—Right lateral incision into the colon.

HUNT—Technique of inguinal herniorrhaphy.

HUNTER—Operation for relief of aneurysm with ligation of the vessel proximal to the defect.

HUNT-TONSLEY—Repair of ptosis of the eyelid.

HYMENOTOMY—Incision with enlargement of the hymenal ring in an imperforate hymen (membranous tissue covering the external vaginal orifice).

HYPOPHYSECTOMY—Excision of the pituitary body.

HYSTERECTOMY—Removal of the uterus, totally or partially, either through an abdominal or vaginal route.

HYSTEROTOMY—Incision into the uterus.

GLOSSARY OF OPERATIVE TITLES (Continued)

ILEECTOMY—Surgical resection of the distal portion of the small intestine (ileum). DO NOT CONFUSE WITH ILIUM (hip bone).

ILEOCECOSTOMY—Formation of a surgical communication between the ileum and cecum.

ILEOCOLOSTOMY—Formation of a surgical communication between the ileum and colon.

ILEOILEOSTOMY—Formation of a communication between two parts of the ileum.

ILEOSIGMOIDOSTOMY—Formation of the communication between the ileum and sigmoid flexure.

ILEOSTOMY—A surgical opening made into the ileum.

IMPLANT OPERATION—Insertion of a prosthesis to simulate a normal anatomic structure or contour.

IMRE—Procedure for correcting ectropion and repair of lid notch.

INCUDECTOMY—Surgical removal of the incus (one of the three ossicles of the middle ear, often referred to as the "anvil").

INDIAN OPERATION—Plastic operation for covering a nasal defect with a flap taken from the forehead.

INGUINAL HERNIORRHAPHY—Repair of a hernia in the groin.

ITALIAN OPERATION—Plastic operation for repair of a nasal defect with a flap taken from the arm.

INTERCRICOTHYROTOMY—Inferior laryngotomy; incision into the larynx through the cricothyroid membrane.

INTERPOSITION—Suspension operation on the uterus for correction of a positional defect; hysteropexy.

IRIDECTOMY—Excision of a portion of the iris (pigmented circular band around the pupil).

IRIDENCLEISIS—Displacement of the pupil by constriction of a portion of the iris in an incision of the cornea.

IRIDODIALYSIS—Detachment of the outer edge of the iris from its ciliary attachment.

IRIDOTASIS (Borthen Operation)—Stretching operation of the iris performed in glaucoma.

IRIDOTOMY—Incision into the iris.

GLOSSARY OF OPERATIVE TITLES (Continued)

ISCHIATIC HERNIOPLASTY—Repair of a hernia in the hip region.

ISTHMECTOMY—Excision of the isthmus of the thyroid gland; median strumectomy.

JABOULAY—Interpelvi-abdominal amputation.

JACOBAEUS—Endoscopic examination for pleural adhesions followed by lysis of adhesions with electrocautery.

JANSEN—Operation on the frontal sinus with scraping of the mucous membrane.

JARVIS—Snare removal of hypertrophic area on the lower turbinate.

JASCHE-ARLT—Procedure for entropion repair.

JAYAPATHY—Repair of tympanic membrane perforation.

JEJUNECTOMY—Resection of all or a portion of the small intestine known as the jejunum.

JEJUNOCECOSTOMY—Formation of a communication between the jejunum and the cecum.

JEJUNOCOLOSTOMY—Formation of a communication between the jejunum and the colon.

JEJUNOILEOSTOMY—Formation of a surgical communication between continuous portions of the jejunum.

JEJUNOJEJUNOSTOMY—Formation of a communication between two non-continuous portions of the jejunum.

JEJUNORRHAPHY—Repair of a wound or perforation of the jejunum.

JEJUNOSTOMY—Formation of a surgical opening into the jejunum through the abdominal wall.

JEJUNOTOMY—Incision into the jejunum.

JELK—Incisions made on both sides of the anus with incision of the rectum for relieving rectal stricture.

JIANU-BECK—Gastrostomy for carcinoma of the stomach.

JOBERT de LAMBELLE—Closure of vesicovaginal fistula.

JOLY—Total hysterectomy (panhysterectomy) for uterine prolapse.

JONNESCO—Excision of sympathetic ganglion on both sides of the neck for exophthalmic goiter.

JUDD—Pyloroplasty.

GLOSSARY OF OPERATIVE TITLES (Continued)

JUMP GRAFT—Transferring a pedicle graft from one location to another in stages.

JUDIN—Closure of duodenal stump.

KADER—Gastrostomy for carcinoma of the stomach.

KADER-SENN—Surgical formation of a gastric fistula.

KEEGAN—Plastic operation for reconstruction of the nose utilizing tissue from one side of the forehead for the flap.

KEEN—Excision of the umbilicus (navel).

KEHR—Resection of the gallbladder and cystic duct followed by drainage of the hepatic duct.

KEHRER—Correction of an inverted nipple.

KELLY—Fixation of the uterus to the anterior abdominal wall for correction of retroversion.

KERATECTOMY—Excision of a portion of the cornea of the eye.

KERATOCENTESIS—Puncture of the cornea.

KERATOPLASTY—Plastic operation on the cornea; e.g., corneal grafting, trephination, tissue replacement, etc.

KERATOTOMY—Surgical incision into the cornea.

KILLIAN—Operation on the frontal sinus with removal of the anterior wall, mucous membranes and ethmoid cells. The upper wall of the orbit is also removed with formation of a communication to the nose.

KING—Fixation of the arytenoid cartilage or muscle.

KIRMISSON—Operation for clubfoot with transplantation of the Achille's tendon to the Peroneus longus muscle.

KIRSCHNER—Operation for ruptured spleen.

KJELLAND—Cystocele repair.

KNAPP—Cataract removal without iridectomy.

KOCHER—Excision of ankle joint with suturing of the peroneal tendons.

    Resection of pylorus.
    Thyroidectomy technique.
    Reduction of dislocated humerus.
    Resection of the tongue.
    Resection of the wrist.

GLOSSARY OF OPERATIVE TITLES (Continued)

KOCK—Corrective operation for uterine prolapse or retroversion with shortening of the base of the broad ligament via a vaginal approach.

KOEBERLE—Fixation of the uterus to the anterior abdominal wall for the correction of retroversion.

KONDOLEON—Therapeutic operation in elephantiasis consisting of removal of strips of subcutaneous connective tissue.

KÖNIG—Operation for correction of congenital dislocation of the hip with reduction of the dislocation and formation of a ring-like projection on the upper border of the acetabulum, fashioned from osteoperiosteal flap taken from the ilium.

KÖRTE-BALLANCE—Operation for relief of facial paralysis consisting of anastomosis of the hypoglossal and facial nerves.

KORTZEBORN—Lengthening of extensor tendons of thumb and formation of a fascial attachment of the thumb to the ulnar side of the hand to relieve "ape hand" deformity.

KRASKE—Surgical approach to the rectum by resection of the coccyx and portion of the sacrum.

KRAUSE—Gasserian ganglionectomy in trigeminal neuralgia.

KRAUSE-WOLFE GRAFT—Full-thickness skin graft.

KRIMER—Palatoplasty; uranoplasty.

KRÖNLEIN—Removal of a portion of the lateral wall of the orbit for removal of tumor without sacrificing the eye.

KUHNT—Frontal sinus operation with resection of the anterior wall and scraping of the mucous membrane.

KUHNT-HELMHOLD—Repair of atonic ectropion of the eyelid.

KUHNT-SZYMANOWSKI—Operation for repair of atonic ectropion of eyelid.

KUSTER—Drainage procedure in mastoiditis with exposure of the antrum, attic and tympanum.

LABBE—Incision into the stomach utilizing a parietal incision along the border of the lowest left rib.

LABYRINTHECTOMY—Excision of the internal ear (labyrinth).

LAGLEYZE—Eyelid repair.

LAGRANGE—Establishment of a filtering scar in glaucoma through a combination sclerectomy and iridectomy.

GLOSSARY OF OPERATIVE TITLES (Continued)

LAHEY—Anterior gastrojejunostomy.

LAMINECTOMY—Excision of the flattened posterior aspect of the vertebral arch from which the spinous processes project.

LANDOLT—Plastic construction of the lower eyelid, the upper eyelid acting as the donor site for the skin graft.

LANE—A short-circuit type operation in which the ileum is attached to the lower portion of the sigmoid, circumventing the colon.

LANE-LANNELONGUE—Decompression of the brain with removal of sections of the bone from the roof of the skull.

LANGE—Implantation of silk strands to simulate tendon transplantation.

LANNELONGUE—Method of craniotomy employed where the head is abnormally small.

LANZ—Insertion of strips of fascia lata into the femur for relief of elephantiasis of the leg.

LAPAROTOMY—Incision through the abdominal wall usually performed for exploration of the abdominal contents.

LAROYENNE—Incision into the uterosacral excavation (pouch of Douglas) for the purpose of permitting drainage of purulent matter.

LARRY—Operation for amputation of the arm by disarticulation of the humerus at the shoulder joint.

LARYNGECTOMY—Removal of the larynx (voice organ).

LARYNGOCENTESIS—Incision into the larynx.

LARYNGOPHARYNGECTOMY—Excision of the larynx and pharynx.

LARYNGOPLASTY—Plastic repair of the larynx.

LARYNGOSCOPY—Endoscopic examination of the inner larynx by means of a laryngoscope.

LARYNGOTRACHEOTOMY—Surgical incision of the larynx and the respiratory tube (trachea) situated just below it.

LATZKO—Extraperitoneal cesarean section.

LAUREN—Plastic closure of defect remaining following mastoidectomy.

LEFEVRE—Method of esophagojejunostomy.

LEFORT—Operation for correction of prolapse of the uterus.

GLOSSARY OF OPERATIVE TITLES (Continued)

LEGG—Tensor fascia transplantation into the femur.

LENNANDER—Operation for dissecting out the inguinal glands.

LERICHE—Periarterial sympathectomy.

LEUCOTOMY—Prefrontal lobotomy of the brain.

LEXER—Resection of gasserian ganglion of the trigeminal nerve.

LIGATION—Operation for tying off a segment of a vascular channel or tubular structure.

LIPECTOMY—Excision of adipose tissue.

LISFRANC—Amputation of the foot with incision between the tarsus and the metatarsus.

LISTON—Method of resection of the upper jaw.

LITHOLAPAXY—Crushing of a calculus within the bladder with a cystoscopic approach followed by irrigation and flushing out of the fragments.

LITHOTOMY—Incision into an organ for removal of a calculus.

LITHOTRIPSY—Procedure for crushing a calculus in the bladder or urethra.

LITHOTRITY—Procedure for crushing a stone situated in the urinary bladder or urethra.

LITTRE—Method of incision into the colon through an inguinal incision.

LIZAR—Operation for resection of the upper jaw.

LOBECTOMY—Excision of a projecting part of an organ or gland such as a lobe of the lung or lobe of the thyroid gland.

LOBOTOMY—Cutting into a nerve tract in the cerebrum of the brain. An incision into a lobe.

LONGMIRE—Surgical connection of an intrahepatic biliary duct to the jejunum after partial removal of the left lobe of the liver to relieve obstruction of the hepatic duct or common bile duct.

LONGUET—Transplantation operation of testicle in the presence of varicocele and hydrocele.

LORENZ—Operation for congenital dislocation of the hip consisting of reduction of dislocation and fixing femur in position until a proper socket can be formed in the acetabulum.

LORETA—Gastrotomy with dilation of stenotic stomach opening. Also: Treatment of aneurysm by insertion of wire and electrolysis.

GLOSSARY OF OPERATIVE TITLES (Continued)

LOSSEN—Resection of the second division of the fifth nerve.

LUC (Caldwell-Luc Operation)—Incision into the maxillary sinus antrum (antrum of Highmore) for the purpose of drainage.

LUND—An operation for correcting a clubfoot (talipes) deformity by removal of the talus bone (astragalus or ankle bone).

LUDLOFF—An operation for correcting a hallux valgus deformity by an oblique incision into the first metatarsal bone.

LYMPHATICOSTOMY—Surgical opening made into a lymphatic duct.

LYON-HORGAN—An operation performed for the relief of angina pectoris consisting of severance and ligation of the superior and inferior thyroid arteries, bilaterally.

MACDOWELL—Resection of an ovary by abdominal section.

MACEWEN—An operation for knock-knee consisting of supracondyloid incision into the femur.

MACHEK-BLASKOVICS—Procedure for correcting entropion.

MACHEK-GIFFORD—Procedure for correction of ptosis of the eyelid.

MACKENRODT—Corrective operation for retrodisplacement of the uterus involving vaginal fixation of round ligaments.

MADELUNG—Incision into the colon through a lumbar incision with detachment and invagination of the distal colon.

MADLENER—Ligation of the oviducts and removal of the fimbriated ends in the female for the purpose of sterilization.

MAKKA—Utilization of the cecum as a bladder and the appendix as the ureter in cases of ectopia of the urinary bladder.

MAMMECTOMY—Excision of the breast.

MAMMILLIPLASTY—Plastic operation of the breast nipple; thelyplasty.

MAMMOTOMY—Incision into the breast.

MANCHESTER—Operation for correcting a prolapsed uterus by amputation of the cervix and fixation of the cardinal ligaments (Fothergill operation).

MARCKWALD—Operation to relieve stenosis of the external os of the uterus by excision of wedge-shaped pieces of tissue from opposite sides of the vaginal section of the cervix.

MARIAN—An operation through a median perineal route for urinary bladder calculus removal.

GLOSSARY OF OPERATIVE TITLES (Continued)

MARSHALL-MARCHETTI—Plication of the urethra for correction of urinary stress incontinence.

MARSUPIALIZATION—Incision into a cystic lesion with evacuation of its contents and approximation of the walls of the cyst to those of the external incision to permit drainage and closure by granulation of the wound.

MARWEDEL—Gastrotomy.

MASTECTOMY—Amputation of the breast.

MASTOIDECTOMY—Scraping of the mastoid area of the temporal bone and curetting out the osseous partitions which form the mastoid cells.

MASTOPEXY—Plastic corrective operation for sagging breasts; mazopexy.

MASTOPLASTY—Plastic operation of the breast; mammoplasty.

MATAS—Corrective operation for aneurysm consisting of opening the defect and resuturing the walls in such a manner as to restore a normal cylindrical lumen.

MAXILLARY ANTROTOMY—Incision into the maxillary antrum (antrum of Highmore).

MAYDL—Colostomy operation in which an open wound is maintained until adhesions are formed. A glass rod is placed beneath the exteriorized colon while it remains out of the abdominal cavity.

MAYO—Technique for posterior gastrojejunostomy involving excision of the pylorus and closure of the proximal end of the duodenum.
Also: Bunionectomy with arthroplasty of 1st metatarsophalangeal joint.

MCARTHUR—Catheterization of the common bile duct.

MCBURNEY—Technique for radical cure of inguinal hernia.

MCGILL—Suprapubic prostatectomy technique.

MCKEEVER—Arthrodesis for correction of hallux rigidus or hallux valgus of the metatarsophalangeal joint of the great toe.

MCREYNOLD—Procedure for correction of strabismus.

MEATOTOMY—Incision to enlarge the external opening of the urethra or meatus; porotomy.

MELLER—Operative technique for excision of the tear sac.

MENGE'S—Resection of the fallopian tube brought out through an inguinal incision and eventuating in sterilization of the female.

MENISCECTOMY—Excision of the fibrocartilage of the knee joint.

GLOSSARY OF OPERATIVE TITLES (Continued)

MERCIER'S—Prostatectomy technique.

MESOPEXY—Attachment or fixation of an incised or torn mesentery (mesenteriopexy).

METATARSECTOMY—Excision of the metatarsus, that portion of the foot skeleton situated between the toes and instep, consisting of five long bones.

MIKULICZ—An operation performed for wry neck (torticollis) involving excision of the sternocleidomastoid muscle.

MIKULICZ-VLADIMIROFF—Resection of the ankle which includes excision of the talus and calcaneus plus removal of the articulating surfaces of the tibia, fibula, cuboid and scaphoid. The patient thereafter has to walk on tiptoe.

MILES'—Proctosigmoidectomy; abdominoperineal resection of the rectum for carcinoma.

MINGAZZINI-FOERSTER—Cutting the 7, 8 and 9th dorsal nerve roots intradurally for locomotor ataxia.

MIRAULT—Cleft lip repair.

MOORE'S—Operation for producing coagulation in an aortic aneurysm by means of a small wire coil inserted into the aneurysmal sac.

MORESTIN'S—Intracondyloid division of the femur with disarticulation of the knee.

MOSCHCOWITZ'S—Femoral herniorrhaphy via an inguinal incision.

MOTAIS'S—An operation performed for ptosis of the eyelid in which the middle third of the tendon of the superior rectus muscle of the eyeball is transplanted into the upper lid, for the purpose of augmenting the action of the levator muscle.

MOYNIHAN—Anterior gastrojejunostomy.

MULE'S—Enucleation of the eyeball followed by insertion of a prosthesis.

MULLER'S—Technique for vaginal hysterectomy.
Sclerectomy performed for detachment of the retina.
Technique for cesarean section involving an incision into the uterus after it is brought up out of the pelvis.

MUSTARD'S—Transfer of the Iliopsoas muscle.
MYECTOMY—Resection of a muscle.

MYOMECTOMY—Excision of tumors with muscular tissue components, most commonly used to refer to excision of myomas of the uterus.

GLOSSARY OF OPERATIVE TITLES (Continued)

MYOPLASTY—Plastic operation on a muscle.

MYORRHAPHY—Repair of a muscle.

MYOTENOTOMY—Division of the tendon of a muscle.

MYOTOMY—Incision into a muscle.

MYRINGOTOMY—Surgical incision of the tympanic membrane.

NAFFZIGER'S—Operation for exophthalmos (protrusion of eyeballs) which includes resection of the super and lateral orbital walls for decompression.

NARATH'S—Operation performed in portal obstruction for the purpose of creating a collateral circulation. This is accomplished by means of fixation of the omentum to the subcutaneous tissue of the abdominal wall.

NEBINGER-PRAUN'S—Operation on the frontal sinus with removal of the anterior bony wall.

NEEDLING OF LENS—An operation for opening the capsule and breaking up the soft or secondary cataract; discission of lens.

NELATON'S—Utilization of a transverse incision to remove the shoulder joint.

NEPHRECTOMY—Excision of the kidney.

NEPHROLITHOTOMY—Removal of a kidney calculus.

NEPHROLYSIS—Lysis or breaking up of the adhesions formed about the kidney.

NEPHROPEXY—Fixation or suspension of a mobile kidney.

NEPHRORRHAPHY—Suture of the kidney.

NEPHROSTOMY—Creation of an opening from the kidney pelvis to the outside of the body.

NEPHROTOMY—Incision into the kidney.

NEUBER—Operation for obliterating a bone cavity with skin flaps developed from the sides of the wound.

NEURECTOMY—Resection of a segment of nerve.

NEUROLYSIS—Lysis or destruction of perineural adhesions.

NEUROPLASTY—Plastic repair of a nerve.

NEURORRHAPHY—Suture of a nerve.

NEUROTOMY—Surgical division of a nerve.

GLOSSARY OF OPERATIVE TITLES (Continued)

NEUROTRIPSY—Operation for crushing of a nerve.

NICOLA—Operation for dislocated shoulder.

OBER'S—Cutting of a joint capsule; capsulotomy.

OBERST'S—An operation for providing drainage of abdominal ascites by burying an abdominal wall skin flap in the abdomen.

OGSTON'S—An operation for the development of an arch in flatfootedness by removing a wedge of the tarsus bone.
An operation for relieving knock-knee by excision of the inner condyle of the femur.

OGSTON-LUC—Frontal sinusotomy.

OLLIER-THIERSCH—A very thin skin graft including the epidermis and some of the dermis.

OLSHAUSEN'S—A corrective operation for retroversion of the uterus consisting of fixation of the uterus to the abdominal wall.

OMBREDDANE—Transscrotal suspension of the testes.
A corrective operation for hypospadius (defect where urethra opens on the undersurface of the penis).
An operative procedure wherein the structures operated upon are exposed to the air.

OMENTECTOMY—Resection of the omentum (membrane enclosing the bowels).

OMPHALECTOMY—Excision of the umbilicus.

ONYCHECTOMY—Removal of a toenail or fingernail.

ONYCHOTOMY—Cutting into a fingernail or toenail.

OOPHORECTOMY—Excision of one or both ovaries.

OOPHOROPEXY—Fixation of a wandering ovary; oothecopexy.

OOPHOROPLASTY—Plastic repair of an ovary.

OOTHECECTOMY—Removal of an ovary.

OPEN REDUCTION—Reduction of a fracture by manipulation performed after incision of the tissues overlying the fracture.

ORBITOTOMY—Surgical entry into the orbit.

ORCHIDECTOMY—Removal of one or both testes.

ORCHIDORRHAPHY—Suspension of the testes in the scrotum by suturing; orchiopexy.

GLOSSARY OF OPERATIVE TITLES (Continued)

ORCHIDOTOMY—Incision into the testis.

ORCHIECTOMY—Same as orchidectomy.

ORCHIOPEXY—Suspension of undescended testis or testes.

ORCHIOPLASTY—Plastic surgery on the testes; orcheoplasty.

ORD'S—An operation for division of fresh adhesions in a joint.

OSSICULECTOMY—Removal of the small bones of the middle ear (incus, malleus or stapes); otectomy.

OSTECTOMY—Removal of a portion of a bone.

OSTEOPERIOSTEAL GRAFT—Graft involving bone and the underlying periosteal membrane.

OSTEOPLASTY—Plastic operation on a bone.

OSTEORRHAPHY—Repair of a bone by wiring the fragments.

OSTEOSYNTHESIS—Bringing pieces of a fractured bone into apposition.

OSTEOTOMY—Cutting into a bone.

OTOPLASTY—Plastic surgery of the auricle (external projection of the ear on each side of the head).

OTOSCOPY—Examination of the ear by means of an instrument (scope).

OVERHOLT'S—Thoracoplasty with replacement of inverted ribs.

PACI'S—Modified Lorenz operation for reduction of congenital dislocation of the hip.

PALATOPLASTY—Plastic repair of the palate (uraniscus) which is the roof of the mouth. Uranoplasty; uraniscoplasty.

PALLIATIVE—A noncurative operation designed for relieving the severity of symptoms.

PANAS'—An operation for ptosis (drooping) of the upper eyelid wherein the upper eyelid is attached to the Occipitofrontalis muscle.
An operation for incision into the rectum.

PANCOAST'S—Transection of the 5th cranial nerve (trigeminal) at the level of the foramen ovale.

PANCREATECTOMY—Resection of the pancreas, a gland which secretes pancreatic juices containing enzymes discharged into the digestive tract and also secretes insulin.

GLOSSARY OF OPERATIVE TITLES (Continued)

PANCREATICODUODENOSTOMY—Creation of a surgical continuity between the pancreas and the duodenum.

PANCREATICOGASTROSTOMY—Continuity established between the stomach and a fistula of the pancreas.

PANCREOLITHOTOMY—Removal of a calculus of the pancreas; pancreatolithotomy.

PANHYSTERECTOMY—Removal of the uterus with the cervix. If salpingo-oophorectomy was also performed, this should be specified since the term panhysterectomy does not include removal of the tubes and ovaries.

PARATHYROIDECTOMY—Resection of the parathyroid glands situated adjacent to the thyroid gland.

PAROTIDECTOMY—Resection of the parotid or salivary gland situated in the upper neck, behind the lower ear.

PEAN'S—Vaginal hysterectomy performed in a piecemeal fashion.
Operation for amputation of the lower extremity at the hip joint.

PEDICLE GRAFT—Preparation of skin for grafting by forming a tubular structure which may be moved to another site on the body which requires the graft.

PERICARDIECTOMY—Resection of a portion of the membrane enveloping the heart particularly in cases where the membrane is constricting the heart as following pericarditis. Pericardectomy.

PERICARDIOCENTESIS—Incision into the pericardium (membrane enveloping the heart) for the purpose of removing purulent secretions. Pericardiostomy.

PERIER'S—Removal of an everted uterus utilizing an elastic ligature.

PERINEOPLASTY—Plastic repair of the perineum. Perineorrhaphy.

PERIOSTEAL GRAFT—Graft consisting of the fibrous membrane which covers the bone.

PERIOSTEOTOMY—Incision through the membranous covering of the bone.

PERITECTOMY—Excision of the pannus (ring of conjunctiva) surrounding the cornea. Peritomy.

PERITONEOCENTESIS—Aspiration of ascitic fluid from the abdomen. Paracentesis; abdominoparacentesis.

PHARYNGECTOMY—Resection of the pharynx (portion of digestive canal situated above the esophagus).

GLOSSARY OF OPERATIVE TITLES (Continued)

PHELP'S—An operation for correcting clubfoot.

PHLEBECTOMY—Resection of a segment of vein.

PHLEBORRHAPHY—Repair of a vein.

PHLEBOTOMY—Incision into a vein usually for the purpose of withdrawing blood.

PHRENICECTOMY—Resection of a portion of phrenic nerve for permanent interruption.

PHRENICO-EXERESIS—Excision of phrenic nerve.

PHRENICOTRIPSY—Crushing operation on the phrenic nerve. Phrenemphraxis.

PHYSICK'S—Iridectomy with removal of a circular section of iris.

PINCH GRAFT—Insertion of small bits of skin into a denuded area.

PINEALECTOMY—Excision of the pineal body.

PIROGOFF AMPUTATION—Technique for amputation of the foot.

PLEURACOTOMY—Incision into the pleural cavity for drainage purposes.

PLEURECTOMY—Resection of the serous membrane covering the lungs.

PLEUROCENTESIS—Puncture of the pleura.

PLEUROLYSIS—Separating the pleura from the fascia of the thoracic wall to permit collapse of lung.

PLICOTOMY—Incision into the plica membranae tympani (posterior tympanic membrane).

PNEUMONECTOMY—Total or partial resection of a lung.

PNEUMONOLYSIS—Same as pleurolysis.

PNEUMONOTOMY—Incision into the lung.

POLLOCK—Amputation at the level of the knee leaving the patella.

POMEROY—Sterilization operation on the female with ligation and resection of the fallopian tubes.

PONCET—Operation for relief of talipes equinus (walking on the toes) by lengthening of the Achilles tendon.

PORRO—Technique for cesarean section with hysterectomy. Celiohysterectomy.

GLOSSARY OF OPERATIVE TITLES (Continued)

PORTACAVAL ANASTOMOSIS—Formation of a communication between the portal and caval veins surgically.

POTTS—Aorticopulmonary shunt (diverting operation).

POTTS-SMITH-GIBSON—Operation performed in pulmonary stenosis consisting of an anastomosis between the pulmonary artery and aorta.

PRESACRAL NEURECTOMY—Resection of a nerve plexus (hypogastric) located before the sacral promontory.

PROCTECTOMY—Resection of the rectum.

PROCTOPEXY—Fixation operation designed to correct prolapse of the rectum.

PROCTOPLASTY—Plastic repair of the rectum and/or anus.

PROCTORRHAPHY—Suture repair of the rectum.

PROCTOSCOPY—Endoscopic examination of the rectum with the aid of a scope.

PROCTOSIGMOIDECTOMY—Resection of the sigmoid colon and rectum.

PROCTOSTOMY—Establishment of an opening into the rectum.

PROCTOTOMY—Incision into the rectum or anus.

PROSTATECTOMY—Resection of the prostate gland.

PROSTATOLITHOTOMY—Incision into the prostate for removal of a calculus.

PROSTATOTOMY—Incision into the prostate gland.

PTYALECTASIS—Dilation of a salivary duct.

PUBIOTOMY—Surgical division of the pubic bone.

PUUSSEPP—Surgical treatment of syringomyelia by division of the central canal of the spinal cord.

PUTTI-PLATT—Capsulorrhaphy of the shoulder.

PYELOLITHOTOMY—Removal of calculus from the renal pelvis.

PYELOPLASTY—Plastic operation of the kidney pelvis.

PYELOSTOMY—Incision into the renal pelvis and drainage of urine by a route other than the ureter.

PYELOTOMY—Incision into the kidney pelvis.

GLOSSARY OF OPERATIVE TITLES (Continued)

PYLOROMYOTOMY—Incision of the muscles of the pylorus; Ramstedt operation.

PYLOROPLASTY—Plastic revision of the pylorus, particularly enlarging a stenotic opening.

PYLOROSTOMY—Surgical opening created through the abdominal wall and pyloric portion of the stomach for feeding purposes.

QUAGLINO—Sclerotomy.

QUENU-MAYO—Resection of the rectum and local lymph glands in cases of malignancy.

RACHIOCENTESIS—Spinal tap.

RADICOTOMY—Surgical division of nerve roots; rhizotomy.

RAMSTEDT—Incision of the muscles of the pylorus performed for congenital pyloric stenosis. Same as Fredet-Ramstedt.

REGNOLI—Excision of the tongue.

REVERDIN GRAFT—Graft utilizing epidermis.

RHINOPLASTY—Plastic repair or reconstruction of the nose.

RHINOSCOPY—Examination of the nose with a speculum.

RHIZOTOMY—Division of the roots of the spinal nerves.

RIDELL—Resection of the walls (anterior and inferior) of the frontal sinus for chronic sinusitis.

RIGAUD—Repair of urethral fistula.

ROBERTS—Pinning operation for correction of a deviated nasal septum.

ROSE—Gasserian ganglionectomy.

ROUGE—Operation for entering the nasal cavities (sinuses).

ROUX-en-Y—Anastomosis between the stomach and distal end of the severed jejunum. The proximal end of the jejunum is anastomosed to jejunum below the first anastomosis.

SAENGER—Technique for cesarean section.

SALPINGECTOMY—Resection of the fallopian tube(s).

SALPINGO-OOPHORECTOMY—Resection of the tube and ovary unilaterally or bilaterally.

SALPINGOPLASTY—Plastic repair of the fallopian tube (oviduct).

GLOSSARY OF OPERATIVE TITLES (Continued)

SALPINGOSTOMY—Incision and drainage of the fallopian tube.

SAUCERIZATION—Formation of a saucer-like depression in a bone.

SCALENECTOMY—Excision of the scalenus muscle.

SCANZONI—Obstetrical forceps delivery of an infant from an occiput posterior position.

SCAPULOPEXY—Fixation of the scapula to the ribs.

SCHAUTA—Vaginal hysterectomy for carcinoma of the cervix uteri.

SCHAUTA-WERTHEIM—Cystocele repair.

SCHUCHARDT—Hysterectomy (removal of uterus) using a paravaginal incision.

SCHWARTZE—Operation performed for drainage of matter in cases of mastoiditis.

SCHWARTZE-STACKE—Operation for mastoiditis.

SCLERECTOMY—Excision of the sclera of the eye.

SCLEROPLASTY—Plastic repair of the sclera covering the eye.

SCLEROSTOMY—Surgical opening through the sclera in glaucoma.

SCROTECTOMY—Resection of a portion of the scrotum.

SEPTECTOMY—Removal of a portion of the nasal septum.

SEQUESTRECTOMY—Removal of a fragment of dead bone which has broken off the normal bone.

SHUNT OPERATION—An operation performed for the purpose of diverting the flow of blood, urine or other body fluid through a route other than the normal anatomic one.

SIALOADENECTOMY—Excision of a salivary gland.

SIALODOCHOPLASTY—Plastic repair of the salivary ducts.

SIALOLITHOTOMY—Removal of calculus from the salivary gland.

SIGMOIDECTOMY—Resection of the sigmoid colon.

SIGMOIDOPEXY—Fixation of the sigmoid to the abdominal wound for repair of rectal prolapse.

SIGMOIDOPROCTOSTOMY—A surgical opening made at the junction of the sigmoid colon and rectum.

SIGMOIDORECTOSTOMY—Same as sigmoidoproctostomy.

GLOSSARY OF OPERATIVE TITLES (Continued)

SIGMOIDOSCOPY—Endoscopic examination of the sigmoid colon.

SIGMOIDOSIGMOIDOSTOMY—Formation of a connection between two parts of the sigmoid colon.

SIGMOIDOSTOMY—Formation of an opening into the sigmoid colon.

SPENCER-WATSON—Operation to relieve ingrowing eyelashes.

SPHENOID SINUSOTOMY—Incision into the sphenoid sinus, one of the accessory sinuses communicating with the nasal cavity.

SPHINCTEROPLASTY—Surgical repair of a circular constricting muscle situated at the mouth of natural orifices such as the bladder, anus, pylorus, ampulla of Vater, etc.

SPHINCTEROTOMY—Incision or division of a sphincter.

SPINAL FUSION—Surgical immobilization of the spine through formation of a bony union; spondylosyndesis.

SPINELLI—Restoration of a prolapsed uterus.

SPLANCHNICECTOMY—Resection of the greater splanchic nerve; splanchnic neurectomy.

SPLENECTOMY—Removal of the spleen.

SPLENOPEXY—Attachment of a mobile spleen to the abdominal wall for purposes of immobilization.

SPLENORENAL ANASTOMOSIS—Surgical connection of the renal vein and splenic vein.

SPLENORRHAPHY—Repair of injury to the spleen.

SPLENOTOMY—Incision into the spleen.

STACKE—Removal of the contents of the middle ear and the mastoid.

STAPEDECTOMY—Removal of the stapes, one of the three tiny bones of the middle ear.

STERNOTOMY—Incision into or through the sternum (breast bone).

STOMATOPLASTY—Plastic operation of the mouth (stoma).

STREATFIELD-SNELLEN—Operation for repair of cicatricial entropion of the eyelid.

STURMDORF—Technique for amputation of the cervix.

SUBMUCOUS RESECTION—Resection of the nasal septum; septectomy.

GLOSSARY OF OPERATIVE TITLES (Continued)

SUSPENSION—Suturing or fixation of a structure to an anatomic site such as the abdominal wall for the purpose of restoring normal anatomic position and relieving malposition or ptosis.

SYMPATHECTOMY—Division of sympathetic nervous pathway.

SYMPATHICOTRIPSY—Crushing operation performed on a ganglion, nerve or plexus of the (involuntary) sympathetic nervous system.

SYNCHONDROTOMY—Incision or division of an articulation which has no appreciable motility and in which cartilage is the intervening connective tissue.

SYNOVECTOMY—Excision of the membrane lining the joint capsule (synovial membrane).

TAIT—Utilization of flaps for closure of a perineal laceration.

TARSECTOMY—Excision of the tarsal bones located in the heel area of the foot.
Excision of the tarsal cartilage of the eyelid.

TARSOPLASTY—Plastic repair of the tarsus (firm outline of the eyelid which gives it shape) of the eyelid.

TARSORRHAPHY—Suturing together, partially or totally, the upper and lower eyelid margins.

TENODESIS—Suturing of the proximal portion of a tendon to the bone or reattachment of it at another site.

TENOPLASTY—Plastic operation of the tendons.

TENORRHAPHY—Restoration of continuity to a severed tendon.

TENOSYNOVECTOMY—Resection of a tendon sheath.

TENOTOMY—Incomplete or complete division of a tendon.

THELEPLASTY—Plastic revision or reconstruction of the nipple of the breast.

   Also: thelyplasty or mammilliplasty.

THIERSCH-OLLIER GRAFT—Thin split skin graft.

THORACOPLASTY—Plastic surgery of the chest (thorax).

THORACOTOMY—Surgical incision of the chest wall.

THROMBECTOMY—Excision of a blood clot from a vein.

THYMECTOMY—Resection of the thymus gland situated in the anterior mediastinal cavity.

GLOSSARY OF OPERATIVE TITLES (Continued)

THYROCHONDROTOMY—Incision into the thyroid cartilage.

THYROCRICOTOMY—Surgical opening into the trachea made through the cricothyroid membrane.

THYROIDECTOMY—Resection of the thyroid gland.

THYROIDOTOMY—Surgical incision into the thyroid.

TONSILLECTOMY—Removal of the tonsils.

TOPECTOMY—Removal of a small area of the frontal cortex in the therapy of mental disease.

TOREK—Suspension of an undescended testicle.

TORKILDSEN—Ventriculocisternostomy utilizing plastic tubing.

TOTI—Dacryocystorhinostomy; passage of a probe through the lacrimal sac and into the nasal cavity for purposes of drainage.

TRACHELECTOMY—Excision of the cervix uteri.

TRACHELOPLASTY—Plastic repair of the cervix uteri.

TRACHELORRHAPHY—Suturing operation of the cervix uteri.

TRACHEOPLASTY—Plastic operation on the trachea.

TRACHEORRHAPHY—Suturing operation of the trachea.

TRACHEOSTOMY—Surgical opening into the trachea made through the neck for relief of severe respiratory distress.

TRACHEOTOMY—Surgical opening made in the trachea.

TRACTOTOMY—Division of a nerve tract.

TRANSDUODENAL CHOLEDOCHOLITHOTOMY—Removal of a common duct stone through a duodenal incision.

TRANSURETHRAL RESECTION OF PROSTATE—Resection of the prostate gland from below with a resectoscope. Also: TUR.

TRENDELENBURG—Excision of varicose veins.

TREPHINATION—Opening made in the skull with an instrument called a trephine. Also: craniotomy.

TURBINECTOMY—Excision of turbinated bone.

TYMPANOPLASTY—Plastic repair of the tympanic membrane and structures of the middle ear. Classified as Type I, II, III, IV and V.

TYMPANOTOMY—Surgical rupture of the tympanic membrane.

GLOSSARY OF OPERATIVE TITLES (Continued)

UMBILECTOMY—Excision of the navel (umbilicus).

UMBILICAL HERNIORRHAPHY—Repair of hernia in the umbilical region.

URACHUS LIGATION—Closure of a passage through the umbilicus, from the urinary bladder to the outside. This passage is present in the fetus and closes off after birth. Sometimes its lumen remains patent requiring surgical closure.

URANOPLASTY—Plastic repair of the palate (roof of the mouth). Also: palatoplasty.

URETERECTOMY—Resection of the ureter, a tube-like structure extending from the kidney to the urinary bladder for the passage of urine.

URETEROCENTESIS—Aspiration or drainage of a ureter.

URETEROCOLOSTOMY—Interruption of the normal course of the ureter to the urinary bladder and implantation of the ureter into the colon.

URETEROCYSTOSTOMY—Reimplantation of the ureter from its normal site to another site in the bladder. Also: ureteroneocystostomy.

URETEROLITHOTOMY—Removal of a calculus from the ureter.

URETEROLYSIS—Freeing (lysis) of adhesions of the ureter.

URETEROPLASTY—Plastic operation on the ureter.

URETEROPYELOSTOMY—Creation of a surgical passage from the renal pelvis to the ureter. Also: ureteroneopyelostomy.

URETERORRHAPHY—Suturing of the ureter for closure of a defect in its wall.

URETEROSIGMOIDOSTOMY—Implantation of the ureter into the sigmoid colon.

URETEROSTOMY—Surgical opening made in the ureter for drainage of urine.

URETEROTOMY—Incision into the ureter.

URETEROURETEROSTOMY—Connection of interrupted segments of the same ureter or one ureter to another.

URETHROPLASTY—Plastic operation on the urethra.

URETHRORRHAPHY—Surgical repair of the urethra.

URETHROSCOPY—Examination of the inside of the urethra with the aid of a scope.

GLOSSARY OF OPERATIVE TITLES (Continued)

URETHROSTOMY—Surgical opening made in the urethra for passage of urine in cases of persistent stricture.

URETHROTOMY—Incision into the urethra for surgical treatment of urethral stricture.

VAGINOTOMY—Incision of the vaginal wall.

VAGOTOMY—Division or partial transection of the vagus nerves. This operation is used in the treatment of duodenal ulcer.

VALVOTOMY—Incision of a valve.

VALVULOTOMY—Same as valvotomy.

VAN MILLINGEN—Entropion operation of the eyelid.

VARICOCELECTOMY—Resection of a portion of the scrotum and enlarged veins for relief of varicocele (varicose veins of the spermatic cord).

VASECTOMY—Resection of the vas deferens (excretory duct of the testicle).

VASOLIGATION—Ligation of the vas deferens. Sterilization operation on the male.

VASOTOMY—Incision of the vas deferens.

VENECTOMY—Resection of a vein. Also: phlebectomy.

VENOTOMY—Puncture or incision into a vein.

VENOVENOSTOMY—Connection of one segment of a vein with another.

VENTRAL HERNIORRHAPHY—Repair of a hernia of the belly wall.

VENTRICULOCISTERNOSTOMY—Surgical connection of the third ventricle of the cerebrum and the cisterna.

VENTRICULOSTOMY—Operation used in the treatment of hydrocephalus in which an opening is formed between the third ventricle floor and the cisterna situated just below it.

VENTROFIXATION—Fixation of the displaced uterus to the abdominal wall.

VERSION—Change in direction of the fetus within the uterus from an abnormal plane to a normal one for purposes of delivery.

VESICULECTOMY—Resection of the seminal vesicle. Sterilization operation on the male.

VESICULOTOMY—Incision into the seminal vesicles.

VESTIBULOTOMY—Opening made in the vestibule of the inner ear.

GLOSSARY OF OPERATIVE TITLES (Continued)

VON HABERER—Method of Billroth I gastrectomy.

VON HABERER-AGUIRRE—Method of Billroth I gastrectomy.

VON HABERER-FINNEY—Method of Billroth I.

VON HACKER—Posterior gastrojejunostomy.

VON EISELBERG—Modification of Billroth II gastrectomy.

VULVECTOMY—Resection of the vulva (external female genitalia).

WARDILL—Technique for palatoplasty.

WATKINS—Interposition operation for correction of uterine prolapse and procidentia uteri.

WATKINS-WERTHEIM—Suspension of the uterus.

WEIR—Operation on the nose performed with a rhinoplasty.

WEIS—Lid fracturing operation.

WERTHEIM—Radical hysterectomy (removal of the uterus, adjacent tissues and wide portion of the vagina) performed for uterine malignancy.

WHARTON-JONES—V-Y procedure for cicatricial ectropion.

WHIPPLE—One stage pancreaticoduodenectomy.

WICHERKIEWICZ—Upper eyelid reconstruction.

WITZEL—Gastrostomy for carcinoma of the stomach.

WÖLFLER—Anterior gastrojejunostomy.

Z-PLASTY—Relaxing incision used for correcting contractures; made in the shape of a Z.

INDEX

A

Abbreviations, medical, 649-654
Abdomen, X-ray of, 77
Abdomino-perineal resection, 335-337
Abell-Gilliam suspension, 364
Abortions, 412-413
   therapeutic, request form, 14
Abraders, 121
Abruptio placenta, 416
Abscess, I & D, 274
Acetone, urinary, 50
Acid phosphatase, 50
ACTH test, 50
Adams-Stokes disease, 636
Addis count, 50
Adenotomes, 121
Adrenal glands, 294-295
   diseases of, 295
   operations of, 295
A/G ratio, 50
A-K amputation, 459
Albumin
   blood, 51
   urine, 51
Aldolase, 51
Aldosterone test, 51
Alkaline phosphatase, 51
Alpha amino nitrogen, 51
Amebiasis, 41
Amniotomes, 121
Amputations, 456
   A-K report, 459-460
   humerus, report, 459
   index finger, report, 460
   techniques, 456
Amylase test
   blood, 52
   urine, 52
Anal sphincterotomy, 335
Anastomosis apparatus, 121
Anastomosis, types, 319-320
Anatomic position, 642
Anchors, 121
Andrews Bottle operation, 597
Anesthesia, 91-93
   induction methods, 93
   listing of, 91-92
   ophthalmic, 92
   preparations used with, 92-93
Angiocardiography, 610
Angiotribes, 121
Ankle
   anatomy illust., 474
   Charnley arthrodesis, 461
   Watson-Jones operation, 480
Anoscopes, 122
Antistreptolysin O titer, 52
Antroscope, 122
Anuria, 27
Anus
   anatomic structures, 330
   circulation, 330
   diseases listed, 333
   illustrated, 332
   operations listed, 333-334
Aorta, 615-616
   Crafoord operation, 619
   insufficiency of, 623
   stenosis of, 628
   valve prostheses, 616
Aortogram, 613
   transbrachial arch, 614
   translumbar, 614
Aortography, 78
Aponeuroses, 240
Apparatus, 122
Appendectomy, 328-329
   incisions, 329
   operative report, 329
   terms used in, 329
Appendix, vermiform, 328
   illustrated, 327
Applicators, 122
Approaches, orthopedic, 455
Arteries, 214-217
   abdomen and pelvis, 223
   head and neck, 221
   lower extremity, 225
   principal, illustrated, 220
   thorax and axilla, 222
   upper extremity, 224

INDEX (Continued)

Arteriogram, 78
  femoral, 613
  subclavian, 612
Arteriography, 78
  femoral, 80-81
  renal, 84
Arteriotomy, report, 620-621
Arthrodesis, 460-461
  ankle, report, 461
  Charnley, report, 461
  hip, report, 462
  ischiofemoral, report, 462
  shoulder, report, 462
  vertebral at L-4, report, 467-468
Arthrography, 78
Arthroplasty, 470
  Austin-Moore report, 471-472
  knee, report, 470-471
  Magnuson report, 472-473
Arytenoidectomy, 523
Ascariasis, 44
Ascheim-Zondek test, 52
Ascorbic acid test, 52
ASO titer, 52
Aspirators, 122
Atrial septal defect, 627
Austin-Moore arthroplasty, 471-472, 485
Authorization for surgery, 5
Autografts, 531
Autotomography, 78
Awls, 123

B

Bacteremia, 32
Bacterial
  agglutinations, 52
  examinations, 31-33
  organisms listed, 33-35
Balloons, 123
Bandages listed, 117-119
Bands, 123
Bankart operation, 480
Barium examinations, 78-79

Bars, 123
Basiotribes, 123
Basophiles, 20
Bassini herniorrhaphy, 266-267
BEI test, 52, 54
Bell's Palsy operation, 538
Bence-Jones protein, 53
Bile test, 53
Biliary tract, 338-347
  diseases listed, 339
  illustrated, 338
  operations listed, 341
Bilirubin test, 53
Bladder, urinary, 585-586
  anatomic features of, 587-588
  arteries, 588
  biopsy report, 589
  calculus removal report, 589
  cystoscopy report, 589-590
  diseases listed, 602-605
  malignant tumors, 586
  operations listed, 605-606
Blades, 123
Bleeding time, 53
Blepharoplasty, 540
  anatomic features, 541
  operative report, 542-543
  ptosis corrections, 542
  techniques listed, 541
Blepharoptosis repair, 542
  techniques listed, 542
Blood
  circulation, 213-214
  examinations, 17-25
    color index, 19
    hematocrit, 19
    hemoglobin, 19
    mean corp. hemoglobin, 19
    red blood count, 17-19
    saturation index, 19
    white blood count, 19-20
  groups, 22-23
  pressure, 214
  production, 17
  Rh factor, 23-25

INDEX (Continued)

transfusion, 22
transfusion refusal form, 10
typing and cross matching, 22
volume, 17
BMR, 53
Body section radiography, 84
Bolts, 123
Bone grafts, 475-478
  femur report, 476
  iliac, 467
  removal of tibial, 477
  techniques listed, 476
  tibial, report, 477
  types listed, 476
Bone marrow, 25-26
  differential, 26
  function, 25
  studies, 25
Bones, 230-232
  diseases listed, 491-494
  listed, 235
  operations listed, 494-499
  skeleton illustrated, 229, 234
Bougies, 123-124
Bovies, 124
Braces, 124
Brachial arteriography, 79
Bradycardia, 637
Brain
  anatomy, 386
  arteries, 388
  exploration, 393-394
  illustrated, 389-390
  structures listed, 387-388
  trauma illustrated, 395
Breasts, 275-280
  anatomy, 277, 279
  arteries, 279
  cancer of, 275-278
  diseases of, 278-279
  illustrated, 277
  operations on, 279
    biopsy, 280
    radical mastectomy, 280
Breech extraction, 427

Breech presentation, 420, 423, 424
  illustrated, 423
  incidence, 420
  types, 420
Brittain arthrodesis, 462
Broaches, 124
Bronchial tree, 558
  illustrated, 560
Bronchography, 79
Bronchoscopes, 124-125, 567
Bronchoscopy, 557-558, 566
  operative report, 567
Bronchus
  anatomy, 558, 559-560
  diseases listed, 573-574
  divisions of, 558
  illustrated, 560
  operations listed, 574-575
BUN, 54
Bunionectomy, 485-486
Burs, 125
Buttons, 125

C

Calcium test, 54
Caldwell-Luc report, 529, 530
Calipers, 125
Cannulae, 125-126
Canthoplasty, 444-445
Capillary fragility test, 55
Capitalization, 656-657
Capsulotomes, 127
Cardiac catheterization, 609, 610
Cardiac massage, report, 571
Cardio-angiography, 79
Carotid angiography, 79
Carotid artery ligation, 622
Cataract, extraction
  extracapsular, 438
  intracapsular, 440
Catecholamines test, 55
Catheters, 127-128
Cautery, 128
Cecil procedure, 554-555
Cecum, illustrated, 327

INDEX (Continued)

Cephalic presentation, 420-424
Cephalin-cholesterol
  flocculation, 55
Cerclage operation, 372
Cerebrospinal fluid, 29-30
  examinations, 30
Cervical fistula, 360
Cervix uteri
  cancer of, 370-372
    stages, 371-372
  diseases of, 377-380
  effacement, 418-419
  electrocoagulation, 374
  fistulas, 360-362
  incompetence, 372
    Cerclage operation, 372
    Lash operation, 373
    Shirodkar operation, 373
  insertion of radium, 374
  operations listed, 381-383
Cesarean section, 429-430
  cervical, report, 430-431
Chalazion excision, 442
Charnley, arthrodesis, 461
Cheiloplasty, 543
  techniques listed, 544
  Tennison report, 545
Chest X-ray, 79
Chisels, 128-129
Chlorides test, 55
Cholangiography, 79-80
Cholecystectomy, 341
  anatomic features, 341
Cholecystography, 80
Cholesterol esters, 55
Cholesterol test, 55
Cholinesterase, 55
Chordotomy, 405
Cimino shunt, 233
Cineradiography (cine), 611
Circulation, blood, 213-214
Circumcision, male, report, 593
  consent form, 12
Cistern puncture, 397
Clamps, 129-133

Cleft palate repair, 549-551
  von Langenbeck, 549-550
  Wardill, 550-551
Clipping middle cerebral artery, 397
Clips, 133
Clot retraction time, 56
Clotting time, 56
CO_2 combining power, 55
Coagulation time, 56
Coagulators, 133
Coarctation of aorta, 619, 628
Cobalt-60, 87-89
Colectomy, report, 328
Collectors, 133
Colloidal gold test, 56
Colon, 323-329, 332
  anatomic features, 324
  arterial supply, 324
  cancer of, 323-324
  diseases listed, 326
  excision (colectomy), 328
  illustrated, 325, 327
Color index, blood, 19
Colostomy, 324
Colporrhaphy, 357
  A & P, 358
Common duct stone removal, 341
Compressors, 133
Conductors, 134
Congo red test, 56
Conization, cervix, 370
Conjunctival flapping, 441
Consent forms
  circumcision, ritual, 12
  cosmetic surgery, 8
  delivery by alternate physician, 7
  eye donation, 10
  grafting of tissue, 9
  motion pictures, 12
  observers, 11
  operation, 5-6
    form, 6
  photographs, 11
  refusal of treatment, 10
  refusal of blood transfusion, 10

INDEX (Continued)

removal of tissue for grafting, 9
televising operation, 11
tissue grafting, 9
valid consent, 5
Contractors, 134
Contrast media
  radiographic, 74-77
  vascular exams, 612
Coombs test, 24-25, 56
Coproporphyrin test, 57
Coronary artery perfusion, 626
Cosmetic operation
  consent form, 8
Costotomes, 134
Counterbores, 134
Crafoord operation, 619-620
Craniectomy, 394
Cranioclasts, 134
Craniotomes, 134
Craniotomy, 391, 393
  instruments, 391-392
C-reactive protein, 57
Creatine
  blood serum, 57
  urine, 57
Creatinine
  blood serum, 57
  urine, 57
Cryoextractors, 134
Cryogenic eye surgery, 439
Cryoglobulin, 57
Cryophakes, 134
Cryoptors, 134
  photograph of, 439
Cryostylet, 134
Cryosurgery, 257, 439
Cryptotomes, 134
Culdoscopes, 134
Curettes, 135-136
Cutters, 136
Cystometers, 136
Cystoscopes, 136, 588-589
  accessories, 136-137
Cystoscopy, report, 588-590
Cystotomes, 137

Cystourethrography, 80

D

D & C, 363
  instruments used in, 363
  operative report, 363
Dacryocystography, 80
Dacryocystorhinostomy, 444
Debriders, 137
Decompression, subtemporal, 396
Decortication, lung, 570-571
Deep therapy, 87
Delivery by another
  physician, form, 7
Delivery, obstetrical
  types, 426-427
Dermabraders, 137
Dermabrasion, facial, 552-553
Dermatomes, 137
Diacetic acid test, 57
Diagnex blue, 57
Dialysis unit, 233
Diaphragmatic hernia, 269
  report, 269-270
Dick test, 58
Dilators, 137-139
Directors, 139
Disc, ruptured, 400-405
  cervical, 404-405
  illustrated, 403
  lumbar, 402-404
Discission of lens, 443
Discography, 80
Dislocations
  Bankart operation, 480
  illustrated types, 479
  operations listed, 478
  Watson-Jones report, 480
Dissectors, 139
Donor of eyes form, 10
Drains, 139-140
Dressings, 117-119
  eyelid, 542
Drills, 140
Drivers, 140-141

INDEX (Continued)

d-Xylose test, 72
Dyspareunia operation, 359
Dystocia, 415

E

Ear
  anatomic features
    external ear, 539
    middle ear, 503-504
  diseases listed, 517
  illustrated, 502
  operations listed, 517
  otoplasty report, 540
  otoplasty techniques, 539
  tympanoplasty, 506-512
Ear, nose and throat, 501-530
  illustrated, 502
ECG, 58
Eclampsia, 415
Ectropion of eyelid report, 441
E.D.C. determination, 414
E.E.G., 58
Effacement of cervix, 418-419
EKG, 58, 611
Elbow anatomy, 464
Electricator, 141
Electrocardiogram, 58, 611
  fetal, 414
Electrocoagulation of cervix, 374
Electrodes, 141-142
Electrodiaphake, 142
Electrophoresis, 67
Electroscopes, 142
Electrosurgical units, 142
  accessories, 142
Electrotomes, 143
Elevators, 143-144
Ellsworth-Howard, 58
Emboli removal, 620-621
Encephalography, 80
Endocrine glands
  illustrated, 293
Endolymphatic-subarachnoid shunt, 505
Endometrium, cancer of, 362

ENT, 501-530
Enterobiasis, 44
Enteroscopes, 144
Enucleators, 144
Eosinophiles, 20
Episiotomy, 426
Erisophakes, 144
Erythroblastosis fetalis, 24
  vaccine RhoGAM, 24-25
Erythrocyte uptake of I-131, 58
Esophagectomy, 571-572
Esophagogastroscopy, 305-306
Esophagoscopes, 144, 305
Esophagoscopy, 306
Esophagus, 302-306
  cancer of, 304
  diseases listed, 304
  esophagectomy report, 571-572
  operations listed, 305
Estrogen levels, 58
ET_3, 58
Ethmoidectomy report, 530
Evacuators, 145
Excavators, 145
Excision
  scar, 537
  skin graft, 537
Exophthalmometer, 145
Exploration
  extracerebral hematoma, 394
Expressors, 145
Exton-Rose test, 60
Extractors, 145
Eye, 433-454
  abbreviations, 437
  accessory structures, 434
  anatomic features, 436-437
  anatomy of, 433
  authorization to use form, 10
  cryogenic surgery on, 439
  diseases listed, 445-451
  donation of, form, 10
  evisceration of, report, 443
  illustrated, 435
  insertion of implant, 443
  medications in surgery, 437

INDEX (Continued)

operations listed, 451-452
  by eponymic title, 452-454
  removal of eye implant, 443
Eye implants, 145-146
Eyelids, 540
  anatomic features, 541
  anesthetics, 542
  dressings, 542
  ptosis repairs, 542
  repair techniques, 541, 542

F

Face
  dermabrasion of, 552-553
  lift operation, 553
Facial fracture appliance, 146
Fallopian tubes, 354, 375-376
  diseases listed, 378
  operations listed, 381-383
Fascia, 240
Fascia lata graft, 538
Fascia stripper, 202
Fasciatomes, 146
Female genitalia, 349-356
  diseases listed, 377-380
  external features, 349-352
  external, illustrated, 351
  internal features, 349-350, 352-356
    illustrated, 353
  operations listed, 381-383
Femoral hernia, 267-268
  anatomic structures, 268
  herniorrhaphy report, 268
  techniques listed, 268
Femoropopliteal by-pass, 617
Femur, bone graft to, 476
Fenestration
  semicircular canal, 515-516
Fertility study, 59
Fetal electrocardiogram, 414
Fiberscopes, 146
Fibrinogen, 59
Fibrinolysin, 59
Filariasis, 45
Finger, index, revision, 460
Fishberg's

concentration, 59
dilution, 59
Fistula
  rectovaginal, 360
  ureterovaginal, 360-361
  vaginoperineal, 361
  vesicocervical, 361
  vesicovaginal, 361-362
Flanges, 146
Flapping of conjunctiva, 441
Fluorescent treponemal antibody, 59
Fluoroscopy, 85
  diagram of, 85
Foot
  anatomy of, 458
Forceps, 146-156
Forcep delivery, 426
Formol gel, 60
Fracture appliance, 157
Fracture frames, 157
Fractures
  reduction techniques, 483
  types illustrated, 482
  types listed, 481
Frei skin test, 60
Friedman test, 60, 413
Frog test, 60
FTA test, 59
Fungi, 38-41
  infections, 38-39
  listing of organisms, 39-41

G

Gallbladder, 339-341
  cholecystectomy, 341
    anatomy in, 341
  diseases listed, 339-340
  operations listed, 340
Galli-Mainini test, 413
Gastrectomy, 309-313
  anatomic features in, 311
  instruments, 310
  operative reports
    Billroth I, 311-312
    Billroth II, 312-313

INDEX (Continued)

techniques defined, 309
techniques listed, 310
Gastrojejunostomy, 320-323
    anatomic features in, 321
    operative report, 320-322
    techniques, 321
Gastroscopes, 157, 314
Gastroscopy, 314
Gastrostomy, 315
    techniques listed, 315
Gauze packers, 157
Genitalia, female, 349-356
    external features, 350-352
        illustrated, 351
        listed, 349
    internal features, 352-356
        illustrated, 353
        ligaments, 355-356
        ovaries, 354-355
        tubes, 354
        uterus, 352-353
        vagina, 352-354, 356
Genitalia, male, 577, 591-606
    illustrated, 594-595
    penis, 592-593
    prostate, 599-601
    testes, 593-598
Glossary of operative titles, 659-698
Glucose test, 60
Glucose tolerance test, 60-61
Glutamic oxalacetic transaminase, 61
Glutamic pyruvic transaminase, 61
Gold, radioactive, 89
Gonadotrophic hormone, 61
Goniometers, 157
GOT test, 61
Gouges, 157-158
GPT test, 61
Grafts, tissue, 535-536
    bone, 535
        iliac, 467
    cartilage, 535
    cornea, 535
    fascia, 536
    fascia lata report, 538
    hair, 536

    mucous membrane, 536
    nerve, 536
    skin, 531, 533-534
    tendon, 536
    vein, 615, 617
Gravindex test, 61
Groin dissection, radical, 271-272
Guides, 158
Guillotines, 158
Guthrie test, 61
Gynecology, 349-383

H

Halters, 158
Hammer toe correction, 485-486
    Jones operation, 486
Hammers, 159
Hand, anatomy illustrated, 457
Hand pieces, 159
Hanger's test, 55, 61
Harelip repair, 545
    Tennison, 545
Harrington operation, 468-470
Hauser procedure, 487
Head holders, 159
Heart
    anatomy of, 626-627
        illustrated, 623
    block, 636, 639
    defects
        aortic insufficiency, 628
        aortic stenosis, 628
        atrial septal, 627
        coarctation of aorta, 628
        mitral insufficiency, 628
        mitral stenosis, 629
        patent ductus arteriosus, 629
        pulmonic stenosis, 629
        Tetralogy of Fallot, 629
        tricuspid stenosis, 629
        ventricular septal defect, 630
    diagnostic examinations, 610-611
        angiocardiography, 610
        cardiac catheterization, 610
        cineradiography, 611
        electrocardiography, 611

INDEX (Continued)

phonocardiography, 611
roentgenography, 610
donors, 607-608
pacemaker, 636-637
surgery, 624-626
  heart lungs by-pass, 624
    illustrated, 625
  hypothermia in, 626
  transplant technique, 607-608
Heart lungs by-pass, 624-626
  illustrated, 625
Hematocrit, 19, 61
Hematuria, 28
Hemilaminectomy, 400-405
  cervical, 404-405
  lumbar, 402-404
Hemodialysis unit, photo, 233
Hemoglobin, 17, 19
  mean corpuscular, 19
Hemorrhoidectomy, 331
Hemorrhoids, 332
Hemostatic agents
  neurosurgical, 392
Hemostatic bags, 159
Hemostats, 159
Hernias, 260-271
  diaphragmatic, 269
  femoral, 267-268
    anatomic features, 268
    type repairs, 268
  inguinal, 264
    anatomic features, 265
  types illustrated, 260
  types listed, 262-264
  umbilical, 270
Heterophile antibody, 62
5-HIAA, 62
Hibbs technique, 467-468
Hip
  anatomy illustrated, 466
  Austin-Moore prosthesis, 485
  Brittain arthrodesis, 462
  Lawson-Thornton plate, 484-485
  open reduction, 484-485
  Smith-Petersen nailing, 484-485
Hippuric acid test, 62

Hirst operation, 359
Hogben test, 62, 413
Homogentisic acid test, 62
Homografts, 531
Hooks, 159-161
Hookworm, 45
Howard test, 62
Humerus
  amputation, 459
  open reduction, 484
Hydroelectomy, 597
17-Hydroxycorticosteroids, 62
5-Hydroxyindoleacetic acid, 62
Hyfrecators, 161
Hyphenation, 657-658
Hypospadias, 554-555
  Cecil procedure, 554
  repair techniques, 554
Hypothermia
  in heart surgery, 626
Hysterectomy, 366-367
  abdominal, total, 368-369
  types, 367
  vaginal, 367-368
Hysteropexy, 364-365
  Abell, 364-365
  Gilliam, modified, 365-366
Hysterosalpingography, 81

I

Icterus index, 62
Indican, 63
Immune response, 532-533
  in heart transplants, 608
Immunologic test, 414
Immuno-suppressive agents, 532-534
Implant materials, 161
Incisions
  appendectomy, 329
  Heerman stapedectomy, 514
  types listed, 96-99
Incision and drainage
  buttocks, 274
  hand, 274
  ischiorectal abscess, 330
Index finger, amputation closure, 460

INDEX (Continued)

Information, medical
  request form, 14-15
Inguinal hernia, 264-267
  anatomic features in, 265
  Bassini repair, 266-267
  McVay repair report, 265
  repair techniques listed, 264
  types illustrated, 260
Instruments, surgical, 121-210
Insufflators, 161
Insulin tolerance, 63
Interatrial septal defect closure, 632
Intervertebral disc, ruptured, 403
Intimectomy
  femoral, report, 618
  for Leriche syndrome, 621
Inulin clearance, 63
Inverters, 162
Iodine-131, 89
Iridectomy
  peripheral, 438
  simple, 437
Iridencleisis, report, 438
Iridium, 192
Iron binding capacity, 63
Iron, inorganic, 63
Irrigators, 162
Ischiorectal abscess, 330
Isoiodeikon test, 63
Isotopes, radioactive, 88-89

J

Jejunostomy, 322
  Marwedel, report, 322-323
  techniques, 322
Joints, bony, 232-236
  diseases listed, 491-494
  operations listed, 494-499
Jones hammer toe operation, 486

K

Kahn test, 63
Keratomes, 162
17-Ketosteroids, 64
Kidneys, 577-578
  anatomic features listed, 578
  artificial, machine, 486
  cancer of, 579
  diseases listed, 602-605
  hemodialysis, 233
  incisions, 582
  nephrectomy report, 582
  nephropexy report, 583
  operations, 584
    listed, 605-606
  transplants, 579-581
    complications, 581
    rejection, 580-581
Knee
  anatomy illustrated, 473
  arthroplasty, 470-471, 472, 475
Knives, 162-165
KUB film, 81
Kuhnt-Szymanowski operation, 441
Kupperman test, 413
Kymography, 86

L

Labor in obstetrics, 416
  induction, 425-426
    indications for, 425
  stages of, 417-418
Laboratory examinations, 17-72
  automated, 48-49
  bacteriologic, 31-35
  blood, 17-25
  blood groups, 22-25
  bone marrow, 25-26
  cerebrospinal fluid, 29-30
  fungi, 38-41
  listing of lab tests, 50-72
  protozoa, 41-44
  richettsias, 36
  sputum, 31
  urine, 26-29
  viruses, 36-38
  worms, 44-48
Labyrinthotomy, transmeatal, 505
Lacrimal tract
  diseases listed, 451
  operations listed, 452
Lactic acid test, 64

INDEX (Continued)

Lactic dehydrogenase test, 64
Laminectomy, 400
  also see: hemilaminectomy
Laryngectomy, total, 522-523
Laryngoplasty, 523-524
Laryngoscopes, 165, 519
Laryngoscopy report, 522
Laryngostats, 165
Larynx, 518
  anatomic features of, 518
  diseases listed, 521
  illustrated, 520
  instruments, 519
  muscles, 518
  operations listed, 521
  tubes, 519
Laser, 258-259
  photocoagulator, 259
Lash operation, 373
Latex slide agglutination, 64
Latzko high colpocleisis, 362
LDH test, 64
L.E. test, 64
Leishmaniasis, 42
Lens, discission of, 443
Lens expressors, 165
Lens loupes, 166
Leriche syndrome, 621
Leucine aminopeptidase, 64
Leukopenia, 20
Leukotomes, 166
Levinson test, 65
Levulose tolerance, 65
Lid everters, 166
Lids: see eyelids
Ligaments, 237-240
  transverse carpal section, 490
  uterine, 355-356
Ligation
  external carotid artery, 622
  patent ductus arteriosus, 632
  saphenous vein, 621
Lights, 166
Lipase test, 65
Lipids, total, 65
Lips, 543

  anatomic features of, 544
  arteries of, 544
  cheiloplasty techniques, 544
  deformities, 544
    Tennison repair, 545
Litholapaxy urinary bladder, 589
Lithotrites, 166
Lithotriptoscopes, 166
Liver, 343-344
  diseases listed, 343
  operations listed, 344
Lobectomy of lung, 568-569
Longitudinal lie, 421, 424
  illustrated, 421
Loops, 166
Lottes nailing of tibia, 483
Lumen finders, 166
Lungs
  anatomic features, 558-559, 561
  cancer of, 563
  decortication, 570-571
  diseases listed, 573-574
  lobectomy of, 568-569
  operations listed, 574-575
  pneumonectomy, 569-570
Lymphangiography, 81
Lymphocytes, 21

M

Magnesium test, 65
Magnets, 166-167
Magnuson arthroplasty, 472-475
Malaria, 42
Malarial film, 65
Male genital system, 577, 591-606
  diseases listed, 602-605
  illustrated, 594, 595
  operations listed, 605-606
Mallein test, 65
Mallets, 167
Mammoplasty
  augmentation, 551-552
Marginal sinus rupture, 416
Marrow, bone
  differential, 26
  studies on, 25

INDEX (Continued)

Mastectomy
  incisions, 280
  radical, report, 280
Mastic test, 65
Mastoid searcher, 167
Mastoids, 81
Mayo-Fueth inversion, 362
McLaughlin canthoplasty, 444
McVay inguinal herniorrhaphy, 265
Meatoantrotomy, 508
Meatoscopes, 167
Meatotomes, 167
Mechanical finger, 167
Mediastinoscopes, 167
Mediastinum, 562
Medical information
  request form, 14-15
Medical terminology, 641-654
  abbreviations, 649-654
  combining forms, 644-647
  elements of, 643
  prefixes, 644-647
  suffixes, 647-648
  symbols, 654
Melanin test, 65
Meniscectomy, medial, 488
Meniscotomes, 167
Metal locators, 167
Metamyelocytes, 20
Micro-mike, 168
Microscopes, 168
Microsurgery, 640
Miles operation, 335-337
Mitral insufficiency, 628
Mitral stenosis, 629
Mobilizers, 168
Monocytes, 21
Motion pictures in OR
  consent form, 12
Mouth gags, 168-169
Mouth, illustrated, 282
Mucoproteins, 65
Mucotomes, 169
Muscles, 240-250
  diseases listed, 491-494
  illustrated, 246
  listing of, 241-245, 247
    of arm and shoulder, 250
    forearm and hand, 249
    head and face, 245, 248
    hip and knee, 249
    leg and foot, 250
    neck, 248
    perineum and pelvis, 249
    trunk, 248
  operations listed, 494-499
Musculoplasty report, 512-513
Musculoskeletal diseases listed, 491-494
Musculoskeletal operations listed, 494-499
  by eponymic title, 496-499
Myelocytes, 21
Myelography, 81
Myringoplasty, 507
Myringotomy report, 512

N

Nails, 169
Nails of fingers and toes, 273
  anatomic structures of, 273
  diseases listed, 273
  radical toenail excision, 273
Nasopharyngoscopes, 169
Neck
  anatomy illustrated, 285
  dissection, 286-287
Needles listed, 170-172
Nephrectomy
  instruments, 582
  report, 582
  techniques listed, 582
Nephrolithotomy report, 584-585
Nephropexy, 583
  report, 583
  techniques listed, 583
Nephrostomy report, 584
Nerves listed, 251-253
  cranial, 251
Nervous system, 250-253
  diseases listed, 407-409
  operations listed, 409-410
Neurosurgery, 385-410

INDEX (Continued)

diseases listed, 407-409
hemostatic agents, 392
operations listed, 409-410
Neurotomes, 172
Neutrophiles
  band (stabs), 20
  juvenile (polys), 20
  mature, 21
  segmented, 21
Nocturia, 27
Nose and sinuses, 525, 545
  anatomic features, 527, 545-546
  arteries of, 527, 546
  diseases listed, 528
  nerves of, 529, 546
  operations listed, 528
  polypectomy report, 529
  rhinoplasty, 546-547
  submucous resection, 529-530, 546-547
NPN test, 66

O

Observers in OR form, 11
Obstetrics, 411-432
  abortions, 412-413
  cesarean section, 429-431
    complications, 415-416
  definitions in, 411
  delivery, 426-427
  diagnoses in, 413
  E.D.C., 414
  effacement of cervix, 418-419
  fetal lie, 419
  labor in, 416-417, 425-426
  multiple pregnancy, 414
  pelves in, 417
  placenta, 427-429
  positions, 424-425
  prematurity, 412
  presentation, 419-420
    illustrated, 421-423
  station, 418-419
  terms used in, 411-412
  tests in, 413-414
  version in, 425

Obturators, 172
Ocular muscle, recession, 440-441
17-OHCS, 62
Oliguria, 27
Open reduction
  hip, 484
  humerus, 484
Operative consent, 5
Operative report
  content, 3
  copies of, 3
  form, 4
  format, 3
Ophthalmodynamometers, 172
Ophthalmology, 433-454
Orchiectomy, bilateral, 597
Orchiopexy, first stage, 598
Organs, internal
  illustrated, 303
Orthopedic surgery, 455-499
  approaches in, 455
  diseases listed, 491-494
  operations listed, 494-496
    by eponymic title, 496-499
Osteoclast, 172
Osteotomes, 172
Otolaryngology, 501-530
Otoplasty, 539-540
  operative report, 540
  techniques listed, 539
Otoscopes, 173
Ovaries, 354-355, 375-376
  diseases listed, 378-379
  operations listed, 381-382
Oxyuriasis, 44

P

Pacemaker, cardiac, 636-637
  battery change, 639
  illustrated, 638
  types listed, 637
Palate, 548-551
  anatomic features, 548-549
  cleft repair, 549-550
    von Langenbeck, 549-550

INDEX (Continued)

Wardill, 550-551
  repair techniques, 549
Palatoplasty
  von Langenbeck, 549-550
  Wardill, 550-551
Pancreas, 344-348
  diseases listed, 347-348
  operations listed, 348
Pancreatoduodenectomy
  techniques, 345
  Whipple operation, 345-346
Pancytopenia, 20
Panendoscope, 173
Paranasal sinuses, 81, 525-530
  anatomic structures, 527
  diseases listed, 528
  illustrated, 526
  operations listed, 528
Parathyroids, 298
  diseases listed, 298
  operations listed, 298
Parotid gland, 283-286
  excision, report, 284
Parotidectomy, 284-286
Patent ductus arteriosus, 629, 632
PBI test, 66
Pelves, types illustrated, 417
Pelvimeters, 173
Pelvimetry, 82
  illustrated, 82-83
Pencils, 173
Penis, 592
  anatomic features, 592-593
  circumcision report, 593
  diseases listed, 602-605
  operations listed, 605-606
Perforators, 173
Perfusion, coronary, 626
Periosteal elevators, 173-174
Periosteotomes, 174
Pessaries, 174
Pharynx
  anatomic features, 548-549
Phenylketonuria, 66
Phonocardiography, 611
Phospholipids, 66
Phosphorus, 67

Phosphorus-32, 89
Photographing consent form, 11
Picks, 175
Pilonidal cyst excision, 274
Pineal gland, 298-299
  diseases of, 299
  operations of, 299
Pins, 175
Pituitary gland, 296-298
  diseases listed, 297-298
Placenta, 427-428
  abruptio, 416
  previa, 416
  types listed, 428-429
Platelets, 21-22
Plates, 175-176
Pleura, 562
  diseases listed, 573-574
  operations listed, 574-575
Pliers, 176
Plugs, 176
Plurals, formation of, 655-656
Pneumoencephalography, 83
Pneumonectomy, 569-570
Pneumothorax apparatus, 176
Polypectomy
  nasal, 529
  rectal, 331
Polyuria, 27
Porphobilinogen, 67
Porphyrins, 67
Portal venography, 83
Positions
  examining, 93-96
  illustrated, 94
  obstetrical, 424-425
  references to, 642
  surgical, 93-96
Potassium, 67
Pott's shunt, 630
Pre-eclampsia, 415
Prefixes, medical, 644-647
Pregnancy, 411-432
  antepartum complications, 415-416
  diagnoses in, 413
    listed, 431-432
  E.D.C. determination, 414

INDEX (Continued)

multiple, 414
operations listed, 432
tests for, 413-414
Prematurity
classification of, 412
Presentation in obstetrics
abbreviations, 424-425
breech, 420, 423
cephalic, 420-422
illustrated
breech, frank, 423
breech, full, 423
breech, single footling, 423
brow, 422
face, 422
knee breech, 423
longitudinal lie, 421
parietal, 422
transverse lie, 421
vertex, 422
lateral, 420-421
Probes, 176-177
Proctoscopes, 177
Proctosigmoidectomy, 335
Profilometers, 177
Progesterone test, 414
Prolapse of uterus, 364
Prostate, 599
anatomic features, 600
diseases listed, 602-605
malignant tumors, 599
operations listed, 605-606
Prostatectomy
suprapubic, 600-601
Prostheses, 177-178
aortic valve, 616
ear piston, 514
vascular, 616
Proteins, total, 67
Prothrombin time, 67
Protozoa, 41-44
listing, 44
PSP, 66, 68
Pterygium, transplant, 442
Pulmonic stenosis, 629, 630-631
Punches, 178-179
Purines, 68

Pyelography, 83-84
Pyelolithotomy, report, 584-585
Pyloromyotomy report, 316
Pyloroplasty, 316
anatomic features in, 316
Ramstedt report, 316
techniques listed, 316

R

RA test, 68
Radiation machines, 87
Radioactive iodine uptake, 62
Radioactive isotopes, 88-89
Radiology (also see: X-ray)
deep therapy, 87
therapeutic, 86-88
Radium, 87
cervical insertion, 374
therapy, 87-88
Radon seeds, 88
Ramstedt pyloromyotomy, 316
Raspatories, 180-181
Rasps, 180
Reamers, 181
Recession, ocular muscles, 440
Rectovaginal fistula, 360
Rectum
anorectal circulation, 330
anorectal structures, 330
cancer of, 332
diseases listed, 333
illustrated, 332
operations listed, 334
Rectum and anus, 330-337
Red blood count, 17-19
differential, 18
Refusal, blood transfusion form, 10
Refusal of treatment form, 10
Rejection, tissue, 532-533
Request for medical information, 14-15
Resectoscopes, 181
Retina
reattachment of, 442-443
Retinoscopes, 181
Retractors, 181-186
Rh factor, 23-25

INDEX (Continued)

erythroblastosis fetalis, 24
   in mothers, 24
   vaccine, 24
Rhinoplasty, 546-547
   Weir operation, 547
Rhizotomy, trigeminal, 392-393
RhoGAM vaccine, 24
Rib contractors, 187
Rib shears, 187
Rib spreaders, 187
Rickettsias, 36
   listing of organisms, 36
Rings, 187
Rod, 187
Roentgenography, cardiac, 610
Rollers, 188
Rongeurs, 188-189
Rulers, 189
Ruptured disc, 400, 402-405
   cervical, report, 404-405
   illustrated, 403
   lumbar, 402-404
Rush rod insertion, 484

S

Safety pin closer, 189
Salivary glands, 283-289
   diseases listed, 288
   operations listed, 289
   parotid gland, 283-284
   sublingual gland, 288
   submaxillary gland, 287-288
Saphenous vein ligation, 621
Saturation index, blood, 19
Saws, 189-190
Scalene node biopsy, 557
Scarifier, 190
Schick test, 68
Schistosomiasis, 45-46
Scissors, 190-192
Sclera marker, 192
Sclerotomes, 192
Scoops, 192-193
Screw drivers, 193
Screws, 193
Scribner shunt, 233

Scrub soaps, 93
Sedimentation rate, 68
Semicircular canal
   fenestration, 515-516
Separators, 194
Septicemia, 32
Septum
   nasal, resection, 529
   straighteners, 194
Serology tests, 69
Serotonin test, 69
Serum transaminase, 71
SGOT, 71
SGPT, 71
Shears, 194
Shirodkar operation, 373
Shoulder
   anatomy illustrated, 463
   arthrodesis, 462-463
   Bankart operation, 480
Shunt
   Cimino in hemodialysis, 233
   endolymphatic-subarachnoid, 505
   mechanisms, 194
   Pott's report, 630
   Scribner in hemodialysis, 233
Sialography, 84
Sickle cell test, 18, 69
Sigmoidoscopes, 194
Sigmoidoscopy, 331
Silastic injection
   malar area, 551
Sims-Huhner test, 59, 69
Sinography, 84
Sinuses, paranasal, 525, 545-546
   anatomic structures, 527, 545-46
   diseases listed, 528
   Caldwell-Luc report, 529-530
   ethmoidectomy report, 530
   illustrated anatomy, 526
   operations listed, 528
   sphenoidotomy report, 530
Skeleton, 229, 234
   bones of, 229-235
Skids, 194
Skin flaps, 534-535

INDEX (Continued)

nasolabial, report, 537
types, 534-535
Skin grafts, 531, 533-534
  chessboard, 533
  excision, 537-538
  free, 533
  full thickness, 533
  Gabarro, 533
  pedicle, 533
  pinch graft, 533
  Reverdin, 533
  split thickness, 533
    report, to auricular area, 537
    report, to finger, 490
  techniques, 534
  tube pedicle, 533
  Wolfe graft, 533
Skull fracture elevation, 396
Slings listed, 119
SMA 12, 48-49
  report form, 49
Small bowel, 318
  diseases of, 318-319
  operations of, 319-323
Smith-Petersen nailing, 484
SMR operative report, 529
Snares, 195
Sodium test, 69
Sounds, 195
Spatulas, 195-196
Specula, 196-198
Sphenoidotomy report, 530
Sphere introducer, 198
Sphincterotome, 198
Sphincterotomy, anal, 335
  of Oddi, 341-342
Spinal cord, 398
  anatomic features, 402
  illustrated, 399
Spinal fluid, 29-30
  examinations, 30
Spinal fusion report, 468-470
Spleen, 299-302
  anatomic features, 300
  diseases listed, 301
  operations, 302

Splenectomy
  operative report, 300-301
  techniques listed, 300
Splenoportography, 83
Splines, 198
Splints, 198-200
Spoons, 200
Spreaders, 201
Spuds, 201
Spur crushers, 201
Sputum examinations, 31
Stabs, 20
Stapes, 514-516
  stapedectomy report, 514-515
  techniques, 514
Staphylococci, 32
Staples, 201
Station in obstetrics, 418-419
Stereoscopy, 86
Sterilization, 13-14
  request form, 14
Sternal approximators, 201
Stomach, 307
  diseases listed, 307-308
  gastrectomy, 309-310
  illustrated anatomy, 307
  operations defined, 309
  operations listed, 308
Stone baskets, 201
Stone dislodgers, 201-202
Strabismus correction, 440-441
Streptococci, 32
Strippers, 202
Stripping
  saphenous vein, 621-622
  vocal cord, 522
Strongyloidiasis, 46
Strontium-90, 89
Subdural hematoma, removal, 393
  illustrated, 395
Sublingual gland, 288
  anatomic features of, 288
Submaxillary gland, 287
  circulation of, 288
  structures of, 287
Submucous resection, 529-530, 546-547

INDEX (Continued)

Suction tubes, 202-203
Suffixes listed, 647-648
Sulkowitch test, 54
Surgical instruments, 121-210
Suspension apparatus, 203
Suspension of the uterus, 364
Suture materials, 99-101
   vascular, 616
Suture methods, 102-115
Suture needles, 115-117
Suture techniques, 109-115
Symbols, medical, 654
Sympathectomy
   cervical, 405
   lumbar, 406

T

T-3 uptake, 70
Tachycardia, 637
Takata-Ara test, 70
Tamps, 203
Tantalum-182, 89
Tapeworms, 46
TBI, 70
Teeth and mouth, 282
Telescopes, 203
Televising operation form, 11
Tenaculums, 203
Tendon graft report, 488
Tendon lengthening, 489
Tendon passers, 204
Tendon shortening, 489
Tendons, 240
   diseases listed, 491-494
   operations listed, 494-499
   tendon graft report, 488
   tenorrhaphy report, 488
Tennison harelip repair, 545
Tenorrhaphy, 488
Tenotomes, 204
Terminology, medical, 641-654
   abbreviations, 649-654
   combining forms, 644-647
   elements of, 643
   prefixes, 644-647

suffixes, 647-648
symbols, 654
Testes, 593
   anatomic features of, 596-597
   diseases listed, 602-605
   hydrocelectomy report, 597
   illustrated, 594
   malignant tumors, 596
   operations listed, 605-606
   orchiectomy report, 597
   orchiopexy, 598
   Torek operation, 598
Tetralogy of Fallot, 629
TGT, 70
Thermopores, 204
Thermosectors, 204
Thoracic diseases, 562-563
   listed, 573-574
Thoracic surgery, 557-575
   diseases, 562-563
   diseases listed, 573-574
   operations listed, 574-575
Thoracoscopes, 204
Thoracotomes, 204
Thoracotomy report, 568, 571
Thorn test, 70
Thornton plate, hip, 484
Thrombocytes, 21
Thrombocytopenia, 22
Thrombocytosis, 22
Thymol turbidity, 70
Thyroid gland, 289-293
   anatomic features, 291
   circulation in, 291
   diseases of, 290-291
   illustrated, 293
   operations, 291
   thyroidectomy report, 292
   uptake, 291
Thyroidectomy, subtotal, 292
Tibia
   bone graft to, 477
   Hauser operation, 487
   Lottes nailing, 483
   removal of bone graft, 477-478

INDEX (Continued)

Tissue banks, 536-537
Tissue grafts
  bone, 535
  cartilage, 535
  cornea, 535
  fascia, 536
  fascia lata report, 538
  hair, 536
  mucous membrane, 536
  nerve, 536
  tendon, 536
Tissue transplants, 531-533
Toenail excision, radical, 273
Tongs, 204
Tongue, 281-282
  depressors, 204
  diseases of, 281
  mouth illustrated, 282
  operations on, 281
Tonometers, 205
Tonsillectomes, 205
T & A, 524-525
Tonsillectomy, 525
Torek operation, 598
Toti operation, 444
Tourniquets, 205
Toxemia, 415
Toxoplasmosis, 43
Trachea, 559, 564-566
  anatomy of, 558-559, 564
  diseases listed, 566, 573-574
  illustrated, 560
  instruments, 564
  operations listed, 566, 574-575
  tracheotomy, 564
    illustrated, 565
  tubes, 564
Trachelotomes, 205
Tracheoscopes, 206
Tracheotomes, 206
Tracheotomy, 523-524, 564
  illustrated, 565
Traction bows, 206
Tractors, 206
Transaminase test, 71

Transcription
  measurement of, 2
  references for, 1
Transilluminators, 206
Transplants
  heart, 607-608
  kidney, 579-581
Transposition of great vessels, 630
Transverse lie
  illustrated, 421
Treacher-Collins syndrome, 551
Trephine operation, 393
Trephines, 206-207
Trichinosis, 46
Trichomoniasis, 43
Tricuspid stenosis, 629
Triiodothyronine, 70
Trocars, 207-208
Trypanosomiasis, 43
Trypsin test, 71
Tuberculosis tests, 33
Tubes, 208-209
  laryngeal, 519
Tuckers, 209
Tunnelers, 209
Turnbuckles, 209
Tympanoplasty, 506-512
  Type I report, 507
  Type II report, 508
  Type III report, 508-509
    revision of, 510-511
  Type IV report, 511
  Type V report, 511-512
  types defined, 506-507

U

Ultrasound, 413
Umbilical hernia, 270-271
  herniorrhaphy report, 270-271
  repair techniques, 270
Urea test, 71
Urea clearance test, 71
Uretero-vaginal fistula, 360
Ureters, 577-578

INDEX (Continued)

anatomic features of, 578
diseases listed, 602-605
operations listed, 605-606
Urethra
  anatomic features of, 587-588
  biopsy report, 589
  diseases listed, 602-605
  operations listed, 605-606
Urethroplasty, 590
  approaches, 590
  operative techniques, 590
Urethroscopy report, 589-590
Urethrotomes, 209
Uric acid test, 71
Urinary bladder, 585
  anatomic features, 587-588
  arteries of, 588
  biopsy, transurethral, 589
  calculus removal, 589
  diseases listed, 602-605
  litholapaxy, 589
  malignant tumors of, 586
  operations listed, 605-606
Urinary diseases, 602-605
Urinary operations, 605-606
Urine, 26-29
  bacteriologic exam, 29
  casts, 28
  color, 27
  disorders of, 27
  examinations, 26-29
  microscopic exam, 28-29
  odor, 27
  secretion rate, 26
  specific gravity, 28
Urobilinogen test, 71
Urology, 577-606
  diseases listed, 602-605
  operations listed, 605-606
Uterine ligaments, 355-356
Uterosalpingography, 81
Uterus, 352, 353
  diseases listed, 377-380
  operations of, 362-374
  operations listed, 381-383
  prolapse operations, 364

V

Vagina, 352
  diseases listed, 380
  operations listed, 381-383
  operations on, 356
Vaginal wall prolapse, 357
Vagino-perineal fistula, 361
Vaginoscopes, 209
Vagotomy, abdominal, 317
Valvulotomes, 210
van den Bergh test, 53
Vascular
  aortic valve prostheses, 616
  prostheses, 616
  surgery, 607-640
  sutures, 616
VDRL, 69, 72
Vectis, 210
Vein by-pass, 618
Vein graft report, 617
Veins, listed, 217-219
  extremities, illustrated, 228
  head and neck, illustrated, 227
  principal, illustrated, 226
Venography, 84
Ventricular septal defect, 630
  closure report, 633-634
Ventriculography, 84
Version in obstetrics, 425
Vertebral column, 400
  illustrated, 401
Vesicocervical fistula, 361
Vesicovaginal fistula, 361
Vesiculography, 84
Viruses, 36-38
  listing, 37-38
VMA test, 72
Vocal cord stripping, 522
von Langenbeck cleft palate repair, 549-550

W

Wardill cleft palate repair, 550-551
Watson-Jones operation, 480
Weir operation, 547

INDEX (Continued)

Whipple operation, 345-346
Whistles, 210
White blood count, 19-21
  differential, 20-21
Wire crimpers, 210
Wires, 210
Worm parasites, 44-48
  listing of, 47-48
Wrenches, 210
Wrist, anatomy illustrated, 465

X

X-ray
  contrast media listing, 74-77
  examinations
    abdomen, 77
    aortography, 78
    arteriography, 78
    arthrography, 78
    autotomography, 78
    barium examinations, 78
    body section radiography, 84
    brachial arteriography, 79
    bronchography, 79
    cardio-angiography, 79
    chest, 79
    cholangiography, 79
    cholecystography, 80
    cystourethrography, 80
    dacryocystography, 80
    discography, 80
    encephalography, 80
    femoral arteriography, 80
    fluoroscopy, 85
    hysterosalpingography, 81
    KUB, 81
    kymography, 86
    lymphangiography, 81
    mastoids, 81
    myelography, 81
    paranasal sinuses, 81
    pelvimetry, 82
      illustrated, 82, 83
    pneumoencephalography, 83
    portal venography, 83
    pyelography, 83
    renal arteriography, 84
    sialography, 84
    sinography, 84
    stereoscopy, 86
    venography, 84
    ventriculography, 84
    vesiculography, 84

Z

Zinc flocculation test, 72
Zoografts, 531